Textbook of Influenza

Textbook of Influenza

Edited by

Robert G. Webster, PhD, FRS
Rose Marie Thomas Chair
Division of Virology, Department of Infectious Diseases
St Jude Children's Research Hospital
Memphis, TN, USA

Arnold S. Monto, MD
Thomas Francis, Jr. Collegiate Professor of Epidemiology
School of Public Health
University of Michigan
Ann Arbor, MI, USA

Thomas J. Braciale, MD, PhD
Director, Beirne B. Carter Center for Immunology Research
Beirne B. Carter Professor in Immunology
Professor of Pathology and Microbiology, Immunology, and Cancer Biology
University of Virginia School of Medicine
Charlottesville, VA, USA

Robert A. Lamb, PhD, ScD
John Evans Professor of Molecular and Cellular Biology
Howard Hughes Medical Institute
Department of Molecular Biosciences
Northwestern University
Evanston, IL, USA

2nd Edition

WILEY Blackwell

This edition first published 2013 © 2013 by John Wiley & Sons, Ltd.

Registered office: John Wiley & Sons, Ltd, The Atrium, Southern Gate, Chichester, West Sussex, PO19 8SQ, UK

Editorial offices: 9600 Garsington Road, Oxford, OX4 2DQ, UK

The Atrium, Southern Gate, Chichester, West Sussex, PO19 8SQ, UK

111 River Street, Hoboken, NJ 07030-5774, USA

For details of our global editorial offices, for customer services and for information about how to apply for permission to reuse the copyright material in this book please see our website at www.wiley.com/wiley-blackwell

Library of congress cataloging-in-publication data

Textbook of influenza / edited by Robert G. Webster, Arnold S. Monto, Thomas J. Braciale, Robert A. Lamb. – 2nd edition.
    p. ; cm.
  Includes bibliographical references and index.
  ISBN 978-0-470-67048-4 (hardback : alk. paper) – ISBN 978-1-118-63681-7 – ISBN 978-1-118-63682-4 (eMobi) – ISBN 978-1-118-63683-1 (ePub) – ISBN 978-1-118-63684-8 (ePDF)
  I. Webster, Robert G., 1932- editor of compilation.   II. Monto, Arnold S., editor of compilation.   III. Braciale, Thomas J., editor of compilation.   IV. Lamb, Robert A., editor of compilation.
  [DNLM: 1. Influenza, Human. WC 515]
  RC150
  616.2'03–dc23
                        2013010901

A catalogue record for this book is available from the British Library.

Wiley also publishes its books in a variety of electronic formats. Some content that appears in print may not be available in electronic books.

Cover image: © Science Photo Library/Coloured TEM of a single influenza virus
Cover design by Meaden Creative

Set in 9/11.5 Sabon by Toppan Best-set Premedia Limited
Printed and bound in Singapore by Markono Print Media Pte Ltd

01 2013

Contents

List of Contributors

Dennis J. Alexander, OBE, PhD, FSB, FRCPath, DSc
Formerly Head, Virology Department
Animal Health and Veterinary Laboratories
Weybridge, Addlestone, Surrey, UK

Rilwan A. Balogun
Microbiology, Immunology and Molecular Genetics
David Geffen School of Medicine
University of California, Los Angeles; *and*
California NanoSystems Institute (CNSI)
Los Angeles, CA, USA

Nicole Baumgarth, DVM, PhD
Professor, Center for Comparative Medicine and
Department of Pathology, Microbiology and
Immunology, University of California
Davis, CA, USA

Thomas J. Braciale, MD, PhD
Director, Beirne B. Carter Center for Immunology
Research, Beirne B. Carter Professor in Immunology
Professor of Pathology and Microbiology,
Immunology, and Cancer Biology
University of Virginia School of Medicine
Charlottesville, VA, USA

Joseph Bresee, MD
Chief, Epidemiology and Prevention Branch
Influenza Division
Centers for Disease Control and Prevention
Atlanta, GA, USA

Carolyn B. Bridges, MD, FACP
CAPT USPHS, Associate Director for Adult
Immunizations, Immunization Services Division
National Center for Immunizations and Respiratory
Diseases
Centers for Disease Control and Prevention
Atlanta, GA, USA

Ilaria Capua, DVM, PhD
Director, OIE/FAO Reference Laboratory for Avian
Influenza and Newcastle Disease
OIE Collaborating Center for Diseases
at the Human-Animal Interface
Istituto Zooprofilattico Sperimentale delle Venezie
Padua, Italy

Michael C. Carroll, PhD
Professor, Department of Pediatrics
Harvard Medical School; *and*
Program in Cellular and Molecular Medicine
Children's Hospital, Boston, MA, USA

Thomas M. Chambers, PhD
Professor, Gluck Equine Research Center
Department of Veterinary Science
University of Kentucky
Lexington, KY, USA

Nancy J. Cox, PhD
Director, Influenza Division
National Center for Immunization and Respiratory
Diseases
Centers for Disease Control and Prevention
Atlanta, GA, USA

Menno D. de Jong, MD, PhD
Professor in Clinical Virology
Head of Department of Medical Microbiology
Academic Medical Center
University of Amsterdam, Amsterdam
The Netherlands

Peter C. Doherty, PhD, FRS
Department of Microbiology and Immunology
The University of Melbourne, Melbourne, VIC,
Australia; *and*
Department of Immunology
St Jude Children's Research Hospital
Memphis, TN, USA

Ruben O. Donis, DVM, PhD
Centers for Disease Control and Prevention
Atlanta, GA, USA

Edward J. Dubovi, PhD
Director, Virology Section
Animal Health Diagnostic Center
College of Veterinary Medicine
Cornell University
Ithaca, NY, USA

Damian C. Ekiert, PhD
Department of Integrative Structural and
Computational Biology
The Scripps Research Institute
La Jolla, CA, USA

Ervin Fodor, DPhil
Professor of Virology
Sir William Dunn School of Pathology
University of Oxford, Oxford, UK

Ron A. M. Fouchier, PhD
Professor in Molecular Virology
Department of Viroscience
Erasmus MC Rotterdam, The Netherlands

Steven J. Gamblin, PhD, FRS, FMedSci
MRC, National Institute for Medical Research
London, UK

Adolfo García-Sastre, PhD
Professor, Department of Microbiology
Fishberg Professor, Department of Medicine
Division of Infectious Diseases; *and*
Director Global Health and Emerging Pathogens
Institute
Icahn School of Medicine at Mount Sinai
New York, NY, USA

Wolfgang Garten, PhD
Professor, Institut für Virologie
Philipps-Universität Marburg
Marburg, Germany

Santiago Gonzalez, PhD
Institute for Research in Biomedicine
Bellinzona, Switzerland

Yi Guan, PhD, MD
Director, State Key Laboratory of Emerging
Infectious Diseases
The University of Hong Kong; *and*
Professor, Centre of Influenza Research
and School of Public Health
Li Ka Shing Faculty of Medicine
The University of Hong Kong
Hong Kong SAR, China

Alan J. Hay, PhD
Virology Division, MRC National Institute
for Medical Research, London, UK

Frederick G. Hayden, MD
Professor of Medicine
Stuart S. Richardson Professor of Clinical Virology
University of Virginia School of Medicine
Charlottesville, VA, USA

Michael G. Ison, MD, MS, FIDSA
Associate Professor of Medicine and Surgery
Divisions of Infectious Diseases and Organ
Transplantation, Northwestern University
Feinberg School of Medicine
Chicago, IL, USA

Akiko Iwasaki, PhD
Professor, Department of Immunobiology
Howard Hughes Medical Institute
Yale University School of Medicine
New Haven, CT, USA

Daniel B. Jernigan, MD, MPH
Deputy Director, Influenza Division, National
Center for Immunization and Respiratory Diseases
Centers for Disease Control and Prevention
Atlanta, GA, USA

Yoshihiro Kawaoka, DVM, PhD
Professor of Virology, Influenza Research Institute
Department of Pathobiological Sciences
School of Veterinary Medicine
University of Wisconsin-Madison, Madison
WI, USA; *and*
Department of Special Pathogens
International Research Center for Infectious
Diseases
Institute of Medical Science
University of Tokyo; *and*
Division of Virology
Department of Microbiology and Immunology
Institute of Medical Science
University of Tokyo; *and*
ERATO Infection-Induced Host Responses Project
Saitama, Japan

Wendy A. Keitel, MD
Kyle and Josephine Morrow Chair in Molecular
Virology and Microbiology; *and*
Professor, Molecular Virology and Microbiology
and Medicine, Baylor College of Medicine
Houston, TX, USA

Anne Kelso, PhD
Director, WHO Collaborating Centre for
Reference and Research on Influenza
North Melbourne, VIC, Australia

Hans-Dieter Klenk, MD
Professor Emeritus, Institut für Virologie
Philipps-Universität Marburg
Marburg, Germany

Robert M. Krug, PhD
Professor and Chair
Department of Molecular Genetics and
Microbiology
Fellow, Mr. and Mrs. Corbin J. Robertson
Sr. Regents Chair in Molecular Biology
Institute for Cellular and Molecular Biology
University of Texas at Austin
Austin, TX, USA

Robert A. Lamb, PhD, ScD
John Evans Professor of Molecular and Cellular
Biology, Howard Hughes Medical Institute
Department of Molecular Biosciences
Northwestern University
Evanston, IL, USA

Gwendolyn Lee
Microbiology, Immunology and Molecular Genetics
David Geffen School of Medicine
University of California, Los Angeles; *and*
California NanoSystems Institute (CNSI)
Los Angeles, CA, USA

Marc Lipsitch, DPhil
Professor of Epidemiology
Center for Communicable Disease Dynamics
Harvard School of Public Health
Boston, MA, USA

Chunlong Ma, PhD
Research Associate, Department of Neurobiology
Department of Molecular Biosciences
Northwestern University, Evanston, IL, USA

Mikhail Matrosovich, PhD
Group Leader, Institut für Virologie
Philipps-Universität Marburg
Marburg, Germany

Jonathan A. McCullers, MD
Dunavant Professor and Chair
Department of Pediatrics
University of Tennessee Health Sciences Center; *and*
Pediatrician-in-Chief
Le Bonheur Children's Hospital, Memphis; *and*
Member, Department of Infectious Diseases
St. Jude Children's Research Hospital
Memphis, TN, USA

Andrew Mehle, PhD
Assistant Professor
Department of Medical Microbiology and
Immunology
University of Wisconsin Madison
Madison, WI, USA

Martin I. Meltzer, MS, PhD
Senior Health Economist and
Distinguished Consultant
Lead, Health Economics and Modeling Unit
(HEMU)
Division of Preparedness and Emerging Infections
National Center for Emerging and Zoonotic
Infectious Diseases
Centers for Disease Control and Prevention
Atlanta, GA, USA

Arnold S. Monto, MD
Thomas Francis, Jr. Collegiate Professor
of Epidemiology
School of Public Health
University of Michigan
Ann Arbor, MI, USA

Gary J. Nabel, MD, PhD
Senior Vice President, Chief Scientific Officer
Sanofi, Cambridge, MA, USA

Debiprosad Nayak, BVSc, PhD
Distinguished Professor Emeritus
Microbiology, Immunology and Molecular Genetics
David Geffen School of Medicine
University of California
Los Angeles, CA, USA

Gabriele Neumann, PhD
Research Professor, Influenza Research Institute
Department of Pathobiological Sciences
School of Veterinary Medicine
University of Wisconsin-Madison
Madison, WI, USA

Kathleen M. Neuzil, MD, MPH
Director, Vaccine Access and Delivery Global
Program, PATH, Clinical Professor
Departments of Medicine and Global Health
University of Washington
Seattle, WA, USA

Jonathan S. Nguyen-Van-Tam, MBE,
BMedSci, BM BS, DM, FFPH, FRSPH, FSB
Professor of Health Protection
Health Protection and Influenza Research Group
University of Nottingham Medical School
City Hospital, Nottingham, UK

Peter Palese, PhD
Professor and Chair, Department of Microbiology
Department of Medicine
Mount Sinai School of Medicine
New York, NY, USA

Samuel K. Peasah, PhD, MBA
Health Economist
Epidemiology & Prevention Branch
Influenza Division/NCIRD/Centers for
Disease Control and Prevention
Atlanta, GA, USA

Malik Peiris, PhD, MD
Centre of Influenza Research and School of Public
Health, Li Ka Shing Faculty of Medicine
The University of Hong Kong
Hong Kong SAR, China

Lawrence H. Pinto, PhD
Professor Emeritus
Department of Neurobiology
Northwestern University
Evanston, IL, USA

Juergen A. Richt, DVM, PhD
Regents Distinguished Professor
Kansas State University
Manhattan, KS, USA

Rupert J. Russell
University of St Andrews, Fife, UK
[Deceased]

Sir John J. Skehel, PhD, FRS, FMedSci
MRC, National Institute for Medical Research
London, UK

Sakar Shivakoti, PhD
Microbiology, Immunology and Molecular Genetics
David Geffen School of Medicine
University of California, Los Angeles
CA, USA; *and*
California NanoSystems Institute (CNSI)
Los Angeles, CA, USA

Derek Smith, BTech, MSc, MA, PhD
Professor of Infectious Disease Informatics
Center for Pathogen Evolution
WHO Collaborating Centre for Modeling Evolution
and Control of Emerging Infectious Diseases
Department of Zoology
University of Cambridge
Cambridge, UK

Klaus Stöhr, PhD, DVM
Vice-President, Head, Global Policy
Novartis Vaccines and Diagnostics, Inc
Cambridge, MA, USA

John Treanor, MD
Professor of Medicine, Microbiology and
Immunology, University of Rochester Medical
Center
Rochester, NY, USA

Stephen J. Turner, PhD
Professor, Department of Microbiology and
Immunology, The University of Melbourne
Melbourne, VIC, Australia

Taia T. Wang, MD, PhD
Instructor in Clinical Investigation
Laboratory of Molecular Genetics and Immunology
Rockefeller University
New York, NY, USA

Richard Webby, PhD
Division of Virology
Department of Infectious Diseases
St. Jude Children's Research Hospital
Memphis, TN, USA

Robert G. Webster, PhD, FRS
Rose Marie Thomas Chair
Division of Virology
Department of Infectious Diseases
St Jude Children's Research Hospital
Memphis, TN, USA

Chih-Jen Wei, PhD
Associate Director for Research
Virology Laboratory and Vector Core Section
Vaccine Research Center
NIAID, National Institutes of Health
Bethesda, MD, USA

Marc-Alain Widdowson, VetMB, MA, MSc
Lead, International Epidemiology and Research
Team, Epidemiology and Response Branch
Influenza Division
Centers for Disease Control and Prevention
Atlanta, GA, USA

Ian A. Wilson, DSc, FRS
Professor, Department of Integrative Structural
and Computational Biology; *and*
IAVI Neutralizing Antibody Center and
Scripps Center for HIV/AIDS Vaccine Immunology
and Immunogen Discovery
The Scripps Research Institute
La Jolla, CA, USA

Maria Zambon, BSc, BM, BCh, PhD, FRCPath,
FMedSci
Director of Reference Microbiology
Public Health England
London, UK

Z. Hong Zhou, PhD
Professor, Microbiology, Immunology
and Molecular Genetics
David Geffen School of Medicine
University of California, Los Angeles; *and*
California NanoSystems Institute (CNSI)
Los Angeles, CA, USA

Foreword to the Second Edition

In the Foreword to the First Edition of the *Textbook of Influenza*, David Tyrrell, one of the early expert researchers on influenza virus, wrote that although there were many original articles, review articles, and book chapters on both clinical and laboratory aspects of influenza, there was a need for a comprehensive book covering influenza from the bedside to basic molecular biology of virus to antiviral drug development. Such a book would enable investigators in the various fields of research to benefit from up-to-date knowledge in areas of research other than theirs. The First Edition was written to meet that need and I think that readers would agree that it indeed did so.

It is also clear, that in the years since that edition, there has been an extraordinary accumulation of knowledge on all aspects of influenza, and that progress is continuing at a rapid pace. Thus, the Second Edition is needed. A look at the titles and authors of the chapters of that edition attests to that. It is noteworthy that in addition to a large number of experts that contributed to the First Edition there are also new editors and new authors in the Second. This is in keeping with the fact that the topics are so important, new approaches and techniques have been developed, and the progress made so great. There is ample reason to believe that the Second Edition will meet the needs as well as, or better than, the First. In addition, it is very likely that, because of rapid advances, in several years a Third Edition will also be needed. It is also possible another reason will be that the virus still has some more surprises up its sleeve!

If one were to judge viruses on the basis of cleverness, it is fair to say that influenza virus would be among the most clever. If a virus's goals were to survive and infect the maximum number of hosts and individuals, to maintain large reservoirs in hosts with the ability to move between hosts, to evade immune responses, either natural, through previous exposure, or vaccination, influenza virus does all of the above very well. A short incubation period and replication in the respiratory tract also help. Compare it to its fellow RNA viruses, measles and yellow fever, which are still preventable by vaccines that have been avail-

able for many years. Also think about features of the structure and replication of the influenza virus. It is a great advantage for the virus to survive change and avoid immune responses if its genetic material is in not one but several pieces that can be exchanged within infected hosts, to have receptors widely available on host cells, and because the virus particle is assembled at the cell surface, to have an enzyme that can destroy the receptors and thus enable the virus to leave the cell surface and spread more easily. For all these reasons and more, the battle with influenza viruses will require continued research using a wide variety of current and new approaches and techniques and the publication of these results in volumes such as this Second Edition of the *Textbook of Influenza*.

I arrived at the Rockefeller Institute (soon to change its name to the Rockefeller University) in the summer of 1957 to begin a postdoctoral fellowship. This was a very fortunate time and place for me for several reasons. First, I joined the laboratory of Frank Horsfall and Igor Tamm, two very distinguished virologists and excellent mentors. In addition, also still active there were several other giants in virology. Peyton Rous, discoverer of the Rous sarcoma virus, the first virus to be shown to cause cancer, Richard Shope, who isolated both swine influenza virus, the first influenza virus to be isolated from a mammal, and the Shope papilloma virus, the first to be shown to cause a tumor in a mammal. Thomas Rivers, though not still active in the laboratory was very much around and editing. He was considered by many to be the Dean of Virology from the 1920s to the 1950s. In 1928 he edited the first comprehensive book on viruses, *Filterable Viruses*, and, in 1948, 1952, and 1959, three comprehensive and excellent editions of *Viral and Rickettsial Diseases of Man*; the third of these was co-edited by Frank Horsfall. A Fourth Edition was edited by Horsfall and Tamm. These volumes might be considered in a way as predecessors of the *Textbook of Influenza*.

The timing for me to arrive at the Rockefeller Institute in 1957 was very good because the Asian influenza pandemic had begun that spring in the Far East, and reached the United States that summer. It was caused by a virus that came to be known as H2N2. From September to November of 1957, I isolated six strains of influenza virus from patients at the Hospital of the Rockefeller Institute, the fifth of which I isolated from my own throat washing during my bout with influenza. That strain, named RI/5/57, became very useful to me and colleagues in the laboratory for many years, and also was used by investigators elsewhere. We used it in studies of the structure, absorption, penetration, replication, and assembly of the virus, including the isolation of and characterization of several previously unrecognized structural and nonstructural proteins of the virus.

In light of the origin of RI/5, it could be said that, to paraphrase David Tyrrell's words in the Foreword to the First Edition of the *Textbook of Virology* mentioned above, these studies in our laboratory went from *bed* to bedside to basic molecular biology.

Purnell W. Choppin
President Emeritus
Howard Hughes Medical Institute
Chevy Chase, MD, USA

Preface to the second edition

The second edition of the *Textbook of Influenza* has been completely revised and reflects the integration of disciplines concerning the emergence, evolution, pathogenesis, and control of influenza viruses in the field of veterinary and human public health with growing acceptance of the "One World–One Health" concept. This is reflected in consolidation of cross-disciplinary interests with a reduction in the number of chapters from 41 in the first *Textbook of Influenza* to 29 chapters in the current edition. Additionally, co-authorship of chapters by experts from complementary disciplines provides new insight. The textbook is aimed at students, researchers, and decision-makers across the "One Health" spectrum including ecologists, clinical and basic scientists, molecular and structural virologists, immunologists, public health officials, economists, and global pandemic control planners.

As predicted in the first *Textbook of Influenza*, the world has experienced another pandemic of influenza – the H1N1 pandemic of 2009. What was not predicted was that the pandemic would be caused by a subtype (H1N1) already circulating in the human population. This edition of the textbook examines the lessons learned and deals with the state of knowledge of many yet unresolved issues of severity and pathogenesis to improve preparation for future pandemics.

The advances in influenza genomics and reverse genetics now permits reconstruction of influenza viruses such as the 1918 Spanish influenza, and provides unique insight into innate immune-based pathogenesis. These strategies also permit studies on the interplay between the virus and the host, with potential for development of novel control strategies. They also bring us face to face with the future where we have the potential to generate influenza viruses that may or may not exist in nature. The textbook provides the background to these advances and the experiments that raise the issue of dual-use research of concern (DURC). The textbook does not attempt to resolve these issues, for resolution of these important issues were ongoing at the time of writing.

The text is divided in to eight sections: 1 A perspective on influenza; 2 Virus structure and replication; 3 Evolution and ecology; 4 Epidemiology and surveillance; 5 Immunology; 6 Vaccines and vaccine development; 7 Antivirals and 8 The outbreak of H7N9.

In the 15 years since publication of the first edition major advances have been made in each of these areas. The chapters in each of these sections are co-authored by leading influenza experts and are original contributions. Because of the desire to keep chapters concise the number of references has been restricted and authors have covered the major contributions in each field, but these are by no means all inclusive. The extent of overlap between chapters is limited and reflects different perspectives on each topic.

A very exciting advance in the section on vaccine development is understanding the molecular basis of antibody cross-reactivity between all of the known influenza hemagglutinin subtypes. These cross-reactive epitopes located in the stalk and receptor binding domains of the hemagglutinin molecule offer the possibility of a universal vaccine – the "Holy Grail" of influenza vaccinologists. The continued circulation and evolution of highly pathogenic H5N1 avian influenza in multiple endemic sites in Eurasia with sporadic spillover into humans and other mammals is a continuing threat to veterinary and human public health. The persistence of the highly pathogenic H5N1 virus in the wild bird reservoir is an unresolved question as is the potential for acquisition of human-to-human transmissibility. The H1, H2, and H3 subtypes are the only subtypes in the past century that have established stable lineages in humans, raising the possibility that only these subtypes can infect humans. However, it is wise to remember that all subtypes of influenza A that become established in mammals emerge from natural reservoirs including the stable H7N7 lineage that infected horses.

History has repeated itself. As was the case during production of the first edition of this textbook, a novel avian H7N9 influenza virus with high virulence for humans emerged in Asia as the second edition was going to press. Proving once again, influenza will continue to challenge us not only as scientists but also as authors. To that end, we have added an Appendix on H7N9 influenza that provides the available preliminary information to meet these challenges.

Robert G. Webster
Arnold S. Monto
Thomas J. Braciale
Robert A. Lamb

Acknowledgments

The contributing authors of the second edition of the *Textbook of Influenza* are the real heroes of this project; they are all extremely busy people but they found the time to make this book what was envisioned – a textbook at the cutting edge of knowledge. We are extremely grateful to every one of the authors and say thank you for a job superbly done. We thank the entire staff of Wiley Blackwell involved in this project, from the initial meeting with Maria Kahn over a cup of tea at The Royal Society for accepting the need for a second edition of the textbook. Rebecca Huxley, Aileen Castell, Claire Brewer, Kate Newell, Lucinda Yeates, and Deidre Berry all played important parts in bringing the book to completion, especially Elisabeth Dodds who handled the entire submission process and Jan East for careful copyediting and adding the final touches. We are especially pleased with the acceptance of the need for color illustrations throughout. Purnell Choppin provides personal insight into influenza in his foreword and James Knowles (St. Jude), Shawn Wood (University of Virginia), Susan H. Dara (University of Michigan), and Barbara St. Cyr (Northwestern University) provided outstanding administrative assistance throughout the project with continuing communication between the authors, editors, and publishing staff. We acknowledge the support of our institutions and funding agencies which are given at the end of each chapter and most importantly we thank our wives, Marjorie Webster, Reay Paterson (Lamb), Ellyne P. Monto, and families for their support and encouragement.

Robert G. Webster
Arnold S. Monto
Thomas J. Braciale
Robert A. Lamb

1

Human influenza: One health, one world

Daniel B. Jernigan and Nancy J. Cox

National Center for Immunization and Respiratory Diseases, Influenza Division, Centers for Disease Control and Prevention Atlanta, GA, USA

Introduction

Influenza viruses know no boundaries, circulating within species and occasionally jumping between them, causing infections around the globe. The impact of influenza is also wide-ranging, and the growing interconnectedness and complexity of the world presents an increasing challenge to influenza prevention and control. As people and the animals that support them increase in numbers and interactions, the opportunities for virus adaptation and cross-species transmission increases as well. An undetected exchange of viruses among humans and animals in a rural village may eventually manifest as a global pandemic. Within this interconnected context, opportunities are also emerging for coordinated, collaborative, innovative, and integrated efforts to focus new technologies and approaches in a shared response to the global challenges of influenza.

Global impact of influenza

Influenza causes significant human illness and death each year. The actual global impact of seasonal influenza is difficult to determine due to incomplete surveillance data; however, the World Health Organization (WHO) has estimated that around 1 billion cases of seasonal influenza infection occur each year, with around 3–5 million cases of severe illness, and 300 000–500 000 deaths [1]. The global financial costs of seasonal influenza are also not well known. In the United States, where data collection is robust, estimates of the costs of influenza have been reported to be an average of $10.4 billion per year for direct medical costs and $87.1 billion for the total economic burden of annual influenza epidemics [2].

Influenza infection in birds and other animals also has a substantial impact. Since the detection and reporting of highly pathogenic avian influenza (HPAI) A (H5N1) epidemics in 1997, the virus has spread globally with hundreds of millions of birds dying from illness or culling. Costs for the international response since 2003 have been estimated to be at least $2 billion [3]. The presence of ongoing outbreaks in South-East Asia has damaged trade potential and has shifted exporting of poultry away to other nonaffected regions. For resource-challenged communities in HPAI H5N1 endemic regions, the loss of protein nutrition from decimated domestic flocks and the drop in income from lost poultry sales is significant. Swine are also infected by influenza viruses, but the burden of illness and death for swine is considerably less than that seen for HPAI viruses in domestic poultry. Influenza illness in swine is often considered by pork producers to have considerably less of an impact on production than on the potential downside for pork consumption and global export which might

---

Textbook of Influenza, Second Edition. Edited by Robert G. Webster, Arnold S. Monto, Thomas J. Braciale, and Robert A. Lamb.
© 2013 John Wiley & Sons, Ltd. Published 2013 by John Wiley & Sons, Ltd.

be prompted by public concerns about swine influenza infecting people. From a human health perspective, the greatest impact of influenza from swine and birds is their important role as sources of novel influenza viruses capable of causing pandemics.

In the last 100 years, there have been four instances where influenza viruses with genes originating from avian or swine reservoirs emerged (either with or without reassortment with human influenza viruses) with sustained, efficient, human-to-human transmission, spreading around the world [4]. The impact from these pandemics has been substantial, most notably with the 1918 H1N1 virus. It has been estimated that, globally, there were around 50 million human deaths due to infection with the 1918 pandemic virus [5]. Estimates of the 2009 pandemic were substantially lower, with 151 700–575 400 deaths globally [6]. If a severe pandemic were to arise from the H5N1 virus, the World Bank has estimated a cost of up to three trillion dollars [7]. For past pandemic viruses, it is not known exactly where or when the interchange of virus occurred from swine or bird to humans, but the subsequent impact from these pandemics was extensive. What are the factors that contribute to emergence of these viruses? What can be done for early detection and prevention?

Influenza in a crowded, connected, and converging world

Increasingly crowded

Over the last two centuries, the world's population has increased dramatically. The number of people on earth reached 1 billion sometime around 1804 [8]. After 123 years of growth, the population rose to 2 billion in 1927. Since then, the numbers have increased substantially, reaching 7 billion in 2011 (Figure 1.1). If the population continues to grow at the current rate, there could be around 11 billion people on the planet by 2050. The exponential explosion in numbers has not been uniform across the globe. Importantly, over 80% of the population increase has occurred in less developed countries. Currently, about 60% of the world's population resides in Asia, 15% in Africa, 11% in Europe, 7% in Latin America and the Caribbean, and 5% in Northern America [9]. By 2050, 83% are projected to reside in Asia and Africa.

Much of this growth has occurred in large, dense, population centers. These communities, where the population exceeds 10 million inhabitants, are referred to as "urban agglomerations" or "megacities." In 1970, there were only two such megacities, but in 2011, there were 23 [10]. Those most recently added to the list of "megacities," and most likely to accelerate in size, including Lagos, Dhaka, Shenzhen, Karachi, Mexico City, Cairo, and São Paolo, are in developing countries and in tropical and subtropical regions. Residents of these urban agglomerations are, on average, much poorer and younger than in developed settings. Many of these megacities are facing a number of infrastructure and societal challenges, some of which also have implications for the control of influenza in humans and animals. These challenges include healthcare and public health infrastructure limitations, air pollution as a significant contributor to respiratory diseases, concentrations of the poorest of the population living in very crowded conditions, and stressed agricultural supply chains attempting to meet a growing appetite for protein [11,12].

Consider Bangladesh for example. In 2010, there were around 150 million people, a number just under half the population of the United States, living on land the size of the state of Iowa [13]. The population of the capital, Dhaka, was 1.4 million in 1970 [10]. It expanded 11-fold to 15.4 million by 2011. In 2025, this megacity is estimated to increase by another 1.5-fold to around 23 million residents. Dhaka currently is one of the world's most crowded cities. On average, the population density of Dhaka is around 32 600 persons/km^2 (84 500/mi^2) [14]. In some exceptionally dense areas, such as the slums of Kamalapur, the density rises to 111 325/km^2 (288 332/mi^2) [15]. Many of the residents in the area are recent immigrants from the countryside, and 44% are under the age of 20 years. In this crowded context with many children, respiratory infections abound. Studies have shown that childhood pneumonia occurs frequently among young children in Dhaka, and influenza and other viral pathogens are identified as the primary cause of these episodes [16,17]. In settings such as these, with the combined contribution of multiple socioeconomic factors and a considerable burden of respiratory illness, seasonal influenza has been identified as an important, and preventable, cause of illness and death.

Dhaka is not alone. Similar megacities are emerging where the promise of employment and a better quality

Global Population and Travel Trends, 1961-2010

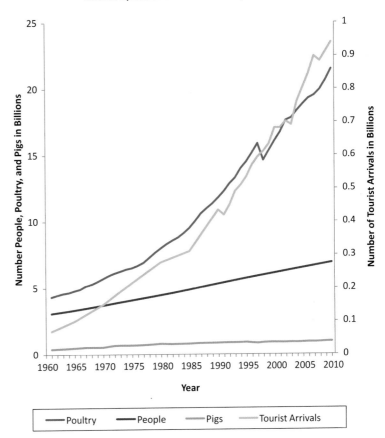

Figure 1.1. Global population and travel trends, 1961–2010. Data sources include: United Nations Food and Agricultural Organization for poultry and pig population estimates [40], United Nations Department of Economic and Social Affairs for human population estimates [9], and United Nations World Tourism Organization for tourist arrival estimates [23].

of life continue to draw people to these exceptionally crowded conditions. What does all this mean for influenza among humans? As population density increases, infection transmission potential increases [18]. With a growing number of crowded urban settings, large numbers of younger individuals, and a high frequency of interaction among the population, influenza viruses are given all the right circumstances for efficient and sustained transmission. This is annually evident for seasonal influenza with high attack rates among schoolchildren, college students, military recruits, cruise ship passengers, nursing home residents, and others in densely populated settings. This is also the case with pandemic influenza. Crowded conditions were identified as a significant contributing factor for the 1968 H3N2 pandemic emergence

in Hong Kong [19]. Population density and urbanization have been associated with pandemic spread and increased mortality for the 1918 pandemic in the United Kingdom [20]. An increasing population density not only provides an opportunity for influenza to be shared *within* a community, it also provides opportunities for influenza to be carried to *other* communities through travelers.

Increasingly connected

The world is more crowded but, just as importantly, it is also more connected. A person can travel to almost any major urban center in the world within the incubation period of influenza [21]. People travel for various reasons, and people are traveling more

5

than ever. For 2011, the projected number of airline passengers was a record-setting 2.75 billion, over 600 million more than in 2006 [22]. Businesses now routinely utilize suppliers and services from distant locations, requiring more global travel. Tourism is also on the rise. From 1950 to 2011, the world's population increased by 2.5-fold, but the number of tourist arrivals increased over 37-fold [8,23] (Figure 1.1). Most increases were in tourists from Asia, and most tourists visited a few highly frequented locations.

The interconnection between communities has an important role in influenza epidemiology. Whereas influenza transmission within communities is predominantly driven by children, transmission between communities is predominantly driven by those who travel frequently, predominately adults. Travelers have been identified as a major contributing factor to the annual cycle of seasonal influenza. In one study, researchers used antigenic and genetic analyses to demonstrate that influenza A (H3N2) virus epidemics for the years 2002–2007 were initiated by influenza viruses originating from East/South-East Asia [24]. The researchers attributed the high frequency of travel and trade from East/South-East Asia to Oceania, North America, and Europe as a likely contributor to the migration of influenza A (H3N2). A lack of travel and trade with South America was suggested to account for the lag in appearance of new viruses to that region.

Tourists have also been identified to contribute to the spread of seasonal influenza. In one report, older travelers from Australia flew to New York City for a cruise to Montreal, likely carrying the influenza A/Sydney/5/97 virus with them [25]. Although this virus had begun to circulate in the Southern Hemisphere, it had not been detected previously in the Northern Hemisphere. The travelers likely infected cruise ship crew members who then infected at least two subsequent cohorts of travelers on the cruise ship. This report demonstrated the potential for travelers to contribute to the global spread of influenza.

Travel has also contributed to the spread of emerging pandemic influenza viruses. Various factors during the 1918 pandemic demonstrate the role of inter-community connections in maintaining the progression of the pandemic. Large-scale movements of military recruits within the United States, and between Europe and the United States, carried the emerging

pandemic strain to other naïve populations [26]. Introduction of the virus to crowded military barracks in the United States and in Europe had a devastating impact on the troops. In the Pacific, ship passengers introduced pandemic influenza to remote islanders with substantial impact; Western Samoa suffered the loss of 19–22% of its population [27,28]. Isolated locations in North America were greatly impacted by introduction of the virus [26]. Native Americans had high case fatality rates, reportedly up to 9%. Remote areas of Alaska worked hard to prevent infection from arriving transport ships, but asymptomatic influenza in sailors on departure from Seattle or Vancouver allowed for introduction in port towns throughout the Alaskan peninsula with devastating outcomes. Even infrequent interaction between fur traders and remote Canadian communities was associated with introduction and spread of pandemic H1N1 in 1918 [29].

Almost a century after the 1918 pandemic, the 2009 pandemic H1N1 (A(H1N1)pdm09) influenza virus emerged and its spread was accelerated by international travel. Soon after the detection of the first two recognized cases of A(H1N1)pdm09 in southern California in the United States, additional cases were rapidly reported from Texas, Chicago, Arizona, and New York [30]. In the first reported case series, 18% of patients with A(H1N1)pdm09 in the United States had traveled to Mexico within 7 days of illness onset [31]. Subsequent travel from Mexico, and onward, especially from the United States, led to the spread of A(H1N1)pdm09 to multiple other countries. Researchers have used statistics of airline travel between Mexico and other countries for the 1 March to 30 April 2008 timeframe to see if the locations of the most frequent destinations predicted sites of earliest recognition of A(H1N1)pdm09 in 2009 [32]. During that time period, 2.35 million people traveled from Mexico to over 1000 cities globally. Countries that had received more than 1400 travelers from Mexico were at a significantly elevated risk of importation of A(H1N1) pdm09. Over 80% of travelers from Mexico flew to the United States and Canada. The three most common destinations were Los Angeles (221 494 people), New York City (126 345), and Chicago (111 531).

For many US college students, and families with children in school, travel to Mexico for spring break provided the opportunity for the virus to infect travelers who then returned home and disseminated the novel virus within their communities. One example from early in the 2009 pandemic is from the University of Delaware [33] where a small number of students traveled to Mexico for spring break and were infected with A(H1N1)pdm09. After returning to school, these travelers introduced the virus to their naïve classmates and provided the virus an opportunity to spread rapidly through the campus over the subsequent two weeks. While the initial number of introductions from travelers was low, transmission of infection increased considerably due to significant person-to-person interaction at "Greek Week". This fraternity and sorority event had a number of social and athletic activities which were apparently quite favorable to virus transmission.

Periodically, some events serve to combine extreme crowding and travel, such as the World Cup football match or the Olympic Games. These events have the potential to be a "perfect storm" for influenza transmission. One of the most dense and traveled mass gatherings is the Hajj, the annual Muslim pilgrimage to Mecca in Saudi Arabia [34]. At its most concentrated point during the one-week event, the crowd compresses to a density of around seven people per square meter as pilgrims circle the kaba sharif. Respiratory infections are common, with influenza frequently identified [35]. In the past, travelers returning from the Hajj have initiated outbreaks of cholera and, most recently, meningococcal meningitis. For past influenza pandemics in 1957 and 1968, the number of visitors was considerably smaller (215 000 and 318 000) and few traveled by air. In 2009, only months after the emergence of A(H1N1)pdm09, over 2.5 million people from 160 countries converged on holy sites in and around Mecca. To minimize the impact of A(H1N1)pdm09, Saudi public health officials screened all arriving travelers for fever and symptoms, and isolated ill persons, established laboratory testing and disease surveillance, utilized treatment centers and clinical algorithms, and encouraged persons at high risk of severe illness to postpone their pilgrimage for a year [36]. Over the summer of 2009, some Muslim countries recommended against attending the Hajj completely. Following the event, surveillance identified no increased illness rates among Hajj attendees and no evidence of significant acceleration of the pandemic attributed to the Hajj [36,37].

Convergence: poultry, pigs, people, and pandemics

The world's population is increasing in megacities, and, for many of these urban residents, the potential for wealth is also increasing. The greater buying power of these residents has led to a rising demand for meat. From the mid-1960s until the mid-1990s, the global consumption of meat rose by 150% [38]. By 2030, the appetite for meat is anticipated to rise an additional 44%; poultry consumption is expected to have the greatest increase. Greater consumption of livestock protein improves overall nutrition and is an efficient food source for urban dwellers [39]. When one considers which source of protein is most efficient for supplying the urban appetite of megacities in the developing world, poultry and pigs are the clear winners; cattle have space and feed requirements that make them less practical. Poultry and pigs, referred to as "monogastrics," can be raised in very animal-dense settings and can be more easily transported to urban markets. One additional important characteristic of both poultry and pigs is their role as predominant animal reservoirs of influenza.

To keep pace with the rising population and growing demand for meat protein, the numbers of monogastrics have risen as well. According to the Food and Agriculture Organization of the United Nations (FAO), in 2010, there were an estimated 21.5 billion poultry (91% are chickens), up from 4.3 billion in the early 1960s [40] (Figure 1.1). That equates to around three birds for every person on the planet. There are around 1 billion pigs as well. Over the 40 years from 1967 to 2007, the amount of available protein from poultry meat (grams per person per day) increased 3.4-fold [41]. For pig meat, it increased 1.6-fold. As the population and demand for meat continues to increase in megacities in the developing world, the infrastructure and biosecurity needed to support livestock commerce will need to be drastically altered.

For urban settings in developing countries, where refrigeration is not widely available, poultry and other meat sources must be transported into cities through wholesale and retail live animal markets. Large cities require a constant source of birds from producers in and around the city at large-scale facilities as well as small village farms. This "poultry commerce" has led to significant increases in urban and peri-urban livestock density and has generated a complicated network of poultry suppliers [42]. Take Jakarta, Indonesia, as an example. It has a population of almost 10 million people who consume around 1 million birds each day [43]. Birds originate from multiple locations on the islands of Java and Sumatra and are carried to Jakarta traveling on over 500 trucks making multiple runs back and forth daily. These birds are handed from wholesaler to retailer, and are made available at over 200 live bird markets in and around the city. A similar situation exists in many other locations around the globe, including Dhaka, Mumbai, Cairo, Lagos, São Paolo, Guangzhou, and many others. In these resource-limited settings, it is challenging to prevent the emergence and spread of avian influenza.

A number of factors have been associated with the emergence, spread, and maintenance of highly pathogenic avian influenza (HPAI) H5N1 viruses in domestic poultry [44]. The cycle of infection first starts with wild migratory birds. Waterfowl are a natural reservoir for low pathogenic influenza viruses, and rivers and lakes, where wild birds congregate with domesticated ducks and geese, promote the exchange of avian influenza viruses. Low pathogenic H5 and H7 viruses may become highly pathogenic as they replicate in domestic birds and, in turn, transmit HPAI to migrating birds that can spread avian influenza viruses across vast distances where domestic poultry, such as chickens, ducks, ostriches, and other domestic fowl, can be infected along the flyways. Once introduced into domestic flocks, other manmade factors lead to further disease: (i) poultry kept in dense conditions where viruses are easily shared among birds; (ii) national highway networks which allow for rapid transport of birds during incubation and infectious periods; (iii) live bird markets which serve as nodes where transmission of HPAI can occur and spread onward; (iv) communities with a high density of homes where people live in close proximity to one another and to flocks of poultry; (v) low literacy rates which are associated with decreased recognition of HPAI and lower rates of reporting infected flocks to authorities; and (vi) practices in low-income communities that depend almost entirely on poultry as a source of protein where diseased poultry are used for their own consumption or are sent to markets.

People and poultry exist in close proximity; however, human infection with avian influenza viruses appears to be rare. Influenza seemingly circulates in parallel, but separate, human and avian epidemics. The same is not the case with pigs. Influenza viruses from birds and people converge in swine as a common basin or "mixing vessel" where adaptation and reassortment are a frequent occurrence. This convergence is most exemplified at a genetic level with the A(H1N1)pdm09 influenza virus [45]. Immediately after detection of the first two recognized cases of pandemic influenza in April 2009, genetic sequencing revealed that the eight gene segments of the virus were from a mix of avian, human, and swine origin from both North America and Eurasia. The mixed lineage of the virus, evident at a molecular level, is a direct reflection of the co-mingling of poultry, pigs, and people at a macro level in farms and live markets throughout the world. Recent experience with a newly recognized H3N2 variant (H3N2v) influenza virus in the United States further reveals the interconnection of animals and humans and the importance of surveillance in swine [46].

In August 2011, routine surveillance for influenza in Pennsylvania and Indiana in the United States detected two unassociated human cases of infection due to an influenza A (H3N2)v virus with genes from avian, swine, and human influenza viruses [46]. Over the subsequent year, hundreds of additional infections from many states were detected primarily among young children who had frequent and prolonged contact with swine, notably at county and state agricultural fairs. This virus was first detected in swine in November 2010 but had not been detected yet in humans. The virus had two interesting features: (i) the hemagglutinin gene was similar to seasonal H3 genes from viruses that circulated among humans in the early to mid-1990s; and (ii) the matrix (M) gene was the M gene of the 2009 H1N1 pandemic virus. Using available sequence data from swine and human influenza surveillance, the natural history of the virus could be deduced. Human H3N2 viruses had been introduced into the swine population in the 1990s. Gene exchange among viruses in swine produced a reassortant virus between (i) the human H3N2 virus which provided the HA and NA genes; and (ii) a common swine influenza virus containing a group of genes referred to as the Triple Reassortant Internal Gene (TRIG) constellation which provided: the PB1,

HA, and NA genes from human influenza origin; the NP, M, and NS genes from swine influenza origin; and the PB2 and PA genes from avian influenza origin. This TRIG-containing virus circulated among pigs since at least 1998. Following the introduction of the 2009 pandemic virus into the swine population in 2009–2010, a further reassortment occurred with the swine H3N2 virus accepting the M gene from the A(H1N1)pdm09 virus to produce the new H3N2v virus which caused hundreds of infections in humans in direct contact with swine in the United States. The H3N2v virus has been shown to be transmissible in ferrets similar to human seasonal viruses [47]. It also appears that people born after the late-1990s have low levels of or no detectable serum antibodies that would be expected to provide cross-protective immunity to the virus. Will this virus take off like the 2009 pandemic H1N1 virus, rapidly traveling to large urban centers around the globe? Even though there appears to be a greater amount of cross-protective immunity in the population than for the 2009 H1N1 pandemic virus prior to its global spread, close monitoring of influenza in human and swine populations is needed to detect any change in virus transmission characteristics, and appropriate swine and human control measures that should be implemented.

Global interconnectedness requires global coordination and response

Global challenges for surveillance

The prevention and control of influenza is impossible without ongoing monitoring of human and animal influenza viruses. Virologic surveillance for human influenza is critical for (i) situational awareness of circulating viruses for directing clinical management; (ii) detection of novel influenza viruses which may indicate emerging and potentially pandemic threats; (iii) acquiring representative influenza viruses for use in vaccines; (iv) monitoring influenza virus resistance to antiviral drugs; and (v) evaluation of the antigenic properties of circulating viruses to detect antigenic drift from currently available vaccines. While it is important to know these characteristics of influenza viruses, many countries have not implemented comprehensive human influenza surveillance programs. A number of challenges face public health authorities:

lack of sustainable funding for surveillance programs; training and maintaining epidemiology and laboratory staff; and justifying influenza surveillance in the context of other public health priorities. For example, many countries in sub-Saharan Africa prior to 2007 had no human influenza surveillance at all; many concluded that influenza only rarely was present and causing disease. With additional resources as a part of global pandemic preparedness, surveillance was initiated and revealed unexpectedly high levels of influenza illness and associated child disease burden [48].

Influenza surveillance in humans is patchy, with some regions of the globe covered much more than others. Animal influenza surveillance, on the other hand, is either poor or nonexistent in most countries. Monitoring influenza viruses in poultry and swine is important for determining causes of illness, targeting control measures, developing appropriate animal vaccines to prevent illness and loss of production, and identifying and sequencing genes of emerging influenza viruses with pandemic potential. The number of gene sequences from avian influenza surveillance has not kept pace with the global increase in the population of poultry [49]. Importantly, sequences from swine influenza viruses were difficult to find in 2009 when the pandemic influenza A(H1N1)pdm09 virus emerged. Gene sequences from the first two recognized human cases were posted as soon as testing and analysis had been completed, and comparison of the novel influenza sequences to those from thousands of recent and historic human influenza viruses immediately demonstrated that the illnesses from California were due to a reassortant virus that previously had not been detected in humans. Comparison with available animal virus sequences revealed clear similarity to sequences from swine viruses, but a significant divergence from the relatively few swine influenza sequences that were available for analysis. This significant evolutionary distance between the new pandemic virus and its closest relatives was attributed to a lack of swine surveillance and to the paucity of posted swine influenza sequence data [45]. Although contributions of animal influenza virus sequences have improved recently, most information in publicly available databases are not geographically representative and are often only deposited years after collection of the specimen. However, sequences from swine influenza viruses in the United States have increased substantially during 2011–2012 in response to the emergence of H3N2v [50].

Surveillance of animal influenza viruses is challenging on a number of levels. First, there are resource challenges. For many countries, there may be difficulties prioritizing resources for animal influenza surveillance over other needs. Establishing and maintaining specimen collection systems and laboratory testing infrastructure requires funding and technical expertise that may be difficult to find. Second, competing interests can be a challenge. In many countries, there are longstanding differences in the mission and priorities of human health authorities and agriculture authorities which often lead to constrained communication and limited collaboration. For instance, Ministries of Health (MoHs) prioritize limiting human illness from zoonotic infections and detecting novel influenza virus infections early to prevent, or at least prepare, for potential pandemics. Ministries of Agriculture (MoAgs), however, often promote swine and poultry production for feeding the population or to increase sales and exports. Differences in missions and priorities between these governmental agencies may be difficult to harmonize.

A third challenge for surveillance of influenza in animals is the designation of a virus as intellectual property [51]. As the world gets smaller, and as companies become more global, the protection of proprietary business information and adherence to international patent law is paramount. As major exporters of emerging technologies, Europe and North America have pushed for greater enforcement of intellectual property rights in other countries. Pirating of movies and computer software are considered theft of intellectual property which should be stopped. What about animal influenza viruses? Are they similar to software? In the United States, and in many other countries, the answer is yes. Patents can be granted for genes, proteins, engineered animals, bacteria, nonhuman influenza and other viruses, and just about anything in the life sciences except humans. This is most relevant to influenza prevention and control in the manufacture of vaccines. A novel animal-origin influenza virus may be detected first in South-East Asia, but production and profit from vaccines using the virus may occur among manufacturers in Europe. Whose property is the virus? It is good to have pre-pandemic vaccines, but should not the country where the virus originated also benefit? Alter-

natively, a veterinary laboratory in the United States or elsewhere may identify a novel H2N3 among swine and consider the virus as a business trade secret with manufacturing potential for vaccinating swine. Profits from use of the virus will allow continued laboratory testing and identification of other viruses; but should not public health have access to the virus and use of the genetic information it contains? When viral genes are considered to be intellectual property, there may be an incentive to delay or withhold public notification of the discovery and details of the virus. Innovation and discovery are the soul of biotechnology and should be protected; however, there is something about influenza viruses that requires a different and more dynamic approach. The influenza virus continually reinvents itself as it travels around an increasingly connected world, and global systems for surveillance and information sharing need to be just as flexible, dynamic, and nimble.

Global regulations for detection and control

Influenza viruses do not respect jurisdictional boundaries. International efforts for mandating common approaches for detecting and responding to influenza epidemics and pandemics are challenging. Starting with cholera in the mid-1800s, global regulations for control of human infectious diseases had various different iterations; however, it was not until 1951 that a formal set of International Health Regulations (IHR) were developed [52]. The IHR were subsequently updated in 1969 and remained unchanged for years. Following eradication of smallpox, the regulations essentially only applied to the traditional quarantinable diseases of cholera, plague, and yellow fever. Over the subsequent decades, the world changed, becoming more crowded and more connected. Notably with the recognition of emerging infections in the 1990s and with severe acute respiratory syndrome (SARS) and avian influenza in the early 2000s, the existing IHR were in need of an update. Global control and response measures needed to be rapid, and existing systems for detecting and reporting important events were inadequate.

In 2005, after years of development and revision by Member States, WHO announced the new IHR which differed dramatically from the 1969 update. The new regulations attempted to address the dynamic nature of emerging infections and the existing resource and political challenges of detection and reporting. One important difference in IHR 2005 was the development of a "public health emergency of international concern" (PHEIC). In bright distinction to the previous, limited list of three quarantinable pathogens, IHR 2005 required reporting of an "extraordinary event" which is determined: (i) to constitute a public health risk to other States through the international spread of disease; and (ii) to potentially require a coordinated international response [53]. A PHEIC could be an event within a country's boundaries, but also could be an event that has had spillover into a country from abroad. This part of the new regulation helped to address the issues of emerging infections in an increasingly interconnected world. In addition to the broad event of a PHEIC, the IHR 2005 lists certain diseases for which a case *may* need to be reported (e.g., cholera, plague, yellow fever). For both the diseases in that list, as well as for the PHEICs, the IHR 2005 provided a decision tool to help Member States determine whether or not an IHR report should be sent to the WHO. The algorithm requires a Member State to ask the following questions: (i) is the public health impact of the event serious; (ii) is the event unusual or unexpected; (iii) is there a significant risk for international spread; and (iv) is there a significant risk for international travel or trade restrictions. If two or more of the questions are answered as yes, then a report of either the PHEIC or the listed disease is required. One important exception to this new framework, however, is that four diseases are required to be reported within 48 hours of their detection without use of the decision algorithm and with no Member State consideration as to whether an IHR is necessary. Those four diseases are smallpox, wild-type poliomyelitis, SARS, and human influenza caused by a new subtype.

What does all this mean for influenza? For one thing, it means that influenza is a central concern for global public health disease control. If a human infection with a new subtype, such as H5N1 or H9N2 occurs, cases must be reported quickly to remain in compliance with the new IHR. But with the addition of the PHEIC concept, there are further implications for the reporting of human infections with other novel influenza viruses. For example, in April 2009, the first two recognized cases of infection with the A(H1N1)pdm09 virus were identified in the United States. This virus did not represent a "new subtype"

of influenza in humans, but was a significantly drifted subtype for which much of the world's population had little to no immunity. Under the expanded definition of an emergency as defined in a PHEIC, the first cases of the 2009 pandemic clearly constituted a "public health risk" requiring a "coordinated international response." For this reason, it was reported immediately as a PEHIC to WHO as required by the IHR. Thus, IHR 2005 provided a framework for reporting and communication that facilitated notification of the world's public health community of the emerging pandemic very early and throughout the course of the event.

Regulations for reporting animal influenza viruses follow a different approach. The World Organization for Animal Health (OIE) maintains a list of notifiable animal diseases to ensure transparency and enhance knowledge about zoonoses around the globe [54]. The FAO enforces international regulations for food security, and requires countries to report the animal diseases on the OIE list [55]. For poultry, this translates to reporting any infection due to avian influenza A H5 and H7 viruses with high or low pathogenicity. When these viruses are detected, there are immediate measures that should be taken, including culling the flock. This focus on H5 and H7 in poultry aligns well with the IHR and human health priorities for preventing illness in people exposed to these birds and for monitoring for the emergence of potentially pandemic viruses. For swine, on the other hand, there is no notifiable influenza disease on the OIE list. Influenza viruses in pigs may cause mild illness or no illness at all. Herein lays a predicament. Human public health authorities want to know when viruses of concern are appearing in swine populations so that pre-pandemic vaccines can be made and diagnostic tests can be optimized for detecting the new viruses. More importantly, human public health authorities are required to submit IHR reports of novel influenza infections to WHO. From the agriculture side, there is no requirement to look for swine influenza, and there is no required intervention if it is detected. Surveillance for swine influenza viruses may, in fact, only serve to frighten the public and lead to decreased pork sales and exports. This disproportionality makes coordinated pandemic preparedness and response very challenging. Any attempt to improve monitoring of novel influenza viruses in swine must address this disparity in regulated reporting between human and agriculture authorities. Unless there is a coincident robust system for detecting swine influenza in pigs, even upgraded regulations to improve reporting of cases are of little value.

Global network for surveillance

Following the discovery of the viral cause of influenza in the 1930s, researchers in London, New York, and elsewhere developed laboratory methods for culturing and characterizing the viruses. As the tools for detecting influenza improved, the potential for monitoring influenza through virologic surveillance was realized. Outbreaks of respiratory disease could be shown to be caused by influenza, and with viruses available for study, vaccines were then possible. Successful efforts to develop an inactivated influenza vaccine in the early 1940s by the US military led to establishment of a small US network of laboratories for isolating the viruses [56]. In 1947, significant antigenic drift in circulating influenza viruses rendered the influenza vaccine ineffective and raised the specter of another pandemic. This event was, in part, the inspiration in 1948 for the WHO Interim Commission to establish the World Influenza Centre in London and propose the organization of a laboratory network that would be coordinated by WHO to monitor influenza viruses infecting humans. By 1949, 38 countries had WHO-designated regional influenza laboratories and it was proposed that all countries eventually might have their own National Influenza Centers (NICs). In 1962, this nascent network of laboratories had grown to include two Collaborating Centers (CCs) for influenza (at the National Institute for Medical Research in London, United Kingdom and the Centers for Disease Control in Atlanta, United States) and 59 NICs. A third CC for the Ecology of Influenza in Animals (Memphis, Tennessee) was initiated in 1976, and by 1984, 108 NICs had been established worldwide. This Global Influenza Surveillance Network (GISN) included five CCs for Influenza (with the addition of CCs at the Victorian Infectious Diseases Reference Laboratory in Melbourne, Australia, and the National Institute for Infectious Diseases in Tokyo, Japan) and 134 National Centers in 2010. In 2011, a sixth CC was established at the Chinese Center for Disease Control and Prevention in Beijing and the name of the WHO network was changed from GISN to the Global Influenza Surveillance and Response System (GISRS) following discussions among Member States at the World Health Assembly. As of July 2012 there were 6 WHO CCs for influenza and 140 NICs in 110 WHO Member States (Figure 1.2).

In an increasingly connected world, a highly connected influenza laboratory network is necessary. From its inception in 1947, the proposed design for the global network of influenza laboratories was for NICs within countries to collect respiratory specimens from clinical encounters, isolate the viruses in culture, and send the grown viruses of interest to the CCs [56]. This basic model has persisted since that time. Many NICs have been added in the last 5 years, especially an encouraging increase of NICs in Africa [57]. The capability of NICs varies considerably; some have high-throughput capacity and others maintain only limited laboratory testing. WHO recognizes this disparity and works through CCs to provide training, laboratory test guidance, and quality assessment in order to have a more standardized laboratory approach across the network. One way WHO has attempted to achieve lab standardization is through distribution of common protocols and reagents. Since the 1970s, standard reference reagents for antigenic testing have been distributed to each WHO-recognized NIC by the WHO CC at Centers for Disease Control (CDC) in the United States. With the availability of molecular testing using real-time reverse transcription polymerase chain reaction (PCR) assays, CDC also began providing molecular test kits to all NICs in 2008. NIC summary reports for virologic surveillance initially were sent weekly by post to WHO in Geneva, and reporting migrated over time to telex, fax, and finally the internet. Currently, data are collected weekly through the WHO FluNet web site and are made publicly available. The amount of testing and reporting of information increased significantly in 2009 with the emergence of the A(H1N1)pdm09 virus and the availability of PCR reagents. By use of the internet, and through training and use of standardized laboratory testing, GISRS was able to rapidly ramp up to provide near real-time tracking of the 2009 pandemic virus. Since then, over 3 million specimens were tested and reported by NICs, with 1.4 million in 2009, 730 000 in 2010, and 930 000 in 2011.

Viruses and specimens first tested at NICs are sent to one of the five CCs that characterize human influenza viruses. NICs are asked to forward representative

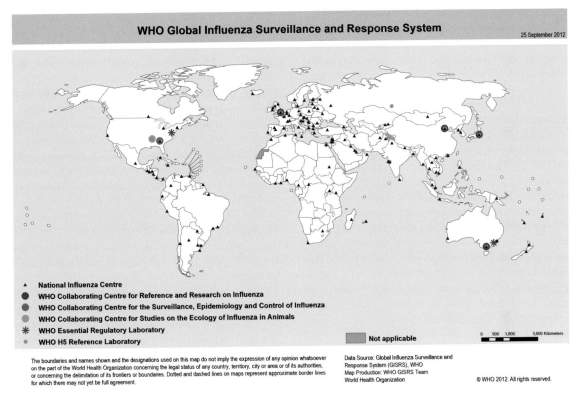

Figure 1.2. Global Influenza Surveillance and Response System, World Health Organization. Established in 1952, the network currently comprises six WHO Collaborating Centers, four WHO Essential Regulatory Laboratories, and 140 institutions in 110 WHO Member States, which are recognized by WHO as National Influenza Centers, in addition to ad hoc groups established to address specific emerging issues [57]. © WHO 2012. All rights reserved.

virus isolates as well as any low-reacting viruses based on antigenic testing. These viruses represent a subset of all tested specimens and are further characterized at the CCs both antigenically and genetically. Collection of specimens and testing at NICs along with comprehensive laboratory testing at the CCs provides critical information for influenza prevention and control: tracking of antiviral resistance, detection of drifted or novel viruses, measurement of the degree of match between circulating and vaccine viruses, and identification of the best vaccine viruses for upcoming vaccine manufacturing. The WHO recommended vaccine viruses are provided to manufacturers who then produce vaccine for use for the Northern and Southern Hemisphere seasons. The WHO GISRS network of NICs and CCs serves to connect across great distances

such that a virus causing illness in an isolated part of the world, such as the Solomon Islands, can become a vaccine preventing illness around the globe.

In the past, viruses were freely distributed and shared among members of the WHO surveillance network and with researchers, vaccine manufacturers, and commercial companies with no restrictions. With the emergence of avian influenza A H5N1 in 2003, and with concerns about the availability of vaccine if a pandemic were to occur, many WHO Member States requested a dialogue to re-evaluate the way the WHO global surveillance system managed the sharing of influenza viruses and the benefits accruing from their use in vaccines and other products [58]. The heart of the issue was that some developing countries were concerned about potential difficulties securing H5N1 vaccine developed from their own viruses. Here was the convergence of people, poultry, pandemics, and *property*. Countries participating in the WHO surveillance network contributed avian influenza viruses isolated from their citizens, but believed they were receiving no benefit in obtaining affordable vaccine to prevent illness in their countries during a pandemic. Through extended international negotiations, the World Health Assembly addressed this concern and, in 2011, approved the Pandemic Influenza Preparedness (PIP) Framework [58]. The agreement was designed to achieve a "fair, transparent, equitable, efficient, effective system" for the sharing of H5N1 and other influenza viruses with human pandemic potential and to provide access to vaccines and sharing of other benefits. In particular, the framework requires users of PIP biologic materials which includes "human clinical specimens, virus isolates of wild type human H5N1 and other influenza viruses with human pandemic potential; and modified viruses prepared from H5N1 and/or other influenza viruses with human pandemic potential developed by WHO GISRS laboratories, these being candidate vaccine viruses generated by reverse genetics and/or high growth re-assortment" [58] to agree to benefit sharing with the countries that provide those materials. In an increasingly connected world, where influenza viruses are shared and transformed into vaccines, the PIP Framework attempts to maintain a lasting connection between virus and benefit sharing for resource-challenged countries. Implementation of this global agreement is only beginning but WHO's GISRS laboratories are instituting new systems for virus tracking. In addition, Industry, Ministries of Health, NICs, CCs, and WHO are working to understand and adhere to the framework. The PIP Framework, IHR, and expanding global laboratory networks are some of many changes occurring with influenza surveillance and control. Many other diagnostic, analytic, and information technologies are available or on the horizon with potential benefits for monitoring outbreaks of concern and response to them.

New opportunities in a changing world

New tools for global detection and surveillance

The recognition of an emerging pandemic and the global response in 2009 was vastly different from

efforts for the 1968 H3N2 pandemic and even different from SARS in 2003. The 2009 response took advantage of new molecular technologies, instant information in connected virtual communities, and convergence of multiple data sources to improve forecasting and for focusing interventions. The 2009 pandemic was the first pandemic during the era of molecular diagnostics. Reverse transcription-PCR was first described for use in detecting influenza in 1991, and since then, the method has been gradually adopted and, with standardization of protocols and decreasing costs, has been applied to influenza surveillance. It is now the method of choice in academic medical centers and public health laboratories [59]. The CDC's WHO CC developed a PCR assay to detect influenza A and B, and influenza A subtypes A/H1, A/H3, and A/H5 to support public health surveillance and pandemic preparedness in the United States. The assay was one of the first seasonal influenza PCR assays to be approved by the US Food and Drug Administration, occurring in September 2008, and was subsequently provided to public health laboratories. By April 2009, when the first cases due to the emerging pandemic A(H1N1)pdm09 virus were recognized, 45 US public health laboratories were already using the devices for seasonal influenza surveillance [60]. As part of the pandemic response, an additional 60 US public health laboratories were rapidly added and many NICs in other countries were also equipped. PCR reagents were shipped from CDC to over 150 GISRS laboratories across the globe throughout the response. For many laboratories distant from the North American epicenter of the pandemic, PCR reagents arrived much sooner than cases of pandemic influenza, allowing for early detection and response.

Perhaps the greatest benefit from the "molecular miracle" has been the use of genetic sequencing to rapidly characterize the viruses for directing public health decision-making. Influenza virus sequence data had been increasingly available in GenBank and other public online repositories; however, with the emergence of A(H1N1)pdm09, sequence entries skyrocketed. The WHO CCs posted thousands of sequences during the first year of the response. Sequence submission from GISRS laboratories and other sources made possible the near real-time monitoring of the virus as it emerged and evolved. Early on, epidemiologic surveillance for hospitalizations and deaths demonstrated great differences in disease outcomes in North America; cases in Mexico appeared to be considerably more severe than in the United States. Fortunately, sequencing of the genes of the H1N1 pandemic influenza viruses demonstrated that the viruses circulating in the two countries did not differ from each other, and neither country's viruses carried any known genetic markers associated with increased disease severity. Genetic sequencing provided the capability to monitor for antiviral resistance, identify the emergence of new mutations associated with more severe outcomes, and track any changes that might represent increasing drift from chosen vaccine viruses. Genetic sequencing and monitoring through GISRS provided a platform for global tracking of the emerging virus, connecting the resources of the broad surveillance community together for pandemic response. Although the 2009 pandemic virus was first detected in humans, it contained genes most closely related to swine influenza viruses. Participation from MoAgs and animal health investigators was less critical during the pandemic response given that the virus was widely circulating in humans. Since then, especially with the increasing prevalence of H3N2v in humans and swine, joint monitoring of swine and human influenza viruses has improved with a considerable increase in the numbers of swine influenza sequences appearing in GenBank.

Looking forward, greater access to rapid sequencing capability will transform influenza diagnosis and surveillance. Given the relatively small genome of the influenza virus, routine sequencing of all eight gene segments will allow diagnostic devices to not only detect the presence of influenza virus, but will concurrently reveal additional information for clinical management, such as known markers for antiviral resistance. For human and animal surveillance, greater routine sequencing will allow public health officials to more easily detect and rapidly characterize emerging novel or antiviral-resistant influenza viruses. Sequence information can be combined with other laboratory and epidemiologic findings to help identify animal influenza viruses most likely to emerge as a pandemic in humans. An example of this convergence of information is the Influenza Risk Assessment Tool (IRAT) being developed by influenza experts which combines 10 evaluation criteria characterizing the properties of the virus, human host susceptibility and pathogenesis, epidemiology of infections, and the

ecology of the virus [61]. This tool will be used to prioritize which viruses should be used to make vaccine viruses and whether pre-pandemic lots of vaccine should be produced.

At present, specimens from humans are collected in clinical settings, sent to state or provincial public health laboratories such as GISRS NICs for PCR testing and culture, and forwarded to WHO CCs for sequencing. Implementing sequencing at the hospital or NIC level, and possibly at the point of clinical care, will greatly expand the availability, timeliness, and comprehensiveness of influenza virus genetic data. Nonetheless, even with the promise of next generation sequencing capability, there are some challenges remaining. First, sequencing is not a replacement for culture. Functional viruses are needed for monitoring the antigenic characteristics of the virus and for performing neuraminidase inhibition assays. Second, although sequencing has dropped dramatically in cost and increased considerably in speed and throughput, the data storage and analysis requirements remain daunting. Current sequencing devices generate terabytes of data requiring dedicated servers to support analysis, often taking considerable time to complete. Use of off-site, cloud-based storage and analysis services will be necessary to allow sequencing to be accessible and cost-efficient for influenza detection and surveillance.

Instant and converging information

Just as the world of people, poultry, and pigs is becoming more crowded and connected, the world of information is undergoing similar dynamics. When influenza cases are reported or when genetic and antigenic characterizations of influenza viruses are posted online, cases and viruses essentially become information. Once available on public web sites, the experience from the 2009 pandemic shows that information itself "goes viral," spreading and changing as it is transmitted. Information is now instantaneous, abundant, and interlinked. Typing "influenza" into a commonly used search engine provides about 260 million results in only 0.18 seconds. The 2009 pandemic was the first pandemic, and the first major infectious disease outbreak, to utilize the full potential of the internet and online communities [62]. From the first recognized cases in April 2009, influenza virus sequence information could be accessed virtually from anywhere, anytime, via the internet. Case counts, of varying accuracy, were posted daily on government web sites along with frequently changing recommendations for clinicians, public health officials, and the general public. Online news media sources reported the progression of the pandemic in a 24-hour news cycle. Publications of scientific findings were available online as soon as peer review was completed and were accompanied by continuous threads of commentary and dialogue among experts and others.

These new online tools allowed public health officials to push information as soon as it was available through multiple channels such as RSS feeds, Twitter, Facebook, ProMED, email groups, and other media. The general public was not only passively receiving information, it could also engage or dialogue with public health officials and online information sources: to provide feedback through chat sessions and blogs; to access additional information such as online tools for finding nearest locations to get vaccinated; to monitor indicators of influenza-like illness using internet search terms such as Google Flu Trends; or to conduct online surveys to estimate vaccine coverage among pregnant women. Perhaps the most important information tool from the pandemic was the ability for disparate data to converge in online communities where the public could access free web-based tools for analysis, interpretation, and visualization. Sites such as the Global Initiative on Sharing All Influenza Data (GISAID) endorsed by WHO CCs, or the Influenza Research Database (IRD) and GenBank made available by the US National Institutes of Health [63], brought hundreds of thousands of influenza genome sequences, protein structures, epidemiologic information, and other data together for use by researchers, modelers, vaccine manufacturers, diagnostic test developers, and public health officials. These platforms provided structure and standardization for available information to converge and facilitate influenza prevention and control. Without these tools, the numerous and distributed pockets of available influenza data would be unconnected and unorganized.

Looking forward, connected and converging information may further assist with influenza diagnosis, treatment, prevention, outbreak detection, and pandemic response. As electronic health records are more widely used, surveillance may be greatly facilitated for influenza-like illness, laboratory-confirmed influenza, and influenza-associated hospitalizations and deaths, and may have the potential to be timelier, more representative, and less resource-intensive for public health agencies. Applications on smart phones could provide patients and clinicians with easy to use algorithms for diagnosing influenza, locating sites for antiviral treatment or vaccination, and for connecting to sites for additional information or participating in surveys. After treatment or vaccination, patient follow-up could occur through email, cell phone text messages, Facebook, and other means to remind patients to complete treatment courses and to collect data useful for monitoring adverse events and vaccine effectiveness. Point-of-care and in-home mobile diagnostic devices already connect to the internet for monitoring glucose and hemoglobin A1C results for diabetic patients. Influenza diagnostic test manufacturers are exploring this same approach for clinician offices and pharmacies to diagnose influenza rapidly, upload the results to electronic health records for clinician and patient access online, and send de-identified laboratory results to cloud-based public health agency reporting sites for influenza surveillance. Cell phone coverage is exploding at a rapid pace in resource-limited settings, allowing many of these tools to be accessible in those locations as well. Although there is great promise in the age of information, public health authorities, academic researchers, and others will need to coordinate efforts to assure that information is shared, rapidly available, readily accessible, and well-structured to facilitate prevention and control efforts.

Conclusions

The world of influenza is complex and interconnected. Human influenza viruses carry within them the history of multiple avian, swine, and human gene origins, reflecting a continuous and opportunistic ability of the virus to reinvent itself and reinfect populations. Pandemics, sometimes with tremendous mortality, can arise from changes to influenza viruses circulating back and forth among people and their animals in isolated farming communities and markets around the globe. The opportunities for exchanging viruses between species and for reassortment of their genes have increased as the populations of humans, swine, and birds have increased, all in close proximity to one another in growing urban communities, and living only one flight (and one incubation period) apart from each other.

Influenza is a global challenge, and the prevention and control of influenza requires a commensurate global response. International networks of laboratories and public health agencies have been established, and have also adapted and reinvented themselves by incorporating new technologies, new regulations, and new information sharing tools and platforms. With an increasingly crowded and connected world, influenza viruses have the opportunity to spread and adapt rapidly. To counter that, new molecular diagnostic and genetic sequencing capabilities are available to public health officials, researchers, and clinicians for rapidly determining appropriate treatment, control measures, and prevention strategies. The greatest remaining challenge is maintaining the resources, innovation, and global coordination for responding to influenza viruses.

Acknowledgments

Any views expressed in the Work by contributors employed by the United States government at the time of writing do not necessarily represent the views of the United States government, and the contributor's contribution to the Work is not meant to serve as an official endorsement of any statement to the extent that such statement may conflict with any official position of the United States government.

References

1. World Health Organization. Programmes and projects. Immunization, vaccines and biologicals: influenza. 2008. Available from: http://www.who.int/immunization/topics/influenza/en/index.html (accessed 13 August 2012).

2. Molinari NA, Ortega-Sanchez IR, Messonnier ML, Thompson WW, Wortley PM, Weintraub E, et al. The annual impact of seasonal influenza in the US: measuring disease burden and costs. Vaccine. 2007;25(27):5086–96.

3. McLeod A. The economics of avian influenza. In: Swayne DE, editor. Avian influenza, 1st ed. Ames, IA: Blackwell Publishing; 2008. p. 537.

4. Kilbourne ED. Influenza pandemics of the 20th century. Emerg Infect Dis. 2006 Jan;12(1):9–14.

5. Taubenberger JK, Morens DM. 1918 Influenza: the mother of all pandemics. Emerg Infect Dis. 2006;12(1):15–22.

6. Dawood FS, Iuliano AD, Reed C, Meltzer MI, Shay DK, Cheng PY, et al. Estimated global mortality associated with the first 12 months of 2009 pandemic influenza A H1N1 virus circulation: a modelling study. Lancet Infect Dis. 2012;12(9):687–95.

7. The World Bank. Issue briefs. Animal and pandemic influenza. 2012. Available from: http://go.worldbank.org/E3NZHTSNE0 (accessed 13 August 2012).

8. United Nations Population Fund. State of world population 2011: people and possibilities in a world of 7 billion. 2011. Available from: http://www.unfpa.org/webdav/site/global/shared/documents/publications/2011/EN-SWOP2011-FINAL.pdf (accessed 22 April 2012).

9. United Nations, Department of Economic and Social Affairs. Population division, population estimates and projections section. World Population Prospects, the 2010 Revision. 2011. Available from: http://esa.un.org/unpd/wpp/Documentation/pdf/WPP2010_Highlights.pdf (accessed 22 April 2012).

10. United Nations, Department of Economic and Social Affairs. Population division, population estimates and projections section. World Urbanization Prospects, the 2011 Revision. 2012. Available from: http://esa.un.org/unpd/wup/pdf/WUP2011_Highlights.pdf (accessed 22 April 2012).

11. United Nations Human Settlements Programme. The challenge of slums: global report on human settlements. 2003. Available from: http://www.unhabitat.org/pmss/listItemDetails.aspx?publicationID=1156 (accessed 22 April 2012).

12. United Nations Human Settlements Programme. State of the world's cities, 2006/7. 2006. Available from: http://www.unhabitat.org/pmss/listItemDetails.aspx?publicationID=2101 (accessed 22 April 2012).

13. Central Intelligence Agency, United States of America. World fact book, country comparison, area. Available from: https://www.cia.gov/library/publications/the-world-factbook/rankorder/2147rank.html (accessed 22 April 2012).

14. Banglapedia: National Encyclopedia of Bangladesh. Dhaka division. Available from: http://www.banglapedia.org/HT/D_0157.HTM

15. International Centre for Diarrhoeal Disease Research, Bangladesh (ICDDR,B). Kamalapur 2005–2007 census results. 2008. Available from: https://centre.icddrb.org/images/SP130.pdf (accessed 22 April 2012).

16. Homaira N, Luby SP, Petri WA, Vainionpaa R, Rahman M, Hossain K, et al. Incidence of respiratory

virus-associated pneumonia in urban poor young children of Dhaka, Bangladesh, 2009–2011. PLoS ONE. 2012;7(2):e32056.

17. Brooks WA, Goswami D, Rahman M, Nahar K, Fry AM, Balish A, et al. Influenza is a major contributor to childhood pneumonia in a tropical developing country. Pediatr Infect Dis J. 2010;29(3):216–21.

18. Jones KE, Patel NG, Levy MA, Storeygard A, Balk D, Gittleman JL, et al. Global trends in emerging infectious diseases. Nature. 2008;451(7181):990–3.

19. Chang WK. National influenza experience in Hong Kong, 1968. Bull World Health Organ. 1969;41(3): 349–51.

20. Eggo RM, Cauchemez S, Ferguson NM. Spatial dynamics of the 1918 influenza pandemic in England, Wales and the United States. J R Soc Interface. 2011;8(55): 233–43.

21. Relman DA, Choffnes ER, Mack A. Infectious Disease Movement in a Borderless World. Institute of Medicine. Washington, DC: The National Academies Press; 2010.

22. International Air Transport Association (IATA). Passenger forecast 2007–2011. . Available from: http://www.iata.org/pressroom/pr/pages/2007-24-10-01.aspx (accessed 24 April 2012).

23. UNWTO (United Nations World Tourism Organization). 2008a. Tourism highlights, 2012 edition. Available from: http://mkt.unwto.org/en/publication/unwto-tourism-highlights-2012-edition (accessed 20 April 2012).

24. Russell CA, Jones TC, Barr IG, Cox NJ, Garten RJ, Gregory V, et al. The global circulation of seasonal influenza A (H3N2) viruses. Science. 2008;320(5874): 340–6.

25. Miller JM, Tam TW, Maloney S, Fukuda K, Cox N, Hockin J, et al. Cruise ships: high-risk passengers and the global spread of new influenza viruses. Clin Infect Dis. 2000;31(2):433–8.

26. Byerly CR. The U.S. military and the influenza pandemic of 1918–1919. Public Health Rep. 2010;125(Suppl. 3):82–91.

27. McLeod M, Baker M, Wilson N, Kelly H, Kiedrzynski T, Kool J. Protective effect of maritime quarantine in south pacific jurisdictions, 1918–19 influenza pandemic. Emerg Infect Dis. 2008;14(3):468–70.

28. Crosby AW. Samoa and Alaska. America's Forgotten Pandemic: The Influenza of 1918, 2nd ed. Cambridge, UK: Cambridge University Press; 2003. p. 227.

29. Sattenspiel L, Herring DA. Simulating the effect of quarantine on the spread of the 1918 flu in central Canada. Bull Math Biol. 2003;65:1–26.

30. CDC. Update: novel influenza A (H1N1) virus infections – worldwide, May 6, 2009. MMWR. 2009;58 (17):453–8.

31. Novel Swine-Origin Influenza A (H1N1) Virus Investigation Team, Dawood FS, Jain S, Finelli L, Shaw MW, Lindstrom S, et al. Emergence of a novel swine-origin influenza A (H1N1) virus in humans. N Engl J Med. 2009;360(25):2605–15.

32. Khan K, Arino J, Hu W, Raposo P, Sears J, Calderon F, et al. Spread of a novel influenza A (H1N1) virus via global airline transportation. N Engl J Med. 2009;361 (2):212–4.

33. Iuliano AD, Reed C, Guh A, Desai M, Dee DL, Kutty P, et al. Notes from the field: outbreak of 2009 pandemic influenza A (H1N1) virus at a large public university in Delaware, April–May 2009. Clin Infect Dis. 2009;49(12):1811–20.

34. Memish ZA, McNabb SJ, Mahoney F, Alrabiah F, Marano N, Ahmed QA, et al. Establishment of public health security in Saudi Arabia for the 2009 Hajj in response to pandemic influenza A H1N1. Lancet. 2009; 374(9703):1786–91.

35. Ahmed QA, Arabi YM, Memish ZA. Health risks at the Hajj. Lancet. 2006;367(9515):1008–15.

36. Memish ZA, Ebrahim SH, Ahmed QA, Deming M, Assiri A. Pandemic H1N1 influenza at the 2009 Hajj: understanding the unexpectedly low H1N1 burden. J R Soc Med. 2010;103(10):386.

37. Ebrahim SH, Memish ZA, Uyeki TM, Khoja TA, Marano N, McNabb SJ. Pandemic H1N1 and the 2009 Hajj. Science. Policy Forum. Public Health. 2009;326 (5955):938–40.

38. Joint WHO/FAO Expert Consultation. Diet, nutrition and the prevention of chronic diseases. WHO Technical Report Series 916. Chapter 3: Global and Regional Food Consumption Patterns and Trends. Available from: http://www.who.int/nutrition/topics/3_food consumption/en/index.html (accessed 29 April 2012).

39. Wennemer H, Flachowsky G, Hoffmann V. Protein, population, politics: towards a sustainable protein supply in the 21st century. Duesseldorf, Germany: Degussa; 2006.

40. Food and Agriculture Organization of the United Nations. FAOSTAT – production – live animals, online database. Available from: faostat.fao.org/ (accessed 29 April 2012).

41. Food and Agriculture Organization of the United Nations. FAOSTAT – food supply – livestock and fish primary equivalent, online database. Available from: faostat.fao.org/ (accessed 29 April 2012).

42. Food and Agriculture Organization of the United Nations. Global Livestock Production and Health Atlas (GLiPHA). World – livestock population – density agric land (LU/sqkm) for 2003 for poultry. Available from: kids.fao.org/glipha (accessed 29 April 2012).

43. Food and Agriculture Organization of the United Nations. Cleaning and disinfection along the Jakarta

poultry market chain to reduce HPAI risk. 2011. Available from: http://www.fao.org/avianflu/en/news/jakarta_market.html (accessed 29 April 2012).

44. Ahmed SS, Ersbøll AK, Biswas PK, Christensen JP, Hannan AS, Toft N. Ecological determinants of highly pathogenic avian influenza (H5N1) outbreaks in bangladesh. PLoS ONE. 2012;7(3):e33938.

45. Garten RJ, Davis CT, Russell CA, Shu B, Lindstrom S, Balish A, et al. Antigenic and genetic characteristics of swine-origin 2009 A(H1N1) influenza viruses circulating in humans. Science. 2009;325:197–201.

46. Lindstrom S, Garten R, Balish A, Shu B, Emery S, Berman L, et al. Human infections with novel reassortant influenza A(H3N2)v viruses, United States, 2011. Emerg Infect Dis. 2012;18(5):834–7.

47. Pearce MB, Jayaraman A, Pappas C, Belser JA, Zeng H, Gustin KM, et al. Pathogenesis and transmission of swine origin A(H3N2)v influenza viruses in ferrets. Proc Natl Acad Sci U S A. 2012;109(10):3944–9.

48. Radin JM, Katz MA, Tempia S, Nzussouo NT, Davis R, Duque J, et al. Influenza surveillance in 15 countries in Africa, 2006–2010. J Infect Dis. 2012;206(Suppl 1): S14–21.

49. Butler D. Flu surveillance lacking. Nature. 2012;483 (7391):520–2.

50. United States Department of Agriculture, Animal and Plant Health Inspection Service. Animal health: swine influenza surveillance. 2012. Available from: http://www.aphis.usda.gov/animal_health/animal_dis_spec/swine/siv_surveillance.shtml (accessed 15 September 2012).

51. Lawson C. Who shall live when not all can live? Intellectual property in accessing and benefit-sharing influenza viruses through the World Health Organisation. J Law Med. 2011;18(3):554–76.

52. Baker MG, Fidler DP. Global public health surveillance under new international health regulations. Emerg Infect Dis. 2006;12(7):1058–65.

53. World Health Organization (WHO): Fifty-eighth world health assembly resolution WHA58.3: revision of the international health regulations. 2005. Available from: http://www.who.int/ipcs/publications/wha/ihr_resolution.pdf (accessed 28 July 2012).

54. World Organization for Animal Health (OIE). OIE listed diseases. 2012. Available from: http://www.oie.int/animal-health-in-the-world/oie-listed-diseases-2012/ (accessed 29 July 2012).

55. Food and Agriculture Organization of the United Nations. Definition and list of notifiable diseases. Chapter 8. Legislation – notifiable diseases. Available from: http://www.fao.org/docrep/U2200E/u2200e0b.htm#notifiable diseases (accessed 29 July 2012).

56. Pereira MS. Global surveillance of influenza. Br Med Bull. 1979;35(1):9–14.

57. World Health Organization. Global influenza surveillance and response system. Available from: http://www.who.int/influenza/gisrs_laboratory/en/ (accessed 29 July 2012).

58. World Health Organization. Pandemic Influenza Preparedness Framework for the sharing of influenza viruses and access to vaccines and other benefits, 2011. WHO Library Catloguing-in-Publication Data.. 2011. Available from: http://apps.who.int/gb/pip/ (accessed 28 July 2012).

59. Kumar S, Henrickson KJ. Update on influenza diagnostics: lessons from the novel H1N1 influenza A pandemic. Clin Microbiol Rev. 2012;25(2):344–61.

60. Jernigan DB, Lindstrom SL, Johnson JR, Miller JD, Hoelscher M, Humes R, et al. Detecting 2009 pandemic influenza A (H1N1) virus infection: availability of diagnostic testing led to rapid pandemic response. Clin Infect Dis. 2011;52(Suppl. 1):S36–43.

61. Centers for Disease Control and Prevention. Influenza Risk Assessment Tool (IRAT), questions and answers. 2012. Available from: http://www.cdc.gov/flu/pandemic-resources/tools/risk-assessment.htm (accessed 12 August 2012).

62. Chew C, Eysenbach G. Pandemics in the age of twitter: content analysis of tweets during the 2009 H1N1 outbreak. PLoS ONE. 2010;5(11):e14118.

63. Squires RB, Noronha J, Hunt V, García-Sastre A, Macken C, Baumgarth N, et al. Influenza research database: an integrated bioinformatics resource for influenza research and surveillance. Influenza Other Respi Viruses. 2012;6:404–16.

2

Influenza pandemics: History and lessons learned

Arnold S. Monto[1] and Robert G. Webster[2]

[1]Department of Epidemiology, University of Michigan School of Public Health, Ann Arbor, MI, USA

[2]Department of Infectious Diseases, Division of Virology, St. Jude Children's Research Hospital, Memphis, TN, USA

Introduction

The highly contagious acute respiratory disease influenza is an ancient disease first described by Hippocrates in 412 BC. Historical descriptions of influenza pandemics in humans indicate that they occurred at irregular intervals, varied in severity, and usually caused highest mortality in the elderly.

Influenza pandemics occur when a novel virus emerges for which a majority of the population has little or no immunity. Global spread follows over a relatively short period of time. The first scientific evidence of influenza pandemics was based on seroarchaeology and the concept of original antigenic sin [1], according to which the first exposure with influenza virus in childhood leaves a lifelong immunologic imprint – the original sin. The most catastrophic pandemic of influenza occurred in 1918 – the so-called Spanish pandemic – which killed an estimated 50 million people globally. General Erich F.W. von Ludendorff attributed the collapse of the German army in 1918 to the introduction of Spanish influenza by doughboys from the United States, a possible unintended use of biologic warfare.

In this chapter, we review the six pandemics of influenza that occurred from 1889 to 2009 and discuss the key lessons learned from these pandemics.

Past and recent influenza pandemics

The 1889 and 1918 pandemics

Historians have been able to track influenza pandemics over the centuries owing to the high morbidity and mortality associated with the disease. However, the virus causing the first well-documented pandemic in 1889 has not been identified, but sera collected from individuals living in that period suggest that it was caused by the H2 or perhaps the H3 subtype of type A influenza [2].

The outbreak appeared to start in Russia and reached St. Petersburg in October 1889. It spread globally thereafter and occurred in repeated waves. As the wave moved through Massachusetts in 1892, a characteristic mortality pattern was observed for the first time – most deaths occurred among the elderly and very young. This pattern has since been seen in subsequent pandemics, except for the one in 1918 [3].

The 1918 pandemic was a watershed event that occurred at the beginning of the twentieth century. The 550 000 deaths in the United States attributed to the various waves after the pandemic has stood the test of time, unlike the global estimate; if the same mortality rates occurred in today's larger population

Textbook of Influenza, Second Edition. Edited by Robert G. Webster, Arnold S. Monto, Thomas J. Braciale, and Robert A. Lamb.
© 2013 John Wiley & Sons, Ltd. Published 2013 by John Wiley & Sons, Ltd.

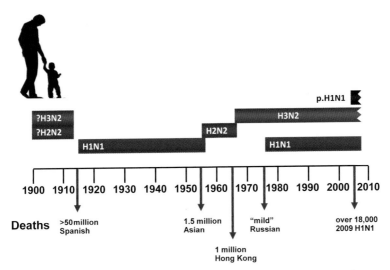

Figure 2.1. Influenza pandemics of the past century. Timeline showing the emergence of pandemic influenza and the timespan of their continued circulation as epidemic strains. Reassortment between influenza viruses circulating in humans with avian influenza viruses (AIVs) from aquatic birds are involved in the emergence of novel pandemic strains, whereas accumulation of point mutations explains antigenic drift and the circulation of epidemic strains. After emergence of a novel pandemic influenza virus, the preceding subtype usually disappears. The exception has been the continued circulation of H3N2 and H1N1 after the reintroduction of the H1N1 virus in 1977.

the number of deaths would be approximately 2 million. In contrast, the global estimates of deaths from the 1918 pandemic rose from the originally reported 20 million to at least 50 million, owing to the original omission of deaths from areas of the world now considered developing. For example, contemporaneous data from India alone revealed that 12.5 million deaths occurred from the pandemic [4] and in Madagascar the death toll was 86 352 (2.65% of the entire population) [5]. Until recently, there were few concrete explanations for the extreme severity of this pandemic. There has been speculation on various epidemiologic, social, and microbiologic factors that might have produced such extreme severity but these factors have been difficult to evaluate. However, cloning of the causative virus strain from archived and other specimens has led to its characterization [6] with clear evidence of its virulence, presented in Chapters 9 and 14.

The place of origin of the viruses of the 1918 pandemic has been debated [7]. There is agreement on the occurrence of a wave of influenza-like illness in many countries across the world in spring 1918. This was considered by contemporaries as the first appearance of the pandemic virus. In most areas, the disease was mild; some studies have suggested that being ill during that period protected against infection with the virus in later waves. Given that the influenza virus responsible for the outbreak could not be identified at the time, the conclusion that the same agent caused waves in the spring and severe episodes later is still open to discussion (Figure 2.1).

The signature of the autumn and later waves was a case fatality rate of 1–2% in 20- to 39-year-olds, an age group in which influenza usually does not cause death. This pattern was also seen in some areas before August–September 1918, which has again led to the suggestion that the virus was circulating during this period [8]. In the United States and United Kingdom, the signature was present through the autumn wave, for which extensive data are available on epidemiologic and pathologic characteristics. In both countries, high fatality rates were seen not only in young adults but also in young children, particularly those younger than 1 year; pregnant women were also at high risk. Data also indicated relative

21

sparing of those above 64 years of age, at least in terms of mortality [9]. In the United States, the epidemic peak gripped the entire country in approximately 10 weeks, at a time when there was little travel except by rail. Island areas such as Australia restricted ship traffic, which delayed the pandemic wave by months. This and other observations from 1918 on social distancing, school closing, and use of face masks were used to make recommendations on use of nonpharmaceutical interventions in recent pandemic planning.

Explanations about the extreme severity of the 1918 pandemic had previously focused on the fact that, as in seasonal outbreaks, bacterial superinfection was involved in many of the deaths. However, why such bacterial infections would have been more lethal in 1918 remains unclear. Recent studies associate the polymerase protein PB1-F2 of the 1918 virus with synergy between bacterial and viral infection. The bacterial agents frequently involved were *Streptococcus pneumoniae, Streptococcus pyogenes*, and *Haemophilus influenzae*. The pathology observed in at least some cases was not seen before in typical bacterial pneumonia; cases in which lungs were fluid-filled and hemorrhagic were particularly novel. "Dusky cyanosis" (purple color of the face) was thought to be unique to this pandemic. At that time these observations were ascribed to a virulent viral infection. A recent review of lung pathology has emphasized the role of bacterial complications, but has not shed light on the primary viral infection that produced these unusual symptoms [10].

The evidence presented in Chapters 9 and 14 that there were unusual virulence makers in the recently recovered viruses is in line with the unique features of the 1918 pandemic. It can be concluded that the tremendous impact of this pandemic was the result of a virus of greater virulence made worse by bacterial superinfections at a time when no antibiotics were available. It should be noted that the recent cases of H5N1 avian infections in humans are also the result of increased virulence associated with specific viral factors; in these cases, severe outcomes are not associated with bacterial involvement [11].

Isolation of influenza viruses and development of vaccine

The first mammalian influenza virus was isolated by Shope from swine in 1931 [12]. Smith et al. [13] recovered the human virus in ferrets and confirmed that the virus produced disease in humans. Subsequently, the virus was adapted to grow in embryonated eggs and agglutination of red cells by virus was noted. Both of these findings made it possible to develop a specific influenza vaccine, which was first shown to be efficacious in 1943.

The vaccine continued to be used annually in the US military, but in 1946–1947 it failed to have a protective effect. A recent study showed very distant serologic relatedness between the new virus, A/FM1/47, and the previous type A viruses which were included in the vaccine [14]. For many years thereafter, this event was viewed as an antigenic shift similar to one that occurs to produce a pandemic. However, a recent molecular analysis showed that the 1947 virus remained in the H1N1 subtype and the episode is now considered to represent a major drift in antigenicity.

The 1957 and 1968 pandemics

In early 1957, a major outbreak of influenza was reported in Hong Kong, and laboratory studies indicated an antigenic shift. We now know that three segments, those coding for the hemagglutinin, neuraminidase, and PB1, had moved from an avian influenza virus (AIV) into the previous A(H1N1) virus, thus producing the new H2N2 subtype [15]. Outbreaks of the new virus had been occurring in mainland China before reaching Hong Kong and further spread throughout the world. Outbreaks in spring 1957 in Japan especially involved school-age children. There was a relatively quiet period over the summer, and outbreaks resumed in the autumn with the opening of schools, particularly in areas spared in the previous spring. In the United States, major outbreaks began in Louisiana when schools opened in mid-August. The national peak of activity was in October 1957, with another wave coming in the winter. The viral seed for the H2N2 vaccine became available in early May, and 6 months later, 49 million doses had been cleared for use in the United States, just after the autumn peak [16].

Mortality characteristics of this pandemic returned to the more expected pattern, being mainly concentrated in the young and the elderly [3]. Those with cardiac abnormalities were also at particular risk of severe disease. Bacterial superinfection was a key feature in those with severe disease, antibiotic-resistant *Staphylococcus aureus* being the predominant pathogen identified. The estimated number of pandemic-related deaths in the United States was 70 000.

Eleven years later, history repeated itself and an outbreak of influenza caused by the H3N2 virus, first occurring in China, was reported in July 1968 from Hong Kong. The virus was again a reassortant, with the hemagglutinin and PB1-coding genes coming from an avian source [15]. Global spread of the virus was well characterized. Increased illnesses in the United States started in the late autumn, with peak transmission in December. The vaccine became available after the pandemic peak. The major increase in the number of individuals with severe disease was delayed in other areas of the world. In Europe, there was moderate spread in 1968–1969, but increases in mortality were not observed until the next year. This may have been the result of the neuraminidase of the virus not changing from the previous subtype, with residual immunity in the population [17]. Clinical characteristics of individuals were similar to those seen in the 1957 pandemic, with high rates of hospitalization and mortality seen in the elderly, young, and those with defined risks such as cardiopulmonary disease. However, not as much attention was given to studies of disease manifestations as in the 1957 pandemic, probably because overall it appeared similar but milder. In the United States, the pandemic caused fewer than half the deaths (34 000) occurring in 1957, despite an increase in the population.

Events in 1976 and 1977

In early 1976, an outbreak of influenza occurred among military recruits in the US military facility at Fort Dix. One of the 230 soldiers infected died, spurring investigation of etiology [18]. Since 1968, two types of influenza viruses, A (H3N2) and B, had been circulating in the world, and the virus isolated from this outbreak did not type as either one of them. The agent, A/New Jersey 76, was finally determined to be an A (H1N1) virus of swine origin. It was known that pandemics were a result of type A animal viruses becoming adapted for human transmission. Past studies of antibodies present in the population had

led to the hypothesis – the recycling theory – according to which A (H2N2) and then A (H3N2) viruses had circulated before, and that the next pandemic virus would be A (H1N1)-like [2]. On the basis of these facts, it was decided that this event likely represented the start of a new pandemic.

The United States started production and careful testing of a specific vaccine for the A/New Jersey virus. Systematic evaluation of the vaccine conducted in the latter half of 1976 was possible only because the virus never returned. A program to vaccinate much of the US population began on 1 October and was terminated on 16 December, because of the appearance of Guillain–Barré syndrome, a rare complication of vaccination.

In subsequent years, there was abortive spread of swine viruses in humans, and it is now our current understanding that this is what happened at Fort Dix. An unanswered question is how to distinguish between such abortive clusters and ones that might result in extensive dissemination. That question reappeared in 2011 when swine origin A (H3N2) was detected in influenza cases in humans.

One year after the 1976 A/New Jersey episode, a second unexpected event took place – the return of type A (H1N1) viruses. Up to that point, whenever a new A subtype had emerged, it replaced the previous one. After the emergence of the A (H3N2) virus in 1968, it became the only subtype circulating. This changed in mid-1977 when A (H1N1) viruses were detected in Siberia [19]. In this outbreak, termed "Russian influenza," the causative agent was remarkably similar to a virus that had circulated in 1950 and was archived in freezer collections. We now know that the virus had circulated in China for months before it appeared in the former Soviet Union. Global spread followed; since the virus was similar to viruses that circulated before 1957, the entire population over approximately 25 years of age was rarely infected. However, major outbreaks of mainly mild disease did occur in those younger age groups, which were well documented in university students. This episode is generally not considered a pandemic, but might be considered a "pseudopandemic," because the A (H1N1) virus has persisted and evolved in subsequent years. Since this point, the influenza vaccine that was bivalent (containing a type A and B strain) became trivalent, with representative A (H3N2), A (H1N1), and type B components.

The threat of an A (H5N1) pandemic

It was originally believed that because of receptor differences (see Chapter 5), AIVs could not transmit directly from birds to humans. In 1997, this concept was shaken by an outbreak of A (H5N1), a highly pathogenic avian virus in humans in Hong Kong [20]. The outbreak was confirmed to be the result of transmission of the viruses from poultry to humans [21]. A total of 18 individuals were infected, of whom 6 died. The world recognized this as a pandemic threat and supported efforts to control the outbreak; it was initially eliminated in Hong Kong by depopulation of live bird markets.

Until 2003, there was little evidence of any further human infections with A (H5N1). The year was notable in terms of respiratory infections, first with the spread of severe acute respiratory syndrome (SARS) through East Asia and in some other parts of the world [22]. As the threat of SARS abated, there were reports that the highly pathogenic avian (H5N1) influenza in humans had returned, with focal transmission from poultry, particularly in Vietnam and Thailand [23]. Details about the severity of disease in humans quickly emerged, including the high case fatality rate of 80% [24]. The major feature of the disease was an acute respiratory disease syndrome (ARDS), with strong evidence of cytokine storm. Viral shedding was prolonged, with some evidence of mitigation with treatment with oseltamivir, although drug-resistant strains emerged [25].

Thereafter, cases of A (H5N1) disease continued to occur in humans in varying numbers. It became clear that despite evidence that the virus was shed from the respiratory and perhaps the enteric tract of those infected, most humans acquired their infection from contact with poultry and not from other humans with infection. However, there were clear examples of unsustained human-to-human transmission [26]. This evidence, when first observed, raised concerns that the virus might be adapting to humans; gradually, however, it was found that this was not the case and that clusters typically occurred among blood relatives, suggesting genetic susceptibility. Strategies were developed to react quickly in the event of human-to-human transmission. One approach was to use antivirals to "quench" the outbreak at its source, which was evaluated in mathematical models and appeared to be successful if begun quickly [27].

Response to the H5N1 threat

Given the experience with avian sources of past pandemic viruses, it was widely believed that the next pandemic might be one caused by H5N1 or a virus derived from it. Before 2003, there was limited national pandemic planning, but it became more general and was accelerated in response to the concern about avian influenza and, indirectly, the experience with SARS. These plans are particularly relevant to the response to the 2009 pandemic. Most pandemic preparation occurred at the World Health Organization (WHO) and in some developed countries. At the WHO, the International Health Regulations (IHR) of 2005 came into effect in 2007 and served as an overall framework for the pandemic response [28].

A critical component developed by the WHO was classification of pandemic phases on the basis of transmission characteristics and extent of spread. This was linked to the kind of response required. The approach used was based on the assumption that the most likely pandemic concern was further spread of an avian virus. The original phases were developed in 2005, revised in 2008, and adopted in early 2009 [29]. The revision was mainly made to reflect the recognition of small clusters of transmission of an H5N1 virus not well adapted to humans; previously, this would have required moving to phase 4, or pandemic alert. The first three phases related to the extent of human transmission of a novel virus, with small, unsustained clusters now being part of phase 3. Phase 4 became the critical phase, to be declared when human-to-human transmission of an animal or hybrid animal–human influenza virus able to cause community-level transmission had been verified. At this point, two important events are likely to occur: switching manufacturing from seasonal to pandemic vaccine and considering an attempt at rapid containment. The rapid containment strategy mainly referred to the use of antivirals in the area where transmission was occurring. The pandemic itself was divided into two phases: (i) phase 5, when the spread was limited to one WHO region, and (ii) phase 6, when two or more regions were involved. Another change in 2009 was separation of the post-pandemic period when the pandemic was ending into two phases: post peak, in recognition of the possible occurrence of later waves, and post pandemic, when activity had returned to seasonal levels. Although it was recognized that severity would be an important component of the response, it was not made part of the definition of a pandemic.

Throughout this time period, nations and the industry were developing vaccines, antivirals, and nonpharmaceutical interventions. Work on vaccine development and evaluation was extensive, and was again mainly directed toward preventing A (H5N1). Initial studies demonstrated that in order to achieve a satisfactory antibody response in humans, much more antigen was necessary than the 15 μg used with seasonal vaccines. Oil-in-water adjuvants were evaluated; they were needed to boost the antibody response, and were actually antigen sparing. Use of the adjuvants allowed as little as 3.8 or 7.5 μg of antigen to be used, but two inoculations were still required.

Antivirals were being employed to treat cases of A (H5N1) and it was clear that oseltamivir in particular reduced viral replication, especially when given early. Studies were undertaken to see whether a higher dose would be more effective. Because antivirals could not be produced in sufficient quantity during a pandemic, many countries began to stockpile them in varying quantities, depending on their populations. Some countries stockpiled oseltamivir only; others such as the United States also stockpiled small quantities of zanamivir, because of the concern of oseltamivir resistance.

Nonpharmaceutical interventions have rarely been used in a systematic way against influenza, but the specter of a H5N1 pandemic that could be more severe than 1918 triggered the study of these options. There were three components to this evaluation. One was historic, examining what interventions were used in 1918 and which ones were successful. Conclusions have influenced recommendations on, for example, social distancing. The second was experimental, focusing on evaluating the role of such interventions as hand hygiene and wearing face masks on acquisition of influenza in seasonal outbreaks. The third was computational modeling, attempting to determine, for example, what effects school closings and border closings would have on the introduction and course of pandemic spread. In the United States, recommendations were developed on specific nonpharmaceutical interventions that would be used; the extent of these interventions would be based on the assessed severity of the pandemic. It was assumed that this could be determined early, and, because infection rates would likely be similar in all pandemics, severity would be driven by differences in case fatality [30].

The 2009 H1N1 influenza pandemic

Despite the knowledge that a pandemic of influenza was overdue and extensive pandemic planning had been carried out for H5N1, the 2009 H1N1 pandemic came as a complete surprise. The emergence of an influenza pandemic virus of the same subtype (H1N1) that was co-circulating with seasonal influenza subtypes (H1N1, H3N2, B) was completely unexpected. There was general acceptance that the pandemic influenza viruses of the past century had emerged by reassortment between influenza viruses in the aquatic bird reservoir and the circulating human influenza virus. As H1N1 viruses that re-emerged in 1977 were still circulating globally in the human population, the human population was considered immunologically "primed" to this subtype and no thought was given to the possibility that this subtype could cause a pandemic. The pandemic H1N1 2009 that emerged in Mexico was first detected in California in April 2009. It is possible that the virus had been circulating in humans for some time before and had not been detected. Initial data on the percentage of young people hospitalized (6.5%) in Mexico, with mortality in this group being 41%, pointed to the possibility of a severe pandemic [31]. Added to this were reports from Canada [32] about the need for high intensive care use among young adults. Antigenic and sequence analysis confirmed that the virus was an H1N1 subtype antigenically related to the 1918 Spanish influenza virus (Table 2.1), further raising the concern of a severe pandemic.

As the pandemic H1N1 2009 influenza virus spread rapidly, nations across the world debated about how to prepare for the pandemic. Past planning helped many countries, but some had prepared only for a catastrophic A (H5N1) event and therefore had difficulty in dealing with one that turned out to be much less severe. The WHO systematically applied the previously devised pandemic phases on the basis of extent of spread. On 25 April 2009, a "public health emergency of international concern" was declared, invoking the IHR. The alert level was immediately moved to phase 5, with spread documented in countries in North America. Phase 6 was declared on 11 June 2009, when the spread was documented in

Table 2.1. Comparison of the properties of the H1N1 influenza pandemic viruses of 1918 and 2009.

Property	Characteristic	1918 Spanish H1N1	2009 H1N1
Biologic	Mortality	20–50 million	Approx. 18 000
	Yield in human airway cells	50×	1×
Virologic	Hemagglutinin structure	Similar	Similar
	Antigenicity	Similar	Similar
	Receptor binding	α2-6 glycans - binds longer chain glycans - binds more strongly	α2-6 glycans
	PB2	Lysine at residue 627	No lysine at residue 627
	PB1-F2	Functional; avian origin	Nonfunctional
	NS1	Not crucial: has PDZ domain	No PDZ domain
Bacterial coinfection		Prevalent (associated with PB1-F2)	Less prevalent

Europe. Along with this official declaration of the pandemic, the WHO stated that the pandemic was of moderate severity. Despite this, questions were later raised on whether the WHO had mishandled the pandemic, leading to an in-depth review of the IHR and the Pandemic Influenza A (H1N1) 2009 [33]. The report concluded that the "WHO performed well in many ways during the pandemic, confronted systemic difficulties and demonstrated some shortcomings. The Committee found no evidence of malfeasance." However, "The world is ill-prepared to respond to a severe influenza pandemic or to any similarly global, sustained and threatening public health emergency."

Characteristics of the 2009 pandemic can be viewed against the background of previous pandemics. The rapid early spread first from Mexico to the United States and Canada and then to Europe could clearly be related to plane travel. However, similar to the seasonal pattern observed in the 1957 pandemic in Japan, only parts of the United States were affected in spring 2009 whereas other parts were affected only in early autumn. An overall observation is that outbreaks in an influenza season can occur outside the typical influenza season.

Because of prior work on vaccines for A (H5N1), the A (H1N1) pandemic vaccine used in most parts of the world was adjuvanted. Many considered the use of adjuvants critical as it allowed antigen sparing, and once started resulted in larger amounts of vaccine being produced. However, other countries used traditional inactivated unadjuvanted vaccines, as much of their population had been previously infected with A (H1N1) viruses and there was no perceived need for adjuvants. In any event, as observed in past pandemics, vaccines arrived late. Although the use of adjuvants resulted in increased production of vaccine, only a limited quantity was used because of various factors.

At the beginning of the pandemic, some countries had large stockpiles of antivirals, again mainly because of concern for A (H5N1). Strategies for antiviral distribution varied significantly. In Japan, large amounts of the antivirals were used, and the lower mortality observed compared with other countries was later attributed to early drug use in treatment. In the United Kingdom, oseltamivir was initially used in prophylaxis to contain spread. When this approach did not succeed, the drug was then employed mainly for treatment. A novel approach was developed to make antivirals available early to ill individuals. Caregivers were required to call a free telephone number to obtain oseltamivir for patient use. In Canada, antivirals were used in the autumn wave in northern communities, which seemed to reduce the severe outcomes previously encountered in the spring. An overall problem in interpreting these results is that nearly all data are observational and do not meet the requirements set by regulatory authorities.

Nonpharmaceutical interventions were rarely used except early in the pandemic when severity had not yet been established. In some countries, school closings were routine during influenza outbreaks, but this was usually not the case in the United States. However, at the start of the pandemic, schools were closed in some regions, especially if there had been a severe outcome locally. Policy recommendations varied over time, leading to confusion; however, by the autumn, it was recommended that schools not be closed, except in extreme circumstances.

The extent of use of nonpharmaceutical interventions was to be driven by the severity of the pandemic, but severity was difficult to establish in the first months. In contrast to the reports from Mexico and the Canadian north, there was extensive morbidity, with little severe disease, in school outbreaks in the United States. It became clear that the characteristics of this pandemic were very different from those seen earlier. Children were frequently infected; some were hospitalized, but deaths were infrequent. Hospitalizations of younger adults were unusual, with approximately 70% occurring in those with pre-existing conditions. Those who were hospitalized often developed ARDS, and, if they survived, remained hospitalized for weeks. There was little evidence of bacterial superinfection. In adults, pregnant women and those with morbid obesity were at high risk of developing severe events. Those older than 64 years were not frequently infected because of immunity from past infections. In typical outbreaks, 90% of mortality occurs in this population, so overall in 2009 deaths occurred less frequently than in seasonal influenza. However, because deaths occurred in mainly younger individuals, in terms of years of life lost the impact of this pandemic was as great as the A (H3N2) pandemic of 1968 [34].

Lessons learned from past influenza pandemics

Pandemics of the past (see earlier sections) can provide an insight into the future. In the following sections, we discuss some of the lessons learned and how they impact future control strategies. Many of the topics are dealt with in detail in later chapters in the textbook.

Zoonotic origins and unpredictability of pandemics

It is now accepted that influenza is a zoonotic infection originating from aquatic birds of the world [35] and probably involves intermediate hosts such as swine to facilitate the genesis of viruses. Of the three types of influenza affecting humans (A, B, C), only influenza A viruses cause pandemics. According to one school of thought, only H1N1, H2N2, and H3N2 influenza viruses have the capacity to cause pandemics in humans [36]. The circulation of H7N7 (equine 1) influenza viruses in horses for many decades supports the notion that AIVs can establish stable influenza virus lineages in mammals. The infrequent infection of humans with H5N1, H7N7, and H9N2 subtypes establishes that these avian subtypes can replicate in humans, but to date have not consistently had human-to-human transmission. There is no known molecular block to the evolution of any of the remaining 13 influenza A subtypes into a pandemic influenza virus infecting humans.

Despite extensive phylogenetic and antigenic analysis of H1N1 and H3N2 influenza viruses, it is currently not possible to predict either the variant of influenza that will produce seasonal outbreaks or the subtype of influenza that will produce the next pandemic. To cope with the problem of continuing evolution of influenza, the WHO has established the Global Influenza Surveillance Response System (GISRS), which continually monitors antigenic and genetic variation worldwide. Recommendations are made annually for vaccine composition for the Northern and Southern Hemispheres to stay abreast of antigenic variation in the circulating viruses (currently H1N1, H3N2, and influenza B). Over the past decade, this network has successfully predicted the dominant influenza virus for most seasons. However, in a few cases the prediction has not been perfect and predictions beyond the immediate season are not possible. Thus, the prediction of what the dominant seasonal influenza viruses for the next season or the next pandemic virus will be is currently not possible and remains a continuing challenge.

Surveillance in swine was inadequate

The importance of influenza surveillance in apparently healthy swine was one of the lessons from the 2009 H1N1 pandemic. Despite the available knowledge on the role of swine as an intermediate host between the aquatic bird reservoir and humans [37], little attention was given to influenza surveillance in apparently healthy swine, as this was considered to provide too little return on the cost. The influenza surveillance program in swine instituted in Hong Kong after the first cases of the highly pathogenic H5N1 avian influenza virus in humans in 1997 established the value of influenza virus surveillance in apparently healthy pigs. Genetic analysis of the influenza viruses from swine in Hong Kong established that the precursors of the pandemic 2009 H1N1 influenza virus had been circulating in swine for 9–17 years [38]. Increased awareness of the importance of influenza surveillance in swine and the wild bird reservoir by national and international programs has culminated in a "One World" approach to influenza in wild birds, domestic animals, and humans. The challenge that remains is to determine which of the myriad of influenza viruses that emerge in swine have the potential for human-to-human transmission and cause a pandemic.

Antigenic and structural similarities are not predictors of severity

An incorrect assumption made in 1977 after the re-emergence of H1N1 influenza virus in humans at Fort Dix, and again in 2009 after emergence of the pandemic H1N1 2009 influenza viruses in Mexico, was that on the basis of antigenic similarities to classical swine influenza and by implication to the 1918 Spanish influenza the ensuing pandemic could be as severe as the 1918 H1N1 Spanish influenza. It is now known that the severity of influenza is a complex combination of viral traits and host factors such as the immune status and susceptibility (see Chapters 9 and 14). Comparison of the biologic and structural features of the 1918 and 2009 H1N1 influenza viruses (Table 2.1) provides insight into why antigenic and structural relationships are insufficient to predict severity. The three-dimensional structures of the hemagglutinin of the 1918 Spanish and 2009 pandemic H1N1 virus were virtually identical and were antigenically closely related [39]. However, the replication rate of the 1918 influenza virus in human bronchoepithelial cells was 50-fold higher [40] than that of pandemic 2009 H1N1 virus. Also, the 1918 influenza virus possessed virulence markers in both the *PB1* and *PB2* polymerase genes (Table 2.1) as well as a nonstructural gene encoding a PDZ domain, but

the pandemic H1N1 2009 influenza virus did not possess these virulence markers.

The association of the PB1-F2 gene product with severe bacterial infections in the 1918 H1N1 Spanish influenza [41] accounts in part for the high percentage of pneumococcal-associated deaths in 1918 [10]. Although the pandemic H1N1 2009 influenza virus was severe in immunologically naïve young adults, pregnant women, and obese persons, lower virus yields and absence of virulence markers explain in part its lower virulence than the 1918 Spanish influenza. The lesson learned is that predictions of influenza severity cannot be made solely on antigenic and structural relationships to earlier pandemics.

An influenza pandemic can arise anywhere in the world

The emergence of the 1957 Asian H2N2 and the 1968 Hong Kong H3N2 pandemics in Asia and the re-emergence of the 1977 Russian strain in northern China has led to the hypothesis that South-East Asia is the epicenter of influenza pandemics [42]. The high density of aquatic birds (ducks, geese), swine, and humans – the three hosts involved in the genesis of influenza – and live poultry markets were considered features supporting this hypothesis. However, the emergence of the 2009 H1N1 pandemic in Mexico emphasizes that pandemic influenza can emerge anywhere in the world, that swine are probably involved in the genesis, and that the ultimate source of each of the eight gene segments is aquatic birds of the world [43]. The precursors of the 2009 H1N1 pandemic virus were the "triple reassortants" from the United States that reassorted with the avian H1N1 viruses that adapted to pigs in Europe prior to 1979.

The high transmissibility of the 2009 pandemic H1N1 in both humans and swine was a novel feature of the 2009 H1N1 virus and offers the possibility of defining the molecular basis of the high transmissibility of this virus. The role of swine in the genesis of this pandemic was again apparent. The lesson learned is that the pandemics of influenza can arise anywhere in the world and that global surveillance is merited.

Pandemic influenza can emerge in any season

In temperate areas of the world seasonal influenza occurs in the cooler months of the year, whereas in the tropics influenza occurs year round but often with peaks in intensity [44]. The Asian H2N2 1957 pandemic was first detected in February 1957 in Guizhou, Southern China, whereas the Hong Kong H2N2 pandemic was first detected in Hong Kong in July 1968. The pandemic H1N1 2009 was first detected in humans in April 2009 but the earliest cases probably occurred in March 2009. Each of these pandemics emerged in the Northern Hemisphere – one in the cooler months (pre-February 1957), one in early spring (March 2009), and one in mid-summer (pre-July 1968). As all these sites of first detections are in the subtropical regions of the world, it is not at variance with the notion of year-round influenza in these regions. The subsequent spread of each pandemic does not follow the expected seasonality of influenza. Thus, the first wave of the 2009 H1N1 pandemic in the temperate regions of the Southern Hemisphere (Australia, New Zealand, Argentina) occurred in the summer months whereas that in the temperate areas of the Northern Hemisphere (Canada, Northern United States, Europe) occurred in the late spring. Data on the seasonal emergence of pandemic influenza are limited but suggest that pandemics can arise in any season and have occurred in subtropical regions of the world. The initial spread of a pandemic influenza in temperate regions of the world can occur in the summer months and does not follow the world pattern of epidemic influenza.

Initial retention of avian receptor binding characteristics in pandemic influenza viruses

Influenza in humans is typically a respiratory tract infection, whereas in avian species low-pathogenicity influenza is typically a gastrointestinal tract infection. The 2009 pandemic H1N1 influenza virus was detected in the stools and urine of patients with the high virus loads [45]. Although the RNA of seasonal influenza in humans has been detected in the stools of patients by reverse transcription polymerase chain reaction (RT-PCR), infectious influenza virus has not yet been isolated. Gastrointestinal symptoms are not frequently (<5%) observed in seasonal influenza.

Because all the gene segments in the 2009 pandemic influenza virus came originally from AIVs, the retention of AIV characteristics during early human transmission is not surprising. Earlier studies reported the detection of AIVs in the intestines and fecal samples of ferrets and pigs after experimental infection [46], indicating that receptors for AIVs are present in ferret and pig intestinal tracts. The detection of α2-3 sialic acid receptors in the lower respiratory tract of humans [47] and the retention of α2-3 sialic acid receptor specificity of early human H1N1 2009 pandemic virus isolates [48] explain in part the initial retention of avian-like receptor binding characteristics of pandemic influenza viruses from humans. The detection of pandemic influenza viruses in the stools and lower respiratory tract of humans is in keeping with the dual receptor specificity of influenza viruses during adaptation to respiratory transmission in a mammalian host.

Vaccines to pandemic influenza viruses are not available during the first wave of infection

Preparation of the inactivated subunit or "intact" influenza vaccines by the current strategy takes approximately 6 months. Live attenuated and inactivated mammalian cell-based influenza vaccines can take slightly shorter times, but in general vaccines made by currently approved methods usually cannot be made in time to prevent the first wave of a novel influenza pandemic. This is illustrated in Figure 2.2, which shows how influenza vaccine shipment and administration in the United States started in late October 2009 just after the peak of the first wave of pandemic H1N1 influenza activity in 2009. As the induction of a protective cellular and/or humoral immune response takes 1–3 weeks, it is likely that vaccine administration had a limited role in controlling the first wave of the H1N1 pandemic in the United States. However, it is possible that the use of vaccine contributed to the reduction in influenza activity and to the absence of a second wave in the cooler months.

Although the production and safety testing of a novel influenza vaccine in less than 6 months is a remarkable achievement, it is usually not fast enough. The time-consuming steps are (i) selection or preparation of a high-yielding vaccine strain in chicken eggs or cell culture; (ii) preparation of high-titer serum to the novel hemagglutinin required for vaccine standardization; (iii) industrial production in embryonated chicken eggs or cell cultures; (iv) inactivation and safety testing; (v) standardization of antigen content; (vi) filling and efficacy testing in animals and humans.

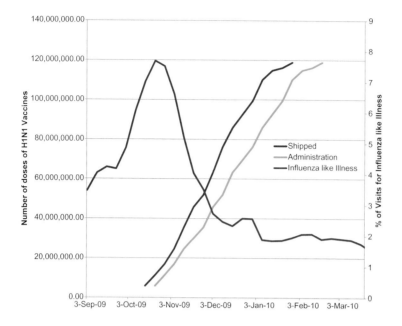

Figure 2.2. The first wave of pandemic H1N1 influenza preceded vaccine availability. Currently available methods for preparing inactivated influenza vaccines take nearly 6 months. As the pandemic influenza virus is already seeded in the human populations, the rate of spread determines how rapidly the peak of the first wave of the pandemic will occur. While vaccination is the best strategy to control influenza, vaccines are usually not available for the first wave and alternative strategies such as antivirals are necessary.

Each of these steps was achieved for the 2009 pandemic H1N1 influenza between April and October 2009. However, despite the best efforts of vaccine manufacturers and regulators, conventional inactivated influenza vaccines still take too long to prepare to have any impact on the first wave of pandemic influenza. This delay has also been seen in Europe, where "mock-up" dossiers had been prepared for a monovalent pandemic vaccine to fast track regulatory checks. Novel strategies to produce influenza vaccines more rapidly, such as pre-pandemic vaccines and universal vaccines, are discussed in Chapter 20, 21, and 29.

The lesson learned is that current strategies for making influenza vaccines are unlikely to provide vaccines in time to have an impact on the first wave of a pandemic. The development of new vaccine methods are needed, as are plans for more rational use of stockpiled antivirals. In many countries there is little or no seasonal use of the drugs, and therefore no past experience based on which drugs can be used in a pandemic.

Antivirals are the first line of defense

Two families of antivirals are approved for use with influenza: (i) adamantanes (amantadine, rimanta-dine), which block the M2 ion channel of the influenza virus; and (ii) neuraminidase inhibitors (oseltamivir (Tamiflu™), zanamivir (Relenza™)), which block virus release (see Chapter 25 on antivirals). In 2009, the antiviral stockpile in the United States that was part of pandemic preparedness for H5N1 contained 50 million regimens, comprising 40 million regimens of oseltamivir and 10 million regimens of zanamivir [49]. Small quantities of rimanta-dine were also available in the stockpile; the mix of drugs was made because of concerns about resistance to oseltamivir, as seen in H1N1 viruses before 2009. The pandemic H1N1 2009 inherited an adamantane-resistant neuraminidase from the European swine lineage, but was sensitive to both the neuraminidase inhibitors. After emergence of the pandemic H1N1 virus, 25% of the US stockpile was deployed to the states in April 2009 for treatment rather than prophylaxis. Because vaccines were not available during the first wave of pandemic H1N1, the antiviral stockpile was the only option for treatment. However, there is little evidence that much of the deployed stockpile was actually used.

One concern about the use of antineuraminidase inhibitors on an H1N1 influenza virus was that in 2007 neuraminidase inhibitor-resistant seasonal

H1N1 emerged in Europe, where little or no neuraminidase inhibitors had been used [50]. The resistant virus had a mutation at residue 274 of the N1 neuraminidase (H274Y) and the sensitivity to oseltamivir was reduced by 200- to 750-fold. The neuraminidase inhibitor-resistant H1N1 virus was surprisingly fit and spread globally in humans in the following year. Although several neuraminidase inhibitor-resistant pandemic H1N1 influenza viruses have emerged with the H274Y mutation to date, consistent human-to-human transmission of resistant virus has not been reported.

The lessons learned were that the stockpile of neuraminidase inhibitors is the first line of defense in the face of an influenza pandemic. However, little of the national stockpile was actually used, indicating the need for improved strategies to distribute the antivirals and implement priorities for use. Neuraminidase inhibitors have been found to be very stable and have a long shelf life (7 years). The continuing concern is that generalized resistance of pandemic H1N1 to neuraminidase inhibitors may emerge, similar to what occurred with the 2007 seasonal H1N1. Additional antiviral drugs directed at different targets are urgently needed, as it is very likely that resistance will emerge to a single antiviral.

Conclusions

Further pandemics of influenza are inevitable, as the ultimate reservoirs of influenza A viruses in wild aquatic birds cannot be eradicated. As we learn more about influenza viruses in wild-bird reservoirs and the genomics of viruses required to transmit to intermediate hosts and ultimately among humans, we may be able to make predictions about which influenza viruses have pandemic potential. From the 1977 and 2009 reintroductions of H1N1 influenza viruses into humans, we have learned that antigenic and structural relationships to the 1918 pandemic do not serve as an indicator of severity. To prevent future ambiguity it is necessary to include a measure of severity in the definition of a pandemic. One possibility is to consider a dual rating of pandemic alerts that includes separate categories for spread and lethality. For example, the 1918 Spanish influenza pandemic might be a 4/5 pandemic (spread/lethality out of 6)

whereas the 2009 H1N1 pandemic might be a 6/2 pandemic.

Although some markers of severity are known, including the role of the polymerase gene products (PB1-F2 and PB2) and the interplay between the hemagglutinin and the neuraminidase as well as the role of NS1 in modulating the innate immune response, we are far from understanding all the complex interactions of gene products of the virus and the host. Pathogenicity and transmissibility are complex issues involving the genomics of both the virus and host. Much remains to be learned in these areas that are relevant to pandemic preparedness. The Holy Grail of influenza control is a universal vaccine; initial studies show promise for the development of universal prophylactic antibodies. It is hoped that the future will hold the development of a universal influenza vaccine as well as the development of new classes of antiviral drugs for use in influenza control and pandemic planning.

Acknowledgments

Arnold S. Monto is supported by U01 IP000474 from the Centers for Disease Control and Prevention. Robert G. Webster is supported by Contract No. HHSN266200700005C with the National Institute of Allergy and Infectious Diseases and by the American Lebanese Syrian Associated Charities (ALSAC). We thank Vani Shanker for editing the chapter and James Knowles for assistance with chapter preparation.

References

1. Francis T Jr. On the doctrine of original antigenic sin. Proc Am Philosoph Soc. 1960;104:572–8.
2. Masurel N, Marine WM. Recycling of Asian and Hong Kong influenza A virus hemagglutinins in man. Am J Epidemiol. 1973;97:44–9.
3. Dauer CC, Serfling RE. Mortality from influenza 1957–1958 and 1959–1960. Am Rev Respir Dis. 1961;83:15–28.
4. Jordan EO. Epidemic Influenza: A Survey. Chicago: American Medical Association; 1927.
5. Rasolofonirina N. The history of flu in Madagascar. Arch Inst Pasteur Madagascar. 2003;69:6–11.

6. Taubenberger JK, Reid AH, Krafft AE, Bijwaard KE, Fanning TG. Initial genetic characterization of the 1918 "Spanish" influenza virus. Science. 1997;275:1793–6.

7. Oxford JS, Sefton A, Jackson R, Innes W, Daniels RS, Johnson NP. World War I may have allowed the emergence of "Spanish" influenza. Lancet Infect Dis. 2002;2: 111–4.

8. Olson DR, Simonsen L, Edelson PJ, Morse SS. Epidemiological evidence of an early wave of the 1918 influenza pandemic in New York City. Proc Natl Acad Sci U S A. 2005;102:11059–63.

9. Nguyen-Van-Tam JS, Hampson AW. The epidemiology and clinical impact of pandemic influenza. Vaccine. 2003;21:1762–8.

10. Morens DM, Taubenberger JK, Fauci AS. Predominant role of bacterial pneumonia as a cause of death in pandemic influenza: implications for pandemic influenza preparedness. J Infect Dis. 2008;198:962–70.

11. Beigel JH, Farrar J, Han AM, Hayden FG, Hyer R, de Jong MD, et al. Avian influenza A (H5N1) infection in humans. N Engl J Med. 2005;353:1374–85.

12. Shope RE. Swine influenza. III. Filtration experiments and etiology. J Exp Med. 1931;54:373–80.

13. Smith W, Andrewes CH, Laidlaw PP. A virus obtained from influenza patients. Lancet. 1933;1:66–8.

14. Kilbourne ED, Smith C, Brett I, Pokorny BA, Johansson B, Cox N. The total influenza vaccine failure of 1947 revisited: major intrasubtypic antigenic change can explain failure of vaccine in a post-World War II epidemic. Proc Natl Acad Sci U S A. 2002;99:10748–52.

15. Kawaoka Y, Krauss S, Webster RG. Avian-to-human transmission of the PB1 gene of influenza A viruses in the 1957 and 1968 pandemics. J Virol. 1989;63: 4603–8.

16. Murray R. Some problems in the standardization and control of influenza vaccine in 1957. Am Rev Respir Dis. 1961;83(2 Pt 2):160–7.

17. Monto AS, Kendal AP. Effect of neuraminidase antibody on Hong Kong influenza. Lancet. 1973;1:623–5.

18. Top FH Jr, Russell PK. Swine influenza A at Fort Dix, New Jersey (January–February 1976). IV. Summary and speculation. J Infect Dis. 1977;136(Suppl.):S376–80.

19. Gregg MB, Hinman AR, Craven RB. The Russian flu. Its history and implications for this year's influenza season. JAMA. 1978;240:2260–3.

20. De Jong JC, Claas EC, Osterhaus AD, Webster RG, Lim WL. A pandemic warning? Nature. 1997;389:554.

21. Bridges CB, Lim W, Hu-Primmer J, Sims L, Fukuda K, Mak KH, et al. Risk of influenza A (H5N1) infection among poultry workers, Hong Kong, 1997–1998. J Infect Dis. 2002;185:1005–10.

22. Lee N, Hui D, Wu A, Chan P, Cameron P, Joynt GM, et al. A major outbreak of severe acute respiratory syndrome in Hong Kong. N Engl J Med. 2003;348: 1986–94.

23. Li KS, Guan Y, Wang J, Smith GJ, Xu KM, Duan L, et al. Genesis of a highly pathogenic and potentially pandemic H5N1 influenza virus in eastern Asia. Nature. 2004;430:209–13.

24. Hien TT, de Jong M, Farrar J. Avian influenza – a challenge to global health care structures. N Engl J Med. 2004;351:2363–5.

25. de Jong MD, Tran TT, Truong HK, Vo MH, Smith GJ, Nguyen VC, et al. Oseltamivir resistance during treatment of influenza A (H5N1) infection. N Engl J Med. 2005;353:2667–72.

26. Wang H, Feng Z, Shu Y, Yu H, Zhou L, Zu R, et al. Probable limited person-to-person transmission of highly pathogenic avian influenza A (H5N1) virus in China. Lancet. 2008;371:1427–34.

27. Ferguson NM, Cummings DA, Cauchemez S, Fraser C, Riley S, Meeyai A, et al. Strategies for containing an emerging influenza pandemic in Southeast Asia. Nature. 2005;437:209–14.

28. World Health Organization. Pandemic influenza preparedness and response: a WHO guidance document. Geneva, Switzerland: World Health Organization; 2009.

29. World Health Organization. International Health Regulations [serial on the Internet]. 2005.24 January 2013]. Available from: http://www.who.int/ihr/en/ (accessed 20 February 2013).

30. Interim Pre-pandemic Planning Guidance: community strategy for pandemic influenza mitigation in the United States. 2007 [cited 24 January 2013]. Available from: http://www.flu.gov/professional/community/community _mitigation.pdf (accessed 20 February 2013).

31. Domínguez-Cherit G, Lapinsky SE, Macias AE, Pinto R, Espinosa-Perez L, de le Torre A, et al. Critically ill patients with 2009 influenza A(H1N1) in Mexico. JAMA. 2009;302:1880–7.

32. Kumar A, Zarychanski R, Pinto R, Cook DJ, Marshall J, Lacroix J, et al. Critically ill patients with 2009 influenza A(H1N1) infection in Canada. Canadian Critical Care Trials Group H1N1 Collaborative. JAMA. 2009;302:1872–9.

33. Report of the Review Committee on the Functioning of the International Health Regulations (2005) in relation to Pandemic (H1N1) 2009. 2011 (Fineberg Report). Available from: http://apps.who.int/gb/ebwha/pdf_files/ WHA64/A64_10-en.pdf (accessed 20 February 2013).

34. Viboud C, Miller M, Olson D, Osterholm M, Simonsen L. Preliminary estimates of mortality and years of life lost associated with the 2009 A/H1N1 pandemic in the US and comparison with past influenza seasons. PLoS Curr. 2010;2:RRN1153.

35. Forrest HL, Webster RG. Perspectives on influenza evolution and the role of research. Anim Health Res Rev. 2010;11:3–18.

36. Alexander DJ. Avian influenza viruses and human health. In: Schudel A, Lombard M, editors. Proceedings of the OIE/FAO International Conference on Avian Influenza. Basel, Switzerland: Developments in Biology; 2006. p. 77–84.

37. Scholtissek C. Pigs as "mixing vessels" for the creation of new pandemic influenza A viruses. Med Principles Pract. 1990/1991;2:65–71.

38. Smith GJ, Vijaykrishna D, Bahl J, Lycett SJ, Worobey M, Pybus OG, et al. Origins and evolutionary genomics of the 2009 swine-origin H1N1 influenza A epidemic. Nature. 2009;25, 459:1122–5.

39. Xu R, Ekiert DC, Krause JC, Hai R, Crowe JE Jr, Wilson IA. Structural basis of preexisting immunity to the 2009 H1N1 pandemic influenza virus. Science. 2010;328:357–60.

40. Zeng H, Pappas C, Katz JM, Tumpey TM. The 2009 pandemic H1N1 and triple-reassortant swine H1N1 influenza viruses replicate efficiently but elicit an attenuated inflammatory response in polarized human bronchial epithelial cells. J Virol. 2011;85: 686–96.

41. McAuley JL, Hornung F, Boyd KL, Smith AM, McKeon R, Bennink J, et al. Expression of the 1918 influenza A virus PB1-F2 enhances the pathogenesis of viral and secondary bacterial pneumonia. Cell Host Microbe. 2007;11:240–9.

42. Shortridge KF, Stuart-Harris CH. An influenza epicenter? Lancet. 1982;9:812–3.

43. Garten RJ, Davis CT, Russell CA, Shu B, Lindstrom S, Balish A, et al. Antigenic and genetic characteristics of swine origin 2009 A(H1N1) influenza viruses circulating in humans. Science. 2009;325:197–201.

44. Moura FEA. Influenza in the tropics. Curr Opin Infect Dis. 2010;23:415–20.

45. To KK, Chan KH, Li IW, Tsang TY, Tse H, Chan JF, et al. Viral load in patients infected with pandemic H1N1 2009 influenza A virus. J Med Virol. 2010;82:1–7.

46. Kawaoka Y, Bordwell E, Webster RG. Intestinal replication of influenza A viruses in two mammalian species. Brief report. Arch Virol. 1987;93:303–8.

47. Nicholls JM, Chan MC, Chan WY, Wong HK, Cheung CY, Kwong DL, et al. Tropism of avian influenza A (H5N1) in the upper and lower respiratory tract. Nat Med. 2007;13:147–9.

48. Ilyushina NA, Khalenkov AM, Seiler JP, Forrest HL, Bovin NV, Majuki H, et al. Adaptation of pandemic H1N1 influenza viruses in mice. J Virol. 2010;84: 8607–16.

49. Patel A, Gorman SE. Stockpiling antiviral drugs for the next influenza pandemic. Clin Pharmacol Ther. 2009;86: 241–3.

50. Meijer A, Lackenby A, Hungnes O, Lina B, van-der-Werf S, Schweiger B, et al. European Influenza Surveillance Scheme. Oseltamivir-resistant influenza virus A (H1N1), Europe, 2007–2008 season. Emerg Infect Dis. 2009;15:552–60.

Structure and replication

Section Editor: Robert A. Lamb

3

Structure, disassembly, assembly, and budding of influenza viruses

Debiprosad Nayak[1], Sakar Shivakoti[1,2], Rilwan A. Balogun[1,2], Gwendolyn Lee[1,2], and Z. Hong Zhou[1,2]

[1]Microbiology, Immunology and Molecular Genetics, David Geffen School of Medicine, University of California, Los Angeles, CA, USA

[2]California NanoSystems Institute (CNSI), Los Angeles, CA, USA

Introduction

Influenza viruses belonging to the *Orthomyxoviridae* family are enveloped, segmented, negative-stranded RNA viruses. They do not form a stable, long-term host–virus relationship within the infected host. Their very survival depends on host-to-host transmission, which, in turn, depends on the cycles of infection and release of progeny viruses from the infected hosts. Thus, influenza virus must find cells with proper receptors and enter the cell by receptor-mediated endocytosis, undergoing disassembly and releasing the viral genome (RNP) into the cytoplasm. Ribonucleoproteins (RNPs) are then transported into the host nucleus for the synthesis of mRNAs and viral RNAs (vRNAs). Translation of viral proteins takes place in the cytoplasm. Nascent RNPs are synthesized in the nucleus, exported out of the nucleus, and transported along with other viral components to the assembly/budding site on the plasma membrane. Finally, the segmented RNPs are assembled, enveloped, and released in the extracellular environment as virions. In this chapter, we review the virion structure and the processes involved in disassembly, assembly, and budding. Readers are advised to refer to several recent reviews for further details and additional references [1–6].

Structure and virus morphology

Structure

Influenza viruses are divided into three types: influenza A, B and C viruses, based on immunologic and biologic properties. Influenza A and B virions contain eight vRNA segments whereas influenza C virus contains seven vRNA segments. A schematic presentation of a typical influenza virus with spheroidal form is shown in Figure 3.1a. Influenza virions possess three subviral components: envelope, matrix layer underneath the lipid bilayers, and RNP core. Unless otherwise specified this chapter deals with influenza A virus.

Envelope

The envelope of influenza A virus consists of a lipid bilayer containing three virally encoded transmembrane proteins HA (hemagglutinin), NA (neuraminidase), and M2 (ion channel) on the outside, and M1 (matrix protein) underneath the membrane. The influenza virus lipid bilayer is mosaic containing both cholesterol-enriched lipid rafts and nonraft lipids derived selectively from the host [3,7]. HA and NA are anchored in the lipid rafts, whereas M2, a cholesterol-binding protein, is not tightly associated with lipid

Textbook of Influenza, Second Edition. Edited by Robert G. Webster, Arnold S. Monto, Thomas J. Braciale, and Robert A. Lamb.
© 2013 John Wiley & Sons, Ltd. Published 2013 by John Wiley & Sons, Ltd.

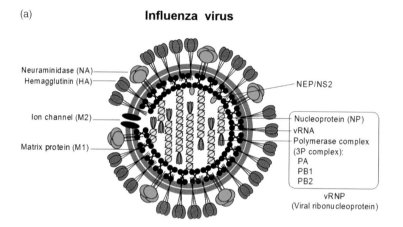

(a)

Influenza virus

Neuraminidase (NA)
Hemagglutinin (HA)
Ion channel (M2)
Matrix protein (M1)

NEP/NS2

Nucleoprotein (NP)
vRNA
Polymerase complex
(3P complex):
  PA
  PB1
  PB2

vRNP
(Viral ribonucleoprotein)

Family: *Orthomyxoviridae*
Genome: (-)ssRNA

Subtype: A (8 RNA segments) eg. WSN
B (8 RNA segments)
C (7 RNA segments)

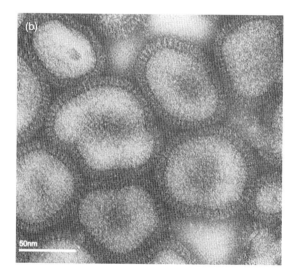

(b)

50nm

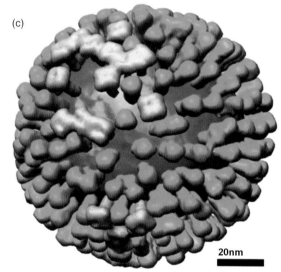

(c)

20nm

Figure 3.1. Influenza virus morphology. (a) A spheroidal influenza virus particle showing the viral components. (b) Transmission electron micrograph of influenza virus type A. Provided by K.G. Murti of St. Jude Children's Research Hospital of Memphis, Tennessee. (c) Artistic rendition of a spheriodal influenza virus based on cryo-electron tomography (cryoET) reconstructions, illustrating the distribution of HA (green), NA in clusters (gold), and lipid bilayers (blue). Reproduced from Harris et al. [12] with permission from National Academy of Sciences, USA. Bar = 20 nm. (d–f) Scanning electron micrographs of virus budding from the host cell. (d) Spheroidal influenza viruses budding in clusters. Provided by David Hockley of the National Institute for Biological Standards and Control, Hertfordshire, UK. (e) Virus particles budding preferentially from filopodia. Bar = 100 nm. Provided by David Hockley of the National Institute for Biological Standards and Control, Hertfordshire, UK. (f) Budding of filamentous virus particles. Provided by David Hockley of the National Institute for Biological Standards and Control at Hertfordshire, UK. Bar = 100 nm.

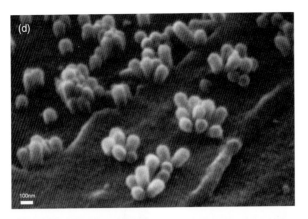

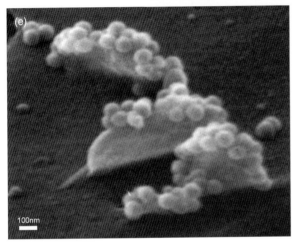

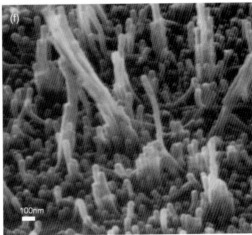

Figure 3.1. (*Continued*)

rafts [2,3,8]. HA is the major envelope protein (~80%) and forms trimeric spikes with receptor-binding sites and epitopes for neutralizing antibodies. NA, the second most abundant (~17%) envelope protein, forms the tetrameric spikes. NA removes the cell surface receptor (sialic acid) and has a critical role in the release of progeny virus particles as well as the spread of virus from host to host. The third envelope protein, the M2 tetramer, is a proton selective ion channel. Although M2 is a minor component (approximately 16–20 molecules/virion), it has a critical role in disassembly as well as in bud release [2,3].

Matrix layer
The matrix layer is composed of M1, the most abundant protein in virions, and a lipid-binding protein

that resides underneath the viral membrane and forms the critical bridge between the viral envelope and the RNP core. M1 interacts with the cytoplasmic tails of HA, NA, and M2 on the outer side and the vRNA and NP [2,3] on the inner side. M1 has a critical role in many stages of the virus replication including regulation of uncoating/disassembly, nuclear import and export of viral RNPs, transcription and replication of vRNA, and, finally, transport and assembly of RNPs and virus budding and morphogenesis [2,3,9].

Virus core
The virus core consists of helical RNP segments containing negative-stranded genomic vRNAs and NP along with minor amounts of the nuclear export

protein (NEP) and 3Pcomplex. The 3Pcomplex is heterotrimeric, composed of basic polymerase protein 1 (PB1), basic polymerase protein 2 (PB2), and acidic polymerase protein (PA). The vRNA in RNP is wrapped around the NP scaffold and exposed outside for gliding interaction with the 3Pcomplex during transcription/replication. In virus particles, the 3Pcomplexes are present only at one end of the RNP and requires primers for transcription-initiation indicating that only transcriptionally inactive RNPs are exported out of nucleus and packaged into virions [2]. Purified RNPs possess a twisted, rod-like structure that is folded back and coiled on itself [4,59,60] and are about 13 nm in diameter but vary in length up to 120 nm, depending on the size of the vRNA segments (see Chapter 4 for details).

Virus morphology

In general, influenza virus particles are pleomorphic and are roughly spheroidal (~100 nm in diameter) but some are filamentous (1 μm or longer). Usually, laboratory adapted viruses, such as A/PR/8, and A/WSN/33 viruses, exhibit spheroidal/ellipsoidal (SE) morphology (Figure 3.1b–e), whereas fresh field virus isolates are more filamentous. However, some virus strains, such as A/Udorn/72 (H3N2) [10], exhibit elongated/filamentous (EF) morphology (Figure 3.1f) even after many passages in the laboratory. Furthermore, the morphology of a specific virus strain can vary depending on how the virus is grown. The polarity of epithelial cells [10] as well as actin microfilaments and lipids (e.g., cholesterol) affect virus morphology [11]. Virus morphology is also determined by specific viral genes (e.g. M1, M2, NA) [2,3].

In the past, the morphology of influenza virus was studied primarily by examination of either negatively stained viral particles or thin sections of virus-infected cells by transmission electron microscopy (TEM) (Figure 3.1b) and scanning electron microscopy (SEM) (Figure 3.1d–f). However, staining by heavy metal salts, exposure to nonphysiologic pH, sample drying, embedding in resins, and sectioning procedures can affect the shape and morphology of virus particles. Influenza viruses are particularly susceptible to these procedures because of their flexible and pH-sensitive envelope and helical RNPs.

Recently, cryo-electron tomography (cryoET) has been used to examine the surface and internal structures of frozen hydrated virions and reconstruct the three-dimensional (3D) structure of virions by combining images of the same virus particles tilted at different angles. Such 3D structures have revealed the arrangement of proteins, nucleic acids, and lipids, as well as interactions among these viral components in their native state. Figure 3.1c shows an artistic rendition of a spheroidal influenza virus based on the cryoET reconstruction of X31 virus (A/Aichi/68, H3N2) [12]. X31 virus exhibited extensive pleomorphism and was divided into five classes of virions based on the shape, size, and arrangement of M1 and RNP. The most abundant particles (~80%) were spheroidal with a mean diameter of 120 nm and an average axial ratio of <1:2. The next predominant class (~14%) had an elongated morphology with an average diameter of 100 nm and an axial ratio of 1:4. The other three classes of virions represented only minor fractions of virions. Approximately, 300 HA (13 nm, triangular in shape) and 40 NA (14 nm, square in shape) spikes were present on the surface of each spheroidal virion. Furthermore, the distribution of HA and NA on the viral surface was not random, but contained local clusters of NA surrounded by more abundant HA spikes [2,12,13]. However, the cause and functional significance of NA clusters remain unclear. These cryoET reconstructions also indicated the presence of M1 beneath the lipid bilayer. Interestingly, some gaps were found in the putative M1 layer, which coincided with the absence of spikes on the outer surface. Authors [12] speculated that these M1 gaps were the pinching off sites for virus release. RNPs were densely packed in the virion interior and had similar dimensions as reported by others [4]. However, the majority of particles contained fewer than eight RNP spots, smaller particles containing fewer RNP spots [12,13].

Later, Calder et al. [13] analyzed Udorn and X31 viruses with cryoET and found that, despite a predominance of EF particles, Udorn viruses exhibited more pleomorphism and virion sizes varied from 120 nm to 1 μm. Filamentous particles were cylindrical in shape with a hemispherical cap at each end and an internal diameter of 55 nm (measured from lipid layer to lipid layer). Spheroidal particles have larger diameter (59 nm). In EF particles, RNPs were parallel and attached to one end of the virus. X31 virus particles mostly exhibited SE forms with hemispherical ends of 70 nm diameters and an axial ratio of 1 : 5; relatively a few EF particles were observed. Virus particles exhibited surface glycoproteins (spikes protruding from the membrane) and a dense M1 layer beneath the membrane. Authors [13] found that some particles lacked RNP but displayed the same morphology as the particles with RNP; they concluded that M1 (not RNP) determined the virus shape and morphology. RNPs had contact with the M1 layer only at the tapered end, and there was no further contact between M1 and RNP. Furthermore, in filamentous particles, NA spikes were found in clusters at the end opposite to RNP attachment.

Nayak et al. [2] have also analyzed PR8 (A/PR/8/34, H1N1), WSN (A/WSN/33, H1N1), and, more recently, Udorn viruses grown in MDCK cells by cryoET. Their analysis yielded essentially similar results as observed by others [12]. In the elongated particles, RNPs were parallel to the surface extending essentially end to end [2]. However, whether the morphology of different classes of virions and their RNP content have any relationship to infectivity remains undetermined. We expect that very small particles containing fewer RNPs are not infectious. Udorn viruses exhibited greater pleomorphism with three major classes of virions. Nearly 60% of virions had SE morphology (Figure 3.2a), similar to that observed by others [12,13]. However, some spheroidal particles (~5%) did not contain any detectable RNP (Figure 3.2a iii, iv). In addition, two classes of filamentous particles were observed (Figure 3.2b–d). One group (Figure 3.2b) of filamentous particles (~22%) had similar dimensions to those observed by others [13], with one set of RNPs lying parallel to each other and suspended from one end of the particle [4,13]. However, some filaments contained RNPs running parallel throughout the length of the particle without any attachment to one end (Figure 3.2b). Interestingly, another group of filamentous particles (~13%) exhibited "beaded" morphology: multiple incomplete spheroidal particles (beads) – up to 15 – connected to each other, resembling beads on a string (Figure 3.2c,d). Each incomplete spheroidal particle contained RNPs, suggesting that these filamentous particles had multiple sets of RNPs. It remains to be seen whether each individual bead of the filamentous particle contains a complete set of RNPs and is infectious. If these particles are produced by incomplete fission during budding, it may provide insight into the budding process and shed light

on the significance of the budding site (see section on bud elongation and closure).

Using longitudinal and transverse serial sectioning, Noda and Kawaoka [4] examined the *in situ* bud morphology on the surface of cells infected by a number of influenza viruses of both spheroidal and filamentous morphologies. They concluded that virus buds had eight RNPs with a 7 + 1 arrangement in transverse sections; none contained more than eight RNP spots. Some contained fewer than eight, depending on the position of the section. By longitudinal sectioning they noted that RNPs were attached to one end of the bud and ran parallel to the surface. The RNPs were ~12 nm in width and varied in length, ranging up to 120 nm. They further noted that all individual RNPs were oriented perpendicular to the cell surface at the budding site (see also Figure 3.2e) and each filamentous bud contained only one set of RNP suspended from the distal end while the rest of the filament remained empty. Recent studies from a number of laboratories support that the majority of RNP-containing virus particles possess eight unique RNP segments in a 7 + 1 arrangement [6,14–16]. It is therefore likely that released particles undergo changes in morphology and arrangement of RNP due to bud fission, causing the variation observed in cryoET reconstruction of released particles versus cell-associated virus buds by thin sectioning.

Disassembly

Steps in the influenza virus life cycle are schematically shown in Figure 3.3a,b. Disassembly is an early event in the virus life cycle following attachment and entry and occurs in the acidic environment of endosome (~pH 5). Disassembly of virions is a complex process involving the coordinated functions of many host and viral components. The first step in the virus life cycle (virus attachment) is brought about by the interaction of ligand (HA) with the cell surface receptor (sialic acid). Both the cell sialic acid receptors and HA present in different virus strains vary and the varying affinity of HA to sialic acid receptors has a critical role in species specificity, zoonoses, pathogenesis, transmission, and pandemic behavior of influenza virus strains. NA co-evolves with the receptor specificity of HA and facilitates infection of ciliated respiratory epithelium [17]. Although NA does not have a major role in clathrin-coated pit (CCP) formation and

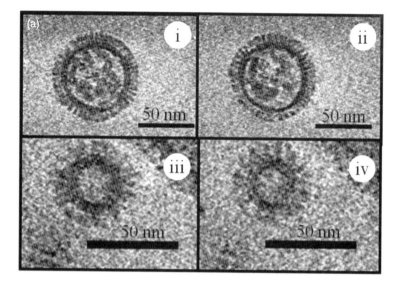

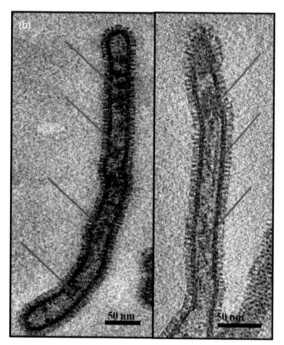

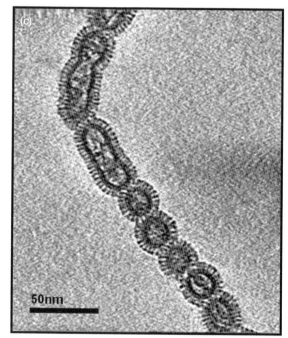

Figure 3.2. CryoET of Udorn (H3N2) virus particles. (a) Spheriodal particles with ribonucleoprotein (RNP) (i and ii) and without RNP cores (iii and iv). Boxes i and ii show an RNP-containing virion at varying heights. RNP can be found throughout the entire particle. In contrast, boxes iii and iv show a particle that lacks an RNP core at varying heights. No electron-dense material was found within the entire particle. (b) RNP distribution in the filamentous phenotype. Two different filamentous particles are shown with electron dense material (RNP), marked by arrows, present throughout the entire particle. (c) Variant form of released virions showing multiple spheroidal particles attached to each other and forming a chain, resembling beads on a string. Bar = 50 nm.

(d)

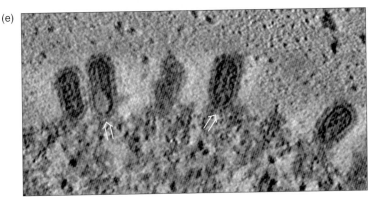

(e)

Figure 3.2. (d) Lack of complete membrane fission in a beaded filamentous particle visualized by cryoET. Four density slices from the cryoET tomogram at varying heights in the Z direction are shown. The varying heights for i, ii, iii, and iv were 62, 75, 83, and 97 out of 256 pixels (units), respectively. Arrows indicate points of junction, where continuous membranes across different "beads" are seen. As exemplified in iii and iv, the particles linked in one portion appear separated in another, depending on the Z height. (e) Virus buds at the cell surface visualized by electron tomography (ET). At 12 hpi, WSN-infected MDCK cells were processed for thin sectioning and examined by ET. The density represents a slice in the three-dimensional volume through the middle of virus buds on the infected cell. One can see the parallel arrangement of the RNPs inside the bud perpendicular to cell surface. The bud neck (indicated by ⇒) has a density gap, suggesting possible absence of M1. HA and NA spikes are seen on the bud envelope. Reproduced from Nayak et al. [2] with permission from Elsevier.

virus entry [18], NA aids influenza virus to get across the sialic acid containing mucin barrier of the respiratory epithelium and facilitates infection of the respiratory epithelial cells in animals. Virus entry is a dynamic process involving both attachment and elution and NA affects virus entry by causing virus elution. It is not clear what fraction of virus enters the cell at the first receptor contact and on an average how many contacts are needed before the virus is engulfed inside the cell by CCP. Once the virus particle becomes entrapped in the endosome, NA plays little part in the process of uncoating.

After binding to the cell surface sialic acid receptors, virions enter the cell via receptor-mediated endocytosis. Using single virus imaging technique, Rust et al. [18] showed that the majority of influenza viruses (~70%) use CCP and the remainder (~30%) use clathrin-independent vesicles for entry. Both pathways lead to viral fusion with endosomal membranes with similar efficiency. However, influenza viruses do not use pre-existing CCP but form *de novo* CCP at the site of attachment. How virus binding attracts clathrin and associated factors to form *de novo* CCP is not clear but most likely multivalent binding of spherical virus particle to the cell surface induces local membrane curvature attracting the Bin/Amphiphysin/Rsv (BAR) domain of amphiphysin to promote CCP formation. Filamentous viruses enter the cell via non-clathrin, non-caveola, dynamin-independant endocytosis [19]. Following entry, virions undergo the processes of uncoating/disassembly which can be separated into two major steps: (i) fusion of the viral and endosomal membranes; and (ii) release of the RNP.

Fusion process

The fusion process between two vesicular membranes is common in eukaryotic cells during many cellular activities such as exocytic transport involving release of extracellular enzymes, synaptic vesicles, and so on. The processes of uncoating/disassembly of parental virus versus assembly/budding of progeny virus represent two opposite poles in virus life cycle; the former requires the dissociation of the virus components in the safe intracellular environment whereas the latter requires the assembly of virus components so that the viral genome is protected in the harsh external environment. Without proper disassembly, synthetic phases of the virus life cycle cannot begin, whereas without proper assembly and release virions cannot find a new host, and continue the infectious cycle. Cycles of assembly and disassembly are repeated not only for the survival of the virus, but also for the development and spread of the disease in and among the infected hosts.

Furthermore, these two opposite processes (i.e., uncoating/disassembly and assembly/budding) occur in the same cell and sometimes in the same compartment of the cell (e.g., plasma membrane in the case of paramyxoviruses); yet these processes are unidirectional and cannot be reversed. From the simplified structural standpoint, three basic structures of both virus entry and exit in opposite directions are shown (Figure 3.3c). At the beginning of the virus life cycle,

these processes are called uncoating/disassembly involving attachment/entry, hemifusion and fusion leading to the release of RNPs inside the cell whereas, at the end of virus life cycle, these reverse processes are called assembly and budding involving bud initiation, hemifission, and fission leading to the release of virus particles. Both fusion and fission involve joining of the lipid bilayers. Uncoating/disassembly requires the fusion of lipid bilayers of one vesicle with another (i.e., lipid bilayers of the virus membrane with the lipid bilayers of the cellular (endosomal) membrane) leading to the formation of one vesicle from two. On the other hand, the virus release requires the fission process where the ends of the lipid bilayers of the same membrane join each other, that is virus membrane joining to virus membrane and cell membrane joining to cell membrane, leading to the formation of two vesicles from one. During fusion, membranes of two heterologous vesicles are joined whereas during fission the ends of the homologous membranes are joined to each other. These processes are unidirectional and not reversible (i.e., fusion cannot be converted into fission or vice versa) because the structural requirements of virus components and involvement of specific host factors for these two events are different. Whether the processes could be made artificially reversible is an intriguing question. Furthermore, it should be noted that although the viral components required for assembly or disassembly are essentially the same, they need not be. For example, although cleaved HA (HA→HA1 and HA2) can function equally in both assembly/budding as well as in uncoating/disassembly, uncleaved HA can function only in assembly/budding but not in uncoating/disassembly. This would suggest that disassembly is not just favoring the reverse processes of assembly/budding but requires additional factors and functions as well as different structures of the same component (e.g., HA) not required in assembly/budding.

Fusion within the endosome

If two lipid vesicles are held together in close proximity within about 1.5 nm, local destabilization of the lipid bilayers occurs and membranes fuse into a single vesicle. Fusion causes mixing of lipids in their bilayers and mixing of their internal contents. This is basically what happens when influenza virus is present in the endosome. When influenza virus binds to the cell surface sialic acid receptor via HA, the distance

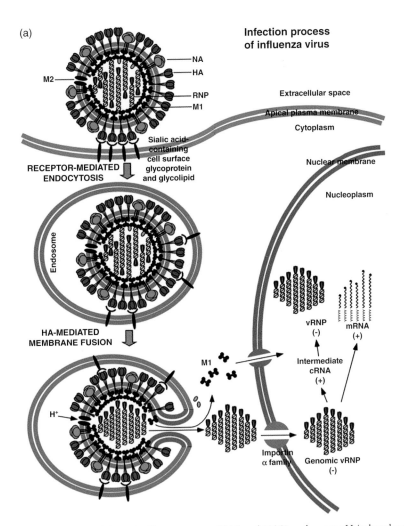

(a)

Infection process of influenza virus

NA
HA
M2
RNP
M1

Extracellular space
Apical plasma membrane
Cytoplasm

Nuclear membrane

Nucleoplasm

Sialic acid-containing cell surface glycoprotein and glycolipid

RECEPTOR-MEDIATED ENDOCYTOSIS

Endosome

HA-MEDIATED MEMBRANE FUSION

H+

M1

vRNP (-)   mRNA (+)

Intermediate cRNA (+)

Importin α family   Genomic vRNP (-)

Figure 3.3. Entry, disassembly, and budding of influenza virus. (a) The attachment, entry, and uncoating steps of the influenza virus infection. Attachment is mediated through HA (red) and sialic acid receptors. The virus enters the cell through the endosome. The HA mediated fusion of virus membrane with endosomal membrane, which occurs at a low pH, results in the release of RNP, transport of RNP into the nucleus, and the transcription (mRNA synthesis) and replication (cRNA and vRNA synthesis) of RNP in the nucleus. (b) Bud closure. The pinching-off region (neck) is shown to consist of membrane devoid of lipid rafts [11], HA and NA spikes, and M1 [12]. However, this region may contain M2 [8]. Reproduced from Nayak et al. [2] with permission from Elsevier. (c) The entry and disassembly as well as assembly, and budding processes within a cell. Note that entry and disassembly require fusion of the membranes, while the same processes in the opposite direction – during budding and bud release – are called fission of the membranes. (d) Boomerang model of HA mediated membrane fusion. (i) Cleaved HA (HA0 becomes

HA1 and HA2) undergoes pH-induced conformational change in the endosome, releasing and inserting the boomerang-shaped fusion peptide into the target (endosome) cellular membrane. (ii) The ectodomain tilts to the plane of the membranes. The boomerangs bring the target membrane close to the viral membrane so that lipid exchange can occur, thereby inducing hemifusion. (iii) In this state, lipids found only on the outer leaflets mix. At the point of hemifusion, the aqueous contents of the two vesicles still remain separated. (iv) Eventually the fusion peptide and the transmembrane domain interact with each other causing the complete fusion of both lipid bilayers, leading to the formation of the initial fusion pore opening. Multiple HA trimers are required in opening the fusion pore [23]. After opening of the initial narrow fusion pore, the pore dilates (not shown) and releases the viral nucleocapsid into the cytoplasm of the infected cell. Reprinted and modified from Tamm [20] with permission from Elsevier.

(b)

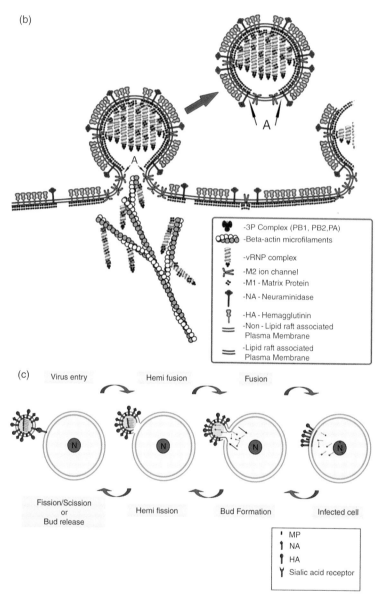

	-3P Complex (PB1, PB2,PA)
	-Beta-actin microfilaments
	-vRNP complex
	-M2 ion channel
	-M1 - Matrix Protein
	-NA - Neuraminidase
	-HA - Hemagglutinin
	-Non - Lipid raft associated Plasma Membrane
	-Lipid raft associated Plasma Membrane

(c)

Virus entry   Hemi fusion   Fusion

Fission/Scission or Bud release   Hemi fission   Bud Formation   Infected cell

	MP
	NA
	HA
	Sialic acid receptor

Figure 3.3. (*Continued*)

between the viral membrane and the cell membrane is approximately 15 nm which is far too great for the fusion of the viral and cell membranes. Influenza viruses have developed a fascinating way to overcome this distance barrier and bring the viral and cellular membranes within the proximity of each other to enable fusion. Because HA is the major barrier separating the two membranes, it has to undergo major structural changes yet hold both membranes and, at the same time, collapse and get out of the way for viral and cellular membranes to meet each other leading to fusion, forming one vesicle and mixing of their content. For HA to undergo such conformational change, two conditions are necessary: HA

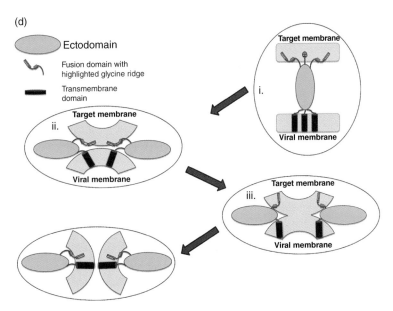

Figure 3.3. (*Continued*)

(HA0) must be cleaved into HA1 and HA2, and be present in an acidic environment (~pH 5). Cleavage of HA generates the fusion peptide (20–24 conserved glycine-rich hydrophobic residues) at the N-terminus of HA2, which is joined to the three-stranded coiled-coil structure by a 28 aa loop and remains buried in the native molecule about 10 nm from the globular head at neutral pH. Acidic pH converts HA into a metastable state in which the loop is converted into a helix and the fusion peptide of the cleaved HA projects upward and is inserted into the target (endosomal) membrane [20–22]. However, despite these dramatic changes, HA remains as a trimer with its globular head bound to its sialic acid receptor and the distance between the endosomal and viral membranes remains around 10 nm (Figure 3.3d i). Next, the coiled-coil stem structure of HA splays apart bringing the viral and endosomal lipid bilayers close to each other for fusion (Figure 3.3d ii). Although the precise mechanisms of these events are unclear, Tamm [20] proposed a spring-loaded boomerang mechanism of influenza-induced membrane fusion. Fusion of the membranes involves the hemifusion state (Figure 3.3d iii) in which one layer of the lipid bilayer undergoes mixing without the mixing of the content. Subsequently, both layers of the lipid bilayers get fused and

a pore is formed mixing the content of both vesicles (Figure 3.3d iv). A number of HA trimers (six or more) are required for the formation of the fusion pore [23]. Because of the low pH induced structural changes in HA, the fusion process is irreversible. Furthermore, both the fusion peptide at the N-terminus and the transmembrane domain (TMD) at the C-terminus of HA2 directly interact with each other and the glycine ridge on the upper face of the N-terminal arm of the fusion peptide is important for helix–helix interaction with the TMD (Figure 3.3d iv) [20]. Lee [21] has proposed that the M1 matrix layer serves as an endoskeleton for the virus and a foundation for HA during membrane fusion. Low pH treatment weakens M1–membrane interaction and renders viral envelope pliable and conducive for fusion [24].

Release of viral RNP

Subsequent to fusion, M1–RNP attachments are disrupted releasing RNP for its transport into the nucleus. M1 becomes disassociated from RNP and the cytoplasmic tails of HA, NA, and M2 in acidic pH. M2, the proton ion channel, present in the virus envelope, remains closed at neutral pH but opens up in acidic pH of the endosome acidifying the virion

47

interior. A few molecules of the M2 tetramer (16–20/virion) are sufficient for acidifying the virion interior and releasing the RNP. Fontana et al. [24] have proposed that the fusion process and RNP release in acidic pH are highly coordinated, otherwise RNPs becomes coagulated and trapped and not released in the cytoplasm. On the other hand, disassociation of RNP from M1 must occur before the complete fusion of the viral membrane with the endosomal membrane, otherwise the neutral pH of the cell cytoplasm will dilute and neutralize the virion interior preventing M1–RNP dissociation. Blocking M2 ion channel by drugs such as amantadine or increasing the endosomal pH prevents virus uncoating and interferes with virus replication (see Chapter 7). M1-free RNPs are then transported into the host nucleus through the nuclear pore complex for transcription and replication of vRNA. In addition to three viral proteins (HA, NA, and M2) and acidic pH, a number of host factors including lipid rafts participate in virus disassembly. Recent genome screens including RNA*i* screens, two hybrid analysis, transcriptome, proteome, reactome and other genome-wide screenings have identified a number of host factors in each step of the viral replication. These include GTPase Rab5, Rab7/protein kinase C Beta (PKCβII) involved in late and early endosomes as well as Rab10 and subunits of cotamer1 (COPI) vesicular complex *(ARCN1, COPA, COPB2, and COPG)*, V-type ATPase, involved in low pH-dependent membrane fusion [25]. However, the precise roles of any of these components in uncoating/disassembly remain undefined.

Transport and assembly

For budding, influenza virus components must be brought and assembled at the budding site for bud initiation and eventual bud release. Therefore, influenza virus budding process can be subdivided into two steps: (i) transport/assembly of viral components at the budding site; and (ii) budding of the progeny particles. During assembly, viral components are transported to the budding site either individually or in the form of complexes which further interact with each other forming higher order of complexes. However, transport/assembly and budding processes are rather a continuum without strong stop–start check points (i.e., completion of the previous step is not required before the initiation of the next step). For example, assembly of viral components into subviral complexes can occur either during transport or during budding; similarly, bud initiation/membrane-bending can occur before all components are brought to the budding site and finally, even bud release can happen in the absence of a complete set of RNPs or without any RNP (Figure 3.2a iii and iv). It is unknown whether there are different requirements for the budding of infectious from noninfectious particles, and whether one is favored over the other.

Assembly and budding require that all three viral components – the viral envelope (with HA, NA, and M2), M1 and RNPs – are brought to the budding site, that is the apical plasma membrane in polarized epithelial cells, whether in cultured cells or in the respiratory epithelium of infected animals. Because complete virus particles are not found inside the infected cell, assembly of virus components into the virus particle must occur at the apical plasma membrane. However, what determines the selection of the apical budding site is unclear. Although influenza virus possesses three transmembrane envelope proteins (HA, NA, and M2) with apical determinants, they may not be sufficient in selecting the apical budding site. For example, apical budding of a mutant HAtyr virus was not significantly affected by basolateral targeting of mutant HAtyr [2]. Over 99% of HAtyr virus particles were released from the apical side even though the majority of HAtyr protein was directed to the basolateral side. Similarly, apical targeting of NA was not sufficient for apical budding of influenza viruses. Therefore other viral components, particularly NP/RNP, may have a significant role in selecting the apical budding site. NP/RNP is transported to the apical plasma membrane independent of the transmembrane viral proteins [2,26]. However, apical determinant(s) of NP/RNP and cellular machinery involved in its apical transport are yet unknown. Cortical actin microfilaments as well as lipid rafts facilitate in apical transport of NP because NP/RNP binds to both [2,26]. For transporting RNP to the budding site, it must be exported from the nucleus into cytoplasm. M1 is critical for nuclear exit of nascent RNPs. M1 enters the nucleus, binds to RNP as well as with NEP, forming the daisy-chain complex of (Crm1 and RanGTP)-NEP-M1-RNP, and mediates nuclear export of RNP [2]. Inhibition of transcription-initiation of RNPs by M1 is critically necessary for nuclear exit and incorporation of RNP into virions because RNPs with the 3Pcomplex present only at one end are found in virus particles [2,27,59,60]. Raf/MEK/ERK-cascade and NF-kappaB modulate nuclear export of RNP [28]. M1 is not known to possess any apical determinants but binds to lipids (but not lipid rafts) and RNA/RNP/NP, and associates with the tails of HA, NA, and M2 [2,29,30]. Therefore, some M1 are transported to the apical budding site on the piggyback of HA, NA, M2, and RNP.

Budding

Virus budding is similar to vesiculation observed in many cell types during growth, cell division, neurotransmission, cell-to-cell communication, and so on. Various types of membrane-bound vesicles including exosomes, microvesicles, and ectosomes (shedding vesicles) are released by living cells. However, these vesicles are different from virus buds in sizes and contents and also in the mechanism of the budding process [31]. Budding is a specialized function of cell in which the cargo is wrapped by a lipoprotein envelope and released in the external environment. In influenza virus budding, RNPs are assembled, packaged, enveloped, and shed from the plasma membrane of infected cells. The budding process involves transport and assembly of viral components to the budding site followed by successive steps involving bud initiation, bud elongation, and bud release. Therefore the size and shape of virus particles may depend on the efficiency of bud release, which in turn follows the orderly progression of successive steps. For example, block or delay in bud release may cause spheroidal particles to turn into elongated or filamentous particles. Below, we review the involvement of viral and host components in influenza virus budding.

Role of viral proteins

Two approaches have been used in defining the role of virus and host components in budding: (i) minimal requirements for budding, that is production of a virus-like particle (VLP); and (ii) mutation(s), deletion(s), and suppression of virus and host components affecting the shape, size, and quantity of released particles. Each assay and procedure can provide useful information but has its limitations. For example, in VLP production using individual or combinations of viral components, the expression level of viral component(s) may not be the same or as regulated as in virus-infected cells. Therefore, when interpreting their functional role in virus budding in infected cells, these limitations should be carefully considered and supported by determining their effect in virus-infected cells [2].

All three TM proteins (HA, NA, and M2) are involved in the assembly and budding processes. However, direct involvement of HA alone in the budding process in virus-infected cells is not clear [3,29]. HA tail-minus mutant viruses did not affect virus budding or the shape and size of released particles [2,30]. Moreover, an engineered WSN-luciferase virus lacking HA RNA released virus particles with equal efficiency form both MDCK-HA and MDCK cells [32]. However, viruses containing specific mutations in the NA cytoplasmic tail (CT) alone or in both HA CT and NA CT affected virus morphology [30]. Also, some mutants with NA CT substitutions and NA TMD replacement produced aberrant and elongated particles [2] indicating a defect in the pinching-off process. Clustering of NA may lead to fission of the bud by uncoupling the matrix layer extension from glycoprotein recruitment and bud extension [13]. Also, YPDX present in the NA ectodomain of some viruses may aid in overcoming tetherin restriction and facilitate virus budding [32] although the precise mechanisms remains undefined.

M2 is a critical component in virus budding. Complete or partial deletion of WSN M2 tail caused attenuation of virus growth, produced elongated, even filamentous particles in some mutants [2,3]. Mutations in Udorn M2 tail affected particle release in VLP assay by cDNA transfection [30]. These M2 mutants were extremely defective in multi-cycle virus growth, and, unlike the wt M2, they were defective in M1–M2 interaction. M2 may facilitate bud scission by bringing the flexible nonraft lipids in the neck region (Figure 3.3b, see section on bud elongation and closure).

M1 also has a critical role in virus assembly and budding processes. M1 affects virus assembly by interacting with the TM proteins (HA, NA, and M2) on the outer side and RNP on the inner side as well as by bringing and concentrating these viral components to the budding site. SUMOylation of M1 at K242 is required for M1–RNP complex formation, export of RNP, transport, assembly, morphogenesis, and budding of influenza [33]. A threshold level of M1 is required for bud release because low levels of M1 and M2 reduced virus release [34]. M1 is critical for maintaining the filamentous morphology of A/Udorn/72 virus particles and a single mutation in M1 (1A variant) caused transformation from filamentous to spheroidal particles [10]. Some M1 mutants also caused budding defects generating elongated buds and releasing elongated particles [2,30,35]. In addition, an influenza C virus M1 mutant containing an M1A24T mutation affected virus morphology by modulating its membrane affinity [36]. Calder et al. [13] have observed Udorn virus particles containing highly ordered helical organization of M1 without any internal RNP and concluded that the helical net of M1 can recruit membrane glycoproteins and drive the budding process.

Role of the eight RNP segments

The role of RNP in the budding process of influenza virus is not clear because both spherical (Figure 3.2a) as well as filamentous particles [13] without RNP are found and because the expression of structural proteins (HA, NA, M1, and M2) can release VLPs [2,30,37,38]. Besides, RNP is found in the distal end of the virus bud away from the fission site [4,13]. However, RNP content may affect the width of the bud and thus may affect virus morphology [13]. Incorporation of all eight (seven for influenza C virus) RNA segments is required for infectivity of virus particles and both M1 and NP have important roles in the incorporation of RNPs [2,3]. However, how these multiple RNP segments are incorporated into virus particles remains unclear. Two models, "random packaging" and "specific packaging," have been proposed for the incorporation of eight specific RNA/RNP segments into virions.

The "random packaging" model predicts the presence of common structural elements in all RNA/RNPs causing them to be incorporated randomly into virions. The incorporation of RNPs in released particles will depend on the concentration of RNPs in infected cells. Support for this model comes from the observation that influenza A virions can possess more than eight RNPs (9–11 RNAs per virion) [2,4,39,40] and at most 1 in 10 or more virus particles are infectious. The "specific

packaging" model predicts that specific structural features are present in each RNA/RNP segment, enabling them to be selectively incorporated into virions. Earlier evidence supporting this model includes the observation that vRNAs are equimolar in virus particles even though vRNA concentrations in infected cells vary [41]. Studies using defective interfering (DI) RNAs support "selective packaging" because small DI RNAs competitively inhibited packaging of their normal counterparts but not other vRNAs [42]. Recent studies from a number of laboratories have shown the presence of segment-specific packaging signal(s) in 3′ and 5′ UTR as well as adjacent coding regions of all eight RNA segments. Furthermore, incorporation of specific RNA segments was critical for the incorporation of other RNA segments indicating a hierarchy RNA incorporation [4,43]. Serial sectioning of influenza A virus infected MDCK cells as well as electron tomography (ET) analysis of released virions also showed that the RNPs of influenza A viruses are organized in a distinct 7 + 1 pattern supporting "specific packaging" ([4,15,44]. Using fluorescence *in situ* hybridization (FISH) analysis Chou et al. [15] observed that the majority of RNP-containing virus particles possess eight unique RNA segments and that PB2, PA, NP, and M RNA segments provide critical roles for genome packaging. They further proposed that genome segments are put together at the same time [43]. However, the fraction of virus particles containing RNP remains to be determined. Such a model predicts that specific RNA–RNA interactions among the RNP segments in *trans* would form multi-segmental RNP complexes and that large RNP complexes containing eight unique RNPs in *trans* are stable. The major weakness of this model is that bud closure and virus release do not depend on the incorporation of eight specific RNA segments because particles with no RNP are found (Figure 3.2a) [13]. However, it is possible that segment-specific complex formation and incorporation of viral RNAs occur but do not affect bud closing and bud release and that RNPs are not active participants in the budding process but passively entrapped and enveloped in the bud and released as virus particles.

Role of host components

Budding of influenza virus also requires the participation of host components [45]. However, the requirements and functions of specific host components in bud maturation and bud release of influenza viruses are poorly understood. Furthermore, different steps of the budding process may be either positively or negatively regulated by host components. Therefore, to facilitate budding, components inhibiting bud release should be removed and components facilitating bud fission be brought to the budding site. However, some component(s) may aid in specific step(s) of budding but may interfere with other steps. For example, cortical actin microfilaments may aid in stabilizing multiple RNPs into complexes, transporting the RNP–M1 complex to the budding site and promoting bud growth and maturation by pushing the RNP complex into the bud. However, actin microfilaments may interfere in the last step of bud fission. Disruption of actin microfilaments facilitates bud release [2,10,46]. Recently, proteomic analysis of purified influenza virus particles suggested incorporation of at least seven host proteins in virions, including β-actin, annexin A5, tubulin, cyclophilin A and A2, colifilin, and glyceraldehyde 3-phosphate dehydrogenase (GAPDH or G3PDH) [47]. Some of these proteins may be involved in the budding process. Rab11 GTPase, a small GTPase binding protein, associates with influenza RNPs and has a critical role in transporting RNPs to the budding site [48,49]. Rab11, which is involved in endocytic recycling, and FIP3 (Rab family interacting protein), which binds to actin and microtubule-based motor proteins, are involved in bud morphogenesis and bud release. RuvB-like protein 2 (RBL2) regulates oligomerization of RNPs and modulates the activity of 3Pcomplex [50]. Chromosome region maintenance 1 (CRM1) forms complexes with RNP for nuclear export. However, influenza virus budding was not affected by either dominant negative VPS4 or by proteasome inhibitors [2,3,51]. The role of tetherin, an interferon-inducible antiviral host factor (also called BST-2), is not clear. It affects VLP production in cells transfected with some NA plasmids but not virus production in virus-infected cells [30,52–54]. Influenza virus budding is also an active energy-dependent process requiring ATP [9,51].

Host lipids, particularly lipid rafts, have critical roles in many aspects of the influenza virus life cycle including assembly and budding [3,7,9]. Lipid rafts are lipid microdomains enriched in sphingolipids and cholesterol-containing lipids in liquid order (l_o) phase and are relatively resistant to nonionic detergent at a low temperature [7]. Lipid rafts are important for transport and assembly of viral components in apical plasma membrane and also facilitate protein–protein interactions of M1 with HA and NA by bringing non-raft-associated M1 RNP to lipid raft microdomains [2]. Lipid rafts function as budding platforms, facilitate membrane bending and bud initiation [7]. Membrane accumulation of HA and its tight association with lipid-raft domains can trigger activation of the MAPK cascade via protein kinase C alpha and induce RNP export from the nucleus into the cytoplasm and thereby coordinate the timing of RNP export to virus budding at the plasma membrane [55]. Also, viperin, an interferon inducible protein, affects influenza virus budding by perturbing lipid rafts in cultured cells but not in infected animals [56]. However, lipid rafts may negatively regulate the final step of bud release. Depletion of cholesterol in infected cells by short MβCD treatment at the late phase of infection facilitated bud completion and increased virus particle release whereas addition of exogenous cholesterol increased the TX-100 insolubility of HA and NA, reduced the release of virus particles, and produced deformed, elongated buds with incomplete buds attached to each other [11]. Thus, lipid rafts have two opposite effects on the influenza virus budding processes. Initially, lipid rafts may facilitate bud formation by bringing and concentrating the viral components at the budding site, as well as causing asymmetry in the lipid bilayers favoring membrane bending and bud initiation [9]. However, at the final stage of bud completion, the lipid rafts may slow down bud closure because of its increased viscosity and rigidity [11]. The mosaic nature of the viral membrane containing both raft-associated and non-raft-associated lipid-microdomains have different functions in the budding processes involving bud initiation and bud closure (see section on bud elongation and closure).

Bud initiation

Budding requires three major steps: bud initiation, bud elongation, and bud completion, releasing the virions from the host cell membrane. Each of these steps involves the interaction of multiple host and viral components. Influenza viruses bud from plasma membranes and more specifically from the apical plasma membrane of polarized epithelial cells. However, even on the plasma membrane influenza viruses do not bud randomly, rather they bud from specific spots or foci as several viruses are seen to bud around the same position on the membrane (Figure 3.1d). Influenza viruses also bud preferably from specific membrane microdomains called filopodia (Figure 3.1e). These membrane projections are enriched in lipid rafts with underlying parallel bundles of actin microfilaments, and function as the sensors for environmental cues. Furthermore, the presence of multiple incompletely separated virus particles with RNP attached to each other (Figure 3.2c) shows that exactly the same spot was used for budding of multiple virus particles and suggests that the transport and assembly machineries are bringing all viral components to the exact same spot multiple times. Such a process would necessitate the supply and coordination of multiple sets of RNPs and other viral components to the same spot at specific intervals and spaghetti-like production and chopping at intervals by bud scission.

Bud initiation requires outward bending of the plasma membrane and involves the transition of a planar membrane structure to a curved structure at the budding site. Although the structural nature and biochemical properties, as well as the physical forces responsible for membrane bending leading to bud initiation remain undefined, most likely both lipid rafts and raft-associated proteins present at the budding site have important roles in membrane curvature and bud initiation. Lipid rafts producing asymmetry of inner and outer lipid bilayers can cause intrinsic curvature of one lipid monolayer relative to the other leading to membrane bending [7]. Selective transfer of lipids between the lipid bilayers, interaction of cholesterol into the budding leaflet as well as hydrolytic cleavage of phosphocholine head groups of sphingomyelin by sphingomyelinase generating smaller head groups can lead to membrane deformation. Additionally, BAR domains have been shown to cause membrane curvature and are known to be present in a number of proteins involved in vesicle formation and recycling [7]. However, their role in influenza virus budding is unknown. In addition to lipid rafts, the presence of specific viral proteins including HA, NA, M2, and M1 proteins further facilitate membrane bending in virus-infected cells [7]. These viral proteins are not passively incorporated in the budding microdomain but actively participate in the budding process. HA TMD peptide assumes a predominantly alpha helical conformation in detergent micelles and phospholipid bilayers and HA TMD, in turn, increases the acyl chain bilayer and packing of lipid bilayer supporting its role in assembling lipid rafts and initiating budding [7]. Specific amino acids in the TMD as well as the CT of HA and NA can affect the helical conformation of HA and NA and thus alter their interaction with lipid rafts [2,3]. In addition, clustering of M1 due to M1–M1 interaction underneath the lipid bilayers causes asymmetry in lipid bilayers producing outward membrane bending and bud initiation [2].

Bud elongation and closure

The factors and forces that regulate bud growth and maturation prior to release are largely undefined. For most viruses, regardless of containing either icosahedral (e.g., SFV) or helical (e.g., VSV) nucleocapsids, the size of the nucleocapsids determines the size of the virions. However, influenza viruses are highly pleomorphic (Figure 3.1a-e and Figure 3.2c) and RNP content is not the major factor in bud growth or bud release because the virus morphology can be maintained entirely by M1 and envelope proteins without any RNP [13].

Basically, two types of particle pleomorphism are observed among influenza viruses: (i) strain-specific, that is strain-to-strain variation which may also vary depending on the host cell; and (ii) variation within the population of plaque-purified viruses. Viral genomic and host factors are important in strain-specific pleomorphism. However, the cause of pleomorphism in plaque-purified influenza viruses is not clear. We propose that the efficiency of bud closure largely determines the shape and size of the released particles; that is, a defect in bud closing will tend to generate more elongated/filamentous than spheroidal particles. This hypothesis provides a simple explanation why mutation(s) in specific viral genes would cause spheroidal particles to become filamentous. This common mechanism also helps to explain the varying sizes and pleomorphism observed among the released virus particles from plaque-purified viruses. However, others [49] have proposed separate pathways and requirements for the generation of spherical versus filamentous particles because depletion of Rab11 in PR/8Mud (PR8 virus containing M RNA of Udorn virus) infected cells produced spheroidal, rather than hyper-filamentous particles attached to the cells. It is possible that Rab11 depletion may have caused other defects including RNP transport, bud initiation, and so on, and bud closing could be one of several factors in influenza virus pleomorphism.

Influenza virus bud growth appears to depend on two forces: pulling and pushing. The pulling force is primarily provided by the transmembrane proteins (HA, NA) along with M1, whereas cortical actin microfilaments which bind to viral RNPs provide the pushing force for incorporating the RNPs and M1 into the bud. These viral and cellular factors may affect bud growth and bud closing and thus determine the shape and size of the virus particles. Finally, bud closure would involve the fusion of two ends of the apposing viral membranes as well as that of the apposing cell membranes leading to the fission of the virus bud from the cell membrane (Figure 3.3b). This would require bringing and holding the apposing membrane ends next to each other in close proximity so that each end can find its counterpart and promote fusion of corresponding lipid bilayers by exchanging lipids so two ends of the viral membrane and two ends of the cellular membrane will fuse with each other causing separation of the virus bud from the membrane of the infected cell.

Bud closing and bud release of influenza virus is very inefficient even in productively infected cells; only a small fraction (~10%) of virus buds are released while the majority of virus buds remain attached to the cell membrane [2] despite their mature appearance (Figure 3.1d,e and Figure 3.2e). The cause of inefficiency in bud release remains unclear. One possibility is that the pinching-off process is energy-dependent [2,51] and limited available energy at the end of the infectious cycle may be responsible for inefficient bud release. Furthermore, host factors including actin microfilaments and lipid rafts may interfere with bud closing [2,10,46].

We proposed that lipid rafts in the neck region, owing to its increased viscosity and rigidity, interfere with bud closure [11]. Presence of M2 protein in the neck region of the bud has been proposed to facilitate bud closing [2,3,8]. Because only a few M2 tetramers are present in virions their presence in the neck region will be infrequent, leading to inefficient bud release. Barman and Nayak [11] proposed that M2 primarily aids in bringing non-lipid-raft lipids in the neck region and thereby facilitates the pinching-off process by inducing the fusion of membranes (Figure 3.3b). They showed that lipid raft disruption by short MβCD treatment, late in the infectious cycle, markedly enhanced virus release [11]. Furthermore, acylation and cholesterol-binding motifs of M2 are not crucial for virus morphology and budding [57]. It is unlikely that the M2 protein could be specifically brought to the neck region for increased bud release by short MβCD treatment [11]. Therfore the major function of M2 in a normal bud session is to bring non-lipid-raft lipids to the neck region. However, Rossman et al. [58] postulated that the amphipathic helix of M2 alters membrane curvature at the neck, thereby facilitating bud fission. It is possible that both functions of M2 may aid in bud fission and further work is needed on the mechanism of bud scission.

Conclusions

Influenza is a worldwide infectious viral disease of great public health concern. Because the host is infected at very low multiplicity of infection, factors contributing to a productive infectious cycle, including the steps of entry, disassembly, assembly, and virus release, are all involved in the development and severity of the disease and in the spread of the disease. Current anti-influenza viral drugs are limited to two families and are based on interfering with the processes of uncoating and releasing the RNP by blocking the M2 proton channel (amantadine and rimantadine) or by preventing the spread of virus particles post-bud completion by inhibiting the enzymatic activity of NA (oseltamivir or Tamiflu®_ by Roche and zanamivir or Relenza® by GlaxoSmithKline). Newly emerging viruses are often resistant to these drugs. A better understanding of each of these steps of the virus life cycle and the identification of specific host and viral components involved in each of these steps may provide newer targets for intervention and lead to the development of newer therapeutic agents. Similarly, because influenza virus bud closing is very inefficient, releasing only a small fraction of virus buds, a process for efficient bud closing and virus release will generate more virus particles for vaccine production. In summary, a more detailed understanding of the influenza virus replication cycle, particularly the steps in budding, will aid both in the treatment of influenza in infected persons and in preventing its spread.

Acknowledgments

Research activities in the authors' laboratories were supported by USPHS grants from NIH/NIAID (AI16348 (DPN), AI41681 (DPN), AI80171 (DPN), AI069015 (ZHZ) and NIGMS GM071940 (ZHZ).

References

1. Nayak DP. Virus morphology, replication, and assembly. In: Hurst CJ, editor. Studies in Viral Ecology, Vol. 2. Animal Host Systems. Hoboken, NJ: Wiley-Blackwell; 2011, pp. 67–130.

2. Nayak DP, Balogun RA, Yamada H, Zhou ZH, Barman S. Influenza virus morphogenesis and budding. Virus Res. 2009;143:147–61.

3. Rossman JS, Lamb RA. Influenza virus assembly and budding. Virology. 2011;411:229–36.

4. Noda T, Kawaoka Y. Structure of influenza virus ribonucleoprotein complexes and their packaging into virions. Rev Med Virol. 2010;20:380–91.

5. Sieczkarski SB, Whittaker GR. Viral entry. Curr Top Microbiol Immunol. 2005;285:1–23.

6. Hutchinson EC, von Kirchbach JC, Gog JR, Digard P. Genome packaging in influenza A virus. J Gen Virol. 2010;91:313–28.

7. Nayak DP, Hui EK. The role of lipid microdomains in virus biology. Subcell Biochem. 2004;37:443–91.

8. Schroeder C, Heider H, Moncke-Buchner E, Lin TI. The influenza virus ion channel and maturation cofactor M2 is a cholesterol-binding protein. Eur Biophys J. 2005;34:52–66.

9. Nayak DP, Hui EK, Barman S. Assembly and budding of influenza virus. Virus Res. 2004;106:147–65.

10. Roberts PC, Compans RW. Host cell dependence of viral morphology. Proc Natl Acad Sci U S A. 1998;95:5746–51.

11. Barman S, Nayak DP. Lipid raft disruption by cholesterol depletion enhances influenza A virus budding from MDCK cells. J Virol. 2007;81:12169–78.

12. Harris A, Cardone G, Winkler DC, Heymann JB, Brecher M, White JM, et al. Influenza virus pleiomorphy characterized by cryoelectron tomography. Proc Natl Acad Sci U S A. 2006;103:19123–7.

13. Calder LJ, Wasilewski S, Berriman JA, Rosenthal PB. Structural organization of a filamentous influenza A virus. Proc Natl Acad Sci U S A. 2010;107:10685–90.

14. Fournier E, Moules V, Essere B, Paillart JC, Sirbat JD, Isel C, et al. A supramolecular assembly formed by influenza A virus genomic RNA segments. Nucleic Acids Res. 2012;40:2197–209.

15. Chou YY, Vafabakhsh R, Doganay S, Gao Q, Ha T, Palese P. One influenza virus particle packages eight unique viral RNAs as shown by FISH analysis. Proc Natl Acad Sci U S A. 2012;109:9101–6.

16. Noda T, Kawaoka Y. Packaging of influenza virus genome: robustness of selection. Proc Natl Acad Sci U S A. 2012;109:8797–8.

17. Matrosovich MN, Matrosovich TY, Gray T, Roberts NA, Klenk HD. Neuraminidase is important for the initiation of influenza virus infection in human airway epithelium. J Virol. 2004;78:12665–7.

18. Rust MJ, Lakadamyali M, Zhang F, Zhuang X. Assembly of endocytic machinery around individual influenza viruses during viral entry. Nat Struct Mol Biol. 2004;11:567–73.

19. Sieczkarski SB, Whittaker GR. Characterization of the host cell entry of filamentous influenza virus. Arch Virol. 2005;150:1783–96.

20. Tamm LK. Hypothesis: spring-loaded boomerang mechanism of influenza hemagglutinin-mediated membrane fusion. Biochim Biophys Acta. 2003;1614:14–23.

21. Lee KK. Architecture of a nascent viral fusion pore. EMBO J. 2010;29:1299–311.

22. Xu R, Wilson IA. Structural characterization of an early fusion intermediate of influenza virus hemagglutinin. J Virol. 2011;85:5172–82.

23. Dobay MP, Dobay A, Bantang J, Mendoza E. How many trimers? Modeling influenza virus fusion yields a minimum aggregate size of six trimers, three of which are fusogenic. Mol Biosyst. 2011;7:2741–9.

24. Fontana J, Cardone G, Heymann JB, Winkler DC, Steven AC. Structural changes in Influenza virus at low pH characterized by cryo-electron tomography. J Virol. 2012;86:2919–29.

25. Watanabe T, Watanabe S, Kawaoka Y. Cellular networks involved in the influenza virus life cycle. Cell Host Microbe. 2010;7:427–39.

26. Elton D, Amorim MJ, Medcalf L, Digard P. "Genome gating"; polarized intranuclear trafficking of influenza virus RNPs. Biol Lett. 2005;1:113–7.

27. Murti KG, Webster RG, Jones IM. Localization of RNA polymerases on influenza viral ribonucleoproteins by immunogold labeling. Virology. 1988;164:562–6.

28. Pinto R, Herold S, Cakarova L, Hoegner K, Lohmeyer J, Planz O, et al. Inhibition of influenza virus-induced NF-kappaB and Raf/MEK/ERK activation can reduce

both virus titers and cytokine expression simultaneously in vitro and in vivo. Antiviral Res. 2011 Oct;92:45–56.

29. McCown MF, Pekosz A. Distinct domains of the influenza a virus M2 protein cytoplasmic tail mediate binding to the M1 protein and facilitate infectious virus production. J Virol. 2006;80:8178–89.

30. Rossman JS, Jing X, Leser GP, Balannik V, Pinto LH, Lamb RA. Influenza virus m2 ion channel protein is necessary for filamentous virion formation. J Virol. 2010;84:5078–88.

31. Camussi G, Deregibus MC, Bruno S, Grange C, Fonsato V, Tetta C. Exosome/microvesicle-mediated epigenetic reprogramming of cells. Am J Cancer Res. 2011;1:98–110.

32. Yondola MA, Fernandes F, Belicha-Villanueva A, Uccellini M, Gao Q, Carter C, et al. Budding capability of the influenza virus neuraminidase can be modulated by tetherin. J Virol. 2011;85:2480–91.

33. Wu CY, Jeng KS, Lai MM. The SUMOylation of matrix protein M1 modulates the assembly and morphogenesis of influenza A virus. J Virol. 2011;85:6618–28.

34. Bourmakina SV, Garcia-Sastre A. The morphology and composition of influenza A virus particles are not affected by low levels of M1 and M2 proteins in infected cells. J Virol. 2005;79:7926–32.

35. Burleigh LM, Calder LJ, Skehel JJ, Steinhauer DA. Influenza a viruses with mutations in the m1 helix six domain display a wide variety of morphological phenotypes. J Virol. 2005;79:1262–70.

36. Muraki Y, Murata T, Takashita E, Matsuzaki Y, Sugawara K, Hongo S. A mutation on influenza C virus M1 protein affects virion morphology by altering the membrane affinity of the protein. J Virol. 2007;81:8766–73.

37. Gomez-Puertas P, Albo C, Perez-Pastrana E, Vivo A, Portela A. Influenza virus matrix protein is the major driving force in virus budding. J Virol. 2000;74:11538–47.

38. Latham T, Galarza JM. Formation of wild-type and chimeric influenza virus-like particles following simultaneous expression of only four structural proteins. J Virol. 2001;75:6154–65.

39. Bancroft CT, Parslow TG. Evidence for segment-nonspecific packaging of the influenza a virus genome. J Virol. 2002;76:7133–9.

40. Enami M, Sharma G, Benham C, Palese P. An influenza virus containing nine different RNA segments. Virology. 1991;185:291–8.

41. Smith GL, Hay AJ. Replication of the influenza virus genome. Virology. 1982;118:96–108.

42. Nayak DP, Chambers TM, Akkina RK. Defective-interfering (DI) RNAs of influenza viruses: origin, structure, expression, and interference. Curr Top Microbiol Immunol. 1985;114:103–51.

43. Gao Q, Chou YY, Doganay S, Vafabakhsh R, Ha T, Palese P. The influenza A virus PB2, PA, NP, and M segments play a pivotal role during genome packaging. J Virol. 2012;86:7043–51.

44. Noda T, Sugita Y, Aoyama K, Hirase A, Kawakami E, Miyazawa A, et al. Three-dimensional analysis of ribonucleoprotein complexes in influenza A virus. Nat Commun. 2012;3:639.

45. Konig R, Stertz S, Zhou Y, Inoue A, Hoffmann HH, Bhattacharyya S, et al. Human host factors required for influenza virus replication. Nature. 2010;463:813–7.

46. Simpson-Holley M, Ellis D, Fisher D, Elton D, McCauley J, Digard P. A functional link between the actin cytoskeleton and lipid rafts during budding of filamentous influenza virions. Virology. 2002;301:212–25.

47. Shaw ML, Stone KL, Colangelo CM, Gulcicek EE, Palese P. Cellular proteins in influenza virus particles. PLoS Pathog. 2008;4:e1000085.

48. Eisfeld AJ, Kawakami E, Watanabe T, Neumann G, Kawaoka Y. RAB11A is essential for transport of the influenza virus genome to the plasma membrane. J Virol. 2011;85:6117–26.

49. Bruce EA, Digard P, Stuart AD. The Rab11 pathway is required for influenza A virus budding and filament formation. J Virol. 2010;84:5848–59.

50. Kakugawa S, Shimojima M, Neumann G, Goto H, Kawaoka Y. RuvB-like protein 2 is a suppressor of influenza A virus polymerases. J Virol. 2009;83:6429–34.

51. Hui EK, Nayak DP. Role of ATP in influenza virus budding. Virology. 2001;290:329–41.

52. Bruce EA, Abbink TE, Wise HM, Rollason R, Galao RP, Banting G, et al. Release of filamentous and spherical influenza A virus is not restricted by tetherin. J Gen Virol. 2012;93:963–9.

53. Watanabe R, Leser GP, Lamb RA. Influenza virus is not restricted by tetherin whereas influenza VLP production is restricted by tetherin. Virology. 2011;417:50–6.

54. Mangeat B, Cavagliotti L, Lehmann M, Gers-Huber G, Kaur I, Thomas Y, et al. Influenza virus partially counteracts restriction imposed by tetherin/BST-2. J Biol Chem. 2012;287:22015–29.

55. Marjuki H, Alam MI, Ehrhardt C, Wagner R, Planz O, Klenk HD, et al. Membrane accumulation of influenza A virus hemagglutinin triggers nuclear export of the viral genome via protein kinase Calpha-mediated activation of ERK signaling. J Biol Chem. 2006;281:16707–15.

56. Wang X, Hinson ER, Cresswell P. The interferon-inducible protein viperin inhibits influenza virus release by perturbing lipid rafts. Cell Host Microbe. 2007;2:96–105.

57. Thaa B, Tielesch C, Moller L, Schmitt AO, Wolff T, Bannert N, et al. Growth of influenza A virus is not

impeded by simultaneous removal of the cholesterol-binding and acylation sites in the M2 protein. J Gen Virol. 2012;93:282–92.

58. Rossman JS, Jing X, Leser GP, Lamb RA. Influenza virus M2 protein mediates ESCRT-independent membrane scission. Cell. 2010;142:902–13.

59. Arranz R, Coloma R, Chichón FJ, Conesa JJ, Carrascosa JL, Valpuesta JM, et al. The structure of native influenza virion ribonucleoproteins. Science. 2013;338:1634–37.

60. Moeller A, Kirchdoerfer RN, Potter CS, Carragher B, Wilson IA. Organization of the influenza virus replication machinery. Science. 2013;338:1631–34.

4

The virus genome and its replication

Robert M. Krug[1] and Ervin Fodor[2]

[1]Department of Molecular Genetics and Microbiology, Institute for Cellular and Molecular Biology, University of Texas at Austin, Austin, TX, USA

[2]Sir William Dunn School of Pathology, University of Oxford, Oxford, UK

The segmented RNA virus genome of influenza A and B viruses

The influenza A virus genome is comprised of eight segments of single-stranded RNA (ssRNA) (Table 4.1). The three largest viral RNA (vRNA) segments encode the three polymerase proteins: PB2 (segment 1), PB1 (segment 2), and PA (segment 3). Segment 2 also encodes two other proteins: PB1-F2, a proapoptotic virulence factor (discussed in Chapter 8), and PB1-N40, a recently identified N-terminally truncated variant of the PB1 protein [1]. Segment 3 also encodes another protein via ribosomal frameshifting, PA-X, which modulates virulence [2]. Segments 4, 5, and 6 each encode a single protein: hemagglutinin (HA), nucleocapsid protein (NP), and neuraminidase (NA), respectively. HA, the major surface protein of the virus, binds to sialic acid-containing receptors on host cells, and is the protein against which neutralizing antibodies are produced. NP binds to the vRNA segments at regular intervals along the entire length, and also has an important role in vRNA replication (as described later). The NA virion surface protein largely functions to remove sialic acid during virus budding from the cell surface and from the HA and NA of the newly assembled virions, thereby obviating aggregation of the budding virions on the cell surface. Genome segments 7 and 8 each encode mRNAs that

undergo splicing, and both the unspliced and the spliced mRNAs are translated [3,4]. Segment 7 unspliced mRNA encodes the matrix protein (M1), which underlies the virion lipid membrane, while the spliced mRNA encodes the M2 ion channel protein that is essential for the uncoating of the virus. Segment 8 unspliced mRNA encodes the multifunctional nonstructural (NS1) protein (discussed in Chapter 7), while the spliced mRNA encodes the nuclear export protein (NS2/NEP) (discussed below).

The influenza B virus genome is also comprised of eight segments of ssRNA (Table 4.1). Most segments encode a single protein, but segments 6, 7, and 8 encode two proteins each. Segment 6 mRNA encodes the NA and NB proteins. NB, an accessory protein dispensable for virus growth in cell culture, is translated from a −1 open reading frame starting seven nucleotides upstream of the NA coding frame. Segment 7 mRNA encodes the M1 and BM2 proteins by using a "stop–start" translation mechanism with the termination codon for M1 (. . .UAAUG) overlapping with the initiation codon for BM2 (UA<u>AUG</u>. . .) [5]. The BM2 protein is the B virus ion channel protein that serves functions similar to those of the influenza A virus M2 protein. Segment 8 mRNA of influenza B viruses, similarly to that of influenza A virus, encodes the NS1 and NEP/NS2 proteins from unspliced and spliced versions, respectively. The NS1

Textbook of Influenza, Second Edition. Edited by Robert G. Webster, Arnold S. Monto, Thomas J. Braciale, and Robert A. Lamb.
© 2013 John Wiley & Sons, Ltd. Published 2013 by John Wiley & Sons, Ltd.

Table 4.1. Genomic RNAs of influenza A and B viruses.

Influenza A virus (A/PR/8/34)

Segment	Length (bases)	Polypeptide	Polypeptide (amino acids)	Function
1	2341	PB2	759	Polymerase subunit, cap-binding
2	2341	PB1	757	Polymerase subunit, nucleotide addition
		N40	718	Unknown function
		PB1-F2	87	Apoptosis regulator/virulence factor
3	2233	PA	716	Polymerase subunit, endonuclease
		PA-X	252	Modulates host response
4	1778	HA	566	Surface glycoprotein, receptor binding
5	1565	NP	498	Major RNP component, viral RNA replication
6	1413	NA	454	Surface glycoprotein, neuraminidase
7	1027	M1	252	Matrix protein
		M2	97	Ion channel protein
8	890	NS1	230	Nonstructural protein, multifunctional
		NS2/NEP	121	Nuclear export protein

Influenza B virus (B/Lee/40)

Segment	Length (bases)	Polypeptide	Polypeptide (amino acids)	Function
1	2369[a]	PB2	770	Polymerase subunit, cap-binding
2	2368	PB1	752	Polymerase subunit, nucleotide addition
3	2245[a]	PA	726	Polymerase subunit, endonuclease
4	1882	HA	584	Surface glycoprotein, receptor binding
5	1841	NP	560	Major RNP component, viral RNA replication
6	1557	NA	486	Surface glycoprotein, neuraminidase
		NB	100	Membrane protein, unknown function
7	1180[a]	M1	248	Matrix protein
		BM2	109	Ion channel protein
8	1096	NS1	281	Nonstructural protein, multifunctional
		NS2/NEP	122	Nuclear export protein

[a]Genome segments from B/Memphis/12/97.

protein of the B virus shares some, but not all functions with the A virus NS1 protein (discussed in Chapter 7).

The coding regions in all genome RNA segments are flanked with noncoding regions at both 5′ and 3′ termini, which are longer in the influenza B virus genome than in the influenza A virus genome. The extreme termini are conserved among all segments in both influenza A and B virus genomes which are followed by segment-specific noncoding regions. The 5′ and 3′ termini of each segment, including the noncoding regions as well as parts of the coding regions, contain signals required for the specific packaging of each of the eight genome segments into virions.

Viral mRNA synthesis (transcription) and viral RNA replication

Most of our knowledge about the molecular mechanisms of viral mRNA synthesis and viral RNA replication is derived from studies of influenza A virus, so the following sections focus on influenza A virus. Given the similar genome organization of influenza B virus and the presence of polymerase proteins that show extensive sequence identity and homology to those of influenza A virus, it is presumed that influenza B virus uses similar transcription and replication mechanisms.

In the virions as well as in infected cells the vRNA segments exist as ribonucleoprotein (RNP) complexes, which contain the trimeric RNA-dependent RNA polymerase complex, consisting of the PB1, PB2, and PA proteins, and multiple copies of NP. The RNA polymerase associates with the partially double-stranded panhandle structure that is formed by the conserved 5′ and 3′ termini of each segment. All the vRNA segments contain the same 13 nucleotides at the 5′ end, and 12 nucleotides at the 3′ end (Figure 4.1), which are partially complementary. The rest of the vRNA segments are associated with NP molecules that are spaced at 24 nucleotide intervals along the vRNA chain. The crystal structure of NP shows that it is a crescent-shaped molecule comprised of two major domains, denoted as head and body domains [6,7]. The RNA-binding surface is the grove between these two domains. An important feature of RNA binding is that the bound RNA is on the outside surface of NP, rendering the NP-associated vRNA susceptible to ribonuclease digestion. NP can also homo-oligomerize through the tail loop of one NP molecule being inserted into a cavity in the body domain of a neighboring NP molecule [8].

Influenza viruses are unusual among negative sense RNA viruses in that they transcribe and replicate their genomes in the nucleus of infected cells. Transcription is initiated with a 10- to 13-base-long capped RNA primer excised from cellular pre-mRNAs in the nucleus by the intrinsic endonuclease of the viral polymerase (Figure 4.2) [9,10]. Cleavage in the infected cell occurs predominately after a CA sequence [11,12]. The cap-dependent endonuclease that cleaves after CA is activated by the binding of the 5′ end of vRNA to a site on the PB1 subunit [13]. The 5′ cap of the pre-mRNA binds to a site on the PB2 subunit [14,15], and is cleaved by the endonuclease that is located in the N-terminal domain of the PA subunit [16,17]. The viral polymerase is associated with the cellular polymerase (polymerase II) that synthesizes capped pre-mRNAs, and this association might be expected to facilitate the access of the viral polymerase to the 5′ cap of nascent pre-mRNAs [18]. By snatching a host cap-1 structure, that is a cap containing a 2′-O-methyl on the penultimate base, influenza A virus acquires resistance to the group of interferon (IFN)-induced proteins that contain tetratricopeptide repeats [19]. In contrast, viruses whose mRNAs lack a 2′-O-methyl on their caps (cap-0 structure) are sensitive to the antiviral action of these IFN-induced proteins. The influenza virus polymerase preferentially uses cap-1-containing RNA primers *in vitro* [20], consistent with the cap usage *in vivo*.

The 3′ end of vRNA (3′-UCGUUU. . .), the template for transcription, also binds to the PB1 subunit [21,22], and transcription is initiated by the addition of a G residue to the 3′ CA end of the capped primer,

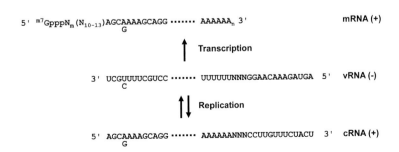

Figure 4.1. Transcription and replication of influenza virus genome segments.

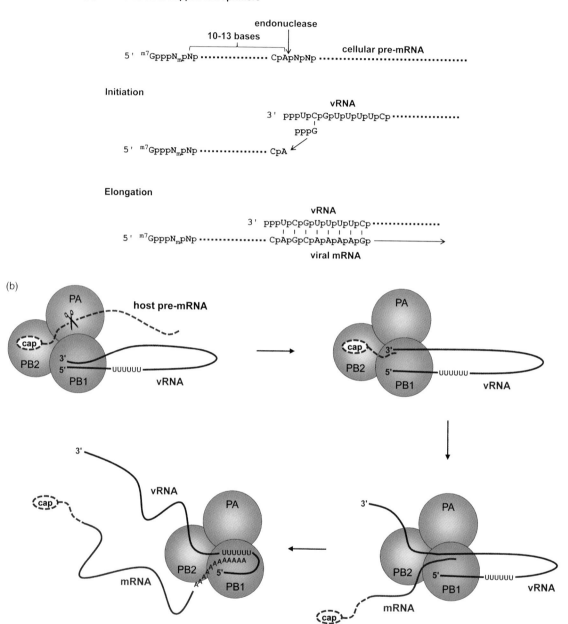

Figure 4.2. Mechanism of viral mRNA synthesis. (a) Generation of capped RNA primers for the initiation of viral mRNA synthesis. (b) Proposed model for the initiation, elongation, and termination of transcription.

directed by the penultimate C residue in the vRNA template. When both the 5′ and 3′ ends of the vRNA are bound to the PB1 subunit, they form several base pairs with each other. The formation of this double-stranded region is required for the initiation of viral RNA transcription [13,23–25]. The active site for nucleotide addition is most likely in the PB1 subunit, which contains a S-D-D motif characteristic of polymerase active sites. Transcription elongation proceeds until the polymerase reaches a sequence of 4–7 uridine (U) residues located 16–20 nucleotides from the 5′ end of the vRNA template, where the polymerase reiteratively copies the U sequence ("stutters"), thereby adding a poly(A) tail to the nascent transcript [26]. It is thought that this "stuttering" occurs because the polymerase remains associated with the 5′ end of the vRNA template throughout elongation while the template is threaded through its active site in a 3′ to 5′ direction [23,24]. When the U sequence reaches the active site of the polymerase, the template cannot proceed further because of steric hindrance caused by the 5′ end of vRNA being bound to the polymerase. This leads to template slipping and repeated copying of the U sequence by the polymerase. Proof that the U sequence acts as a template for polyadenylation came from the finding that replacing the U sequence with an A sequence resulted in viral mRNAs with poly(U) tails. The poly(U)-tailed mRNAs were retained in the nucleus of infected cells, confirming that the poly(A) tail is required for the nuclear export of mRNAs [26,27].

Replication of vRNA consists of two stages. During the first stage, genomic vRNA is replicated into a full-length copy, denoted as complementary RNA, or cRNA, and during the second stage cRNA is copied into vRNA. Because cRNA is a full-length copy of vRNA, anti-termination at the poly(A) addition site has to occur. Both cRNA and vRNA contain a 5′ triphosphate end, indicating that their synthesis is initiated *de novo* in a primer-independent manner. Primer-independent initiation for cRNA synthesis occurs at the 3′ terminus of the vRNA, giving rise initially to the dinucleotide pppApG, immediately followed by elongation. It has been reported that initiation of vRNA synthesis is different. Specifically, pppApG is synthesized internally by copying the bases at positions 4 and 5 at the 3′ end of cRNA, followed by realignment with the 3′ terminal cRNA bases at positions 1 and 2 for subsequent elongation [28].

Various mechanisms have been proposed for cRNA and vRNA synthesis, which involve roles for viral (NP, viral RNA polymerase proteins, NS1, NEP/NS2, small viral RNAs (svRNAs)) and host factors (e.g., MCM, UAP65, tat-SF1, availability of capped RNA primers and ribonucleoside triphosphates; reviewed in [29,30]). However, no mechanism has been definitively established.

According to one model, the viral polymerase has the inherent capacity to initiate unprimed cRNA and vRNA synthesis, but synthesizes only short transcripts (approximately 22 bases long) that do not extend past the surface of the polymerase [31]. Because vRNA synthesis predominates over cRNA synthesis during infection (discussed below), these short transcripts may correspond to the svRNAs detected in infected cells [32,33]. The viral NP protein binds to both the polymerase and the emerging nascent transcript, enabling elongation of these transcripts, a process analogous to the "promoter clearance" mechanisms of other polymerases [31]. Successive targeting of NP monomers to the elongating RNA through the interaction between NP and the viral polymerase would result in the encapsidation of vRNA and cRNA chains by NP during synthesis. This encapsidation would be facilitated and stabilized by NP–NP oligomerization. Consistent with this mechanism, oligomerization and RNA-binding mutants of NP do not support the replication of genome-length vRNA templates [34]. This mechanism predicts that NP together with the viral polymerase would stabilize vRNA and cRNA by preventing nuclease digestion in infected cells, as has been reported [35]. In addition, the binding of NP molecules to elongating cRNA chains could also be responsible for overcoming the steric block that results in poly(A) addition during viral mRNA synthesis, thereby enabling the polymerase to copy the 5′ end of vRNA.

Several alternative mechanisms have been proposed. For example, it has been proposed that mRNA synthesis is performed *in cis* by the RNA polymerase that forms part of the vRNP, while replication is performed *in trans* by an RNA polymerase that is distinct from the RNP-associated polymerase [36]. During mRNA synthesis, the transcribing RNP-associated polymerase would remain associated with the 5′ end of the vRNA template resulting in steric hindrance and termination by polyadenylation. In contrast, no such a steric block would occur during replication by the *trans* polymerase, and polyadenylation would be avoided. Thus, newly synthesized RNA polymerase, distinct from the polymerase in RNPs introduced into cells by the infecting virions, would be required for replication. This *trans*-acting RNA polymerase might already contain the 22–27 nucleotide-long svRNAs that have been identified in infected cells [32,33].

Regulation of viral RNA synthesis in infected cells

The vRNPs of the infecting virus are released into the cytoplasm and are transported into the nucleus, where the vRNA segments are transcribed into viral mRNAs, a process denoted as primary transcription. The proteins encoded by these primary transcripts (mRNAs) include NP and polymerase (PB1, PB2, and PA) proteins, which are required for the onset of cRNA synthesis. It has been observed that at early times specific cRNAs, notably the NP and NS1 cRNAs, are selectively copied into vRNAs, which are then transcribed to generate the NP and NS1 mRNAs, accounting for the early synthesis of the NP and NS1 proteins [37,38]. In contrast, the synthesis of the other viral structural proteins, particularly the M1 protein, appears to be delayed because the copying of their cRNAs into vRNAs is delayed. However, no regulatory mechanisms to describe this phenomenon have yet been identified. Overall, during the course of infection cRNA reaches a plateau early and remains at low levels. Synthesis of vRNA starts at approximately 2 hours after infection, and during the early phase of infection this synthesis generates additional vRNA templates that are required for amplified transcription (secondary transcription), that is the high level of mRNA synthesis needed to synthesize the high level of viral proteins [37,39].

Viral mRNA synthesis increases concomitantly with vRNA synthesis for the first several hours. At about 3.5–4 hours after infection viral mRNA synthesis sharply decreases. In contrast, vRNA synthesis continues at a high rate to produce the vRNA molecules that will be incorporated into progeny virions [37,40]. Several mechanisms have been proposed for the sharp decrease in viral mRNA synthesis: (i) the inhibition and degradation of the host polymerase II (see below) leads to a sharp decline in the availability of newly synthesized capped RNA primers to initiate viral mRNA synthesis; and/or (ii) the increased level of the M1 protein depletes the nuclear pool of vRNA templates for viral mRNA synthesis by mediating (along with the NS2/NEP protein) the export of vRNPs into the cytoplasm (see below). Indeed, the vRNAs (vRNPs) that are synthesized at later times are efficiently transported to the cytoplasm for packaging into new virions.

The role of host factors in viral RNA synthesis

The viral polymerase interacts with cellular nuclear enzymes that function in the production of cellular mRNAs. The viral polymerase binds to the C-terminal domain (CTD) of the large subunit of the cellular Pol II enzyme, which synthesizes the transcripts that are processed to form cellular mRNAs [18]. The CTD is comprised of 52 heptad repeats (Tyr–Ser–Pro–Thr–Ser–Pro–Ser). The viral polymerase preferentially binds to the form of CTD that is phosphorylated on serine 5 of the heptad repeats, the form that is involved in transcription initiation and activation of the capping machinery of the host. Association of the viral polymerase with host Pol II may therefore improve the availability of capped RNA primers for viral transcription. In addition, the viral polymerase is found in a macromolecular complex that contains the viral NS1 protein and at least one cellular 3′ end processing factor, the 30-kDa subunit of the cleavage and polyadenylation specificity factor (CPSF30) [41]. It is not known whether these two viral polymerase interactions with host factors are related to each other, for example, via the association of 3′ end processing factors, including CPSF, with the CTD of the cellular Pol II.

Several studies have been directed at identifying other host factors that interact with the influenza virus polymerase [42–46]. Many studies have used either plasmids or viral vectors to generate influenza virus polymerase complexes in cells, and then identified cellular proteins that co-purify with these complexes. In addition, one study used a bioinformatics approach, coupled with siRNA knockdowns, to identify host proteins that interact with the viral polymerase. The proteins identified in these studies include several DEAD box RNA helicases, heterogeneous nuclear RNP proteins (hnRNP proteins), and heat shock proteins.

Transcription and replication of the viral genome by the viral polymerase and NP are host-dependent processes (reviewed in [47]). The viral polymerase and NP undergo adaptive changes upon transmission of influenza viruses from one species to another, that is from birds to mammals. These adaptive changes include amino acid changes in the PB2 subunit of the polymerase (e.g., E627K, D701N), which enable the virus to replicate efficiently in mammalian systems, often leading to increased virulence in mammals [48,49]. One study implicated the DEAD box RNA helicase 17 (DDX17) in the species-specific regulation of the H5N1 viral polymerase that depended on the identity of the PB2 amino acid at position 627 [44]. In addition, the differential use of α-importin isoforms in the nuclear import of NP and PB2 has been implicated in host adaptation [50].

Splicing and nuclear export of viral mRNAs

Splicing of the viral M1 and NS1 mRNAs is catalyzed by the host splicing machinery. Access to this splicing machinery is probably facilitated by the association of the viral polymerase with the CTD of host Pol II. Unlike the splicing of host pre-mRNAs, the splicing of the viral M1 and NS1 mRNAs is incomplete, such that the amounts of the spliced M2 and NS2/NEP mRNAs are only about 10–15% of the amounts of the respective unspliced M1 and NS1 mRNA precursors [4,51]. The rate of NS1 mRNA splicing is the same whether it is synthesized by the viral polymerase in influenza A virus-infected cells or is synthesized by host Pol II in cells infected by an adenovirus expressing the NS gene [52]. Consequently, inefficient splicing of NS1 and M1 mRNAs in influenza virus-infected cells probably results from decreased association with the host splicing machinery, possibly because of the requirement for co-transcriptional recruitment of the splicing machinery during Pol II transcription and/or because of efficient nuclear export of the NS1 and M1 mRNA precursors.

Nuclear export of influenza A viral mRNAs is apparently mediated at least in part by host factors, specifically, the transcription-export (TREX) complex and NXF1/TAP [53–55]. Access to this host cell machinery would also be facilitated by the association of the viral polymerase with the CTD of host Pol II

and possibly the binding of the nuclear cap-binding complex (CBC) to the 5' cap of viral mRNAs [53]. The viral polymerase was also shown to associate with viral mRNAs, binding to the 5' cap and a common 5' terminal sequence present in all viral mRNAs *in vitro* [56]. This may selectively protect viral mRNAs from cap-snatching carried out by other viral polymerases. Binding of the viral polymerase to the 5' ends of viral mRNAs may also occur in the cytoplasm, as it has been reported that such binding could promote translation that is independent of the cap-binding eIF4E translation initiation factor [57]. However, association of viral mRNAs with eIF4E has also been reported [53]. Viral mRNAs would not have to compete with a significant number of host mRNAs for cellular splicing, transport, and translation factors, because the generation of processed, polyadenylated host mRNAs is inhibited by the viral NS1 protein. In addition, it has been reported that the viral NS1 protein has a role in the nuclear export and translation of viral mRNAs [54,58].

Splicing of M1 mRNA is also regulated by additional mechanisms. M1 mRNA has two alternative 5' splice sites: a strong distal 5' splice site producing mRNA3 that has the coding potential for nine amino acids and a weak proximal 5' splice site producing M2 mRNA encoding the M2 ion-channel protein. The distal mRNA 5' splice site is the only one used when a DNA plasmid encoding the M1 gene is transfected into cells, indicating that this strong 5' splice site would have to be blocked in influenza virus-infected cells to enable the weak M2 5' splice site to be utilized [59]. The tripartite viral RNA polymerase probably carries out this function: it binds to the 5' cap and the first 12 5' bases of the M1 mRNA *in vitro*, thereby blocking the mRNA3 5' splice site, which is at position 11 [59]. The cellular splicing machinery can then switch to the downstream (proximal) M2 5' splice site. Utilization of this weak M2 5' splice site requires its activation by the cellular SF2/ASF protein, which binds to a purine-rich splicing enhancer sequence that is located in the 3' exon of M1 mRNA [60]. During virus infection of several cell lines M2 mRNA and the M2 ion channel protein are produced in amounts that are proportional to the different expression levels of the SF2/ASF protein. A regulatory role for NS1 has also been proposed [61].

Nuclear export of viral RNPs

Late in infection newly synthesized vRNA genomes, in the form of viral ribonucleoprotein complexes (vRNPs), are exported from the nucleus and travel across the cytoplasm to the site of budding at the cell membrane. According to the current model, the viral M1 and NEP/NS2 proteins direct the nuclear export of vRNPs by M1 directly interacting with vRNPs, while NEP/NS2 acts as a bridge between M1 and the cellular export receptor, Crm1 [62–64]. Accordingly, the nuclear export of vRNPs can be blocked by leptomycin B, an inhibitor of Crm1. Alternative models, involving a direct interaction between Crm1 and NP leading to M1 and NEP-NS2-independent export have also been proposed, suggesting that redundant pathways might exist [65]. Influenza vRNPs may gain preferential access to the cellular export machinery through chromatin targeting [66].

References

1. Wise HM, Foeglein A, Sun J, Dalton RM, Patel S, Howard W, et al. A complicated message: Identification of a novel PB1-related protein translated from influenza A virus segment 2 mRNA. J Virol. 2009;83(16): 8021–31.

2. Jagger BW, Wise HM, Kash JC, Walters KA, Wills NM, Xiao YL, et al. An overlapping protein-coding region in influenza A virus segment 3 modulates the host response. Science. 2012;337(6091):199–204.

3. Lamb RA, Choppin PW. Segment 8 of the influenza virus genome is unique in coding for two polypeptides. Proc Natl Acad Sci U S A. 1979;76(10):4908–12.

4. Lamb RA, Choppin PW, Chanock RM, Lai CJ. Mapping of the two overlapping genes for polypeptides NS1 and NS2 on RNA segment 8 of influenza virus genome. Proc Natl Acad Sci U S A. 1980;77(4):1857–61.

5. Shaw MW, Choppin PW, Lamb RA. A previously unrecognized influenza B virus glycoprotein from a bicistronic mRNA that also encodes the viral neuraminidase. Proc Natl Acad Sci U S A. 1983;80(16):4879–83.

6. Ng AK, Zhang H, Tan K, Li Z, Liu JH, Chan PK, et al. Structure of the influenza virus A H5N1 nucleoprotein: implications for RNA binding, oligomerization, and vaccine design. FASEB J. 2008;22(10):3638–47.

7. Ye Q, Krug RM, Tao YJ. The mechanism by which influenza A virus nucleoprotein forms oligomers and binds RNA. Nature. 2006;444(7122):1078–82.

8. Chan WH, Ng AK, Robb NC, Lam MK, Chan PK, Au SW, et al. Functional analysis of the influenza virus H5N1 nucleoprotein tail loop reveals amino acids that are crucial for oligomerization and ribonucleoprotein activities. J Virol. 2010;84(14):7337–45.

9. Plotch SJ, Bouloy M, Ulmanen I, Krug RM. A unique cap(m7GpppXm)-dependent influenza virion endonuclease cleaves capped RNAs to generate the primers that initiate viral RNA transcription. Cell. 1981;23(3): 847–58.

10. Bouloy M, Plotch SJ, Krug RM. Globin mRNAs are primers for the transcription of influenza viral RNA in vitro. Proc Natl Acad Sci U S A. 1978;75(10): 4886–90.

11. Beaton AR, Krug RM. Selected host cell capped RNA fragments prime influenza viral RNA transcription in vivo. Nucleic Acids Res. 1981;9(17):4423–36.

12. Shaw MW, Lamb RA. A specific sub-set of host-cell mRNAs prime influenza virus mRNA synthesis. Virus Res. 1984;1(6):455–67.

13. Rao P, Yuan W, Krug RM. Crucial role of CA cleavage sites in the cap-snatching mechanism for initiating viral mRNA synthesis. EMBO J. 2003;22(5): 1188–98.

14. Guilligay D, Tarendeau F, Resa-Infante P, Coloma R, Crepin T, Sehr P, et al. The structural basis for cap binding by influenza virus polymerase subunit PB2. Nat Struct Mol Biol. 2008;15(5):500–6.

15. Ulmanen I, Broni BA, Krug RM. Role of two of the influenza virus core P proteins in recognizing cap 1 structures (m7GpppNm) on RNAs and in initiating viral RNA transcription. Proc Natl Acad Sci U S A. 1981;78(12):7355–9.

16. Dias A, Bouvier D, Crepin T, McCarthy AA, Hart DJ, Baudin F, et al. The cap-snatching endonuclease of influenza virus polymerase resides in the PA subunit. Nature. 2009;458(7240):914–8.

17. Yuan P, Bartlam M, Lou Z, Chen S, Zhou J, He X, et al. Crystal structure of an avian influenza polymerase PA(N) reveals an endonuclease active site. Nature. 2009;458(7240):909–13.

18. Engelhardt OG, Smith M, Fodor E. Association of the influenza A virus RNA-dependent RNA polymerase with cellular RNA polymerase II. J Virol. 2005;79(9): 5812–8.

19. Daffis S, Szretter KJ, Schriewer J, Li J, Youn S, Errett J, et al. 2′-O methylation of the viral mRNA cap evades host restriction by IFIT family members. Nature. 2010;468(7322):452–6.

20. Bouloy M, Plotch SJ, Krug RM. Both the 7-methyl and the 2′-O-methyl groups in the cap of mRNA strongly influence its ability to act as primer for influenza virus RNA transcription. Proc Natl Acad Sci U S A. 1980; 77(7):3952–6.

21. Li ML, Ramirez BC, Krug RM. RNA-dependent activation of primer RNA production by influenza virus

polymerase: different regions of the same protein subunit constitute the two required RNA-binding sites. EMBO J. 1998;17(19):5844–52.

22. Gonzalez S, Ortin J. Distinct regions of influenza virus PB1 polymerase subunit recognize vRNA and cRNA templates. EMBO J. 1999;18(13):3767–75.

23. Fodor E, Pritlove DC, Brownlee GG. The influenza virus panhandle is involved in the initiation of transcription. J Virol. 1994;68(6):4092–6.

24. Hagen M, Chung TD, Butcher JA, Krystal M. Recombinant influenza virus polymerase: requirement of both 5′ and 3′ viral ends for endonuclease activity. J Virol. 1994;68(3):1509–15.

25. Flick R, Neumann G, Hoffmann E, Neumeier E, Hobom G. Promoter elements in the influenza vRNA terminal structure. RNA. 1996;2(10):1046–57.

26. Poon LL, Pritlove DC, Fodor E, Brownlee GG. Direct evidence that the poly(A) tail of influenza A virus mRNA is synthesized by reiterative copying of a U track in the virion RNA template. J Virol. 1999;73(4): 3473–6.

27. Poon LL, Fodor E, Brownlee GG. Polyuridylated mRNA synthesized by a recombinant influenza virus is defective in nuclear export. J Virol. 2000;74(1): 418–27.

28. Deng T, Vreede FT, Brownlee GG. Different de novo initiation strategies are used by influenza virus RNA polymerase on its cRNA and viral RNA promoters during viral RNA replication. J Virol. 2006;80(5): 2337–48.

29. Resa-Infante P, Jorba N, Coloma R, Ortin J. The influenza virus RNA synthesis machine: Advances in its structure and function. RNA Biol. 2011;8(2):207–15.

30. Nagata K, Kawaguchi A, Naito T. Host factors for replication and transcription of the influenza virus genome. Rev Med Virol. 2008;18(4):247–60.

31. Kawaguchi A, Momose F, Nagata K. Replication-coupled and host factor-mediated encapsidation of the influenza virus genome by viral nucleoprotein. J Virol. 2011;85(13):6197–204.

32. Umbach JL, Yen HL, Poon LL, Cullen BR. Influenza A virus expresses high levels of an unusual class of small viral leader RNAs in infected cells. MBio. 2010;1(4): e00204–10.

33. Perez JT, Varble A, Sachidanandam R, Zlatev I, Manoharan M, Garcia-Sastre A, et al. Influenza A virus-generated small RNAs regulate the switch from transcription to replication. Proc Natl Acad Sci U S A. 2010;107(25):11525–30.

34. Vreede FT, Ng AK, Shaw PC, Fodor E. Stabilisation of influenza virus replication intermediates is dependent on the RNA-binding but not the homo-oligomerisation activity of the viral nucleoprotein. J Virol. 2011;85: 12073–8.

35. Vreede FT, Jung TE, Brownlee GG. Model suggesting that replication of influenza virus is regulated by stabilization of replicative intermediates. J Virol. 2004;78 (17):9568–72.

36. Jorba N, Coloma R, Ortin J. Genetic trans-complementation establishes a new model for influenza virus RNA transcription and replication. PLoS Pathog. 2009;5(5):e1000462.

37. Shapiro GI, Gurney T Jr, Krug RM. Influenza virus gene expression: control mechanisms at early and late times of infection and nuclear-cytoplasmic transport of virus-specific RNAs. J Virol. 1987;61(3):764–73.

38. Smith GL, Hay AJ. Replication of the influenza virus genome. Virology. 1982;118(1):96–108.

39. Kawakami E, Watanabe T, Fujii K, Goto H, Watanabe S, Noda T, et al. Strand-specific real-time RT-PCR for distinguishing influenza vRNA, cRNA, and mRNA. J Virol Methods. 2011;173(1):1–6.

40. Vreede FT, Chan AY, Sharps J, Fodor E. Mechanisms and functional implications of the degradation of host RNA polymerase II in influenza virus infected cells. Virology. 2010;396(1):125–34.

41. Kuo RL, Krug RM. Influenza a virus polymerase is an integral component of the CPSF30-NS1A protein complex in infected cells. J Virol. 2009;83(4):1611–6.

42. Jorba N, Juarez S, Torreira E, Gastaminza P, Zamarreno N, Albar JP, et al. Analysis of the interaction of influenza virus polymerase complex with human cell factors. Proteomics. 2008;8(10):2077–88.

43. Mayer D, Molawi K, Martinez-Sobrido L, Ghanem A, Thomas S, Baginsky S, et al. Identification of cellular interaction partners of the influenza virus ribonucleoprotein complex and polymerase complex using proteomic-based approaches. J Proteome Res. 2007;6 (2):672–82.

44. Bortz E, Westera L, Maamary J, Steel J, Albrecht RA, Manicassamy B, et al. Host- and strain-specific regulation of influenza virus polymerase activity by interacting cellular proteins. MBio. 2011;2(4): e00151–11.

45. Bradel-Tretheway BG, Mattiacio JL, Krasnoselsky A, Stevenson C, Purdy D, Dewhurst S, et al. Comprehensive proteomic analysis of influenza virus polymerase complex reveals a novel association with mitochondrial proteins and RNA polymerase accessory factors. J Virol. 2011;85(17):8569–81.

46. Deng T, Engelhardt OG, Thomas B, Akoulitchev AV, Brownlee GG, Fodor E. Role of ran binding protein 5 in nuclear import and assembly of the influenza virus RNA polymerase complex. J Virol. 2006;80(24): 11911–9.

47. Naffakh N, Tomoiu A, Rameix-Welti MA, van der Werf S. Host restriction of avian influenza viruses at the level of the ribonucleoproteins. Annu Rev Microbiol. 2008;62:403–24.

48. Hatta M, Gao P, Halfmann P, Kawaoka Y. Molecular basis for high virulence of Hong Kong H5N1 influenza A viruses. Science. 2001;293(5536):1840–2.

49. Steel J, Lowen AC, Mubareka S, Palese P. Transmission of influenza virus in a mammalian host is increased by PB2 amino acids 627K or 627E/701N. PLoS Pathog. 2009;5(1):e1000252.

50. Gabriel G, Klingel K, Otte A, Thiele S, Hudjetz B, Arman-Kalcek G, et al. Differential use of importin-alpha isoforms governs cell tropism and host adaptation of influenza virus. Nat Commun. 2011;2:156.

51. Lamb RA, Lai CJ, Choppin PW. Sequences of mRNAs derived from genome RNA segment 7 of influenza virus: colinear and interrupted mRNAs code for overlapping proteins. Proc Natl Acad Sci U S A. 1981;78(7): 4170–4.

52. Alonso-Caplen FV, Krug RM. Regulation of the extent of splicing of influenza virus NS1 mRNA: role of the rates of splicing and of the nucleocytoplasmic transport of NS1 mRNA. Mol Cell Biol. 1991;11(2):1092–8.

53. Bier K, York A, Fodor E. Cellular cap-binding proteins associate with influenza virus mRNAs. J Gen Virol. 2011;92:1627–34.

54. Wang W, Cui ZQ, Han H, Zhang ZP, Wei HP, Zhou YF, et al. Imaging and characterizing influenza A virus mRNA transport in living cells. Nucleic Acids Res. 2008;36(15):4913–28.

55. Read EK, Digard P. Individual influenza A virus mRNAs show differential dependence on cellular NXF1/TAP for their nuclear export. J Gen Virol. 2010;91(Pt 5):1290–301.

56. Shih SR, Krug RM. Surprising function of the three influenza viral polymerase proteins: selective protection of viral mRNAs against the cap-snatching reaction catalyzed by the same polymerase proteins. Virology. 1996;226(2):430–5.

57. Burgui I, Yanguez E, Sonenberg N, Nieto A. Influenza virus mRNA translation revisited: is the eIF4E cap-binding factor required for viral mRNA translation? J Virol. 2007;81(22):12427–38.

58. de la Luna S, Fortes P, Beloso A, Ortin J. Influenza virus NS1 protein enhances the rate of translation initiation of viral mRNAs. J Virol. 1995;69(4):2427–33.

59. Shih SR, Nemeroff ME, Krug RM. The choice of alternative 5′ splice sites in influenza virus M1 mRNA is regulated by the viral polymerase complex. Proc Natl Acad Sci U S A. 1995;92(14):6324–8.

60. Shih SR, Krug RM. Novel exploitation of a nuclear function by influenza virus: the cellular SF2/ASF splicing factor controls the amount of the essential viral M2 ion channel protein in infected cells. EMBO J. 1996; 15(19):5415–27.

61. Robb NC, Fodor E. The accumulation of influenza A virus segment 7 spliced mRNAs is regulated by the NS1 protein. J Gen Virol. 2011;93:113–8.

62. Akarsu H, Burmeister WP, Petosa C, Petit I, Muller CW, Ruigrok RW, et al. Crystal structure of the M1 protein-binding domain of the influenza A virus nuclear export protein (NEP/NS2). EMBO J. 2003;22(18):4646–55.

63. O'Neill RE, Talon J, Palese P. The influenza virus NEP (NS2 protein) mediates the nuclear export of viral ribonucleoproteins. EMBO J. 1998;17(1):288–96.

64. Neumann G, Hughes MT, Kawaoka Y. Influenza A virus NS2 protein mediates vRNP nuclear export through NES-independent interaction with hCRM1. EMBO J. 2000;19(24):6751–8.

65. Elton D, Simpson-Holley M, Archer K, Medcalf L, Hallam R, McCauley J, et al. Interaction of the influenza virus nucleoprotein with the cellular CRM1-mediated nuclear export pathway. J Virol. 2001;75(1):408–19.

66. Chase GP, Rameix-Welti MA, Zvirbliene A, Zvirblis G, Gotz V, Wolff T, et al. Influenza virus ribonucleoprotein complexes gain preferential access to cellular export machinery through chromatin targeting. PLoS Pathog. 2011;7(9):e1002187.

5 Influenza glycoproteins: Hemagglutinin and neuraminidase

Rupert J. Russell[1], Steven J. Gamblin[2], and John J. Skehel[2]

[1]University of St Andrews, Fife, UK

[2]National Institute for Medical Research, MRC, London, UK

HA and NA structures, functions, antigenicity and classification: An overview

The spike-like structures that project about 13 nm from influenza A and B virus membranes (Figure 5.1) are hemagglutinin (HA) and neuraminidase (NA) glycoproteins. On capsular-shaped viruses there are about 500 HA and 100 NA spikes; filamentous viruses contain hundreds more. Both HA and NA spikes are distributed around the membrane but NA appear to be clustered in the region where the budding virus is released from cells [1]. Both glycoproteins are anchored in the membrane through a region of uncharged amino acids, 27–29 residues long, and both extend from the inner surface of the virus membrane to interact with the virus matrix protein, M1 [2]. The inner sequences consist of 11 residues in HA and 6 conserved residues in NA.

HA is a type I membrane glycoprotein that contains an N-terminal signal sequence and a C-terminal membrane anchor. It is a trimer of identical subunits containing 540–550 amino acids [3]. It is synthesized in the endoplasmic reticulum (ER) of the host cell, following recognition of the 16–18 residue signal sequence, and translocation across the ER membrane [4]. During translocation HA is glycosylated at 5–7 sites, some of which are recognized by the ER chap-

erones, calreticulin and calnexin [5]. Subunits and assembled trimers are retained in the ER membrane and subsequently in the cell surface membrane, through the C-terminal membrane anchor sequence. A cysteine residue at the C-terminus of this sequence of HA is palmitoylated, and there are two further conserved cysteines to which palmitate is attached in the inner sequence [6]. These lipids may be involved in anchoring and in concentrating HA in cholesterol- and sphingolipid-rich regions of the membrane from which viruses bud as they are assembled [7].

In contrast to HA, NA is a type II membrane glycoprotein in which an uncharged region close to the N-terminus of each subunit functions as both signal sequence and membrane anchor [8]. The molecule is a tetramer of identical subunits about 470 amino acids long which is also glycosylated at seven sites during translocation (Figure 5.1).

The three-dimensional structures of membrane anchorless HA and NA, obtained by proteolysis of viruses or of detergent-isolated full-length glycoproteins, or by expression in eukaryotic cells, have been determined by X-ray crystallography [9]. The N- and C-termini of HA are positioned together near the virus membrane, as a result of the mechanism of HA synthesis and folding in the ER. From the membrane, HA extends 130 nm, forming a structure that consists of three subdomains: fusion, vestigial esterase, and

Textbook of Influenza, Second Edition. Edited by Robert G. Webster, Arnold S. Monto, Thomas J. Braciale, and Robert A. Lamb.
© 2013 John Wiley & Sons, Ltd. Published 2013 by John Wiley & Sons, Ltd.

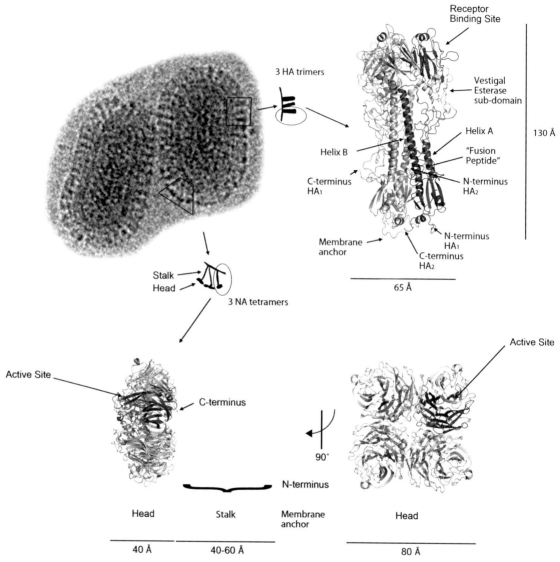

Figure 5.1. The structure of hemagglutinin (HA) and neuraminidase (NA)by electron microscopy on virus, and by X-ray crystallography. A picture of two capsule-shaped viruses seen by cryo-electron microscopy (cryo-EM) [1] with two areas of virus membrane highlighted, containing three HA trimers or three NA tetramers. The structures of HA and NA are from Wiley and Skehel [3] and Colman and Ward [8].

receptor binding, based on similarities to regions of the HEF glycoprotein of influenza C virus, which is an evolutionary precursor of influenza A and B HAs (Figure 5.1) [10]. The fusion sub-domain of each subunit of the trimer consists of two antiparallel, β-strands, the C-terminal of which is linked to a central structure that contains two prominent antiparallel α-helices and a membrane-proximal five-stranded structure. The receptor binding and the vestigial esterase sub-domains form the globular membrane-distal structure. This is attached to two segments of the fusion sub-domain, one extending from the HA

N-terminus to the N-terminus of the vestigial esterase sub-domain, and the other extending from the C-terminus of the vestigial esterase sub-domain to the central part of the fusion sub-domain. The subunits associate throughout the length of the trimer, and a prominent trimeric coiled-coil is formed between the central α-helices (helix B, Figure 5.1) of the fusion sub-domain [11].

NA is a tetramer with a molecular weight of about 240 kDA. Each monomer comprises about 470 amino acids. The membrane anchor and stalk region account approximately for the first 75 residues. The globular head domain, containing the enzyme active site, is attached to the C-terminus of the stalk. The structure of the tetrameric head has been determined for all 9 subtypes by X-ray crystallography [8, 9]. It is a box-like structure, about 8 nm × 8 nm across and 4 nm deep (Figure 5.1). The overall architecture of each subunit is a six-bladed propeller structure with each blade consisting of a beta-sheet of four antiparallel beta-strands. Each propeller blade begins with a strand at the center of the domain which runs approximately parallel with the barrel axis. Each successive β-strand twists in the usual manner so that the fourth strand is roughly perpendicular to the barrel axis. The fourth strand of one blade is connected to the first strand of the next by a long loop. A combination of these inter-strand loops constitutes most of the active site of the enzyme which is located somewhat off-center, on the membrane-distal side of the beta-propeller [12].

The functions of both HA and NA involve recognition of the influenza virus receptor, sialic acid [13, 14]. HA is the receptor binding glycoprotein that binds virus to cell-surface sialylated glycoproteins. The bound virus is taken into cells by endocytosis mainly via clathrin-coated pits [15, 16]. Endocytic vesicles are acidified to about pH 5 by the action of a cellular membrane proton pump. Between pH 5 and 6.4, depending on the virus strain, HA is activated to mediate membrane fusion. This process requires extensive refolding of the molecule and reorganization of virus and endosomal lipid membranes to form a fused single membrane [11]. There are suggestions that NA may also have a role in this function [17], but HA expressed alone appears to be fully functional for membrane fusion.

NA functions in the final stages of infection by removing sialic acid from cellular glycoconjugates and from newly synthesized HA and NA which are sialylated as part of their glycosylation during biosynthesis. As a result, newly made viruses are released from the infected cell to spread the infection [18].

Sixteen subtypes of influenza A HA (H1–H16) and 9 of NA (N1–N9) have been identified and distinguished structurally and antigenically. All are found in numerous combinations in viruses of avian species. Their genetic relationships are shown in Figure 5.9, which also indicates that both HAs and NAs form two groups. Only H1, H2, and H3, and N1 and N2, have, to date, been found as components of epidemic viruses in humans. Viruses with H3 and H7 HAs, and containing N8 and N7 NAs, respectively, have caused outbreaks in horses; viruses containing at least four HA subtypes, H1, H2, H3, and H9, and two NA subtypes, N1 and N2, have been isolated from pigs. Influenza B viruses are mainly found in humans and form a single antigenic group.

Genetic analyses indicate that the HA and NA of human influenza A viruses derive from avian or swine viruses [19], and cross-species transfer is accompanied by changes in the specificities of HA receptor binding and NA-mediated virus release [20].

Antibodies that neutralize virus infectivity recognize HA [21]. In the main, they bind to the surfaces of the membrane-distal, receptor binding and vestigial esterase sub-domains, to block receptor binding or, by cross-linking HA subunits, to block the changes in conformation of HA required for membrane fusion. The sites of antibody binding are known from comparative sequence analyses of monoclonal antibody-selected antigenic mutant HAs [3, 22, 23] and from studies of the structures of complexes formed between HA and monoclonal antibodies, by electron microscopy and X-ray crystallography [21, 24]. Antigenic variation that occurs during pandemic periods results from the selection of mutants under immune pressure from antibodies produced by infected humans. Consistent with *in vitro* selection studies with monoclonal antibodies, the sequence changes in naturally occurring antigenic mutants predominantly involve surface residues of the membrane-distal sub-domains [3, 21]. Rare antibodies have been described that also block virus infection but bind to the fusion sub-domain of HA, nearer the membrane anchor. They have been examined in detail because they bind to HAs of different subtypes [25], in some cases of all subtypes [26], and might be useful in the development of cross-subtype therapies and protective vaccines.

Anti-NA antibodies block the spread of infection by preventing NA activity required for release of newly made virus from infected cells [18]. NA also varies extensively during pandemics [8], indicating that it is also a target for immune pressure. The locations of antibody binding sites on the molecule [27], near the enzyme active site, have also been determined by electron microscopy [28] and X-ray crystallography of complexes between NA and monoclonal antibodies [29, 30].

Recognition of the importance of anti-HA and anti-NA antibodies in immunity to influenza led, in part, to studies of small molecules that can block the functions of HA and NA, with a view to antiviral drug development. For HA, molecules that prevent either receptor binding or membrane fusion have been successfully identified [3], but, in the case of NA, the enzyme inhibitors zanamivir and oseltamivir are already licensed as anti-influenza drugs and widely marketed [31]. Detailed studies of mutants resistant to these drugs, isolated *in vitro* and *in vivo*, have

added to an understanding of their mechanisms of action [31]. They have also provided evidence for the evolution of a balance between NA activity and HA affinity [32].

Functions of hemagglutinin

Receptor binding

Sialic acid receptor binding site
The sialic acid receptor for influenza viruses, *N*-acetyl neuraminic acid, is a terminal saccharide of the carbohydrate side-chains of cell-surface glycoproteins [33]. The structures of receptor analogs complexed with different HAs, determined by X-ray crystallography, show that sialic acid is bound in a shallow pocket of conserved amino acids, at the membrane-distal tip of each HA subunit (Figure 5.1) [3]. One side of the pyranose ring faces the base of the site, as shown in Figure 5.2, as well as the α-anomeric, axial, carboxylate substituent, the nitrogen atom of the acetamido-substituent, and the 8- and 9- hydroxyl groups. The base is formed by a hydrogen-bonded

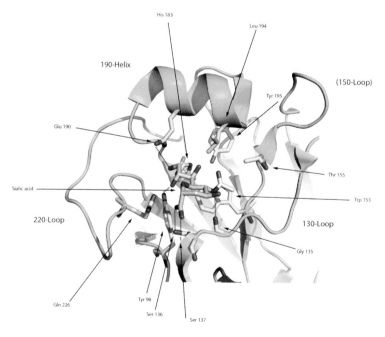

HA Receptor Binding Site

Figure 5.2. The HA sialic acid receptor binding site of avian HA. Conserved residues that form the base of the site, Tyr-98, Trp-153, His-183, Tyr-195 are shown, and conserved residues on the edges of the site, Ser-136 (130-Loop), Glu-190, Leu-194 (190-Helix), and Gln-226 (220-Loop). Bound sialic acid in white is in the α-anomeric conformation, with the axial COOH group pointing downwards towards the base of the site. The four H-bonds made between conserved atoms and sialic acid: Tyr-98 OH and 8-OH of sialic acid, main-chain carbonyl-135 and acetamido N of sialic acid, Ser-136 OH and sialic acid carboxylate, Glu-190 and 9-OH of sialic acid, are indicated by dotted lines.

network of conserved amino acids, Tyr-98, Trp-153, His-183, and Tyr-195, and its edges are three conserved elements of secondary structure, the 130-loop, residues 133–138, the 190-α-helix, residues 189–199, and the 220-loop, residues 220–229.

The mechanism of binding has been investigated by determining the relative affinities of derivatives of sialic acid [34], by site-specific mutagenesis of conserved residues [35], and by X-ray crystallography of complexes formed by soaking HA crystals in solutions of receptor analogs (Figure 5.3) [9, 36]. The sialic acid receptor is bound in a similar way by all HAs, through hydrophobic interactions and by hydrogen bonds to residues in the conserved base and edges of the binding site (Figure 5.2) [3, 11]. Hydrogen bonds are formed between the carboxylate group of sialic acid and the hydroxyl of Ser-136, and with the main chain amide of residue137; between the nitrogen of the sialic acid acetamido substituent and the main-chain carbonyl of residue135; between the 8-OH of the glycerol substituent of sialic acid and Tyr-98; and between the 9-OH of the glycerol substituent and His-183. In addition, the methyl group of the acetamido substituent is in van der Waals contact with the six-membered ring of Trp-153. Interactions with other sugars in the receptor carbohydrate side-chain, important in specificity variation, are variable from strain to strain of virus, and depend on the sequences of the structures that form the edges of the site [9].

Receptor binding specificity

Receptor binding is species specific [20]. Avian and equine viruses prefer to bind sialic acid in α2,3-linkage to galactose, the penultimate saccharide in Asn-linked carbohydrate side-chains of glycoproteins; viruses from humans prefer α2,6-linked sialic acid; and swine viruses appear to bind sialic acid in both linkages. These specificities reflect the relative abundance of sialic acids in the different linkages on cells at different sites of infection, which has been shown by microscopy involving labeling with specific lectins that bind to cells displaying either α2,6-linked sialic acid, *Sambucus nigra* lectin, or α2,3-linked sialic acid, *Maackia amurensis* lectin [37–39]. Human infections involve cells of the respiratory tract; cells of the enteric tract are involved in avian virus infections.

The HA of the three human viruses that caused the pandemics of 1918 (H1), 1957 (H2), and 1968 (H3) have been shown by genetic analyses to derive from avian viruses [19]. Because of the differences in receptor binding specificity of avian and human viruses [20], cross-species transfer requires changes in the properties of the HA of the precursor avian viruses. These occur as a result of mutations in the receptor binding site. The mutations are different in H1 from those in H2 and H3 [40]. In H1, the mutations Ser-138→Ala, and Glu-190→Asp, and Gly-225→Asp, are deduced to be important for cross-species transfer, and the substitution Glu-190→Asp was found in the HA of viruses proposed to be intermediates formed early during transfer [40]. In both H2 and H3, Gln-226→Leu and Gly-228→Ser are the major differences between avian and human HA.

Receptor complexes with pandemic HAs and their avian precursors

The complexes formed by three HAs from human H1, H2, and H3 viruses, and by three potential avian precursor HAs with both the α2,6-linked sialylpentasaccharide, LSTc, as the human receptor analog, and the α2,3-linked sialylpentasaccharide LSTa as the avian receptor analog [9], are shown in Figure 5.3.

Human HA complexes with human receptors

In the complexes formed by all three human HAs with human receptors, the α2,6-linkage between sialic acid and galactose-2 adopts a *cis*-conformation in which the glycosidic oxygen points out of the site. The galactose-2 ring, together with C-6 of galactose-2 in the linkage, presents a nonpolar surface towards the base of the receptor binding site. The receptor analog forms a folded-back structure and exits the site towards the C-terminus of the 190-helix (Figure 5.3).

In the human receptor analog complex with human H1 HA, the LSTc pentasaccharide is not as folded-back as in the H2 and H3 complexes (Figure 5.3). Hydrogen bonds are formed between Lys-222 and the 2-OH and 3-OH groups of galactose-2 and between Asp-225 and the 3-OH of galactose-2. Asp-190 forms a hydrogen bond with *N*-acetyl glucosamine-3. Gln-226 is positioned about 0.1 nm lower in the site than in the complex formed between avian H1 and avian receptor analogs, accommodating the nonpolar

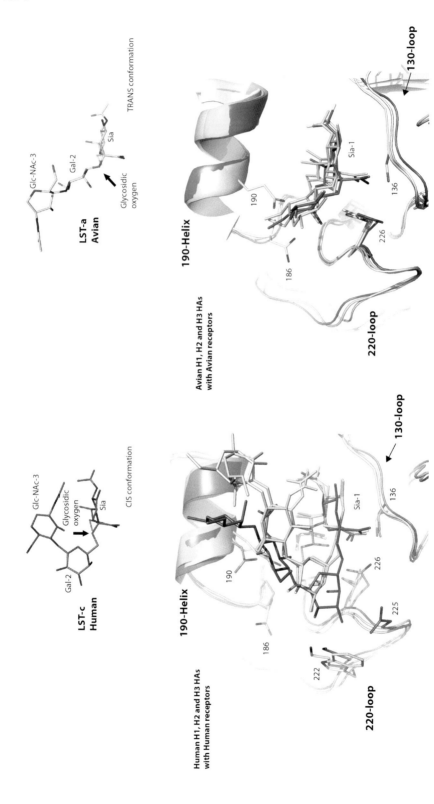

**LST-a
Avian**

TRANS conformation

Glc-NAc-3
Gal-2
Sia
Glycosidic oxygen

**LST-c
Human**

CIS conformation

Glc-NAc-3
Glycosidic oxygen
Gal-2
Sia

190-Helix

190

186

Sia-1

136

226

220-loop

130-loop

**Avian H1, H2 and H3 HAs
with Avian receptors**

190-Helix

190

186

Sia-1

136

226

225

222

220-loop

130-loop

**Human H1, H2 and H3 HAs
with Human receptors**

Figure 5.3. The receptor binding sites of HAs from H1, H2, and H3 pandemic viruses and from avian viruses of the same subtypes. The distinct *cis*- and *trans*- conformations of the human and avian receptor analogs are shown above the structures of complexes formed by soaking crystals of the HAs in solutions of the analogs. H1 blue, H2 yellow, and H3 gray for HAs and bound analogs [9].

C-6 of the glycosidic linkage that faces into the site. This lower positioning of Gln-226 in the human receptor complex and in unliganded H1 is a result of the Glu-190→Asp mutation and the resulting loss of Glu-190 to Gln-226 interaction, mediated through a water molecule.

In the complexes formed by both human H2 and H3 with human receptor analogs, the polar to non-polar substitution, Gln-226→Leu, accommodates the nonpolar surface formed by C-6 and the galactose-2 ring. The Gly-228→Ser substitution, which also occurs in both human H2 and H3, results in Ser-228 forming a hydrogen bond with the 9-OH of sialic acid. This interaction substitutes for one formed through a water molecule between the 9-OH and the carbonyl of Gly-228 in human H1 and in avian H1, H2, and H3 HAs.

Avian HA complexes with avian receptors
In avian H1, H2, and H3 complexes with the avian receptor analog, LSTa, the first three saccharides of the pentasaccharide form an extended structure in which galactose-2 is projected upwards, and the pentasaccharide exits the site over the 220-loop (Figure 5.3). In all three complexes the α2,3-linkage is in a *trans* conformation which directs the oxygen of the glycosidic bond between sialic acid and galactose-2 towards the base of the site. The galactose-2 ring is oriented edge-on to the base of the site. The *trans* conformation allows the formation of additional hydrogen bonds between the side-chain amino and carbonyl groups of Gln-226 with the 4-OH group of galactose-2 and the glycosidic linkage oxygen. This particular binding motif is common to all avian HAs that have been examined [41].

In avian H1 and H2, additional hydrogen bonds are formed between Lys 222 and the 3- and 4-OH of galactose-2. Ser-193 also forms a hydrogen bond with the nitrogen atom of the third saccharide of the receptor, N-acetyl-glucosamine-3.

HAs from other avian viruses have also been shown to demonstrate specificity for additional linkages in sialylated carbohydrate side-chains, and to recognize modifications of N-acetyl glucosamine-3. For example, H5 from chicken viruses prefer the galactose-2 β1,4-N-acetyl glucosamine-3 linkage and the sulfated third saccharide, 6-O-sulfo-GlcNAc, while H5 from ducks prefer the galactose-2 β1,3-GlcNAc linkage [42].

Avian HA complexes with human receptors and human HA complexes with avian receptors
Further information on the molecular basis of receptor binding specificity has been obtained by analyses of avian HA binding to human receptor analogs and vice versa.

The electron density for the human receptor analog in avian H1 and H3 complexes is weak and poorly defined, indicating low affinity. By contrast, in the avian H2–human receptor complex, there is well-defined electron density for sialic acid, galactose-2, and N-acetyl glucosamine-3. In this case, tighter binding appears to be due to interactions made by Asn-186 and Gln-226, through a water molecule, with the 4-OH group of galactose-2. The receptor analog is folded back, as in the human H2 and H3 complexes. Because residue 186 in H1 is proline and in H3 is serine, avian H1 and H3 cannot participate in these interactions and consequently bind human receptors poorly [43].

For human H1 complexed with avian receptor, electron density for the avian receptor is weak because the Glu-190→Asp mutation disrupts the higher position of Gln-226 required for its interactions with the glycosidic oxygen and the 4-OH group of galactose-2 [43]. In the human H2 and H3 complexes formed with the avian receptor, Leu-226 creates a hydrophobic environment that is incompatible with the orientation towards the base of the site, of the glycosidic oxygen of the α2,3-linkage [36, 43].

There is a possible advantage for all three human HAs of this low affinity for the avian receptor because mucins in the human respiratory tract are rich in α2,3-linked sialosides which, if bound tighter, would compete for virus binding to the human, α2,6-linked, cell-surface receptors [44].

Estimating affinity and specificity
Receptor binding specificity and affinity have been estimated in a variety of ways. Initially, the ability of viruses to agglutinate erythrocytes provided estimates of relative affinity and gave the glycoprotein its name [45]. Subsequently, the use of erythrocytes from different species, which have different relative abundance of α2,3- and α2,6-linked sialic acid [46], and the use of specifically re-sialylated erythrocytes that contain either α2,6- or α2,3-linked sialic acid [33], have also given estimates of binding specificity. Solid-phase microplate assays in which ligands are fixed to

the plates through polaccrylamide linkers [47] and ligand microarray procedures [48] have given large amounts of data on the fine-specificity of binding (Figure 5.4) much of which remains to be correlated, for example, to cell-specificity of infection. Quantitative assays of receptor binding using viruses have included surface plasmon resonance [49], interferometry [50], and nuclear magnetic resonance (NMR) [34]. Quantitative estimates of affinity using isolated HA by NMR gave dissociation constants for human H3 of 2.1 mM for α2,6-siallylactose and 3.2 mM for α2,3-siallylactose [34]. These indications of low affinity and small differences in binding specificity imply that the tight binding of viruses to cells during infection and the much greater specificity differences observed in assays of virus binding compared with isolated HA binding result from multiple interactions of virus HAs with receptors.

Receptor binding summary

1. A sialic acid binding site, formed of conserved residues, is located at the membrane-distal tip of each subunit of HA. Avian HAs prefer to bind sialic acid in α2,3-linkage to galactose; human HAs prefer sialic acid in α2,6-linkage.

2. Avian to human cross-species transfer requires a change in specificity for receptor. Viruses that in avians replicate in cells of the enteric tracts, which contain an abundance of sialic acid in α2,3-linkage, need to acquire the ability to replicate in cells of the human respiratory tract, with an abundance of sialic acid in α2,6-linkage.

3. The required changes in binding specificity occur through mutations that create less polar environments in the region of the binding site occupied by the sialic acid–galactose-2 linkage. This was achieved in the 1918 H1 pandemic by repositioning of Gln-226 as a result of the Glu-190→Asp mutation and consequent loss of a hydrogen bond network. In the H2 and H3 pandemics of 1957 and 1968 it was achieved directly as a result of the polar to nonpolar, Gln-226→Leu mutation.

4. Differences in fine specificity between receptor analogs such as 6-O-sulfo-sialyllactosamine, preferred by domesticated birds, result from interactions of other saccharide residues than sialic acid and galactose-2, with different amino acids in the con-

served secondary structure elements that form the edges of the receptor binding site.

5. The binding affinity of individual receptor binding sites can be low, K_D about 2 mM, and specificity differences can also be low, 1.5- to 2-fold affinity differences between α2,3- and α2,6-receptor binding. High binding avidity and specificity of virus–cell surface interactions results from simultaneous binding of about four HA molecules.

Hemagglutinin-mediated membrane fusion

Viruses with membranes, including influenza, deliver their nucleic acids into cells during infection by fusing the virus membrane with a cellular membrane. For infections with many viruses, for example, paramyxoviruses, such as Sendai virus and respiratory syncitial virus, and retroviruses like HIV, fusion is between the virus membrane and the cell-surface membrane. For influenza viruses, fusion is between the virus membrane and the membrane of the endosome into which the sialic acid receptor-bound virus is taken by endocytosis [15, 16].

The membrane fusion potential of virus fusion glycoproteins requires activation. This is achieved for viruses that fuse at the cell surface, HIV for example, as a result of changes in the conformation of its fusion glycoprotein, which are induced by its interaction with the virus receptor, CD4, and the chemokine receptor that serves as virus co-receptor. For influenza HA, activation happens as a result of a pH change in the endosome, brought about by the activity of an endosomal membrane proton pump. At low pH, for many influenza viruses about pH 5.5 at 37°, HA is induced to adopt its membrane fusion active conformation [3, 11]. Because the extensive changes induced in HA structure at fusion pH are required during fusion and are irreversible, premature activation would result in loss of fusion activity. As a consequence, HA is synthesized, transferred to the cell surface, and assembled into virus membranes under conditions where activation is avoided. This is achieved in two ways. First, HA is synthesized as a single polypeptide, HA0, which is refractory to low pH and inactive in membrane fusion. HA0 proteolytic cleavage is required to generate the primed HA that is able to respond to low pH activation [51]. Second, the virus-encoded membrane protein, M2, is

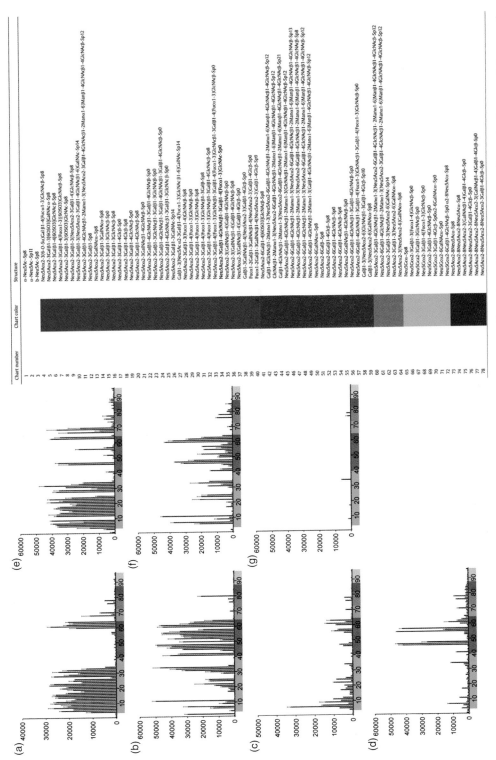

Figure 5.4. Receptor binding preferences of wild-type and mutant H5 viruses. The range of ligands used in microarray experiments is shown and the type of variation in binding signals detected with different mutant viruses. From Maines et al. [142] with permission from Elsevier.

a proton channel that neutralizes low pH compartments in the Golgi network of infected cells by allowing the efflux of protons into the cytoplasm [52]. As a consequence, HAs resulting from HA0 precursor cleavage before or during passage through this network retain their neutral pH conformation.

HA0 cleavage

HA0 is processed proteolytically to form two disulfide-linked polypeptides: HA1 and HA2 [53]. HA1 is larger (328 residues) and has the same N-terminal sequence as HA0 and a novel C-terminus; HA2 (221 residues) has a novel N-terminus and the same membrane anchor sequence at its C-terminus as HA0 (Figure 5.5). The HA2 N-terminal sequence is called the "fusion peptide" largely because synthetic peptide analogs of this conserved, nonpolar sequence, fuse lipid membranes *in vitro* [3].

Cleavage is essential for membrane fusion and hence for infectivity [53]. Cleavage of all H subtypes occurs at an arginine residue between the C-terminus of HA1 and the N-terminus of HA2. In some H5 and H7 viruses, which are primarily isolated from domesticated poultry, HA1 and HA2 are separated by a polybasic sequence, either Arg–X–Lys/Arg–Arg- or Lys–Lys/Arg–Lys/Thr–Arg- [54]. In these cases, cleavage is mediated in the trans Golgi network by a proprotein convertase such as furin, which cleaves preferentially sequences containing arginine four residues from the cleavage site, position 4. Alternatively, cleavage can be mediated by the membrane serine proteases MSPL and its variant, trans membrane protease serine S13 (TMPRSS13), which cleave polybasic sequences with either arginine or lysine at position 4 [55]. Cleavage at the polybasic sequences occurs readily and the viruses produced are highly

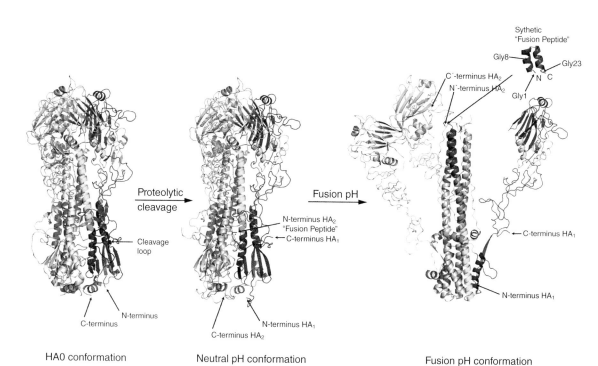

HA0 conformation   Neutral pH conformation   Fusion pH conformation

Figure 5.5. The three conformations of HA, from biosynthesis to membrane fusion. The structures of HA0 and neutral pH conformations are taken from Skehel and Wiley [11] and Wiley and Skehel [3]. The structure of the fusion pH conformation is a composite of structures of fragments of HA described in [66, 68, 86]. The orientations of the HA1 domains and the positioning of the "fusion peptide" are imaginary.

infectious and highly pathogenic [54]. As a consequence, the sequences are used as markers of the high pathogenicity of H5 and H7 virus isolates.

The vast majority of HA0s have a single arginine at the cleavage site and are cleaved at the cell surface or following release of virus from the cell, by secreted trypsin and other enzymes such as tryptase Clara [56]. However, they are also cleaved by the type II membrane anchored trypsin-like serine protease, human airway trypsin-like protease (HAT), and TMPRSS2 [57]. Both types of protease are found in human airway epithelial cells, HAT on ciliated cells of the trachea and bronchi and TMPRSS2 more widely distributed. In MDCK cells TMPRSS2 has been shown to be active in the ER and not at the cell surface, cleaving HA0 within the cell. HAT, however, cleaves at the cell surface and can cleave HA0 either on newly made virus or on newly infecting virus before cell entry [58]. *In vivo*, protease expression is restricted to specific tissues and can therefore restrict the spread of infection. It has also been noted that influenza infection can up-regulate cellular proteases and may influence tissue tropism [59].

Analyses of the structures of uncleaved HA0s show that the uncleaved and cleaved molecules are very similar except for 19 residues at the site of cleavage [11]. The sites are almost circular surface loops, which are readily accessible for cleavage. Once HA0 is cleaved, the C-terminal region of HA1 moves out of a cavity to allow the N-terminal 12 residues of the " fusion peptide," to refold into the HA trimer interface (Figure 5.5). The "fusion peptide" is formed of 23 conserved residues, the 10 N-terminal of which are nonpolar. On insertion into the trimer interface these nonpolar residues bury three ionizable residues, Asp-109 and Asp-112 of HA2, and His-17 of HA1. In this form the fusion potential of HA is "primed" for activation at fusion pH.

Endocytosis
Virus infection begins with recognition by HAs of cell-surface sialylated glycoprotein receptors. Subsequently, receptor bound viruses appear to exploit various endocytic pathways to enter cells [15, 16]. Viewed by fluorescent microscopy, about 60% of bound viruses are seen to enter cells via newly assembled clathrin-coated pits. The remaining 40%, which can be separately observed in mutant cells blocked for clathrin-mediated endocytosis, or in cells incubated in cholesterol-sequestering drugs that interfere with caveolin-mediated uptake, are seen to be taken up by clathrin- and caveolin-independent pathways [60]. Endocytic vesicle formation depends on activation by virus, of cellular signaling pathways and the resulting endosomes are associated with numerous cellular proteins. Among these is the vacuolar- H^+-ATPase responsible for changing endosome pH; pH 6.0–6.5 in early endosomes and pH 5.0–6.0 in late endosomes. Single virus tracking experiments indicate that virus-containing endosomes associate with microtubules and are moved towards the perinuclear region of the cell, the site of the microtubule organizing center [15]. At that site in late endosomes, acidification by the vacuolar ATPase proton pump to about pH 5.5 activates the fusion potential of primed HAs [61]. Influenza viruses that fuse *in vitro* at higher pH presumably are activated in early endosomes.

Fusion activation
Activation of fusion requires the low pH of endosomes, about pH 5.0–6.0, depending on the strain of virus. *In vitro*, activation can also occur at elevated temperature at neutral pH [62]. For example, the 1968 H3 virus fuses membranes at pH 5.6 at 37° and at pH 7.3 at 62°. Recognition of this interdependence of fusion pH and temperature has led to the description of "primed" HA as a metastable structure, particularly in relation to the conformation that HA assumes irreversibly at fusion pH, which is one of much greater stability. For example, the 1968 H3 following incubation at fusion pH has a temperature of denaturation of about 90°.

Fusion pH mutants
In vitro, the pH of fusion is seen to vary from strain to strain of virus mainly between pH 5.0 and 6.0. However, a number of viruses fuse above pH 6.0. To investigate the molecular location of amino acid sequence differences that influence fusion pH, mutant viruses with increased pH of fusion have been selected using the drug amantadine. At higher concentrations than those required for its antiviral activity (millimolar by comparison with micromolar at which amantadine blocks the M2 proton channel) [52], amantadine, which is a base, increases the pH of endosomes, so that only mutant viruses that fuse at higher pH than wild-type can infect treated cells [63]. Similar mutants have also been isolated following multiple passages of

viruses in tissue culture cells which may have late endosomes at higher pH [64]. The majority of mutations increase the pH of fusion from 0.2 to 0.5 pH units although a number increase by up to 0.8 units. The amino acid substitutions that the mutants contain are located in the "fusion peptide" and throughout the length of the molecule, at interfaces between monomers in the HA trimer. All are found to decrease the thermal stability of HA and there is a linear relationship between the decrease in stability and the increase in pH of fusion of the mutants.

The particular residue or residues that are the primary target of low pH activation were not identified in these studies. However, it is notable that the largest increase in pH, 0.8–0.9 pH units, result from substitutions of His-17 in H3 HA, which is buried by the "fusion peptide" when it refolds following HA0 cleavage [11]. Because histidines are the only amino acids that are uncharged at neutral pH and charged below pH 6, they are considered likely mediators of proton-controlled switches at endosomal pH [65]. The location of histidine-17 near the "fusion peptide" makes it a likely candidate for this function in HA, and its changed environment, from solvent accessible to buried, following HA0 cleavage, supports this possibility.

Comparison of the structures of H3 HA0 and cleaved H3 indicates that on cleavage the only residues that change their locations are those in the cleavage loop. Because the structure of HA0 is insensitive to low pH, it seems likely that some new aspect of cleaved HA structure is involved in priming HA for fusion activation. The seven residues of the cleavage loop that form the C-terminus of HA1 are exposed to solvent before and after cleavage. On the other hand, insertion into the HA trimer interphase of the uncharged "fusion peptide," buries residues His-17 of HA1 and Asp-109 and Asp-112 of HA2. In this location protonation of His-17 at fusion pH could destabilize "primed" HA, reinforcing the possibility that His-17 may have a role in activation of H3 HA for fusion.

Structural changes at fusion pH
Details of the changes in structure required for fusion have been determined by electron microscopy of HA in the fusion pH conformation, and by electron microscopy and X-ray crystallography of two protease fragments derived from membrane anchorless

H3 HA following incubation at fusion pH. One fragment consists of the receptor binding and vestigial esterase membrane-distal sub-domains [66] and the other of the F sub-domain from which the "fusion peptide" has been removed for crystallization [67]. A third fragment prepared by expression in *Escherichia coli* of the H3 F sub-domain (HA2 residues 23_2–185_2) yielded similar data to the protease fragment of the F sub-domain but was more complete in the N- and C-terminal regions (Figure 5.5) [68]. The changes in structure observed are not known to occur in any particular order although attempts using antipeptide antibodies to examine the kinetics of exposure of particular regions of HA at fusion pH suggest that there may be an order to them [69]. Structural data indicate that the membrane-distal domain is detrimerized and that the neutral pH structures of the receptor binding and vestigial esterase sub-domains are retained in the monomers. This is consistent with the observed receptor binding ability of fusion pH HA [34]. The "fusion peptide" is extruded from its buried position in the trimer interphase of neutral pH HA and is seen by electron microscopy to associate with the "fusion peptides" of other molecules to form rosettes of up to about 10 HAs [70]. Removal of the N-terminal 37 residues, including the "fusion peptide," by proteolysis allows crystallization of a soluble F sub-domain, residues 38–160. The structure determined by X-ray crystallography (Figure 5.5) reveals that Thr-38 of HA2 forms the N-terminus of the three α-helices in a 10 nm-long coiled-coil. The helices are formed from α-helix-A reoriented through 180°, and the extended chain, HA2 residues 59–74, which at neutral pH connects the C-terminus of a-helix-A to the N-terminus of α-helix-B, which has folded into an α-helix, and is also reoriented through 180°. These are positioned contiguous with the C-terminal portion of helix B. At the C-terminus of the α-helices of this new coiled-coil, two turns of neutral pH α-helix B refold to form a 180° turn. This reorients the C-terminus of neutral pH α-helix B, still associated with a β-sheet hairpin, residues 131–140 of HA2, to pack in the grooves between two of the helices of the coiled-coil (Figure 5.5). The C-terminal membrane-proximal 23-residue α-helical structures of neutral pH HA unfold to cross a neighboring α-helix. They refold to form a 7 nm-long chain that packs into the adjacent groove of the coiled-coil and extends to its N-terminus.

For determination of these structures, both of these regions have been removed to allow crystallization. In the complete structure, the HA2 N-terminal "fusion peptide" would be at the same end of the molecule as the HA2 C-terminal membrane anchor.

In the molecule expressed in *E. coli* which contains extended N- and C-termini by comparison with the proteolytic fragment of HA2 (HA2 residues 23–185 vs. 38–160) three residues conserved in all influenza viruses, HA2 Ala-35, Ala-36, and Asp-37, cap the N-termini. They also make extensive contacts with residues HA2 174–178 at the C-termini, fixing the N- and C-terminal regions together. The significance of these interactions for the process of membrane fusion is not known but site-specific mutation experiments indicate that changes in the conserved N-terminal residues inhibit membrane fusion *in vitro*. The structural consequences of capping the coiled-coil are that the α-helices terminate at the caps and do not extend to the membrane-associated region of the "fusion peptide." The connecting peptides between the N-termini of the coiled-coil and the "fusion peptide" and between the C-termini of the extended chains packed in the grooves of the coiled-coil and the membrane anchor may therefore be flexible.

The fusion process

It is generally assumed that during infection, as a consequence of the structural rearrangements in HA at fusion pH, the "fusion peptide" is inserted into the target endosomal membrane. Consistent with this assumption, experiments with liposomes containing photoreactive hydrophobic labeling reagents indicate that at fusion pH *in vitro* only the "fusion peptide" associates with the liposomes and becomes labeled [71]. At least three possible consequences of these interactions for the mechanism of membrane fusion have been suggested.

First, the target membrane containing the newly inserted "fusion peptide," and the virus membrane containing the HA membrane anchor, are bridged, perhaps by an extended intermediate structure. The intermediate could be about twice as long as the 10 nm-long coiled-coil structure seen by X-ray crystallography, and the ability of HA to form such extended structures was predicted from its sequence. The structures were in fact predicted, partially correctly, to be components of both the neutral pH HA structure and the fusion pH HA structure, before

either of the structures had been determined by X-ray crystallography [72, 73].

Second, the two membranes may be drawn together by formation of the 180° turn at the C-terminus of the coiled-coil (Figure 5.5). Co-location of the "fusion peptide" and the membrane anchor at one end of the fusion pH HA structure is consistent with this suggestion, particularly if the newly formed, 10 nm-long, rod-shaped molecule is eventually positioned parallel with the virus and the endosomal membranes [74].

Third, the structure of the lipid membranes is reorganized so that the outer leaflets of the bilayers fuse to form the highly curved stalk-like structures proposed as hemifusion intermediates in fusion pore formation [75]. X-ray diffraction and differential scanning calorimetry studies of lipid vesicles indicate that addition of synthetic "fusion peptide" analogs to membranes induces the formation of an inverted cubic phase in preference to an inverted hexagonal phase [76]. This is consistent with the possibility that the "fusion peptide," and possibly its interaction with the membrane anchor, directly influences the structure of membranes during fusion.

A number of studies have concluded that single HA trimers are the functional entities of HA involved in fusion [77, 78]. However, the possibility has also been proposed, from estimates of the amount of HA expressed on cell surfaces in relation to fusion activity, that multi-HA complexes are formed and that in some way these complexes are required for fusion pore formation, including the possibility that they may form protein-lined pores [79].

The structures adopted at fusion pH, by either the "fusion peptide" or the membrane anchor as components of HA, are not known. However, it is possible that at an important stage in fusion, the "fusion peptide" and the membrane anchor may associate in a way that is necessary for fusion. Such an interaction could occur early in the fusion process if the "fusion peptide" initially interacts with the virus membrane, or during completion of fusion, if the two regions are brought together as HA refolds. Both possibilities have been considered. However, experiments with fusion-competent HA can contain the membrane anchor of an unrelated membrane protein instead of the HA membrane anchor, indicating that any required interaction between the "fusion peptide" and the membrane anchor need not be sequence-specific [80].

Energy requirements for membrane fusion

In preparation of HA for membrane fusion, two events result in the formation of molecules with different thermal stabilities: HA0 cleavage and fusion-pH activation of HA. HA0 is less stable than HA, and HA is less stable at neutral pH than at fusion pH. The initial change, an increase in temperature of denaturation from 50° to 62°, results from cleavage of the precursor HA0, and burial of the "fusion peptide" in the trimer interface [81]. The second change, an increase from 62° to 90° at fusion pH, results from the formation of the highly stable coiled-coil of fusion pH HA [62]. The free energy available from these cleavage and refolding events is presumably used to overcome the repulsive forces that exist between membranes as they are brought together and the processes involved in maintaining the bilayer structure of the membranes that are reorganized during fusion.

Structure of the "fusion peptide"

"Fusion peptide" analogs have been used in studies to explore the significance of its conserved amino acid sequences for fusion and to determine "fusion peptide" structure [82]. Remarkably, in the former, there is close similarity between the activity of mutant peptides and of viruses with HAs containing the same mutations. However, the low solubility of the peptide analogs can make results difficult to interpret and, in some instances, there is no correlation between fusion activity and properties, such as angle of insertion of peptides into liposomes [83]. Furthermore, the dependence on low pH for the membrane association and fusion activities of peptides also appears contrary to observations that the pH of fusion by HA correlates with the pH of its conformational change; HA mutants that adopt the low pH conformation above pH 6.0 acquire fusion activity at above pH 6.0 [64]. Attention has therefore focused on the effects of site-specific mutation of "fusion peptides" in viruses [84]. From these studies the importance of the length of the "fusion peptide," of the N-terminal glycine residue, and of the glycine residue at position 8, are clearly shown.

Based on these results, together with those obtained with other mutants [82], the N-terminal region of HA2 can be modeled as an α-helical structure with the potential to form a hydrophobic trimer, in which conserved, long side-chain nonpolar residues at positions 2, 6, and 10 are on one face of the α-helix, with conserved glycine residues at positions 4, 8, and 12 on the opposite face [84].

Direct analyses of the structure of "fusion peptide" analogs by NMR also indicate predominantly α-helical structures for both 20 and 23 residue, peptide analogs in dodecylphosphocholine vesicles. However, in the former case, the 20-residue peptide adopts a boomerang-like conformation and, in the latter, the 23-residue peptide forms an α-helical hairpin-like structure (Figure 5.5) [85, 86]. The hairpin-like structure of the more complete 23-residue peptide is stabilized by interactions between the tightly packed α-helices, and in addition by hydrogen bonds made by the amino group of the N-terminal glycine and carbonyl oxygens of residues at the C-terminus. The hairpin-like structure is consistent with the sequence requirements of membrane fusion activity defined by site-specific mutagenesis of virus HA, and, in particular, can explain the strict requirement for glycine at position 8, which is buried in the interhelical interface of the hairpin. A question remains regarding the relationship between the structures of monomer peptides used in the NMR studies, and the structure adopted by the "fusion peptide" in fusion active HA, which may be trimeric, and may be associated with the membrane anchor. Nevertheless, a looped-back structure such as an α-helical hairpin might be similar to the likely structures adopted by "fusion peptides" that are positioned internally in other fusion glycoproteins such as that in influenza C hemagglutinin-esterase-fusion glcoprotein (HEF). In this case the analogous "fusion peptide" begins seven residues from the N-terminus generated by precursor HEF0 cleavage [10].

Membrane fusion summary

1. During virus replication mRNA for hemagglutinin is translated into HA0, a precursor of the two polypeptides HA1 and HA2 that forms the subunits of HA trimers in infectious virus. The proteolytic cleavage of HA0 to produce HA1 and HA2 is required to generate the N-terminus of HA2, a part of HA called the "fusion peptide". Following HA0 cleavage the "fusion peptide" is refolded into the trimer interface.

2. At the beginning of the next cycle of infection, following endocytosis of receptor bound virus, HA mediates fusion of virus and endosomal membranes to deliver the genome transcriptase complex into the cell for virus replication to begin. Activation of HA fusion potential occurs following acidification of endosomes to about pH 5.0 by the action of a cellular proton pump.

3. At low pH, fusion is activated in a process that involves extensive changes in HA structure which include repositioning of the "fusion peptide" to the N-terminus of a newly formed coiled-coil, where it is co-located with the HA membrane anchor. As a consequence of these structural rearrangements the HA forms a bridge between the virus and endosomal membranes. These changes in HA conformation are required during fusion to bring the two membranes together and in some way to reorganize membrane bilayer structure.

Neuraminidase

The activity of an enzyme that eluted influenza viruses bound to erythrocytes was discovered in early experiments on hemagglutination [45]. About 15 years

later, the enzyme was identified as a neuraminidase [13, 14] which was eventually shown to be a component of the virus membrane that is involved in the spread of influenza infection from cell to cell [18, 87].

Neuraminidase active site

The active site is located in a pocket lined with residues that are essentially invariant in all influenza A and B viruses [12, 88]. On the basis of contact with the reaction product, sialic acid, the following residues are considered catalytic: Arg-118, Asp-151, Arg-152, Arg-224, Glu-276, Arg-292, Arg-371, and Tyr-406 (Figure 5.6). Key conserved residues in proximity to the reaction product, but not making direct contact with it, have an important structural role. They have been described as framework residues and include: Glu-119, Arg-156, Trp-178, Ser-179, Asp-198, Ile-222, Glu-227, Glu-277, Asn-294, and Glu-425. There is also strong conservation of a number of proline and cysteine residues important for the overall structural integrity of the molecule.

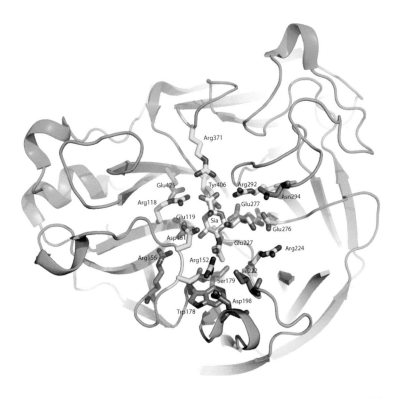

Figure 5.6. The active site of NA. One of the four subunits in the NA head structure (Figure 5.1) is shown. Sialic acid (in white) is modeled in the site to show the positions relative to it of the catalytic residues (yellow) and the framework residues (blue).

The eight conserved catalytic residues are arranged in a series of interconnected pockets that define the way in which the enzyme interacts with sialic acid. One end of the active site is dominated by a triarginyl cluster, comprising Arg-118, Arg-292, and Arg-371. All three residues interact with the carboxylate of the bound sialic acid and probably contribute to the boat geometry it adopts on binding. Also located in this part of the active site is Tyr-406 which appears to have a critical role in catalysis. Adjoining this region is another pocket containing the acidic residues Asp-151 and Glu-119, which interact with the C3 and C4 hydroxyl groups, respectively, and Glu-227, which hydrogen bonds to a water molecule that interacts with the NH group of the C5 acetamido substituent. The carbonyl oxygen of the acetamido substituent hydrogen bonds to Arg-152. On the opposite side of the active site to Asp-151, Glu-276 forms charged hydrogen bonds with the C-8 and C-9 hydroxyl groups of the glycerol side-chain [89].

The mechanism of catalysis

The catalytic mechanism has not been proven but there is a consensus regarding its main features (Figure 5.7) [90, 91]. Binding of substrate to the active site, through the range of interactions described above, and particularly involving salt bridge formation between the carboxylate of the substrate and the triarginyl cluster, leads to a change from the preferred chair conformation (I) to a distorted boat conformation (II). This facilitates formation of a sialosyl cation intermediate (III). The stability of the oxocarbonium ion (III) favors breakage of the glycosidic bond, and the aglycone molecule leaves the active site with the glycosidic oxygen. The proximity of the acidic residues of the active site to the oxocarbonium ion stabilize this positively charged species and maintain the planar carbon at C2. It is thought likely that the neuraminic acid moiety is kept covalently attached to the enzyme at this stage via the hydroxyl group of Tyr-406 and that this covalent species (IV) is characteristic of all exosialidases. The oxocarbonium ion (V) is then hydroxylated from solvent and the product (VI) dissociates.

Enzyme assays and kinetics

Several methods are available for determining the activity of neuraminidases: the periodic acid–thiobarbituric acid assay [92], a coupled enzyme assay in which NADH is produced from NAD+ (with β-galactosidase and glucose dehydrogenase as the coupling enzymes) [93], the MUNANA assay in which the fluorogenic reagent

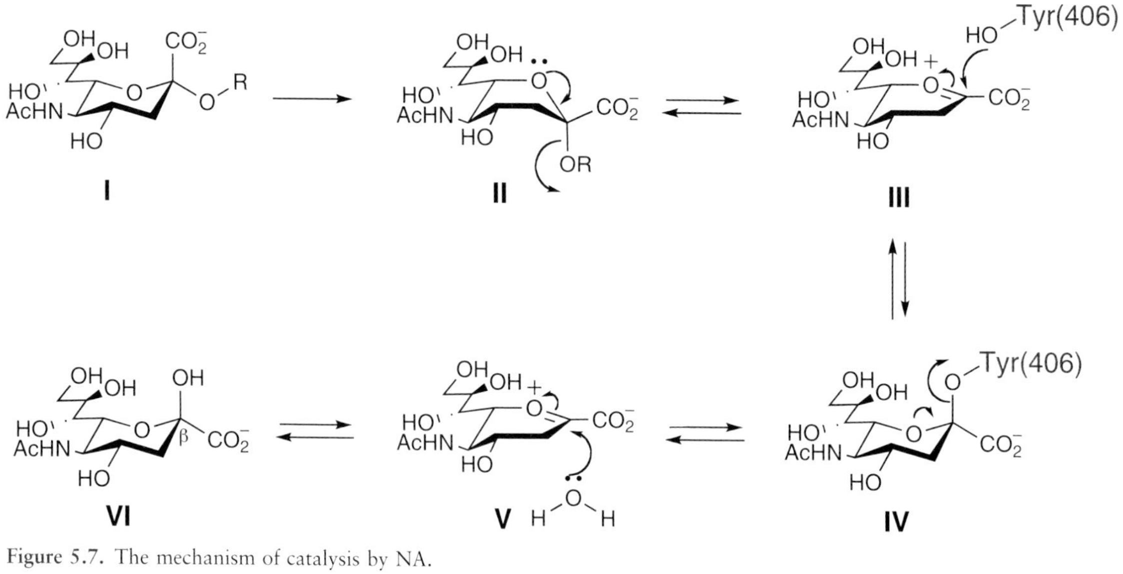

Figure 5.7. The mechanism of catalysis by NA.

2′-(4-methylumbelliferyl)-α-D-N-acetylneuraminic acid is converted to the highly fluorescent 4-methylumbelliferone [94], and a sensitive chemiluminescence assay in which the 1,2-dioxetane derivative of sialic acid (NA-STAR) is used as the substrate [95].

Although neuraminidases of different influenza virus subtypes have different properties there are several common features. They show activity over a broad pH range (4–7) and have temperature optima close to 37°C, with inactivation occurring at temperatures greater than 55°C. Although they do not have an absolute requirement for calcium the addition of this metal ion generally increases V_{max} (two- to five-fold) without affecting the K_m [96]. In most studies, neuraminidases appear to show a preference for the α-2,3-linkage over the α-2,6-linkage (K_m values being typically 100–400 and 300–800 μM, respectively).

Enzyme inhibition assays are ideal for determining the susceptibility of clinical isolates to antiviral drugs. The method currently most widely used for detecting enzyme inhibition is the MUNANA assay which can be used in routine microtiter plate-based assays. The K_i (or IC_{50}) for an inhibitor is easily determined by studying the effect of different inhibitor concentrations on the rate of MUNANA hydrolysis. At low concentrations of inhibitor the approach to the new steady-state inhibited rate following addition of inhibitor is often slow. Analysis of the kinetics of this change can be used to obtain association and dissociation rate constants for inhibitor binding [97].

Association and dissociation rate constants for oseltamivir are typically in the range $1–4\,mmol^{-1}\,s^{-1}$ and $2–8 \times 10^{-4}\,s^{-1}$, respectively. Zanamivir typically binds slightly more slowly with association and dissociation rate constants of $0.5–1.5\,mmol^{-1}\,s^{-1}$ and $0.5–3 \times 10^{-4}\,s^{-1}$, respectively. The decrease in inhibitor affinity observed with oseltamivir resistant mutants (>100-fold) derives from reduced association rate constants (5- to 10-fold) and increased dissociation rate constants (10- to 50-fold).

Inhibitors of HA and NA functions and potential antiviral drugs

Each of the functions of HA and NA represent targets for inhibitory molecules that could potentially be developed as anti-influenza drugs. The identification and investigation of the mechanisms of action of such small molecules can also shed light on the mechanisms of the activities mediated by HA and NA.

For HA both receptor binding and membrane fusion are the obvious targets for inhibitors. The conserved nature of the molecular sites involved in these activities has encouraged studies of their inhibition.

Receptor binding

Inhibition of receptor binding has attracted attention because this is the first step in infection, because the affinity of HA for the receptor sialic acid is low, and because inhibition would involve blocking an activity that occurs extracellularly rather than requiring cross-membrane transport for activity. A number of high affinity sialic acid derivatives have been reported and the structures of complexes that they form with HA have been determined by X-ray crystallography. The highest affinity compound in the main series of inhibitors examined, NeuAc4D2N6 (α-2-O-6-(naphthylmethyleneamidocarboxyhexyl)-4-O dansyl-sialic acid), bound to HA more than 500 times more tightly than α-methyl sialic acid. The naphthyl hydrocarbon extended from the sialic acid binding site, through a hydrophobic channel formed between the 130-loop and the 220-loop [98]. Naturally occurring inhibitors of infectivity such as α-2-macroglobulin, which is rich in α-2,6-linked sialic acid, achieve high affinity binding through multivalent attachment of sialic acids to many HAs. A similar approach using multivalent sialosides has also been used with inhibitors. Bivalent sialosides of the derivatives mentioned above, especially with linkers over 5 nm-long, prevented hemagglutination of viruses about 5000 times more effectively than monovalent α-methyl sialoside. Tetravalent sialosides were more effective and polyvalent compounds containing 60 sialosides were up to 50 000 times as effective, with polymers of particular architecture being more or less effective and more or less toxic to cells [99, 100].

The possibility that sialosides with greater specificity for HA can be identified, to extend these approaches to receptor binding inhibition, is one of the objectives of the detailed analyses of receptor binding specificity using microarrays containing a wide range of natural sialosides [48]. An increased knowledge of receptor specificity, for example, in relation to the infection of cells of particular importance in pathogenesis would be an important contribution to inhibitor development.

Membrane fusion

Inhibition of HA0 cleavage

A number of studies have indicated the feasibility of blocking the enzymes involved in cleavage of HA0 at both polybasic and single arginine residue sites of cleavage.

In vitro and in infected cells, di-basic peptidyl chloroalkyl ketones block cleavage by furin-like enzymes at polybasic sites found in pathogenic H5 and H7 HA0s [101]. Cleavage at single arginine sites by HAT and TMPRSS2 is blocked by peptide mimetic protease inhibitors, both cell-permeable and impermeable. Aprotinin, a 58-residue peptide serine protease inhibitor from bovine lung also prevents cleavage at single arginine sites and has been licensed as an anti-influenza treatment for respiratory tract application and for intravenous administration in severe cases of influenza [59]. Tryptase Clara, a serine protease secreted by Clara cells of bronchiolar epithelium, which specifically recognizes the Gln/Glu-X-Arg sequences at the cleavage sites in H1, H2, and H3 HA0s of three human pandemics, is also inhibited by a protease inhibitor in mucous and by C-terminal fragments derived from it [102]. The contribution of these natural products to drug treatments remains to be determined, not least because the precise nature of the proteases required for cleavage during infection has not been established nor has the potential redundancy between the proteases that have been identified as candidates been assessed.

Inhibition of PH-dependent changes in HA structure

There have been a number of reports of small molecules with the ability to block the low pH-induced changes in HA conformation, required for HA-mediated membrane fusion. Compounds related to podocarpic acid block the conformational change and infection, and selected resistant mutants that had less stable HAs. The pH of change increased by 0.3 to 0.6 as a result of amino acid substitutions in helix B of HA2 and in the HA trimer interface [103]. Screening for antiviral activity also led to the demonstration that N-substituted piperidine blocked infectivity and selected resistant mutations HA2 Phe-110→Ser and Phe-3→Leu, near the N-terminus of the "fusion peptide" [104]. A series of quinolizin-benzamide compounds, one of which was shown by photo-affinity labeling to interact with residues HA2 95, 96, 97, and 103, 104, and 105, also blocked infectivity and selected a resistant mutant containing the substitution HA2 Phe-110→Ser [105]. All of these various compounds, from the molecular locations and the effects of the resistance mutations that they select, may act in a similar, but as yet unknown, way to stabilize HA and prevent the required conformational change at the normal pH of fusion. They have the additional similarity of specifically inhibiting group 1 H1 and H2 viruses but not group 2 H3 viruses. By contrast, a number of benzoquinones and hydroquinones, selected on the basis of modeling studies for binding in a cavity near the "fusion peptide," blocked the infectivity of H3 subtype HA but not H1 and H2 subtype HAs [106]. Selected resistant mutants had amino acid substitutions near the "fusion peptide" that increased the pH of fusion by up to 0.4 units. Analysis by X-ray crystallography of complexes formed by H3 HA with the tert-butylhydroquinone used in these studies [107], indicated that the compound bound near the C-terminus of helix A (Figure 5.1), between helix A and helix B of the neighboring subunit of the trimer. The structure of this region is specifically different between the two groups of HA with group1 HAs having a longer helix A than group2 HAs, and group 2 helix A being linked by a specific salt-bridge to the neighboring helix B. The structure of the complex therefore explained the group-specificity of these compounds. It also suggested a mechanism for the inhibition of the low pH induced conformational change in which group 2 HAs were specifically stabilized by inter- and intra-subunit interactions mediated by the bound compound [107]. The resistance mutations located near the "fusion peptide," rather than preventing inhibitor binding, appear to have destabilized HA and hence reversed the stabilizing effects of the inhibitor.

Anti-NA drugs

By contrast with the lack of progress in development of drugs that target HA, two anti-NA drugs, zanamavir and oseltamivir, have been licensed for therapeutic and prophylactic use [108–110]. They act specifically against all subtypes of influenza A NAs and influenza B NA. They differ in the ring structure of the sialic acid derivative and the active substituents (Figure 5.8), which target different parts of the enzyme and provide the basis for specific resistance profiles. The guanidino group of zanamivir interacts with a pocket in the catalytic site formed by the acidic residues

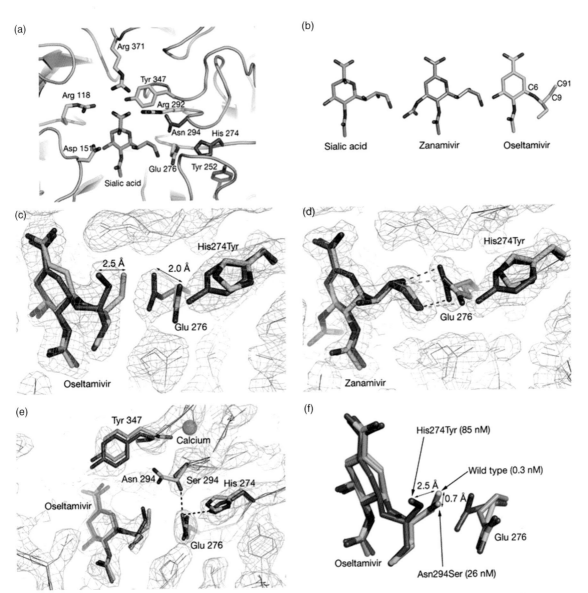

Figure 5.8. The structures of complexes between the NA inhibitors zanamivir and oseltamivir and wild-type and resistant mutant NAs. (a) The position of sialic acid in the NA active site (compare Figure 5.6) and (b) of the structure of sialic acid, by comparison with zanamivir and oseltamivir. The structures are formed by complexes of the resistant mutant NAs with oseltamivir (c) and zanamivir (d) and highlight the amino acid substitution His-274→Tyr in the oseltamivir resistant mutant. They show the effects of the substitution on the position of the Glu-276 side-chain and the oseltamivir pentyl-oxy substituent. (d) The H-bonds formed by both mutant and wild-type Glu-276 with zanamivir, correlating with the lack of resistance of the mutant to zanamivir. (e) Overlaid complexes of the oseltamivir resistant mutant Asn-294→ Ser and wild-type NAs. (f) Conformations of Glu-276 and oseltamivir in the mutant His-274→Tyr and Asn-294→Ser complexes are overlaid on the wild-type complex.

glutamic acid 119, aspartic acid 151, and glutamic acid 227. Zanamivir has an affinity of binding 1000-fold greater than that of the enzyme substrate. The hydrophobic ethylpropoxy moiety of oseltamivir increases affinity by a similar amount by binding to a hydrophobic pocket in the active site, exposed following reorientation of glutamic acid 276 [110]. A third compound, peramivir, which is still under clinical development, possesses both active substituents. All three compounds have K_i values in the nanomolar range. The IC_{50}s reported for inhibition of different NAs vary within the ranges of 2–30 nmol for zanamivir, 2–69 nmol for oseltamivir and 1–4 nmol for peramivir [111]. The IC_{50} for oseltamivir inhibition of influenza B NA is somewhat higher than those for the NAs of human H1N1 and H3N2 viruses, possibly contributing to reduced effectiveness of this drug against influenza B.

Inhibitor binding
Crystal structures of zanamivir, oseltamivir, and peramivir in complex with N2 or N9 NAs showed that only minor conformational changes occur in the active site upon inhibitor binding. For example, in unliganded N9 NA the carboxylate of Glu-276 faces into the active site cavity, but upon oseltamivir binding Glu-276 adopts a conformation that points the carboxylate away from the active site so that it now makes a bidentate interaction with the guanidinium group of Arg-224. In so doing the hydrophobic aliphatic side-chain groups of Glu-276 move towards the C6-linked hydrophobic substituent of oseltamivir.

When N1 and N8 NAs are incubated in zanamivir, oseltamivir, or peramivir, the 150-loop changes its conformation so that it closely resembles the "closed" conformation that N2 and N9 NAs adopt in the presence and in the absence of inhibitors [112]. The presence of the 150-cavity that results from the open conformation of the 150-loop does not significantly influence binding of the drugs. However, it provides the basis for attempts to develop alternative inhibitors with substituents that target the 150-cavity [113].

NA group-specific differences in inhibitor resistant mutants
A number of oseltamivir resistant mutants show NA group specificity because different mutations are principally responsible for resistance in either group 1 or group 2 NAs. Structural analyses of the sites of muta-tion have revealed both a basis for resistance and for the observed group specificity. Two examples are described for which the structures of NA complexed with drugs are available.

The mutation Arg-292→Lys causes high resistance of group 2 NAs to oseltamivir, but has little effect on group 1 NAs. Analysis of the effect of this mutation on N2 revealed that resistance results from the loss of a charged hydrogen bond to the carboxylate group of oseltamivir [109]. The structure of N1 complexed with oseltamivir [97] revealed the likely reason that this mutation does not affect binding to group 1 NAs (Figure 5.8). A conserved tyrosine residue at position 347 in group 1 NAs makes an additional hydrogen bond to the carboxylate group of the inhibitor that cannot be made by the equivalent residues in group 2 NAs. This additional hydrogen bond interaction, possible only in group 1 NAs, probably compensates for the loss of the interaction associated with the Arg-292→Lys mutation.

The mutation His-274→Tyr leads to high resistance of group1 NAs against oseltamivir but has little effect on group2 NAs. Inspection of the structures of the group 1 NAs in complex with oseltamivir, and comparison with equivalent group 2 NA complexes, shows that this behavior is mediated by the differential effect of this mutation on the conformation of Glu-276. There appear to be at least two contributory factors to this mutation being accommodated in group 2 but not in group 1 NAs [97]. First, the 270 loop (approaching residue 273) in group 1 makes a tighter turn than the equivalent loop in group 2. Second, in group 1, but not in group 2, there is a conserved tyrosine residue at position 252 that makes hydrogen bonds to the carbonyl at position 273 and the amide at 250 (NH) and to the histidine side-chain at 274. The histidine also hydrogen bonds through its other side-chain nitrogen with Glu-276 (Figure 5.8). The substitution of the bulkier tyrosine residue at position 274 in group 1 can only be accommodated by the new side-chain moving towards, and partially displacing, Glu276. In contrast, in group 2 NAs, the much smaller threonine residue at position 252 leaves space for the introduced tyrosine to occupy without perturbing Glu276.

Prospects for additional targets for inhibition

One of the objectives of identifying specific cellular molecules that participate in processes required for virus infection [114], such as endocytosis, is to investigate whether the inhibition or removal of their activities might be useful in blocking infection. Inhibition of a protease involved in HA0 cleavage, mentioned above, is one such possibility. The use of a bacterial neuraminidase fused with a respiratory epithelium anchoring sequence to remove cell-surface sialic acids required as influenza receptors is another example that is being actively explored. However, there are hundreds of molecules that might be targets, and the cellular sites of action of HA and NA could make molecules that affect their activities particularly favorable for follow-up studies.

Antigenicity of HA and NA

Influenza viruses are notorious for antigenic variation and the accompanying frequent recurrence of epidemics. The HA and NA glycoproteins are the variable antigens.

Two sorts of antigenic variation occur. In the first, the glycoproteins of a subtype with different antigenic properties from those of the subtypes currently circulating in humans may be transferred into the human population from an animal or avian source. Apart from particular age groups that may have been exposed to similar viruses in the past, such as occurred when H1N1 viruses were introduced in 1977 and 2009, there is no immunity to the new viruses and widespread transmission results in a pandemic. Since the 1918 H1N1 pandemic, the mechanism by which cross-species transfer has occurred has involved reassortment of virus genes from avian or animal viruses

with genes from human viruses, to create pandemic viruses with new HAs and, in 1957, with a new HA and a new NA. The known pandemics were caused by H1N1 viruses, in 1918, 1977, and 2009; an H2N2 virus in 1957; and an H3N2 virus in 1968. In the second type of variation, mutation occurs in the HAs and NAs of a subtype currently circulating in humans. This happened in all three pandemic periods of the twentieth century, on numerous occasions.

Antigenic subtypes were initially defined using serologic tests in which hyperimmune sera were reacted with the HA and NA components of detergent solutions of viruses. Sera prepared using HA or NA of any one subtype only reacted with HA or NA from viruses of the same subtype [115]. The antigenic groupings distinguished in this way are consistent with those subsequently defined by analyses of HA and NA sequences (Figure 5.9). There are 16 H and 9 N subtypes all identified in numerous combinations of HA and NA in viruses isolated from avian species. Viruses containing H17 and N10 have recently been identified in bats.

HA subtypes
For HA, the number of identical amino acids in different subtypes varies from 40% to 70% and within subtypes from 80% to 100%. On the basis of sequence similarity the subtypes form five clades and two groups (Figure 5.9).

The overall structures of all HAs from the two groups are very similar (Figure 5.10) [116, 117]. They differ in the orientation of the membrane-distal subdomains relative to the central B α-helices of the F

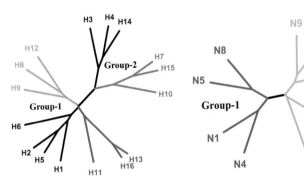

Figure 5.9. The phylogenetic relationships between the subtypes and groups of HAs and NAs.

Haemagglutinin (H1–H16) **Neuraminidase (N1–N9)**

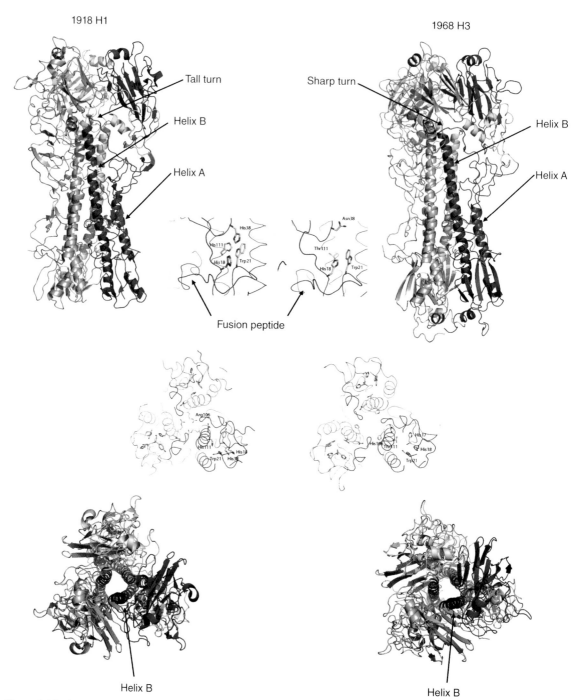

Figure 5.10. A comparison of the structures of 1918 H1 and 1968 H3 HAs as representatives of group 1 and 2 HAs. Structural differences are highlighted between the HAs, in the lengths of helix A, the conformation of the turn at the N-terminus of helix B, and in the structure near the "fusion peptide," (inserts). The two views down the threefold axis of symmetry show the difference in orientation (about 30°) between the membrane-distal sub-domains relative to the F sub-domain.

sub-domain. The two groups are distinguishable by a number of structural features, in positions that are prominent in the structural changes required for HA-mediated membrane fusion. Three of these positions are indicated in Figure 5.10. They include group-specific differences in structure at the C-terminus of α-helix A, the shorter α-helix of the HA2 part of the F sub-domain; at the C-terminus of the extended chain that links α-helix A with α-helix B; and near the N-terminus of HA2, at the site of insertion of the "fusion peptide" following its generation by cleavage of the precursor, HA0. A functional significance for these group-specific differences in structure is not known but they may have been selected during evolution in different environments to favor different pathways of refolding HA for membrane fusion.

NA subtypes

For NA, the nine N subtypes share 50–70% sequence identity. They also form two groups genetically (Figure 5.9) (unconnected to the two groups of HA) that have distinctive group-specific, structural features. The most prominent of these is the 150-loop, which in the group 1 NA apo-structure is in an open conformation [112]. The loop is closed on ligand binding to form a similar structure to that formed by group 2 NAs. The proximity of the 150-loop and the 150-cavity, created in the open conformation, to the enzyme active site is consistent with the possibility that the two groups of NA may have evolved as a result of selective pressure imposed on the site, perhaps by the availability of different sialylated oligosaccharides as receptors and substrates.

Intra-subtype variation in HA

The identities of the regions of HA and NA that form the subtype-specific antigenic regions recognized by hyperimmune sera in the subtype classification procedure have not been described. However, the major differences between subtypes in the two clades of group 2 HAs are in their surface structures (unpublished data), and the possibility of a similar situation for NA subtypes has been suggested [8]. Surface changes certainly seem to be responsible for the intra-subtype antigenic variation that has occurred during the H1, H2, and H3 pandemic periods 1918–1957, 1957–1968, and from 1968 to date, respectively [43, 118, 119]. In the H3N2 pandemic period, from 1968

to the present, nucleotide sequence analyses indicate that all of the amino acid substitutions that are retained in HAs of viruses isolated in subsequent years involve surface residues, many closely surrounding the receptor-binding site. Of the sporadic changes, which are not retained, over 60% are in buried locations in HA. The surface amino acid substitutions include changes in residue side-chain length and polarity and, in a number of cases, lead to the formation of new sites for glycosylation [3]. In one period of the H3N2 pandemic, between 1968 and the mid-1980s, there was an accumulation of basic residues in the membrane-distal sub-domains, as a result of amino acid substitutions which have been retained and which may, in some way, facilitate cell association of the mutant viruses. In the same period and since, there has been an accumulation of new carbohydrate side-chains in the same sub-domains, and between 1968 and 2005 the number has increased from 6 to 11.

The molecular locations of the retained substitutions are similar to those of amino acid substitutions detected in antigenic mutants selected by growth of virus in the presence of different anti-HA monoclonal antibodies. This supports the interpretation that the retained surface residues have also been selected because they prevent antibody binding and are therefore responsible for antigenic variation [21].

Intra-subtype variation in NA

Unlike antibodies that bind to HA, anti-NA antibodies do not neutralize virus infectivity. However, they are able to prevent the release of newly assembled viruses by blocking NA activity, and they prevent the spread of infection in this way. Antigenic mutant NAs that are able to release virus in the presence of antibodies are selected at this stage of infection.

Consistent with the ability of anti-NA antibodies to block the spread of infection, the frequency of sequence changes, known mainly from studies of H2N2 and H3N2 viruses isolated since 1957, is similar to the frequency of changes in HA during the same period, at about three amino acid residues per year [8]. Among the changes involved, as in HA, side-chain length and polarity, and also a new site for carbohydrate side-chain addition, at residue 329 [120], is observed. Most of the changes (about 70%) are located on the upper surface of NA primarily on prominent loop structures surrounding the active site

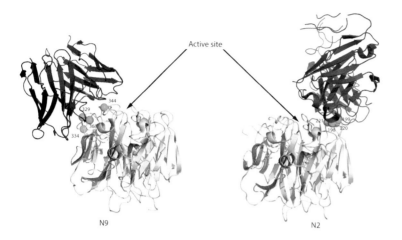

Figure 5.11. The structures of two complexes formed by monoclonal antibodies against the group 2 NAs, N2, and N9 [29, 30]. The antibodies are bound on opposite sides of the enzyme active site, in positions where variation occurs in natural N2 variants from 1957 to date.

of the enzyme. Among these the region containing residues 328–370 is most variable early in the N2 period [8]. The remainder of the amino acid substitutions are located on the sides and membrane-facing surface of NA. The basis of selection pressure for changes at these sites is not known.

Remarkably, comparison of two N9 viruses, one isolated from a tern, the other from a whale, revealed that 14 of the 17 amino acid sequence differences between them were located on the membrane-facing side of NA and the other three were on the membrane-associated stalk. The length of time over which such differences occurred is of course unknown [8].

Amino acid substitutions in N2 NA mutants selected by monoclonal antibodies are located in the same regions of the NA surface as the retained changes in sequences detected in NAs from viruses isolated during the pandemic period. Two major groups of mutations in upper surface loops on opposite sides of the enzyme active site have been identified (Figure 5.11), involving residues 198, 199, 220, and 221, and 329, 334, 344, and 368. These findings clearly support the proposed antigenic significance of the sequence changes in these regions, which were identified in the intrapandemic antigenic mutants [30].

Structures of complexes formed by HA and NA with antibodies

Electron micrographs of complexes formed between HA and NA with different monoclonal antibodies directly indicate the locations of antibody binding sites [24, 28]. The sites of amino acid substitutions in mutant HAs that the antibodies select coincide with these locations. The conclusions are supported by structural analyses of monoclonal antibody-selected mutant HAs and NAs by X-ray crystallography. These studies showed that only local changes in HA structure could be detected in the mutant glycoproteins [21, 121, 122] and that these were at the sites of the selected amino acid substitutions. Subsequently, these conclusions were verified by X-ray crystallography of the structures of complexes formed between different monoclonal antibodies with either NA or HA (Figure 5.11 and Figure 5.12).

Monoclonal Fab-NA complexes were in fact, among the earliest antibody–protein complexes to be examined in detail and they allowed a number of general properties of the interactions between antigens and antibodies to be proposed. In particular they addressed the sizes of the interacting surfaces, the requirement for the surfaces to have complementary shapes, the importance of local structures at the sites of amino acid substitutions, and the consequences of substitutions for the energetics of antigen–antibody interactions [31]. The overall conclusion in relation to the mechanism of infection blocking by anti-NA antibodies is that by binding in the region of the enzyme active site, enzyme activity is blocked by restricting access of substrate or by directly interacting with residues involved in enzyme activity.

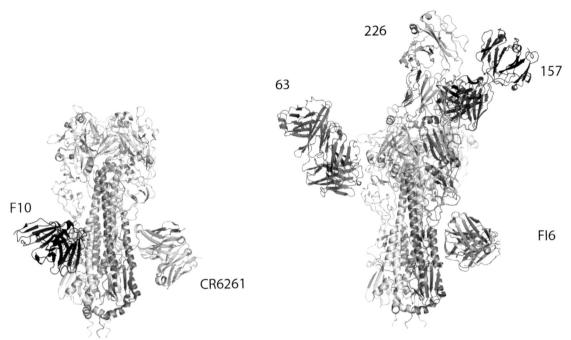

Figure 5.12. The binding locations n HA of Fabs from six monoclonal antibodies. Fabs 63, 157, and 226 are from mouse antibodies that select binding-resistant mutations at HA1 residue 63, 157, and 226, respectively [21]. F16 is from a human cross-reactive monoclonal antibody that binds to HAs of all 16 subtypes [130]. CR6261 [135], and F10 [137] are from antibodies that bind to all group 1 HAs.

Infectivity neutralization

Assays of inhibition of virus binding to cells and of virus infectivity neutralization by a number of anti-HA monoclonal antibodies indicate that both occur at the same antibody concentrations [21]. This correlation supports the proposal that antibodies prevent infection by blocking receptor binding. It is also consistent with the membrane-distal location of the antibody binding sites, many of which are close to the conserved receptor binding site. The structures of two monoclonal antibody complexes indicate that the antibodies interact directly with conserved residues in the receptor binding site (Figure 5.12) [21]. Because the antibody affinities are much greater than the affinity of the site for the sialic acid receptor, binding at these sites would effectively block receptor binding and consequently infection.

One of the complexes with HA that has been studied (Figure 5.11) in addition to blocking receptor binding also cross-bridges two of the HA subunits in the trimer. *In vitro*, this prevents the changes in conformation required for HA-mediated membrane fusion and mimics the inhibition of fusion by mutant HAs in which the subunits of the trimer were cross-linked by disulfide bonds [123]. For subunit cross-bridging to be an effective mechanism for antibody-mediated neutralization of infectivity, it would have to occur at an antibody concentration at which virus binding to cells was not prevented, because membrane fusion follows virus binding and endocytosis. A clearer understanding of the mechanistic details of HA-mediated membrane fusion, particularly in relation to the number of HA molecules involved in a fusion event, is required before this possibility can be properly assessed.

The amounts of different anti-HA antibodies required for infectivity neutralization [124] depend on the geometries of antibody binding and on the location of the antibody binding sites. Those antibodies that extend directly from the top of HA neutralize viruses at concentrations lower than those needed to saturate the virus. Other antibodies that bind to the sides of

91

HA occupy more space on the viral surface and neutralize at concentrations similar to those at which saturation occurs [21]. Estimates of the affinities of anti-HA antibodies for isolated HAs by comparison with their affinities for HAs on viruses led to the following observations. The affinities of different antibodies for HA were similar, irrespective of their sites of binding. By contrast, the affinities for HAs on viruses of antibodies that bound to sites at the membrane-distal tips of HA were higher than the affinities of antibodies that bound to sites closer to the virus membrane [21].

Variation of HA and NA

Differences in the extent of HA and NA variation compared with the surface proteins of many other viruses may be caused by the existence of the animal and avian reservoirs of influenza viruses. From these sources, viruses are transferred into humans at irregular intervals, as on the three occasions of the pandemics of the twentieth century; 1918, 1957, and 1968. Once introduced into the human population HAs and NAs of the new subtypes could presumably continue to vary until the viability of the virus is compromised. This could occur by deleterious effects on receptor binding or membrane fusion or receptor destroying ability. The selection of new sites for glycosylation may be especially important in this regard. This is because, unlike those sites at which multiple amino acid substitutions can be selected, sites modified by glycosylation are not under immune pressure to change because they are recognized as self. Their accumulation may limit the extent of antigenic variation and eventually viability. On the other hand, the extent of glycosylation may itself be limited as a consequence of its deleterious effects on HA and NA functions [125].

Effects of HA and NA glycosylation

Glycosylation of HA and NA involves normal cellular enzymes except for the removal of terminal sialic acid residues which is done by the virus NA. The attached carbohydrate side-chains influence the functions and the antigenicity of HA, and there may be a similar effect of glycosylation on NA antigenicity.

During biosynthesis in the ER, the lectin chaperones calnexin and calreticulin, which recognize glucosylated carbohydrate side-chain intermediates, are both required for correct HA folding [126]. They presumably bind to conserved carbohydrate side-chains near the N-terminus in the case of ER membrane-bound calnexin, and in the membrane-distal esterase and receptor binding sub-domains in the case of the ER lumenal, calreticulin. In this way, by holding sub-domains apart until synthesis is completed, the required disulfide bond formation and association of N- and C-terminal regions of HA0 appear to be facilitated. Similar details are not available for the role of chaperones in NA biosynthesis. However, carbohydrate side-chains attached at the three glycosylation sites on the NA stalk near the membrane anchor may be recognized by calnexin. Carbohydrate side-chains on the upper and lower surface of the NA membrane-distal structure may be recognized by calreticulin.

Effects of glycosylation on HA receptor binding affinity were initially observed in studies of differences in the antigenic properties of viruses isolated from humans and then grown in either hens' eggs or in MDCK cells. H1 viruses glycosylated at residue HA1 156, near the receptor binding site, were produced in MDCK cells but not in eggs [127]. They were antigenically distinguishable from egg-grown viruses in hemagglutination inhibition and infectivity neutralization tests and had different receptor binding affinities. Such changes can have an important bearing on optimum vaccine strain selection if viruses from different cell sources are compared in the process of selection. They could also affect vaccination efficiency if glycosylation mutant viruses are selected in the eggs or cells used in vaccine production.

The proximity of the receptor binding site to many antigenic sites is reflected in the fact that inhibition of receptor binding is the major mechanism of virus infectivity neutralization. In addition to selection for an effect on receptor-binding properties, glycosylation can also result from antibody-mediated selection of antigenic mutants. During the H3 pandemic period, between 1968 and 1985, four additional sites for glycosylation accumulated in the receptor binding and vestigial esterase sub-domains of HA. Glycosylation at one of these sites, which was also detected in a monoclonal antibody-selected mutant, was shown to be directly responsible for preventing antibody binding *in vitro* because inhibition of glycosylation allowed the antibody to bind to the mutant HA [128]. Site-specific mutagenesis to remove specific glycosylation sites has given similar information [129]. Carbohydrate side-chains on HA and NA are not recognized as foreign and are not antigenic. However, the protein surface that they cover can be considerably greater than an amino acid side-chain and their ability to inhibit antibody binding can be significant. This is presumably the case for the four naturally occurring mutant H3 HAs and also for an N2 mutant NA that had an additional glycosylation site.

Interestingly, however, a carbohydrate side-chain normally positioned in a site recognized by an antibody has been observed by X-ray crystallography of HA complexed with the antibody to have rotated out of its normal position, allowing antibody to bind [130].

HA0 cleavage is essential for virus-mediated membrane fusion and for virus infectivity. Cleavage of some H5 and H7 HAs, which contain polybasic amino acid cleavage sites, is efficient and contributes to the high pathogenicity of the viruses. This is in part due to the recognition of the cleavage site by intracellular proteases and in part to the accessibility of the site because of its exposure in a prominent surface loop of HA0 [53]. The HA0s of other H5 viruses contain a single arginine residue at the site of cleavage. They are not readily cleaved and the viruses are not pathogenic. They are rendered pathogenic by mutation that results in removal of a conserved carbohydrate side-chain adjacent to the site of cleavage that otherwise restricts proteolysis [131].

Loss of a carbohydrate side-chain, as in this case and in the example of the receptor binding-site mutant in egg grown virus, influences HA function. As a consequence it can be selected during virus growth under appropriate conditions. Gain of a side-chain may also be a selective advantage when it results in antigenic change, by preventing antibody binding. Loss of a side-chain, however, because it is not antigenic, is unlikely to be selected for antigenic change.

Cross-reactive anti-HA antibodies

The ability to subtype influenza viruses using hyper-immune antisera prepared against HA and NA demonstrated that cross-subtype reactive antibodies are induced at relatively low frequency. Nevertheless, anti-HA antibodies have been characterized that are not only highly cross-reactive within a subtype, but also some that have the ability to bind to HAs of all 16 subtypes.

The existence of antibodies of the first sort, those that react widely within a subtype, has been noted for a number of monoclonal antibodies that bind in, or near to, the receptor binding sites of H1, H3, or H5 viruses [132–134]. In neither H1 nor H5 cases was it possible to determine binding specificity by sequencing antibody-resistant HA variants. However, by X-ray crystallography of complexes formed between H1 HA and Fab fragments prepared from antibodies from infected humans [134], the CDR3 of the Fab heavy chain is seen to bind in the sialic acid receptor binding pocket, with HCDR3 aspartic acid and valine residues making similar contacts with conserved site residues as those made by sialic acid. By electron microscopy the anti-H5 antibody was also shown to bind to the membrane-distal tip of the receptor binding sub-domain [133]. In both cases, therefore, the antibodies neutralize virus infectivity presumably by blocking receptor binding as was observed for the anti-H3 antibody [132].

The sites of antibody binding and the molecular basis of binding specificity of a number of antibodies that bind to HAs of multiple subtypes have also been determined by X-ray crystallography. Two sorts of antibodies have been analyzed, one reacting exclusively with HAs of either group 1 or 2 [135–137], the other reacting with HAs of both groups [130]. In all cases the Fabs are bound to the F sub-domain of HA near the position where the "fusion peptide" is buried in the trimer interface (Figure 5.5). These antibodies block virus infection and can be shown, *in vitro*, to prevent the low pH-induced changes in conformation required for membrane fusion. They may neutralize virus infectivity by this mechanism or they may interfere with assembly or release of virus at later stages of virus replication. Because it is unnecessary *in vivo* for infection-blocking antibodies to inhibit a specific function of HA or NA, it is also possible that cell-associated HA–antibody complexes may target infected cells for lysis by Fc-receptor-bearing cells.

HA/NA co-variation of activity and specificity

Recognition of sialic acid by HA as virus receptor and by NA in virus release from infected cells leads to the evolution of balances in their specificities and affinities, which optimize virus replication [138]. Both HA and NA are species specific: all avian virus HAs prefer to bind sialic acid in α2,3-linkage; avian NAs are also

2,3-specific. Equine virus HAs prefer the α2,3-linkage but unlike avian viruses cannot bind 4-O-acetyl sialic acid, despite its abundance in equines; equine virus NA also cannot hydrolyze glycoconjugates containing 4-O-acetyl sialic acid. Infection and transmission in humans of the pandemic viruses H2N2 (1957) and H3N2 (1968), which were derived by reassortment from avian viruses, required changes in H2 and H3, and N2 specificity from α2,3-avian receptor, to α2,6-human receptor preference. Receptor binding specificity changed at the beginning of the pandemics as a result of Gln-226→Leu, and Gly-228→Ser mutations in the 220-loop of the receptor binding site. By contrast, changes in N2 specificity were more gradual, amounting to only about 30% α2,6- and 70% α2,3-linkage preference after 30 years in humans, accompanied by the mutation Ile-275→Val near the enzyme active site [139].

A number of *in vitro* experiments involving, for example, viruses with naturally occurring mutant H7 HA and N7 NA, or H1 viruses with deletion mutant N1, emphasize their required covariation for efficient virus replication [140, 141]. The mutations in H7 HA involved glycosylation near the receptor binding site, which decreased receptor binding affinity, presumably by decreasing receptor access to the site. In N7 NA, deletion of 28 residues from the stalk resulted in a short-stalk NA with lower enzyme activity, probably as a result of restricted access to the cell surface substrates. The reassorted viruses with lower receptor binding affinity were at a disadvantage during infection if sialic acid was removed too quickly from the cell surface by NA. However, they were less dependent on NA activity for release from infected cells. The most effective combinations recorded for virus production were glycosylated HA (low affinity) together with short-stalk NA (low activity), and unglycosylated HA (higher affinity) together with long-stalk NA (higher activity), consistent with the suspected optimum balances. In the H1N1 experiments multiple passage in eggs of an NA deletion mutant virus that was initially unable to replicate led to the selection of two sorts of viable viruses [141]. One sort contained recombinant genes for NA with insertions of fragments of unrelated virus genes that restored the length of the NA stalk. The other sort had decreased HA binding avidity as a result of mutations near the receptor binding site.

Analyses of drug-resistant mutants selected *in vitro* during the development of the anti-NA drugs zanamivir and oseltamivir lead to similar conclusions. They indicate that, *in vitro*, mutations in HA, which decrease receptor binding affinity to the extent that they are released from cells without NA activity, could result in the production of drug-resistant viruses [32, 93]. Additionally, viruses containing mutant HA with lower affinity for receptor were observed to require the presence of drug to block NA activity at the initial stages of infection, in this way ensuring that sufficient sialic acid was available on the surfaces of the cells for the mutant viruses to use as receptor.

References

1. Calder LJ, Wasilewski S, Berriman JA, Rosenthal PB. Structural organization of a filamentous influenza A virus. Proc Natl Acad Sci U S A. 2010;107(23):10685–90.
2. Rossman JS, Lamb RA. Influenza virus assembly and budding. Virology. 2011;411(2):229–36.
3. Wiley DC, Skehel JJ. The structure and function of the hemagglutinin membrane glycoprotein of influenza virus. Annu Rev Biochem. 1987;56:365–94.
4. Gallagher PJ, Henneberry JM, Sambrook JF, Gething MJ. Glycosylation requirements for intracellular transport and function of the hemagglutinin of influenza virus. J Virol. 1992;66(12):7136–45.
5. Daniels R, Kurowski B, Johnson AE, Hebert DN. N-linked glycans direct the cotranslational folding pathway of influenza hemagglutinin. Mol Cell. 2003;11(1):79–90.
6. Chen BJ, Takeda M, Lamb RA. Influenza virus hemagglutinin (H3 subtype) requires palmitoylation of its cytoplasmic tail for assembly: M1 proteins of two subtypes differ in their ability to support assembly. J Virol. [Research Support, N.I.H., Extramural Research Support, Non-U.S. Gov't Research Support, U.S. Gov't, P.H.S.]. 2005;79(21):13673–84.
7. Takeda M, Leser GP, Russell CJ, Lamb RA. Influenza virus hemagglutinin concentrates in lipid raft microdomains for efficient viral fusion. Proc Natl Acad Sci U S A. 2003;100(25):14610–7.
8. Colman PM, Ward CW. Structure and diversity of influenza virus neuraminidase. Curr Top Microbiol Immunol. 1985;114:177–255.
9. Gamblin SJ, Skehel JJ. Influenza hemagglutinin and neuraminidase membrane glycoproteins. J Biol Chem. 2010;285(37):28403–9.

10. Rosenthal PB, Zhang X, Formanowski F, Fitz W, Wong CH, Meier-Ewert H, et al. Structure of the haemagglutinin-esterase-fusion glycoprotein of influenza C virus. Nature. 1998;396(6706):92–6.

11. Skehel JJ, Wiley DC. Receptor binding and membrane fusion in virus entry: the influenza hemagglutinin. Annu Rev Biochem. 2000;69:531–69.

12. Varghese JN, Laver WG, Colman PM. Structure of the influenza virus glycoprotein antigen neuraminidase at 2.9 A resolution. Nature. 1983;303(5912):35–40.

13. Gottschalk A. The influenza virus neuraminidase. Nature. 1958;181(4606):377–8.

14. Klenk E, Faillard H, Lempfrid H. [Enzymatic effect of the influenza virus]. Hoppe Seylers Z Physiol Chem. 1955;301(4–6):235–46.

15. Lakadamyali M, Rust MJ, Babcock HP, Zhuang X. Visualizing infection of individual influenza viruses. Proc Natl Acad Sci U S A. [Research Support, U.S. Gov't, Non-P.H.S.]. 2003;100(16):9280–5.

16. Rust MJ, Lakadamyali M, Zhang F, Zhuang X. Assembly of endocytic machinery around individual influenza viruses during viral entry. Nat Struct Mol Biol. 2004;11(6):567–73.

17. Matrosovich MN, Matrosovich TY, Gray T, Roberts NA, Klenk HD. Neuraminidase is important for the initiation of influenza virus infection in human airway epithelium. J Virol. 2004;78(22):12665–7.

18. Palese P, Tobita K, Ueda M, Compans RW. Characterization of temperature sensitive influenza virus mutants defective in neuraminidase. Virology. 1974;61(2):397–410.

19. Webster RG, Bean WJ, Gorman OT, Chambers TM, Kawaoka Y. Evolution and ecology of influenza A viruses. Microbiol Rev. 1992;56(1):152–79.

20. Rogers GN, Paulson JC. Receptor determinants of human and animal influenza virus isolates: differences in receptor specificity of the H3 hemagglutinin based on species of origin. Virology. 1983;127(2):361–73.

21. Knossow M, Skehel JJ. Variation and infectivity neutralization in influenza. Immunology. 2006;119(1):1–7.

22. Gerhard W, Webster RG. Antigenic drift in influenza A viruses. I. Selection and characterization of antigenic variants of A/PR/8/34 (HON1) influenza virus with monoclonal antibodies. J Exp Med. 1978;148(2):383–92.

23. Gerhard W, Yewdell J, Frankel ME, Webster R. Antigenic structure of influenza virus haemagglutinin defined by hybridoma antibodies. Nature. 1981;290(5808):713–7.

24. Wrigley NG, Brown EB, Daniels RS, Douglas AR, Skehel JJ, Wiley DC. Electron microscopy of influenza haemagglutinin-monoclonal antibody complexes. Virology. [Research Support, U.S. Gov't, Non-P.H.S. Research Support, U.S. Gov't, P.H.S.]. 1983;131(2):308–14.

25. Throsby M, van den Brink E, Jongeneelen M, Poon LL, Alard P, Cornelissen L, et al. Heterosubtypic neutralizing monoclonal antibodies cross-protective against H5N1 and H1N1 recovered from human IgM+ memory B cells. PLoS ONE. [Research Support, Non-U.S. Gov't]. 2008;3(12):e3942.

26. Corti D, Suguitan AL Jr, Pinna D, Silacci C, Fernandez-Rodriguez BM, Vanzetta F, et al. Heterosubtypic neutralizing antibodies are produced by individuals immunized with a seasonal influenza vaccine. J Clin Invest. 2010;120(5):1663–73.

27. Colman PM, Varghese JN, Laver WG. Structure of the catalytic and antigenic sites in influenza virus neuraminidase. Nature. 1983;303(5912):41–4.

28. Tulloch PA, Colman PM, Davis PC, Laver WG, Webster RG, Air GM. Electron and X-ray diffraction studies of influenza neuraminidase complexed with monoclonal antibodies. J Mol Biol. 1986;190(2):215–25.

29. Tulip WR, Varghese JN, Webster RG, Laver WG, Colman PM. Crystal structures of two mutant neuraminidase-antibody complexes with amino acid substitutions in the interface. J Mol Biol. 1992;227(1):149–59.

30. Venkatramani L, Bochkareva E, Lee JT, Gulati U, Graeme Laver W, Bochkarev A, et al. An epidemiologically significant epitope of a 1998 human influenza virus neuraminidase forms a highly hydrated interface in the NA-antibody complex. J Mol Biol. 2006;356(3):651–63.

31. Colman PM. Influenza virus neuraminidase: structure, antibodies, and inhibitors. Protein Sci. 1994;3(10):1687–96.

32. McKimm-Breschkin JL, Blick TJ, Sahasrabudhe A, Tiong T, Marshall D, Hart GJ, et al. Generation and characterization of variants of NWS/G70C influenza virus after in vitro passage in 4-amino-Neu5Ac2en and 4-guanidino-Neu5Ac2en. Antimicrob Agents Chemother. 1996;40(1):40–6.

33. Paulson JC, Sadler JE, Hill RL. Restoration of specific myxovirus receptors to asialoerythrocytes by incorporation of sialic acid with pure sialyltransferases. J Biol Chem. 1979;254(6):2120–4.

34. Sauter NK, Bednarski MD, Wurzburg BA, Hanson JE, Whitesides GM, Skehel JJ, et al. Hemagglutinins from two influenza virus variants bind to sialic acid derivatives with millimolar dissociation constants: a 500-MHz proton nuclear magnetic resonance study. Biochemistry. 1989;28(21):8388–96.

35. Martin J, Wharton SA, Lin YP, Takemoto DK, Skehel JJ, Wiley DC, et al. Studies of the binding properties of influenza hemagglutinin receptor-site mutants. Virology. 1998;241(1):101–11.

36. Eisen MB, Sabesan S, Skehel JJ, Wiley DC. Binding of the influenza A virus to cell-surface receptors: structures of five hemagglutinin-sialyloligosaccharide complexes determined by X-ray crystallography. Virology. 1997;232(1):19–31.

37. Baum LG, Paulson JC. Sialyloligosaccharides of the respiratory epithelium in the selection of human influenza virus receptor specificity. Acta Histochem Suppl. 1990;40:35–8.

38. Shinya K, Ebina M, Yamada S, Ono M, Kasai N, Kawaoka Y. Avian flu: influenza virus receptors in the human airway. Nature. 2006;440(7083):435–6.

39. Matrosovich MN, Matrosovich TY, Gray T, Roberts NA, Klenk HD. Human and avian influenza viruses target different cell types in cultures of human airway epithelium. Proc Natl Acad Sci U S A. 2004;101(13):4620–4.

40. Matrosovich M, Tuzikov A, Bovin N, Gambaryan A, Klimov A, Castrucci MR, et al. Early alterations of the receptor-binding properties of H1, H2, and H3 avian influenza virus hemagglutinins after their introduction into mammals. J Virol. 2000;74(18):8502–12.

41. Ha Y, Stevens DJ, Skehel JJ, Wiley DC. X-ray structures of H5 avian and H9 swine influenza virus hemagglutinins bound to avian and human receptor analogs. Proc Natl Acad Sci U S A. 2001;98(20):11181–6.

42. Gambaryan A, Yamnikova S, Lvov D, Tuzikov A, Chinarev A, Pazynina G, et al. Receptor specificity of influenza viruses from birds and mammals: new data on involvement of the inner fragments of the carbohydrate chain. Virology. 2005;334(2):276–83.

43. Liu J, Stevens DJ, Haire LF, Walker PA, Coombs PJ, Russell RJ, et al. Structures of receptor complexes formed by hemagglutinins from the Asian Influenza pandemic of 1957. Proc Natl Acad Sci U S A. 2009;106(40):17175–80.

44. Couceiro JN, Paulson JC, Baum LG. Influenza virus strains selectively recognize sialyloligosaccharides on human respiratory epithelium; the role of the host cell in selection of hemagglutinin receptor specificity. Virus Res. 1993;29(2):155–65.

45. Hirst GK. Adsorption of Influenza Hemagglutinins and Virus by Red Blood Cells. J Exp Med. 1942;76(2):195–209.

46. Ito T, Suzuki Y, Mitnaul L, Vines A, Kida H, Kawaoka Y. Receptor specificity of influenza A viruses correlates with the agglutination of erythrocytes from different animal species. Virology. 1997;227(2):493–9.

47. Matrosovich MN, Gambaryan AS. Solid-phase assays of receptor-binding specificity. Methods Mol Biol. 2012;865:71–94.

48. Stevens J, Blixt O, Paulson JC, Wilson IA. Glycan microarray technologies: tools to survey host specificity of influenza viruses. Nat Rev Microbiol. 2006;4(11):857–64.

49. Takemoto DK, Skehel JJ, Wiley DC. A surface plasmon resonance assay for the binding of influenza virus hemagglutinin to its sialic acid receptor. Virology. 1996;217(2):452–8.

50. Lin YP, Xiong X, Wharton SA, Martin SR, Coombs PJ, Vachieri SG, et al. Evolution of the receptor binding properties of the influenza A(H3N2) hemagglutinin. Proc Natl Acad Sci U S A. 2012;109(52):21474–9. doi: 10.1073/pnas.1218841110.

51. Steinhauer DA. Role of hemagglutinin cleavage for the pathogenicity of influenza virus. Virology. 1999;258(1):1–20.

52. Hay AJ. The mechanism of action of amantadine and rimantadine against influenza virses. In: Notkins AL, Oldstone MBA, editors. Concepts in viral pathogenesis III. New York: Springer-Verlag; 1989. pp. 561–7.

53. Klenk HD, Garten W. Host cell proteases controlling virus pathogenicity. Trends Microbiol. 1994;2(2):39–43.

54. Rott R, Klenk HD, Nagai Y, Tashiro M. Influenza viruses, cell enzymes, and pathogenicity. Am J Respir Crit Care Med. 1995;152(4 Pt 2):S16–9.

55. Okumura Y, Takahashi E, Yano M, Ohuchi M, Daidoji T, Nakaya T, et al. Novel type II transmembrane serine proteases, MSPL and TMPRSS13, Proteolytically activate membrane fusion activity of the hemagglutinin of highly pathogenic avian influenza viruses and induce their multicycle replication. J Virol. 2010;84(10):5089–96.

56. Kido H, Beppu Y, Sakai K, Towatari T. Molecular basis of proteolytic activation of Sendai virus infection and the defensive compounds for infection. Biol Chem. 1997;378(3–4):255–63.

57. Bottcher E, Matrosovich T, Beyerle M, Klenk HD, Garten W, Matrosovich M. Proteolytic activation of influenza viruses by serine proteases TMPRSS2 and HAT from human airway epithelium. J Virol. 2006;80(19):9896–8.

58. Bottcher-Friebertshauser E, Freuer C, Sielaff F, Schmidt S, Eickmann M, Uhlendorff J, et al. Cleavage of influenza virus hemagglutinin by airway proteases TMPRSS2 and HAT differs in subcellular localization and susceptibility to protease inhibitors. J Virol. 2010;84(11):5605–14.

59. Zhirnov OP, Klenk HD, Wright PF. Aprotinin and similar protease inhibitors as drugs against influenza. Antiviral Res. 2011;92(1):27–36.

60. Sieczkarski SB, Whittaker GR. Influenza virus can enter and infect cells in the absence of clathrin-mediated endocytosis. J Virol. 2002;76(20): 10455–64.

61. Lozach PY, Huotari J, Helenius A. Late-penetrating viruses. Curr Opin Virol. 2011;1(1):35–43.

62. Ruigrok RW, Martin SR, Wharton SA, Skehel JJ, Bayley PM, Wiley DC. Conformational changes in the hemagglutinin of influenza virus which accompany heat-induced fusion of virus with liposomes. Virology. 1986;155(2):484–97.

63. Daniels RS, Downie JC, Hay AJ, Knossow M, Skehel JJ, Wang ML, et al. Fusion mutants of the influenza virus hemagglutinin glycoprotein. Cell. 1985;40(2):431–9.

64. Lin YP, Wharton SA, Martin J, Skehel JJ, Wiley DC, Steinhauer DA. Adaptation of egg-grown and trans-fectant influenza viruses for growth in mammalian cells: selection of hemagglutinin mutants with elevated pH of membrane fusion. Virology. 1997;233(2): 402–10.

65. Rotzschke O, Lau JM, Hofstatter M, Falk K, Strominger JL. A pH-sensitive histidine residue as control element for ligand release from HLA-DR molecules. Proc Natl Acad Sci U S A. 2002;99(26): 16946–50.

66. Bizebard T, Gigant B, Rigolet P, Rasmussen B, Diat O, Bosecke P, et al. Structure of influenza virus haemagglutinin complexed with a neutralizing antibody. Nature. 1995;376(6535):92–4.

67. Bullough PA, Hughson FM, Skehel JJ, Wiley DC. Structure of influenza haemagglutinin at the pH of membrane fusion. Nature. 1994;371(6492):37–43.

68. Chen J, Skehel JJ, Wiley DC. N- and C-terminal residues combine in the fusion-pH influenza hemagglutinin HA(2) subunit to form an N cap that terminates the triple-stranded coiled coil. Proc Natl Acad Sci U S A. 1999;96(16):8967–72.

69. White JM, Wilson IA. Anti-peptide antibodies detect steps in a protein conformational change: low-pH activation of the influenza virus hemagglutinin. J Cell Biol. 1987;105(6 Pt 2):2887–96.

70. Ruigrok RW, Wrigley NG, Calder LJ, Cusack S, Wharton SA, Brown EB, et al. Electron microscopy of the low pH structure of influenza virus haemagglutinin. EMBO J. 1986;5(1):41–9.

71. Tsurudome M, Gluck R, Graf R, Falchetto R, Schaller U, Brunner J. Lipid interactions of the hemagglutinin HA2 NH2-terminal segment during influenza virus-induced membrane fusion. J Biol Chem. 1992;267(28): 20225–32.

72. Carr CM, Kim PS. A spring-loaded mechanism for the conformational change of influenza hemagglutinin. Cell. 1993;73(4):823–32.

73. Ward CW, Dopheide TA. Influenza virus haemagglutinin. Structural predictions suggest that the fibrillar appearance is due to the presence of a coiled-coil. Aust J Biol Sci. 1980;33(4):441–7.

74. Weissenhorn W, Dessen A, Calder LJ, Harrison SC, Skehel JJ, Wiley DC. Structural basis for membrane fusion by enveloped viruses. Mol Membr Biol. 1999;16(1):3–9.

75. Kozlov MM, Chernomordik LV. A mechanism of protein-mediated fusion: coupling between refolding of the influenza hemagglutinin and lipid rearrangements. Biophys J. 1998;75(3):1384–96.

76. Siegel DP, Epand RM. Effect of influenza hemagglutinin fusion peptide on lamellar/inverted phase transitions in dipalmitoleoylphosphatidylethanolamine: implications for membrane fusion mechanisms. Biochim Biophys Acta. 2000;1468(1–2):87–98.

77. Imai M, Mizuno T, Kawasaki K. Membrane fusion by single influenza hemagglutinin trimers. Kinetic evidence from image analysis of hemagglutinin-reconstituted vesicles. J Biol Chem. 2006;281(18): 12729–35.

78. Kim CS, Epand RF, Leikina E, Epand RM, Chernomordik LV. The final conformation of the complete ectodomain of the HA2 subunit of influenza hemagglutinin can by itself drive low pH-dependent fusion. J Biol Chem. 2011;286(15):13226–34.

79. Cohen FS, Melikyan GB. Implications of a fusion peptide structure. Nat Struct Biol. 2001;8(8):653–5.

80. Melikyan GB, Lin S, Roth MG, Cohen FS. Amino acid sequence requirements of the transmembrane and cytoplasmic domains of influenza virus hemagglutinin for viable membrane fusion. Mol Biol Cell. 1999;10(6): 1821–36.

81. Skehel JJ, Wharton S, Calder L, Stevens DJ, editors. On the activation of membrane fusion by influenza haemagglutinin. 2008.

82. Cross KJ, Langley WA, Russell RJ, Skehel JJ, Steinhauer DA. Composition and functions of the influenza fusion peptide. Protein Pept Lett. 2009;16(7): 766–78.

83. Han X, Steinhauer DA, Wharton SA, Tamm LK. Interaction of mutant influenza virus hemagglutinin fusion peptides with lipid bilayers: probing the role of hydrophobic residue size in the central region of the fusion peptide. Biochemistry. 1999;38(45):15052–9.

84. Skehel JJ, Cross K, Steinhauer D, Wiley DC. Influenza fusion peptides. Biochem Soc Trans. [Comparative Study Research Support, Non-U.S. Gov't Research Support, U.S. Gov't, P.H.S. Review]. 2001;29(Pt 4): 623–6.

85. Han X, Bushweller JH, Cafiso DS, Tamm LK. Membrane structure and fusion-triggering conformational

change of the fusion domain from influenza hemagglutinin. Nat Struct Biol. 2001;8(8):715–20.

86. Lorieau JL, Louis JM, Bax A. The complete influenza hemagglutinin fusion domain adopts a tight helical hairpin arrangement at the lipid:water interface. Proc Natl Acad Sci U S A. 2010;107(25):11341–6.

87. Webster RG, Laver WG, Kilbourne ED. Reactions of antibodies with surface antigens of influenza virus. J Gen Virol. 1968;3(3):315–26.

88. Burmeister WP, Ruigrok RW, Cusack S. The 2.2 A resolution crystal structure of influenza B neuraminidase and its complex with sialic acid. EMBO J. 1992;11(1):49–56.

89. Colman PM. Structural basis of antigenic variation: studies of influenza virus neuraminidase. Immunol Cell Biol. 1992;70(Pt 3):209–14.

90. Taylor NR, von Itzstein M. Molecular modeling studies on ligand binding to sialidase from influenza virus and the mechanism of catalysis. J Med Chem. 1994;37(5):616–24.

91. von Itzstein M. The war against influenza: discovery and development of sialidase inhibitors. Nat Rev Drug Discov. 2007;6(12):967–74.

92. Aymard-Henry M, Coleman MT, Dowdle WR, Laver WG, Schild GC, Webster RG. Influenzavirus neuraminidase and neuraminidase-inhibition test procedures. Bull World Health Organ. 1973;48(2):199–202.

93. Baigent SJ, Bethell RC, McCauley JW. Genetic analysis reveals that both haemagglutinin and neuraminidase determine the sensitivity of naturally occurring avian influenza viruses to zanamivir in vitro. Virology. 1999;263(2):323–38.

94. Potier M, Mameli L, Belisle M, Dallaire L, Melancon SB. Fluorometric assay of neuraminidase with a sodium (4-methylumbelliferyl-alpha-D-N-acetylneuraminate) substrate. Anal Biochem. 1979;94(2):287–96.

95. Buxton RC, Edwards B, Juo RR, Voyta JC, Tisdale M, Bethell RC. Development of a sensitive chemiluminescent neuraminidase assay for the determination of influenza virus susceptibility to zanamivir. Anal Biochem. 2000;280(2):291–300.

96. Johansson BE, Brett IC. Variation in the divalent cation requirements of influenza a virus N2 neuraminidases. J Biochem. 2003;134(3):345–52.

97. Collins PJ, Haire LF, Lin YP, Liu J, Russell RJ, Walker PA, et al. Crystal structures of oseltamivir-resistant influenza virus neuraminidase mutants. Nature. 2008;453(7199):1258–61.

98. Watowich SJ, Skehel JJ, Wiley DC. Crystal structures of influenza virus hemagglutinin in complex with high-affinity receptor analogs. Structure. 1994;2(8):719–31.

99. Glick GD, Toogood PL, Wiley DC, Skehel JJ, Knowles JR. Ligand recognition by influenza virus. The binding of bivalent sialosides. J Biol Chem. 1991;266(35):23660–9.

100. Reuter JD, Myc A, Hayes MM, Gan Z, Roy R, Qin D, et al. Inhibition of viral adhesion and infection by sialic-acid-conjugated dendritic polymers. Bioconjug Chem. 1999;10(2):271–8.

101. Garten W, Hallenberger S, Ortmann D, Schafer W, Vey M, Angliker H, et al. Processing of viral glycoproteins by the subtilisin-like endoprotease furin and its inhibition by specific peptidylchloroalkylketones. Biochimie. 1994;76(3–4):217–25.

102. Kido H, Beppu Y, Imamura Y, Chen Y, Murakami M, Oba K, et al. The human mucus protease inhibitor and its mutants are novel defensive compounds against infection with influenza A and Sendai viruses. Biopolymers. 1999;51(1):79–86.

103. Staschke KA, Hatch SD, Tang JC, Hornback WJ, Munroe JE, Colacino JM, et al. Inhibition of influenza virus hemagglutinin-mediated membrane fusion by a compound related to podocarpic acid. Virology. 1998;248(2):264–74.

104. Plotch SJ, O'Hara B, Morin J, Palant O, LaRocque J, Bloom JD, et al. Inhibition of influenza A virus replication by compounds interfering with the fusogenic function of the viral hemagglutinin. J Virol. 1999;73(1):140–51.

105. Cianci C, Yu KL, Dischino DD, Harte W, Deshpande M, Luo G, et al. pH-dependent changes in photoaffinity labeling patterns of the H1 influenza virus hemagglutinin by using an inhibitor of viral fusion. J Virol. 1999;73(3):1785–94.

106. Hoffman LR, Kuntz ID, White JM. Structure-based identification of an inducer of the low-pH conformational change in the influenza virus hemagglutinin: irreversible inhibition of infectivity. J Virol. 1997;71(11):8808–20.

107. Russell RJ, Kerry PS, Stevens DJ, Steinhauer DA, Martin SR, Gamblin SJ, et al. Structure of influenza hemagglutinin in complex with an inhibitor of membrane fusion. Proc Natl Acad Sci U S A. 2008;105(46):17736–41.

108. Colman PM. Neuraminidase inhibitors as antivirals. Vaccine. 2002;20(Suppl. 2):S55–8.

109. Colman PM. New antivirals and drug resistance. Annu Rev Biochem. 2009;78:95–118.

110. Kim CU, Lew W, Williams MA, Liu H, Zhang L, Swaminathan S, et al. Influenza neuraminidase inhibitors possessing a novel hydrophobic interaction in the enzyme active site: design, synthesis, and structural analysis of carbocyclic sialic acid analogues with potent anti-influenza activity. J Am Chem Soc. 1997;119(4):681–90.

111. Gubareva LV, Webster RG, Hayden FG. Comparison of the activities of zanamivir, oseltamivir, and RWJ-270201 against clinical isolates of influenza virus and neuraminidase inhibitor-resistant variants. Antimicrob Agents Chemother. 2001;45(12):3403–8.

112. Russell RJ, Haire LF, Stevens DJ, Collins PJ, Lin YP, Blackburn GM, et al. The structure of H5N1 avian influenza neuraminidase suggests new opportunities for drug design. Nature. 2006;443(7107):45–9.

113. Rudrawar S, Dyason JC, Rameix-Welti MA, Rose FJ, Kerry PS, Russell RJ, et al. Novel sialic acid derivatives lock open the 150-loop of an influenza A virus group-1 sialidase. Nat Commun. 2010;1:113.

114. Konig R, Stertz S, Zhou Y, Inoue A, Hoffmann HH, Bhattacharyya S, et al. Human host factors required for influenza virus replication. Nature. 2010;463 (7282):813–7.

115. A revision of the system of nomenclature for influenza viruses: a WHO memorandum. Bull World Health Organ. 1980;58(4):585–91.

116. Ha Y, Stevens DJ, Skehel JJ, Wiley DC. H5 avian and H9 swine influenza virus haemagglutinin structures: possible origin of influenza subtypes. EMBO J. 2002;21(5):865–75.

117. Russell RJ, Gamblin SJ, Haire LF, Stevens DJ, Xiao B, Ha Y, et al. H1 and H7 influenza haemagglutinin structures extend a structural classification of haemagglutinin subtypes. Virology. 2004;325(2):287–96.

118. Caton AJ, Brownlee GG, Yewdell JW, Gerhard W. The antigenic structure of the influenza virus A/PR/8/34 hemagglutinin (H1 subtype). Cell. 1982;31(2 Pt 1):417–27.

119. Wiley DC, Wilson IA, Skehel JJ. Structural identification of the antibody-binding sites of Hong Kong influenza haemagglutinin and their involvement in antigenic variation. Nature. 1981;289(5796):373–8.

120. Xu X, Cox NJ, Bender CA, Regnery HL, Shaw MW. Genetic variation in neuraminidase genes of influenza A (H3N2) viruses. Virology. 1996;224(1):175–83.

121. Knossow M, Daniels RS, Douglas AR, Skehel JJ, Wiley DC. Three-dimensional structure of an antigenic mutant of the influenza virus haemagglutinin. Nature. 1984;311(5987):678–80.

122. Tulip WR, Varghese JN, Baker AT, van Donkelaar A, Laver WG, Webster RG, et al. Refined atomic structures of N9 subtype influenza virus neuraminidase and escape mutants. J Mol Biol. 1991;221(2):487–97.

123. Godley L, Pfeifer J, Steinhauer D, Ely B, Shaw G, Kaufmann R, et al. Introduction of intersubunit disulfide bonds in the membrane-distal region of the influenza hemagglutinin abolishes membrane fusion activity. Cell. 1992;68(4):635–45.

124. Knossow M, Gaudier M, Douglas A, Barrere B, Bizebard T, Barbey C, et al. Mechanism of neutralization of influenza virus infectivity by antibodies. Virology. 2002;302(2):294–8.

125. Das SR, Hensley SE, David A, Schmidt L, Gibbs JS, Puigbo P, et al. Fitness costs limit influenza A virus hemagglutinin glycosylation as an immune evasion strategy. Proc Natl Acad Sci U S A. 2011;108(51): E1417–22.

126. Molinari M, Eriksson KK, Calanca V, Galli C, Cresswell P, Michalak M, et al. Contrasting functions of calreticulin and calnexin in glycoprotein folding and ER quality control. Mol Cell. 2004;13(1): 125–35.

127. Gambaryan AS, Robertson JS, Matrosovich MN. Effects of egg-adaptation on the receptor-binding properties of human influenza A and B viruses. Virology. 1999;258(2):232–9.

128. Skehel JJ, Stevens DJ, Daniels RS, Douglas AR, Knossow M, Wilson IA, et al. A carbohydrate side chain on hemagglutinins of Hong Kong influenza viruses inhibits recognition by a monoclonal antibody. Proc Natl Acad Sci U S A. 1984;81(6):1779–83.

129. Abe Y, Takashita E, Sugawara K, Matsuzaki Y, Muraki Y, Hongo S. Effect of the addition of oligosaccharides on the biological activities and antigenicity of influenza A/H3N2 virus hemagglutinin. J Virol. 2004;78(18): 9605–11.

130. Corti D, Voss J, Gamblin SJ, Codoni G, Macagno A, Jarrossay D, et al. A neutralizing antibody selected from plasma cells that binds to group 1 and group 2 influenza A hemagglutinins. Science. 2011;333(6044): 850–6.

131. Imai M, Watanabe T, Hatta M, Das SC, Ozawa M, Shinya K, et al. Experimental adaptation of an influenza H5 HA confers respiratory droplet transmission to a reassortant H5 HA/H1N1 virus in ferrets. Nature. 2012;486(7403):420–8.

132. Daniels PS, Jeffries S, Yates P, Schild GC, Rogers GN, Paulson JC, et al. The receptor-binding and membrane-fusion properties of influenza virus variants selected using anti-haemagglutinin monoclonal antibodies. EMBO J. 1987;6(5):1459–65.

133. Hu H, Voss J, Zhang G, Buchy P, Zuo T, Wang L, et al. A human antibody recognizing a conserved epitope of H5 hemagglutinin broadly neutralizes highly pathogenic avian influenza H5N1 viruses. J Virol. 2012;86 (6):2978–89.

134. Whittle JR, Zhang R, Khurana S, King LR, Manischewitz J, Golding H, et al. Broadly neutralizing human antibody that recognizes the receptor-binding pocket of influenza virus hemagglutinin. Proc Natl Acad Sci U S A. 2011;108(34):14216–21.

135. Ekiert DC, Bhabha G, Elsliger MA, Friesen RH, Jongeneelen M, Throsby M, et al. Antibody recognition

of a highly conserved influenza virus epitope. Science. 2009;324(5924):246–51.

136. Ekiert DC, Friesen RH, Bhabha G, Kwaks T, Jongeneelen M, Yu W, et al. A highly conserved neutralizing epitope on group 2 influenza A viruses. Science. 2011;333(6044):843–50.

137. Sui J, Hwang WC, Perez S, Wei G, Aird D, Chen LM, et al. Structural and functional bases for broad-spectrum neutralization of avian and human influenza A viruses. Nat Struct Mol Biol. 2009;16(3):265–73.

138. Wagner R, Matrosovich M, Klenk HD. Functional balance between haemagglutinin and neuraminidase in influenza virus infections. Rev Med Virol. [Research Support, Non-U.S. Gov't Review]. 2002;12(3):159–66.

139. Kobasa D, Kodihalli S, Luo M, Castrucci MR, Donatelli I, Suzuki Y, et al. Amino acid residues contribut-

ing to the substrate specificity of the influenza A virus neuraminidase. J Virol. 1999;73(8):6743–51.

140. Baigent SJ, McCauley JW. Glycosylation of haemagglutinin and stalk-length of neuraminidase combine to regulate the growth of avian influenza viruses in tissue culture. Virus Res. 2001;79(1–2):177–85.

141. Mitnaul LJ, Matrosovich MN, Castrucci MR, Tuzikov AB, Bovin NV, Kobasa D, et al. Balanced hemagglutinin and neuraminidase activities are critical for efficient replication of influenza A virus. J Virol. [Research Support, Non-U.S. Gov't Research Support, U.S. Gov't, P.H.S.]. 2000;74(13):6015–20.

142. Maines TR, Chen LM, Van Hoeven N, Trumpey TM, Blixt O, Belsen JA, et al. Effect of receptor binding domain mutations on receptor binding and transmissibility of avian influenza H5N1 viruses. Virology. 2011;413(1):139–47.

6

Proton channels of influenza A and B viruses

Chunlong Ma[1,2], Lawrence H. Pinto[1], and Robert A. Lamb[2,3]

[1]Department of Neurobiology, Northwestern University, Evanston, IL, USA
[2]Department of Molecular Biosciences, Northwestern University, Evanston, IL, USA
[3]Howard Hughes Medical Institute, Northwestern University, Evanston, IL, USA

Influenza A virus M2 protein

The influenza A virus M2 protein is encoded by a spliced mRNA derived from RNA segment 7 [1]. The M2 protein [2] is a 97 residue integral membrane protein [3] which has a small ectodomain of 23 residues, a 19 residue transmembrane (TM) domain and a 54 residue cytoplasmic tail [3]. The M2 protein is a homotetramer that either forms a completely disulfide-linked homotetramer or a tetramer consisting of a pair of disulfide-linked dimers [4,5]. Adjacent to the cytoplasmic face of the membrane is an amphipathic helix (residues 47–60) which is involved in cholesterol binding, filamentous virus formation, and membrane scission [6–8]. In virus infected cells, M2 is expressed abundantly at the cell surface [3] and is localized to the periphery of lipid rafts [7–10], microdomains that are enriched in sphingomyelin and cholesterol, and it is from these domains that influenza virus buds [11]. Only 15–20 tetramers of M2 on average become incorporated into a spherical virion [12]. A monoclonal antibody (MAb) (14C2) specific for the M2 ectodomain, restricts the growth of some strains of influenza virus [12] and this MAb causes the fragmentation of filamentous particles into spherical particles [7]. The change in curvature of membranes is a property of the M2 amphipathic helix [7]. The M2 ectodomain is fairly well conserved among all influenza A virus subtypes and this raises the possibility that the M2 ectodomain (M2e) is a possible immunogen vaccine candidate [13,14]. The M2 protein has also been implicated in activating inflammasomes [15] and in blocking autophagosome fusion with lysosomes ([16], reviewed in [17]).

The A/M2 protein has ion channel activity that is required for efficient viral replication

A series of studies demonstrated that the M2 protein has a role in the virus life cycle. The antiviral drug amantadine and its analog compound rimantadine inhibit influenza A virus replication [18]. In the presence of the drug, the ribonucleoprotein (RNP)–M1 protein complex was able to be isolated from virions at neutral pH, whereas this complex was not isolated in the absence of the drug [19]. *In vitro* studies showed that acidic treatment (pH 5.5) specifically removes M1 from the RNPs [20]. Studies with amantadine-resistant mutant influenza A viruses showed that the amino acid substitutions mapped to the TM domain of the A/M2 protein, suggesting that amantadine-like drugs target the A/M2 protein [54]. Finally, in some strains of influenza virus, for example H7N1 fowl plague virus, where the hemagglutinin

Textbook of Influenza, Second Edition. Edited by Robert G. Webster, Arnold S. Monto, Thomas J. Braciale, and Robert A. Lamb.
© 2013 John Wiley & Sons, Ltd. Published 2013 by John Wiley & Sons, Ltd.

has a high pH (pH 6) of transition to the low pH induced form of HA, the A/M2 protein equilibrates the pH of the trans-Golgi network with that of the cytoplasm to prevent a premature conformational change in HA [21–25]. In aggregate these data indicated that the A/M2 protein facilitates the dissociation of the RNP–M1 complex by acidifying the interior of virions when they are in endosomes during the uncoating process and also by helping to prevent a premature conformational change in HA by equilibrating the pH of the Golgi lumen with that of the cytoplasm. Both of these findings suggested that the protein possessed proton channel activity ([4]; reviewed in [26]).

Direct experimental evidence that the M2 protein had ion channel activity was obtained by *in vitro* expression of M2 protein in oocytes of *Xenopus laevis* and two electrode voltage clamp measurements [27]. When the A/M2 protein was expressed on the plasma membrane of oocytes, an inward current flowed when the oocytes were exposed to low pH in the bathing solution, analogous to lowering the pH of the medium bathing the ectodomain of the M2 protein in a virion [27]. This inward current was specifically blocked by the antiviral drugs amantadine and rimantadine. Moreover, when the amantadine-resistant mutant A/M2-S31N was expressed in oocytes, amantadine did not block oocyte conductance [27]. M2-specific surface conductances were also observed in mammalian cells [28,29] and artificial lipid bilayers [30,31].

Although a series of studies established that the ion channel activity of the A/M2 protein facilitates influenza virion uncoating in endosomes and equilibrates the pH of the trans Golgi with the cytoplasm, one study reported that influenza A virus can undergo multiple cycles of replication without M2 ion channel activity [32]. An A/M2 protein was found that displayed no detectable ion channel activity after a deletion of three amino acids in TM domain (M2-del29-31) [27], and a mutant virus was recovered containing this mutant A/M2 protein. The growth of this mutant virus was reported to be "very similar" to the growth of wt influenza A virus [32]. This unexpected observation was re-examined by Takeda et al. [33], who found that the rate of growth of the M2-del29-31 virus was comparable with that of the amantadine sensitive N31S M2 A/WSN/33 virus after this virus was inhibited by amantadine. Moreover, in a biologic

fitness assay, in which one genotype of virus was pitted against the other in a competition study, the wt influenza virus completely outgrew viruses containing the M2-del29-31 after 4 days, even though the initial coinfection contained a 100 times greater M2-del29-31 titer.

Taking these results together, we conclude that the M2 channel function is indeed essential for viral replication (Figure 6.1). Spherical influenza A virus particles mostly enter cells via clathrin-mediated endocytosis. While in the endosome, in order to release the M1 protein from the RNPs, the interior of membrane-bound virus must be acidified. M2 proton channels facilitate the flow of protons from the acidic endosome lumen to the interior of the virion to serve this acidification function. This function has been found to be essential in all subtypes of influenza A virus that have been studied.

M2 proton conduction mechanism

The M2 proton conduction mechanism has been studied extensively in oocytes, mammalian cells, and lipid bilayers [27–29,34,35]. When the wt A/M2 protein was expressed on the plasma membrane of oocytes [27] or mammalian cells [29], the channel was activated by lowering the bath solution pH, but it was not activated by changing membrane voltage. His37 is the only residue in the TM domain with a pKa in the relevant pH range. When His37 was replaced by Gly, or Glu, the channel was no longer regulated by pH of the bathing medium (external pH) and was not selective for protons; however, this mutant ion channel was still partially inhibited by amantadine [36]. Recent solid state nuclear magnetic resonance (ssNMR) studies have measured the pKa values for the His37 residues (see below); from these studies, it has been concluded that protonation of His37 is an essential step for both activation of the M2 channel and conducting protons across the channel.

Under normal conditions, the A/M2 protein only conducts protons. This nearly perfect proton selectivity relies on the presence of His37. From the measurement of reversal potential using *in vitro* expression systems, such as oocytes and mammalian cells, the estimated selectivity of protons over Na^+ or K^+ is $>1.5 \times 10^6$ [30,37]. Mutation of His37 to Gly, Ala,

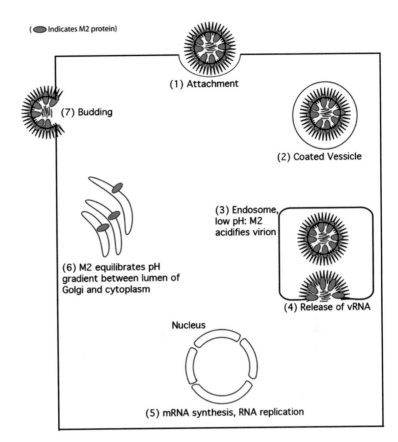

(● Indicates M2 protein)

(1) Attachment

(7) Budding

(2) Coated Vessicle

(3) Endosome, low pH: M2 acidifies virion

(6) M2 equilibrates pH gradient between lumen of Golgi and cytoplasm

(4) Release of vRNA

Nucleus

(5) mRNA synthesis, RNA replication

Figure 6.1. Life cycle of influenza virus showing the steps in which the A/M2 proton channel functions. The life cycle and the role of the A/M2 channel are similar for both influenza A and B viruses. In the endosome (step 3), the A/M2 proton-selective ion channel conducts protons into the interior of virions, facilitating the uncoating process. For certain strains of influenza A viruses, in the trans-Golgi apparatus (step 6), the A/M2 channel also equilibrates the pH gradient to prevent premature conformational changes of hemagglutinin. Reproduced from Pinto and Lamb [76] with permission of The Royal Society of Chemistry (RSC) for the European Society for Photobiology, the European Photochemistry Association, and the RSC.

Glu, Ser, or Thr enables the channel to conduct Na^+ and K^+ [36]. Moreover, when imidazole (the histidine side-chain) was added to the medium bathing the His37 substitution mutants, proton selectivity was partially restored. Thus, the proton conduction mechanism requires the presence of His37 in order to ensure the high proton selectivity.

The A/M2 proton channel rectifies inwardly (protons flow more easily in the inward direction). The opening and closing of the A/M2 channel (channel gating) is exclusively regulated by the external pH (of the medium bathing the ectodomain), but not internal pH (of the medium bathing the endodomain). Cells expressing the wt A/M2 protein bathed in low pH solution displayed inward current, the magnitude of which increased with the decrease of external pH (in the range of pH 7.0–5.0). However, cells did not display outward current even when the internal pH

of cells was deliberately lowered by injection of acidic HCl solution or incubation at lower pH solution for an extended period [34]. Extensive mutagenesis studies indicated that Trp41 in the TM domain functions as a gate. Unlike the case for the wt A/M2 channel, the mutant channel formed when Trp41 was mutated to Ala, Cys, or Phe (but not Tyr), *did* display outward proton current when the internal pH was lowered [34]. Another line of evidence for Trp41 gating function comes from studies with divalent copper ion. Cu^{2+} is able to coordinate His37, and therefore was found to inhibit channel activity when Cu^{2+} was applied externally. On the other hand, when Cu^{2+} was injected into cells, the inhibition was only observed for the W41A mutant channel, but not for the wt A/M2 channel. The simple explanation for this observation is that the bulky Trp41 side-chain blocks the access of Cu^{2+} to His37 residues when Cu^{2+} is

103

applied internally [34]. Furthermore, Raman spectroscopy demonstrated a pH-dependent interaction between Trp41 and His37 [38]. Concerted conformational changes in His37 and Trp41 are thought to constitute the heart of the proton conduction cycle [39].

There is a general consensus that the A/M2 proton channel has a very low conductance [30,35,40]. Indeed, in some reports the A/M2 protein is proposed to be a transporter because of its low conductance. Under the assumption that all A/M2 proteins on the membrane form an open channel, A/M2 is calculated to conduct 1–1000 proton/s/channel under the experimental conditions of external pH between 5 and 7, and electrical gradient between 0 and 130 mV. These rates are much lower than those of K^+ or Na^+ channels under physiologic conditions. The slow conduction rate of the A/M2 channel does not imply that in the proton conduction cycle it must overcome a large energy barrier; it is possibly a simple consequence of very low proton availability under physiologic conditions (pH 5–7). However, the inherent concentration dependence of an ion channel does not ensure that when proton concentration is increased, the channel conduction rate will increase proportionally. One interesting observation is that when the bath solution pH is lowered to below 5, the conduction rate seems to reach a maximal value for some A/M2 variants [28]. Two types of models have been proposed to explain reaching a maximal value.

Both a channel gating model and a shuttle model [41,42] have been proposed to explain the proton conductance of the A/M2 ion channel. Functional studies have established that the motif $H^{37}XXXW^{41}$ is the heart of the proton conduction mechanism, and extensive molecular dynamics(MD) simulations have been carried out to study the proton conduction mechanism. In the channel gating model, the pH-dependent activation of the A/M2 channel is associated with His37 tetrad protonation. When His37 is protonated in the tetrad, the channel is opened by positive electrostatic repulsion, thereby forming a continuous water wire. MD simulation suggested that a small conformational change in the His37 side-chain is enough to open the channel. In this model, the saturation of the conduction rate at lower pH can be explained if the entry of protons into the channel is much faster than the rate at which the proton travels through the channel. In this case the time

taken to travel through the channel is the rate limiting step, and is independent of the bulk proton concentration.

The second explanation for proton transport reaching a maximal value is provided by the shuttle model, which involves the protonation and deprotonation of His37. The initial shuttle model proposed the following steps: His37 side-chain imidazole accepts one proton from the extracellular (ectodomain) side to form a biprotonated intermediate; then the bound proton is released to the intracellular (endodomain) side, and His37 returns to the neutral form [42]. With the availability of high resolution structures in different confirmations as well as dynamic details for these conformations, this model was expanded. Hu et al. [43] reported that the pKa values for successive protonation of four His37 residues in the A/M2 TM domain in the lipid bilayer were 8.2, 8.2, 6.3, and <5.0. Nuclear magnetic resonance (NMR) studies showed that after the third proton binds to the His37 tetrad, the A/M2 channel is much more dynamic than the 0, +1, and +2 states [44]. One recent simulation showed that the +3 state has the lowest free energy barrier for proton permeation [45]. Very recently, Hong et al. [39], in an ssNMR study, proposed a proton conduction mechanism in which His37 dynamically shuttles protons into the virion. In this mechanism, the rate-limiting step is the ring-flip-assisted His37 deprotonation of the imidazole side-chain. This feature of the shuttle model helps to explain the low pH conduction saturation.

Atomic structures of the A/M2 channel

Many structural and biophysical studies were carried out on a peptide corresponding to the M2 protein pore-forming TM domain but some structural studies also included the cytoplasmic amphipathic helix. Prior to the availability of high resolution structures of the A/M2 protein solved by X-ray crystallography [46] and NMR spectroscopy [44,47,48], the first A/M2 TM domain model was constructed by Cys-scanning mutagenesis studies [42]. A series of Cys mutations was successively generated in the TM domain, mutant proteins were expressed in *Xenopus* oocytes, and changes of channel properties (activity, selectivity, and amantadine sensitivity) were measured. Based on the changes in these functional properties with residue number, a three-dimensional structural model was proposed. A continuous channel, enough to accommodate an amantadine molecule, was proposed to exist from the N-terminus to His37. This proposed cavity was largest in the vicinity of Gly34, and the only major occlusion of the channel lay at His37. The key features of this model were confirmed by high resolution structures solved more than a decade later [46].

It is important to consider the minimal size of peptide derived from the M2 sequence that retains the key features of the A/M2 ion channel, proton selectivity and activation, and amantadine sensitivity. This is important because structural studies of the A/M2 channel have in some cases used only the TM domain or in other cases the TM domain plus the amphiphilic domain, and/or nearly the entire protein [39,44,46]. Several lines of evidence indicate that the amphiphilic helix is not required for A/M2 channel function.

1. Synthetic peptides spanning residues 22–46 conducted protons into liposomes in an amantadine-sensitive manner when these peptides were incorporated into liposome bilayers. Parallel studies with oocytes showed that the same length peptide was not expressed at the oocyte plasma membrane; however, a peptide consisting of the TM domain and part of amphiphic helix [21–51] did display amantadine-sensitive inward current in oocytes.

2. When five hydrophobic residues of the amphiphilic helix facing the plasma membrane (Phe47, Phe48, Ile51, Ile51, and Phe55) were mutated to Ala simultaneously, the resulting mutant A/M2 channel displayed indistinguishable channel properties from the wt A/M2 channel. A recent study showed that the amphiphic helix is very important to viron budding and scission from the infected cell [8].

The models of the A/M2 protein structure derived by using different techniques (i.e., X-ray crystallography, solution NMR, and ssNMR) have similar overall features, among which are a left-handed helical TM domain, pore-lining residues that agree with those identified in functional studies, and a water-filled channel (Figure 6.2) [44,46,48,49]. The crystal structure with the highest resolution (1.65 Å

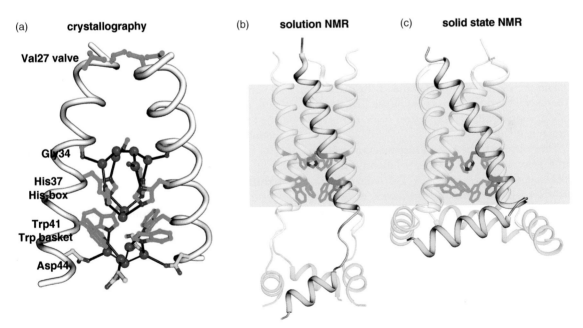

(a) **crystallography** (b) **solution NMR** (c) **solid state NMR**

Val27 valve

Gly34

His37
His box

Trp41
Trp basket

Asp44

Figure 6.2. Comparison of (a) crystal structure (PDB:3LBW), (b) solution NMR structure (PDB: 2RLF), and (c) solid state NMR structure (PDB:2L0J). Critical residue His37 is in cyan, Trp41 is in green [75]. Reproduced from Pielak et al. [74] with permission from Elsevier.

105

in detergent micelles at pH 6.5), (protein data base; PDB 3LBW; Figure 6.2a), shows the channel pore to be lined by ordered water molecules alternating with the side-chains of the pore-lining resides. The channel pore is interrupted by the His37 residue, forming a "His-box." Below this "His-box," Trp41 forms a "Trp-basket." The volume between the "His-box" and the "Trp-basket" are bridged by an ordered water cluster. The conformation of this structure is intermediate between the structures solved at higher and lower pH [46], suggesting a mechanism in which conformational changes facilitate proton conduction through the channel pore.

The A/M2 protein has been extensively studied by ssNMR. Earlier work by Kovacs et al. [50] determined the helix orientation and tilt by measuring orientation-dependent 15N tensors. Recently, tetramer structures (PDB numbers 2KQT, 2L0J) were obtained using the experimental side-chain dihedral restraints, dipolar couplings, NOE signals, or REDOR distances [47,48]. Structure PDB 2KQT by Cady et al. [47] showed a well-defined A/M2–amantadine complex, which provided direct evidence for the location of the amantadine binding site. Sharma et al. [48] also solved the structure for the A/M2 TM domain plus amphipathic helix with ssNMR (PDB 2L0J) (Figure 6.2c). In this structure, they used membrane depth data for the amphipathic helix from a previous electron paramagnetic resonance (EPR) study [51] together with their measured distance restrains to obtain the overall TM-amphipathic helix structure. The overall backbone structure of the TM domain found with NMR [47,48] agrees with the crystal structure (PDB 3LBW) [49].

The structures of the A/M2 TM domain and amphipathic helix were also solved by solution NMR (PDB 2RLF) (Figure 6.2b) [44]. The TM domain of this structure agrees reasonably well with the ssNMR structure. However, the position of the amphipathic helix in the two structures differs significantly: in the ssNMR structure [48], this amphipathic helix is in direct contact with membrane lipid headgroup, while in the solution structure [44] the amphiphic helix forms a bundle extending into bulk aqueous solution.

The A/M2 protein shows extensive pH-dependent conformational changes and dynamics that differ when studied in lipid bilayers versus detergent micelles. Three different crystal structures at three different pH values (5.3, 6.5, and 7.3) displayed significantly different conformations [46,49]. Solid state NMR spectra indicated that the A/M2 TM domain backbone undergoes conformational fluctuations, and pH-dependent motion in critical residues His37 and Trp41 [39,47]. Solution NMR also showed pH-dependent broadening of peaks in the amide region [44]. These observations are in good agreement with the observation that A/M2 channel function is strongly regulated by pH.

The A/M2 conformation is also dependent on the solubilizing environment. X-ray and solution structures were determined in a detergent environment, whereas ssNMR structures were determined in lipid bilayers (Figure 6.2). Structures determined in detergents and detergent micelles have been found to have notable differences from those determined in lipid bilayers (compare Figure 6.2c with 6.2a and 6.2b). Thus, the amphipathic helix as a water-exposed bundle observed in solution NMR structure could possibly be a result of detergent solubilization [52]. Further, the length of the fatty acid chain comprising the lipid bilayer in which the M2 protein is contained has been shown to influence A/M2 conformation, with short chain lipids increasing the TM domain helical tilt; this increase in tilt results in a better match between the length of the hydrophobic portion of the peptide and the thickness of the lipid bilayer [53]. These understandable differences in conformation found among studies with various environments of the M2 protein nevertheless have in common the finding of a four helix TM bundle with increased dynamics within the range of pH over which the activity of the M2 channel is modulated.

Inhibition of the A/M2 channel

Because A/M2 channel function is essential for virus replication, antiviral drugs that inhibit A/M2 channel function also inhibit influenza A virus replication. The FDA-approved antiviral drug amantadine and its analog rimantadine inhibit the wt A/M2 channel, but not the BM2 channel, consistent with amantadine and rimantadine inhibiting replication of influenza A virus, but not influenza B virus. Several observations indicate that amantadine inhibits A/M2 channel activity by physically blocking the channel pore at an outer membrane "pore blocking site."

1. When amantadine-resistant mutant viruses were isolated, the mutations were mapped to the N-terminal portion of A/M2 TM domain at positions 26, 27, 30, 31, and 34. All of these mutations are lining the pore or very close to the pore [54].

2. Amantadine only inhibits the A/M2 channel when it is applied externally. When amantadine is injected into cells expressing A/M2 protein, concentrations as high as 1 mmol/L amantadine did not inhibit the A/M2 channel, probably because of the blockage of access to the outer channel pore by residues His37 and Trp41 [55].

3. Neutron diffraction experiments showed that amantadine lies in the outer leaflet of the membrane [56].

4. The Hill coefficient of amantadine inhibition is very close to 1, which is consistent with amantadine inhibition with stoichiometry 1:1 [55].

5. Amantadine inhibition is not dependent on membrane voltage, a finding inconsistent with the crossing of charged amantadine through the pore [57].

In a solution NMR structure of A/M2 TM domain plus amphipathic helix (residues 18–60) [44], amantadine was found to bind to the A/M2 channel in the region of boundary between the inner face of the lipid bilayer and the amphipathic helix. To determine this structure the A/M2 peptide was in a solution of 40 mmol/L rimantadine and 300 mmol/L dihexanoylphosphatidyl-choline. Four rimantadine molecules were found to be bound on the outside of the protein helix facing the lipid bilayer, interacting with Asp44 via a hydrogen bond, and thus located in the membrane environment at the end of the TM helix. Based on this structure, an allosteric mechanism for amantadine inhibition was proposed, in which internal drug binding to an inner "allosteric site" stabilizes the closed state, making it more difficult to open the channel. Because the allosteric mechanism was proposed, a series of studies were carried out to distinguish "pore-blocking mechanism" from the "allosteric mechanism."

1. If binding to Asp44 is the biologically relevant action of amantadine, then mutation to another residue ought to reduce inhibition. This has not been found to be the case consistently. Pielak et al. [40] found that when Asp44 was mutated to Ala, the resulting D44A mutant channel was insensitive to rimantadine in a liposomal proton flux assay. However, in stark contrast, Jing et al. [58] showed that when the D44A mutant channel was expressed at the surface of the oocyte plasma membrane, the drug sensitivity of the D44A mutant channel was indistinguishable from that of the wt A/M2 channel. Moreover, when the D44A mutation was introduced into the influenza A virus genome using reverse genetics procedures, the resulting mutant virus was as sensitive to amantadine or rimantadine as wt virus [58].

2. The BM2 channel of influenza B virus is not sensitive to amantadine, and therefore replacement of its TM domain with the TM domain of the biologically relevant part of the A/M2 TM domain ought to confer amantadine sensitivity. When the influenza B virus BM2 channel (see below) N-terminal portion (residues 6–18) of the TM domain was replaced with the corresponding portion of A/M2 protein (residues 24–36), which includes the proposed outer "pore blocking" drug binding site, the resulting chimeric protein BM2 (24-36aaA/M2) was inhibited about 50% by 100 μmol amantadine [59]. Moreover, when five extra residues of the ectodomain closest to the A/M2 TM domain were transferred to the BM2 protein, the resulting chimeric protein BM2 (19-36aaA/M2) could be almost completely inhibited by 100 μmol amantadine. Further, when the corresponding residues in the proposed inner "allosteric mechanism" binding site (residues 37–45) were transferred to BM2, the resulting chimeric BM2 (37-45aaA/M2) was as resistant to amantadine as the wt BM2 channel [59].

3. A series of surface plasmon resonance (SPR) experiments showed that amantadine and rimantadine are capable of binding A/M2 protein at both the proposed outer pore blocking site and allosteric inhibition site, but the pore blocking site has approximately three orders magnitude higher affinity than the allosteric site [60].

4. In a recent ssNMR structure with TM domain and amphiphic helix [48], the binding pocket identified in the allosteric inhibition mechanism was filled with side-chains of Ile51 and Phe54, blocking the access to Asp44 at the bottom of pocket from exterior.

5. Cady et al. [47] used perdeuterated amantadine, which enabled them measure the distance between amantadine and 13C-labeled residues in A/M2 protein via 13C{2H} rotational-echo double-resonance (REDOR) NMR spectra. The NMR spectra showed that two amantadine binding sites exist in the A/M2 protein in lipid bilayers. The high affinity site, occupied by a single amantadine, is located in the channel lumen. The low affinity site was observed on the C-terminal protein surface facing the lipid only when the drug reached a high concentration in the bilayer. These observations indicate that the "allosteric site" on the inner face of the lipid bilayer, as observed in the solution NMR structure, is the low affinity binding site and that it is not the primary site associated with the pharmacologic inhibition of the A/M2 ion channel.

New development of A/M2 channel inhibitors

There are two classes of A/M2 channel inhibitors identified so far: amantadine and rimantadine, and the spirene-containing compounds, such as 1 (BL-1743) and its analogs 2 and 3 (Figure 6.3). However, these compounds are only effective against the wt A/M2 channel and are ineffective against amantadine-resistant mutant channels. With wide circulation of amantadine-resistant mutant virus subtypes, the efficacy of amantadine and rimantadine dropped sharply in recent years, prompting the Centers for Disease Control to recommend discontinuing the use of amantadine-based drugs. Thus, there is an urgent need for the development of novel anti-influenza drugs that are effective against the most common amantadine-resistant mutants.

We would like to argue that the search for useful, new inhibitors of the A/M2 channel that is found in currently circulating virus subtypes is tractable. Of

the several amantadine-resistant mutants observed in the last two decades, S31N is found in viruses that are particularly fit [61], being observed in more than 90% of influenza A virus isolates in certain years. More recently, the pandemic H1N1 swine flu virus, which globally caused significant morbidity and mortality, is amantadine resistant, and the M2 protein contains the S31N mutation. Although viruses containing the S31N mutation are particular fit, the current dominance of this mutation is not the result of drug selection pressure [62]. In contrast, another amantadine-resistant mutation, V27A, was identified as the major mutation emerging from drug selection pressure. In some years, V27A mutant virus subtypes were dominant in circulating viruses. Some other amantadine-resistant mutant viruses (e.g., V27D, G34E) have been formed under drug selection pressure in vitro or in vivo but do not appear to be highly transmissible. Systematic mutation of the A/M2 pore-lining residues and functional characterization of the resulting mutant channels has increased our understanding of what functional alterations of the M2 ion channel with single-step mutations are capable of producing a viable proton channel with the properties needed to support virus uncoating [63]. In common among the ion channels of transmissible virus subtypes were two properties that were suggested to be essential criteria for the M2 channel to support the function of a transmissible virus subtype.

1. The mutant ion channel must have similar channel conductance at low pH (pH 5 to 6) to the wt A/M2 channel.

2. The mutant channel must have very low residual conductance at neutral pH (pH 7).

These criteria are consistent with the role of the A/M2 channel function in virus life cycle. On the other hand, the ability to conduct protons across membranes is potentially toxic to the host cell which the virus relies on for replication, therefore at neutral pH, low conductance will minimize the damage to host cell. It is very important to point out that there are very few mutations (i.e., D44F, A30G, G34T) other than those already observed in highly transmissible viruses (i.e., V27A, S31N, and D44N) that meet the two criteria [63]. Moreover, all the mutations at Asp44 are amantadine sensitive [58]. Studies attempting to develop new A/M2 channel inhibitors need to focus on the limited number of mutants that are capable of replacing the wt A/M2 channel.

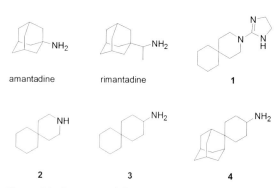

Figure 6.3. Structures of the A/M2 proton channel inhibitors.

With the availability of new high resolution structures of M2 in different conformations and new approaches to drug design (i.e., MD simulation), investigators are able to develop new compounds with improved efficacy against the wt A/M2 channel or new compounds capable of inhibiting the amantadine-insensitive A/M2 channels. Wang et al. [64] showed that compound 2 (Figure 6.3) is capable of inhibiting A/M2 wt channel with an IC_{50} of 0.92 μmol in oocyte two electrode voltage measurements, which represents a more than 10-fold increase in potency compared to amantadine. Solid state NMR data showed that although this compound interacts with the A/M2 TM domain in a similar location to amantadine, it interacts with a longer stretch of the TM helix, induces a more homogeneous conformation of the A/M2 protein, and immobilizes the Gly34-Ile35 region. This immobilization is important because conformational changes are required during the proton conduction process. Furthermore, significant progress has also been made in designing drugs against the amantadine-resistant V27A mutant channel. With the help of MD simulation to probe the different binding modes of various compounds, a compound (4 in Figure 6.3) was identified [65]. Oocyte two electrode voltage measurements and plaque reduction assays confirmed its efficacy against both the V27A mutant channel and the V27A bearing mutant virus [65]. The efficacy of this compound to protect mice from infection with virus containing the M2 V27A mutation has been confirmed in preliminary studies. A few studies have reported successful identification or design of S31N mutant channel inhibitors by various computational methods, but none of these hits were confirmed in any *in vitro* or *in vivo* biologic assay [66]. Nevertheless, with the demonstration of a V27A A/M2 channel inhibitor, the identification of new compounds against the S31N mutant channel will be possible.

Influenza B virus BM2 protein is also a proton channel

It was anticipated that influenza B virus would require an ion channel activity to aid virus uncoating in endosomes, particularly as the influenza B virus M protein can be removed from the RNP core by low pH (5.5) treatment [67,68]. Influenza B virus RNA segment 7 in addition to encoding the M1 protein encodes the BM2 protein [69]. The influenza B virus BM2 protein (109 amino acids) is translated from an open reading frame that is −2 nucleotides with respect to the reading frame of the M1 protein and it is conserved in all isolates of influenza B virus. Analysis of properties of the BM2 protein, including detergent solubility, insolubility in alkali pH 11, flotation in membrane fractions, and epitope tagging immunocytochemistry indicate BM2 protein is an integral membrane protein expressed at the cell surface and it adopts an $N_{out}C_{in}$ orientation with a single TM domain and is the fourth integral membrane protein encoded by influenza B virus in addition to hemagglutinin (HA), neuraminidase (NA), and the NB glycoprotein [70]. Chemical cross-linking and functional studies indicated that the BM2 protein is oligomeric, most likely a tetramer [71]. In comparing the BM2 protein sequence with the A/M2 sequence it is found that the BM2 protein has a shorter N-terminal (7 residues) than A/M2 protein (24 residues), while the BM2 protein has a longer C-terminal cytoplasmic tail (82 residues) than A/M2 protein (51 residues). The A/M2 protein and BM2 protein have very little sequence identity. However, comparison of the sequence of the TM domain of the BM2 and A/M2 proteins indicates that the two key residues for activation and gating, His37 and Trp41 respectively, in the A/M2 ion channel [34,36] are found at the same spacing HXXXW (His19 and Trp23) in the BM2 TM domain [70].

When BM2 was expressed in oocytes or in mammalian cells, BM2 protein is capable of acidifying the interior of oocytes or mammalian cells [68]. Whole-cell membrane current was observed when oocytes expressing BM2 protein or FLAG-tagged protein were bathed at low pH (pH 5.5) [68]. Although detailed ion-selectivity studies were not carried out because of the lack of effective BM2 channel inhibitors, the shift of reversal potential in various bathing pH is consistent with a shift in the proton equilibrium potential [68], suggesting BM2 channel is proton selective. The His and Trp residues in BM2 were shown to be critical for ion channel function [68]. Sequence analysis and Cys-scanning mutagenesis identified that Ser9, Ser12, Ser16, His19, and Trp23 in the TM domain line the channel pore [72].

Recently, a BM2 structure was solved by solution NMR [73]. This full length structure was constructed by two overlapping structures (TM channel domain residues 1–33; cytoplasmic domain residues 26–109), which constitutes a membrane embedded channel domain and cytoplasmic domain. Overall, the BM2 TM domain is very similar to the A/M2 TM domain, that is a left-handed four-helix bundle. However, there is an observable difference in global structure of these two channel domains: A/M2 structures show helical kinks at Gly34 residue, while the BM2 structure shows strong coiled-coil characteristics with heptad repeats. Following the channel domain, residues 47–60 of the A/M2 domain form a membrane surface bound amphiphilic helix [48,51], but the corresponding domain (residues 27–40) of BM2 is at the junction of the two determined structures [73]. Residues 27–30 were shown to form an extension of the channel domain without break, and residues 30–40 were not solved in the structure. There were no structures available for cytoplasmic tail of A/M2 protein (residues 61–97). In the BM2 structure, the cytoplasmic tail (residues 42–109) was found to form mainly a left-handed coiled-coil tetramer [73]. The structural differences between the A/M2 and BM2 channels help explain the differences in their pharmacology.

No effective BM2 channel inhibitor has been found. A few observations possibly will explain why amantadine has low efficacy against the BM2 channel.
1. The BM2 channel pore is lined with polar amino acid serine, not hydrophobic residues found in A/M2. This is expected to reduce affinity for the hydrophobic adamantane cage of the amantadine.
2. BM2 channel adopts a coiled-coil assembly, which greatly reduces the size of channel pore, preventing amantadine drugs from fitting into the pore.

Influenza B virus is a substantial component of the annual seasonal flu. The lack of effective BM2 channel inhibitors presents an important challenge to the field. Possibly a future generation of compounds could target the HXXXW motif, which is conserved among all influenza A and B viruses.

Note added in proof

Recently, Pielak et al. [74], who had proposed an allosteric binding mechanism for amantadine with the drug binding weakly to M2 on the outside of the channel at the cytoplasmic amphipathic helix–membrane region, reported a new solution NMR structure for a chimeric A/M2-BM2 fusion protein,

similar to BM2 (24-36aaA/M2) described in the main text. The new structure of the chimeric channel showed, without any doubt, that rimantadine bound inside the pore. Near the N-terminal end of the channel, methyl groups of Val27 and Ala30 from four subunits form a hydrophobic pocket around the adamantane, and the drug amino group appears to be in polar contact with the backbone oxygen of Ala30 [74]. This new structure effectively ends the controversy about the mechanism of amantadine inhibition of the M2 ion channel.

Acknowledgments

Research in the authors' laboratories was supported by NIH research grants from the National Institute of Allergy and Infectious Diseases, AI-20201and AI-074571.

References

1. Lamb RA, Lai C-J, Choppin PW. Sequences of mRNAs derived from genome RNA segment 7 of influenza virus: colinear and interrupted mRNAs code for overlapping proteins. Proc Natl Acad Sci U S A. 1981;78:4170–4.
2. Lamb RA, Choppin PW. Identification of a second protein (M2) encoded by RNA segment 7 of influenza virus. Virology. 1981;112:729–37.
3. Lamb RA, Zebedee SL, Richardson CD. Influenza virus M2 protein is an integral membrane protein expressed on the infected-cell surface. Cell. 1985;40:627–33.
4. Sugrue RJ, Hay AJ. Structural characteristics of the M2 protein of influenza A viruses: evidence that it forms a tetrameric channel. Virology. 1991;180:617–24.
5. Holsinger LJ, Lamb RA. Influenza virus M2 integral membrane protein is a homotetramer stabilized by formation of disulfide bonds. Virology. 1991;183: 32–43.
6. Schroeder C, Heider H, Moncke-Buchner E, Lin TI. The influenza virus ion channel and maturation cofactor M2 is a cholesterol-binding protein. Eur Biophys J. 2005;34: 52–66.
7. Rossman JS, Jing X, Leser GP, Balannik V, Pinto LH, Lamb RA. Influenza virus M2 ion channel protein is necessary for filamentous virion formation. J Virol. 2010;84:5078–88.
8. Rossman JS, Jing X, Leser GP, Lamb RA. Influenza virus M2 protein mediates ESCRT-independent membrane scission. Cell. 2010;142:902–13.

9. Zhang J, Lamb RA. Characterization of the membrane association of the influenza virus matrix protein in living cells. Virology. 1996;225:255–66.

10. Chen BJ, Leser GP, Morita E, Lamb RA. Influenza virus hemagglutinin and neuraminidase, but not the matrix protein, are required for assembly and budding of plasmid-derived virus-like particles. J Virol. 2007;81: 7111–23.

11. Simons K, Toomre D. Lipid rafts and signal transduction. Nat Rev Mol Cell Biol. 2000;1:31–9.

12. Zebedee SL, Lamb RA. Influenza A virus M2 protein: monoclonal antibody restriction of virus growth and detection of M2 in virions. J Virol. 1988;62:2762–72.

13. El Bakkouri K, Descamps F, De Filette M, Smet A, Festjens E, Birkett A, et al. Universal vaccine based on ectodomain of matrix protein 2 of influenza A: Fc receptors and alveolar macrophages mediate protection. J Immunol. 2011;186:1022–31.

14. Grandea AG 3rd, Olsen OA, Cox TC, Renshaw M, Hammond PW, Chan-Hui PY, et al. Human antibodies reveal a protective epitope that is highly conserved among human and nonhuman influenza A viruses. Proc Natl Acad Sci U S A. 2010;107:12658–63.

15. Ichinohe T, Pang IK, Iwasaki A. Influenza virus activates inflammasomes via its intracellular M2 ion channel. Nat Immunol. 2010;11:404–10.

16. Gannage M, Dormann D, Albrecht R, Dengjel J, Torossi T, Ramer PC, et al. Matrix protein 2 of influenza A virus blocks autophagosome fusion with lysosomes. Cell Host Microbe. 2009;6:367–80.

17. Rossman JS, Lamb RA. Autophagy, apoptosis, and the influenza virus M2 protein. Cell Host Microbe. 2009;6:299–300.

18. Davies WL, Grunert RR, Haff RF, McGahen JW, Neumayer EM, Paulshock M, et al. Antiviral activity of 1-adamantanamine (amantadine). Science. 1964;144: 862–3.

19. Bukrinskaya AG, Vorkunova NK, Kornilayeva GV. Narmanbetova RA, Vorkunova GK. Influenza virus uncoating in infected cells and effects of rimantadine. J Gen Virol. 1982;60:49–59.

20. Zhirnov OP. Solubilization of matrix protein M1/M from virions occurs at different pH for orthomyxo- and paramyxoviruses. Virology. 1990;176:274–9.

21. Sugrue RJ, Bahadur G, Zambon MC, Hall-Smith M, Douglas AR, Hay AJ. Specific structural alteration of the influenza haemagglutinin by amantadine. EMBO J. 1990;9:3469–76.

22. Grambas S, Hay AJ. Maturation of influenza A virus hemagglutinin – estimates of the pH encountered during transport and its regulation by the M2 protein. Virology. 1992;190:11–8.

23. Grambas S, Bennett MS, Hay AJ. Influence of amantadine resistance mutations on the pH regulatory function of the M2 protein of influenza A viruses. Virology. 1992;191:541–9.

24. Takeuchi K, Lamb RA. Influenza virus M2 protein ion channel activity stabilizes the native form of fowl plague virus hemagglutinin during intracellular transport. J Virol. 1994;68:911–9.

25. Sakaguchi T, Leser GP, Lamb RA. The ion channel activity of the influenza virus M2 protein affects transport through the Golgi apparatus. J Cell Biol. 1996; 133:733–47.

26. Lamb RA, Holsinger LJ, Pinto LH. The influenza A virus M_2 ion channel protein and its role in the influenza virus life cycle. In: Wimmer E, editor. Receptor-Mediated Virus Entry into Cells. Cold Spring Harbor, NY: Cold Spring Harbor Press; 1994. pp. 303–21.

27. Pinto LH, Holsinger LJ, Lamb RA. Influenza virus M2 protein has ion channel activity. Cell. 1992;69: 517–28.

28. Chizhmakov IV, Geraghty FM, Ogden DC, Hayhurst A, Antoniou M, Hay AJ. Selective proton permeability and pH regulation of the influenza virus M2 channel expressed in mouse erythroleukaemia cells. J Physiol. 1996;494:329–36.

29. Wang C, Lamb RA, Pinto LH. Direct measurement of the influenza A virus M2 protein ion channel in mammalian cells. Virology. 1994;205:133–40.

30. Lin TI, Schroeder C. Definitive assignment of proton selectivity and attoampere unitary current to the M2 ion channel protein of influenza A virus. J Virol. 2001; 75:3647–56.

31. Tosteson MT, Pinto LH, Holsinger LJ, Lamb RA. Reconstitution of the influenza virus M2 ion channel in lipid bilayers. J Membr Biol. 1994;142:117–26.

32. Watanabe T, Ito H, Kida H, Kawaoka Y. Influenza A virus can undergo multiple cycles of replication without M2 ion channel activity. J Virol. 2001;75:5656–62.

33. Takeda M, Pekosz A, Shuck K, Pinto LH, Lamb RA. Influenza a virus M2 ion channel activity is essential for efficient replication in tissue culture. J Virol. 2002; 76:1391–9.

34. Tang Y, Zaitseva F, Lamb RA, Pinto LH. The gate of the influenza virus M2 proton channel is formed by a single tryptophan residue. J Biol Chem. 2002;277: 39880–6.

35. Ma C, Polishchuk AL, Ohigashi Y, Stouffer AL, Schon A, Magavern E, et al. Identification of the functional core of the influenza A virus A/M2 proton-selective ion channel. Proc Natl Acad Sci U S A. 2009;106: 12283–8.

36. Wang C, Lamb RA, Pinto LH. Activation of the M_2 ion channel of influenza virus: a role for the transmembrane domain histidine residue. Biophys J. 1995;69:1363–71.

37. Mould JA, Drury JE, Frings SM, Kaupp UB, Pekosz A, Lamb RA, et al. Permeation and activation of the M2

ion channel of influenza A virus. J Biol Chem. 2000;
275:31038–50.

38. Okada A, Miura T, Takeuchi H. Protonation of histidine and histidine-tryptophan interaction in the activation of the M2 ion channel from influenza a virus. Biochemistry. 2001;40:6053–60.

39. Hu F, Luo W, Hong M. Mechanisms of proton conduction and gating in influenza M2 proton channels from solid-state NMR. Science. 2010;330:505–8.

40. Pielak RM, Schnell JR, Chou JJ. Mechanism of drug inhibition and drug resistance of influenza A M2 channel. Proc Natl Acad Sci U S A. 2009;106:7379–84.

41. Sansom MSP, Kerr ID, Smith GR, Son HS. The influenza A virus M2 channel: a molecular modeling and simulation study. Virology. 1997;233:163–73.

42. Pinto LH, Dieckmann GR, Gandhi CS, Papworth CG, Braman J, Shaughnessy MA, et al. A functionally defined model for the M2 proton channel of influenza A virus suggests a mechanism for its ion selectivity. Proc Natl Acad Sci U S A. 1997;94:11301–6.

43. Hu J, Fu R, Nishimura K, Zhang L, Zhou HX, Busath DD, et al. Histidines, heart of the hydrogen ion channel from influenza A virus: toward an understanding of conductance and proton selectivity. Proc Natl Acad Sci U S A. 2006;103:6865–70.

44. Schnell JR, Chou JJ. Structure and mechanism of the M2 proton channel of influenza A virus. Nature. 2008;451:591–5.

45. Khurana E, Dal Peraro M, DeVane R, Vemparala S, DeGrado WF, Klein ML. Molecular dynamics calculations suggest a conduction mechanism for the M2 proton channel from influenza A virus. Proc Natl Acad Sci U S A. 2009;106:1069–74.

46. Stouffer AL, Acharya R, Salom D, Levine AS, Di Costanzo L, Soto CS, et al. Structural basis for the function and inhibition of an influenza virus proton channel. Nature. 2008;451:596–9.

47. Cady SD, Schmidt-Rohr K, Wang J, Soto CS, Degrado WF, Hong M. Structure of the amantadine binding site of influenza M2 proton channels in lipid bilayers. Nature. 2010;463:689–92.

48. Sharma M, Yi M, Dong H, Qin H, Peterson E, Busath DD, et al. Insight into the mechanism of the influenza A proton channel from a structure in a lipid bilayer. Science. 2010;330:509–12.

49. Acharya R, Carnevale V, Fiorin G, Levine BG, Polishchuk AL, Balannik V, et al. Structure and mechanism of proton transport through the transmembrane tetrameric M2 protein bundle of the influenza A virus. Proc Natl Acad Sci U S A. 2010;107:15075–80.

50. Kovacs FA, Denny JK, Song Z, Quine JR, Cross TA. Helix tilt of the M2 transmembrane peptide from influenza A virus: an intrinsic property. J Mol Biol. 2000; 295:117–25.

51. Nguyen PA, Soto CS, Polishchuk A, Caputo GA, Tatko CD, Ma C, et al. pH-induced conformational change of the influenza M2 protein C-terminal domain. Biochemistry. 2008;47:9934–6.

52. Cross TA, Sharma M, Yi M, Zhou HX. Influence of solubilizing environments on membrane protein structures. Trends Biochem Sci. 2011;36:117–25.

53. Duong-Ly KC, Nanda V, Degrado WF, Howard KP. The conformation of the pore region of the M2 proton channel depends on lipid bilayer environment. Protein Sci. 2005;14:856–61.

54. Hay AJ, Wolstenholme AJ, Skehel JJ, Smith MH. Molecular basis of resistance of influenza A viruses to amantadine. EMBO J. 1985;4:3021–4.

55. Wang C, Takeuchi K, Pinto LH, Lamb RA. The ion channel activity of the influenza A virus M_2 protein: characterization of the amantadine block. J Virol. 1993; 67:5585–94.

56. Duff KC, Gilchrist PJ, Saxena AM, Bradshaw JP. Neutron diffraction reveals the site of amantadine blockade in the influenza A M2 ion channel. Virology. 1994;202:287–93.

57. Balannik V, Wang J, Ohigashi Y, Jing X, Magavern E, Lamb RA, et al. Design and pharmacological characterization of inhibitors of amantadine-resistant mutants of the M2 ion channel of influenza A virus. Biochemistry. 2009;48:11872–82.

58. Jing X, Ma C, Ohigashi Y, Oliveira FA, Jardetzky TS, Pinto LH, et al. Functional studies indicate amantadine binds to the pore of the influenza A virus M2 proton-selective ion channel. Proc Natl Acad Sci U S A. 2008; 105:10967–72.

59. Ohigashi Y, Ma C, Jing X, Balannick V, Pinto LH, Lamb RA. An amantadine-sensitive chimeric BM2 ion channel of influenza B virus has implications for the mechanism of drug inhibition. Proc Natl Acad Sci U S A. 2009; 106:18775–9.

60. Rosenberg MR, Casarotto MG. Coexistence of two adamantane binding sites in the influenza A M2 ion channel. Proc Natl Acad Sci U S A. 2010;107:13866–71.

61. Abed Y, Goyette N, Boivin G. Generation and characterization of recombinant influenza A (H1N1) viruses harboring amantadine resistance mutations. Antimicrob Agents Chemother. 2005;4:556–9.

62. Furuse Y, Suzuki A, Oshitani H. Large-scale sequence analysis of M gene of influenza A viruses from different species: mechanisms for emergence and spread of amantadine resistance. Antimicrob Agents Chemother. 2009;53:4457–63.

63. Balannik V, Carnevale V, Fiorin G, Levine BG, Lamb RA, Klein ML, et al. Functional studies and modeling

of pore-lining residue mutants of the influenza a virus M2 ion channel. Biochemistry. 2010;49:696–708.

64. Wang J, Cady SD, Balannik V, Pinto LH, DeGrado WF, Hong M. Discovery of spiro-piperidine inhibitors and their modulation of the dynamics of the M2 proton channel from influenza A virus. J Am Chem Soc. 2009;131:8066–76.

65. Wang J, Ma C, Fiorin G, Carnevale V, Wang T, Hu F, et al. Molecular dynamics simulation directed rational design of inhibitors targeting drug-resistant mutants of influenza A virus M2. J Am Chem Soc. 2011;133: 12834–41.

66. Du QS, Huang RB, Wang SQ, Chou KC. Designing inhibitors of M2 proton channel against H1N1 swine influenza virus. PLoS ONE. 2010;5(2):e9388.

67. Zhirnov OP. Isolation of matrix protein M1 from influenza viruses by acid-dependent extraction with nonionic detergent. Virology. 1992;186:324–30.

68. Mould JA, Paterson RG, Takeda M, Ohigashi Y, Venkataraman P, Lamb RA, et al. Influenza B virus BM2 protein has ion channel activity that conducts protons across membranes. Dev Cell. 2003;5:175–84.

69. Horvath CM, Williams MA, Lamb RA. Eukaryotic coupled translation of tandem cistrons: identification of the influenza B virus BM2 polypeptide. EMBO J. 1990;9:2639–47.

70. Paterson RG, Takeda M, Ohigashi Y, Pinto LH, Lamb RA. Influenza B virus BM2 protein is an oligomeric integral membrane protein expressed at the cell surface. Virology. 2003;306:7–17.

71. Balannik V, Lamb RA, Pinto LH. The oligomeric state of the active BM2 ion channel protein of influenza B virus. J Biol Chem. 2008;283:4895–904.

72. Ma C, Soto CS, Ohigashi Y, Taylor A, Bournas V, Glawe B, et al. Identification of the pore-lining residues of the BM2 ion channel protein of influenza B virus. J Biol Chem. 2008;283:15921–31.

73. Wang J, Pielak RM, McClintock MA, Chou JJ. Solution structure and functional analysis of the influenza B proton channel. Nat Struct Mol Biol. 2009;16: 1267–71.

74. Pielak RM, Oxenoid K, Chou JJ. Structural investigation of rimantadine inhibition of the AM2-BM2 chimera channel of influenza viruses. Structure. 2011;19:1655–63.

75. Wang J, Qiu JX, Soto C, DeGrado WF. Structural and dynamic mechanisms for the function and inhibition of the M2 proton channel from influenza A virus. Curr Opin Struct Biol. 2011;1:68–80.

76. Pinto LH, Lamb RA. Influenza virus proton channels. Photochem Photobiol Sci. 2006;5:629–32.

7

The NS1 protein: A master regulator of host and viral functions

Robert M. Krug[1] and Adolfo García-Sastre[2]

[1]Department of Molecular Genetics and Microbiology, Institute for Cellular and Molecular Biology, University of Texas at Austin, Austin, TX, USA

[2]Department of Microbiology and Department of Medicine, Division of Infectious Diseases, Global Health and Emerging Pathogens Institute, Icahn School of Medicine at Mount Sinai, New York, NY, USA

Introduction

All viruses need to deal with the host antiviral response. Cells have been equipped with multiple sensors of viral infection that trigger potent antiviral pathways, including the induction of interferons (IFNs) and IFN-stimulated genes that inhibit viral replication. Conversely, viruses have evolved strategies to counteract the host antiviral pathways by hiding from cellular sensors, by actively inhibiting antiviral pathways, or both. In the case of influenza viruses, the viral NS1 protein has a critical role in preventing the host antiviral response. While this is the case for both influenza A and B viruses, most of the studies have been conducted with the NS1 of influenza A viruses, and so in this chapter we mainly discuss influenza A virus NS1 features and functions, but we also discuss a unique feature of the influenza B virus NS1 protein.

By knocking out the NS1 gene, influenza A viruses become highly attenuated mainly because of the induction of a rapid unchecked type I/III IFN response in infected cells that prevent viral replication [1]. The NS1 protein, by interacting with cytoplasmic and nuclear host factors, significantly attenuates IFN induction and the antiviral effects of IFN. Intriguingly, some of the NS1–host protein interactions appear to be virus strain specific, and this may have important implications in host tropism and virulence. In addition to its IFN antagonistic properties, the NS1 protein regulates several other processes in virus-infected cells, such as the phosphoinisotide 3-kinase (PI3K) cellular pathway, viral RNA synthesis, and viral protein synthesis. The requirement of NS1 for optimal viral replication makes this protein an attractive target for influenza antiviral and vaccine development.

General features and structures of the influenza A virus NS1 protein

The NS1 proteins of wild-type influenza A viruses range in size from 215 to 237 amino acids long, and are comprised of two functional domains: N-terminal RNA-binding domain (RBD) (amino acids 1–73); and C-terminal effector domain (ED) (amino acids 85-end) [2] (Figure 7.1a). These two domains are connected by a short linker. The NS1 proteins of all human influenza A virus strains (H1N1, H2N2, H3N2) isolated between 1950 and 1989 are 237 amino acids long, for example, the NS1 protein of the H3N2 A/ Udorn/72 (Ud) strain shown in Figure 7.1a. The NS1 proteins from all other human H1N1 and H3N2 strains, with the exception of the 2009-derived pandemic H1N1 viruses, for example, the H3N2

Textbook of Influenza, Second Edition. Edited by Robert G. Webster, Arnold S. Monto, Thomas J. Braciale, and Robert A. Lamb.
© 2013 John Wiley & Sons, Ltd. Published 2013 by John Wiley & Sons, Ltd.

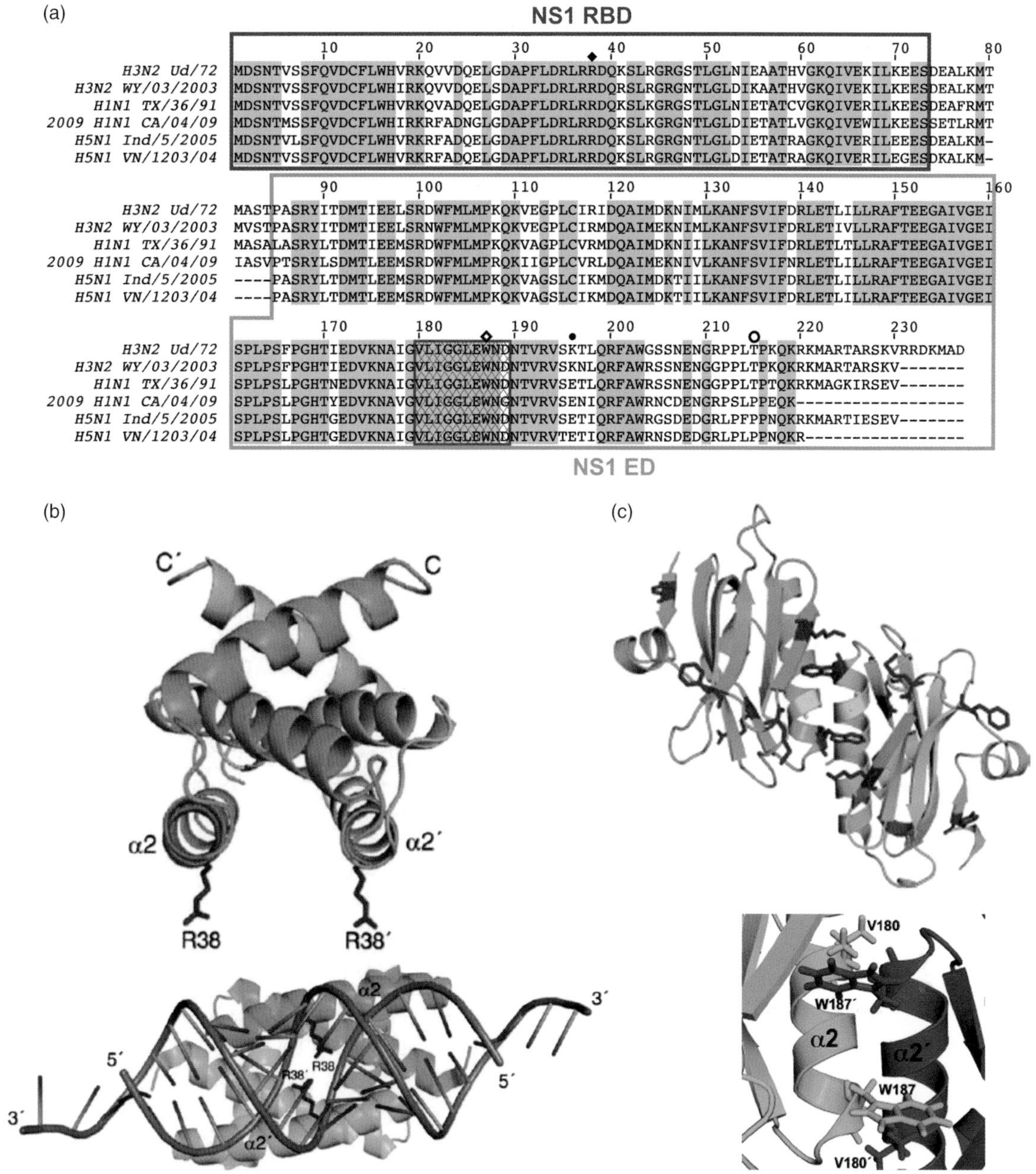

Figure 7.1. Sequences and structures of influenza A virus NS1 proteins. (a) Sequence alignment of the indicated NS1 proteins. Conserved amino acids are shown in light blue. The RNA-binding domain (RBD) and effector domain (ED) domains are outlined in dark blue and orange, respectively. The helix–helix dimer interface is outlined in black, and the W287 amino acid that is critical for dimer formation is denoted. In addition, the R at position 38, the K/E at 196, and the T/P at 215 are also denoted. (b) The structure of the RBD: (Top) the structure of the RBD in the absence of double-stranded RNA (dsRNA). (Bottom) The structure of the RBD bound to a 19 base pair dsRNA. (c) The structure of the ED dimer. (Top) ED dimer of the Ud virus NS1 protein, showing the mutations that verified the helix–helix interface. Side-chains for mutated amino acids are colored as follows: red, mutants that dissociate the dimer; blue, mutants that do not dissociate the dimer; yellow, mutants that partially dissociate the dimer. (Bottom) Close-up view of the helix–helix interface showing W187 from each ED chain jutting into a hydrophobic pocket in the other chain.

A/Wyoming/3/2003 and the H1N1 A/TX/36/91 strains, are 230 amino acids long, and have a C-terminal end of RSKV or RSEV, respectively. In contrast, the NS1 protein of the 2009 H1N1 pandemic virus is only 219 amino acids long and lacks this C-terminus. All the above NS1 proteins contain a 11 amino acid long linker. In contrast, the NS1 proteins of several highly pathogenic avian H5N1 viruses, including those isolated from humans, contain a short 6 amino acid long linker. Most of these H5N1 NS1 proteins are 225 amino acids long (e.g., A/IND/5/2005) and have a C-terminal end of ESEV or ESPV [3], but some of these H5N1 NS1 proteins are only 215 amino acids long and lack the ESEV/ESPV C-terminus (e.g., A/VN/1203/04). The presence of T at position 215 is commonly considered to be a signature for human influenza A virus strains. All influenza A viruses circulating in humans from 1920 to 2008 encode NS1 proteins with T at position 215, whereas the NS1 proteins of avian influenza A viruses, including H5N1 viruses, contain proline (P) at this position. Two viruses that have circulated in humans, the 2009 H1N1 pandemic virus (shown in Figure 7.1a) and the 1918 pandemic virus, encode NS1 proteins with the avian P-215 signature.

Cellular localization of NS1 is regulated at least by one or two nuclear import sequences and a nuclear export sequence. All the NS1 proteins contain a nuclear localization sequence (NLS1) (amino acids 35–41) that overlaps with the sequence required for double-stranded RNA (dsRNA) binding (Figure 7.1a) [4,5]. Consequently, when R38 is replaced with A, not only is dsRNA binding eliminated, but also the NSL1 is inactivated [5,6]. The NS1 protein of the H3N2 Ud virus also possesses a second NLS (NLS2), a bipartite NLS comprised of amino acids 219–232, KRKMARTARSKVRR, a sequence in which two short amino acid sequences (underlined) are separated by a nonspecific 9-amino acid spacer [5]. The bipartite NLS2 is only present in the NS1 proteins that are 237 amino acids long. Whereas NLS1 directs the NS1 protein almost totally to the nucleoplasm, NLS2 directs at least some of the NS1 protein to the nucleolus. The majority of NS1 proteins also contain a nuclear export signal, similar to the Ud NS1 sequence, FDRLETLILL, at positions 138–147 [7]. By gaining access to various cellular compartments, the NS1 protein is able to perform its multiple distinct functions.

Overall, as shown by the sequences highlighted in light blue in Figure 7.1a, there is extensive conservation of sequence between these NS1 proteins from these different virus strains. The largest sequence variations occur in the C-terminal region of the ED. These differences in the C-terminal domain lead to functional differences, as described later in this chapter. There is also similar homology with the NS1 proteins of influenza A viruses that infect horses, pigs, and dogs. The NS1 proteins of these mammalian influenza A viruses constitute the A allele of the NS1 protein. The NS1 A allele is also found in avian influenza A viruses, along with another allele, called the B allele, which has much lower homology to the A allele and which is found exclusively in avian influenza A viruses [2].

The three-dimensional structure of the RBD and of the majority of the ED (e.g., amino acids 85–215 of the Ud NS1 protein) has been determined (Figure 7.1b,c). The C-terminal amino acids appear to be largely unstructured. The linker region is also probably largely unstructured. The isolated RBD forms a unique six-helical head-to-tail homodimer, which binds dsRNA (Figure 7.1b) [6,8,9]. Only one amino acid (R38/R38′) is absolutely required for dsRNA binding [6]. The pocket at the bottom of the structure shown in Figure 7.1b (top) binds the major groove of A-form dsRNA, as shown by the crystal structure of the RBD in complex with a 19-base pair dsRNA (Figure 7.1b, bottom) [10]. The R38/R38′ residues from the two monomers form hydrogen bonds with each other, as well as with the two RNA strands, thereby anchoring the dsRNA. In addition to R38, positively charged residues in the middle of the dsRNA binding surface, such as R35, R37, and K41 make hydrogen bonds and electrostatic interactions with both strands of the dsRNA. The isolated ED of NS1 also forms a homodimer, with each monomer subunit adopting a novel α-helix β-crescent fold (Figure 7.1c). X-ray crystallography and nuclear magnetic resonance (NMR), coupled with mutagenesis, established that the ED dimerizes through the denoted helix–helix interface in which the W187 residue from each monomer juts into a deep hydrophobic pocket in the adjacent subunit [11–14]. Replacing W187 with R or A disrupts the dimer. Whereas the RBD is an extremely stable homodimer (K_d in the very low nM range), the K_d for dimerization of the ED is quite weak, for example, the K_d for dimerization of the Ud virus ED is 90 μmol [11].

Molecular and cellular functions

Inhibition of the RIG-I pathway

RIG-I is a critical cytoplasmic sensor of viral RNA [15], and is required for IFN induction after virus infection of many different type of cells, including epithelial cells and conventional dendritic cells. In the case of influenza virus, RIG-I is essential for IFN induction in epithelial cells, the main targets of infection *in vivo* [16–19]. Influenza viral RNA displays a dsRNA structure adjacent to a 5′-tri-phosphate, characteristics that are associated with optimal recognition by RIG-I and that distinguish viral RNA from host RNA [19]. When RIG-I binds to such RNAs, it undergoes a conformational change associated with the activation of its ATPase activity and translocation on RNA [20]. This change results in exposure of its CARD N-terminal domains, which are K63 polyubiquitinated by TRIM25 [21] and RIPLET [22] ubiquitin ligases and/or bind to K63 polyubiquitin free chains that are also synthesized by TRIM25 [23]. As a result, RIG-I oligomerizes and its CARD domain associates with the CARD domain of the adaptor MAVS, leading to the formation of a signaling platform that activates kinases and transcription factors IRF3 and NFkB [15]. These two activated transcription factors are needed for the activation of IFN transcription. The NS1 protein binds dsRNA, but with low affinity [24], so that it is unlikely that this binding results in sequestration of the viral RNA substrate of RIG-I, thereby inhibiting RIG-I activation. Several groups have reported interaction of RIG-I with the NS1 protein, which may result in direct inhibition of RIG-I activation [16–19]. More recently, Gack et al. [25] reported an association of the PR8 NS1 with the coiled-coil domain of TRIM25. This association does not inhibit TRIM25–RIG-I interactions, but prevents TRIM25 oligomerization, which is required for its E3 ligase activity [25]. Thus, the PR8 NS1 effectively prevents TRIM25 mediated ubiquitination of RIG-I, preventing downstream interactions of RIG-I with MAVS and the initiation of signaling leading to IFN induction (Table 7.1). Mutations in the PR8 NS1 involved in interactions with TRIM25, namely mutations in either R38/K41 (also involved in dsRNA binding) or E96/E97, result in viral attenuation and higher IFN induction [25]. While the NS1–human TRIM25 interactions appear to be highly conserved, differences exist among different influenza virus strains in their ability to prevent RIG-I/MAVS signaling (see section on inhibition of host gene expression) [26]. In addition, the nuclear pool of the NS1 protein can shortcut induction of the IFN response by virtue of its cellular transcriptional and post-transcriptional inhibitory functions, which result in a general inhibition of host gene expression, including the expression of genes involved in the antiviral response.

Table 7.1. Influenza A virus NS1 functions.

	Partner	Function
Inhibitory functions	TRIM25	Inhibition of RIG-I and of IFN promoter activation
	CPSF30	Inhibition of host mRNA polyadenylation
	PAF1	Inhibition of host transcriptional elongation
	PKR	Inhibition of eIF2α phosphorylation and of translational block
	dsRNA	Inhibition of OAS and of RNA degradation
Stimulatory functions	p85β	Activation of PI3K
	eIF4G, PABP1	Stimulation of viral translation
	Viral RNP	Stimulation of viral RNA synthesis

Inhibition of host gene expression

The mature 3′ ends of cellular mRNAs are generated by endonucleolytic cleavage of the primary transcripts (pre-mRNAs), followed by polyadenylation of the upstream cleavage products. This process requires the presence of a conserved AAUAAA sequence in the pre-mRNA that is located 10–30 bases upstream of the cleavage site [27,28]. This sequence is recognized by the cellular CPSF factor. The NS1 protein binds and sequesters the 30 kDa subunit of CPSF (CPSF30), resulting in the inhibition of the 3′ end processing of cellular pre-mRNAs (Table 7.1) [29]. Unprocessed cellular pre-mRNAs accumulate in the nucleus, and the production of mature mRNAs in the cytoplasm is inhibited. A major consequence of this NS1 function is that the production of mature IFN and other antiviral pre-mRNAs is inhibited, thereby countering the host antiviral response [30–32]. In contrast, the polyadenylation of viral mRNAs is not inhibited because it is catalyzed by the viral polymerase [33].

CPSF30 contains five C3H zinc fingers [32,34]. A small (61-amino acid) fragment of CPSF30 comprising zinc fingers 2 and 3 (F2F3) is sufficient for binding the NS1 protein. Expression of F2F3 in virus-infected cells leads to the inhibition of Ud virus and increased production of IFN-β mRNA, presumably by occupying the CPSF30 binding site on the NS1 protein and hence blocking the binding of endogenous CPSF30 to this site. Based on these results, the CPSF30 binding site was identified by determining the X-ray crystal structure of F2F3 in complex with the NS1 ED of the Ud virus [30]. The complex is a tetramer, in which two F2F3 molecules wrap around two NS1 EDs that are interacting with each other in a head-to-head orientation (Figure 7.2a). Consequently, the helix–helix dimer of the ED that forms in the absence of F2F3 (Figure 7.1c), which is largely mediated by W187, is disrupted [30]. In fact, as a result of the rearrangement, W187 becomes part of the two symmetric F2F3 binding pockets (Figure 7.2b). Each of these pockets also contains predominately hydrophobic amino acids that interact with the aromatic side chains of Y97, F98, and F102 of the F3 zinc finger of F2F3 [30]. The NS1 amino acids in the F2F3 pocket are highly conserved among influenza A viruses isolated from humans. Substitution of R for one of the pocket amino acids (G184) eliminates detectable F2F3 binding *in vitro*, and a recombinant Ud virus

that encodes a NS1 protein with this substitution is attenuated, coupled with increased production of IFN-β [30]. Consequently, at least for the Ud virus, NS1 binding of CPSF30 is required for efficient virus replication.

Two NS1 amino acids outside the binding pocket, F103 and M106, have critical roles in the formation of the tetrameric structure (Figure 7.2c) [30]. For example, the side-chain of M106 in one NS1 molecule interacts with the side-chain of M106 (M106′) in the other NS1 protein (NS1′) as well as with residues in both F2F3 and F2F3′. F103 and M106 are highly conserved in seasonal (H1N1, H2N2, H3N2) influenza A viruses, and are conserved in H5N1 viruses isolated since 2003. Although F103L and M106I substitutions eliminate detectable F2F3 binding *in vitro* [35,36], they reduce rather than eliminate CPSF30 binding in infected cells because the viral polymerase proteins bind to, and stabilize the NS1–CPSF30 complex [36,37]. Nonetheless, such reduced binding of CPSF30 attenuates the virulence of the H5N1 viruses isolated in 1997 [38].

There are potentially two major mechanisms by which an influenza A virus NS1 protein may inhibit the antiviral IFN response (Table 7.1): (i) inhibiting the RIG-I/TRIM25 mediated activation of the IRF3 and NFκB transcription factors needed for transcription of the IFN gene (see section on inhibition of the RIG-I pathway); and (ii) inhibiting the 3′ end processing of IFN pre-mRNAs (see section on inhibition of host gene expression). A key question is whether both mechanisms are required for efficient virus replication. Recent results indicate that only one of these mechanisms may suffice for certain virus strains that infect humans. Several H3N2 and H2N2 viruses, as well as a subset of H1N1 viruses, do not inhibit the activation of IRF3 and IFN transcription [26]. This lack of inhibition has been correlated with the presence of a K at position 196 (versus an E) in the NS1 protein. Substituting E for the K at 196 in a H3N2 (Ud 1972 virus) NS1 protein in a recombinant virus restored a substantial amount of the inhibition of IRF3 and IFN-β transcription, and substituting the C-terminal region of a H1N1 NS1 protein (containing E at 196) for the H3N2 C-terminal region restored almost all of the inhibitory activity [26]. The NS1 proteins of all these viruses bind human TRIM25 (see section on inhibition of the RIG-I pathway) [25,26]. These results, as well as other results (see section on

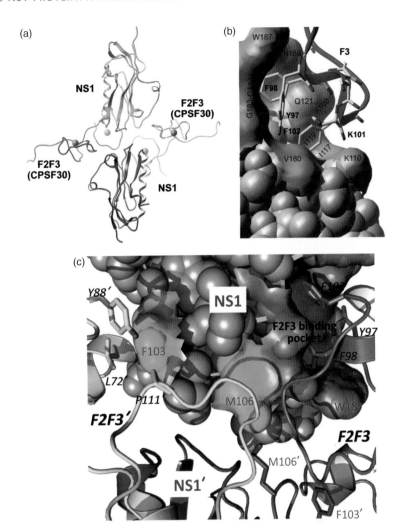

Figure 7.2. Crystal structure of the complex of F2F3 with the Ud NS1 ED (amino acids 85–215). (a) Two NS1 EDs and two F2F3 domains (blue and yellow) of CPSF30 form the tetramer. Both chains of the NS1 ED interact with each F2F3 molecule. (b) Expanded view of the F2F3 binding pocket. The NS1 amino acids labeled in red interact with the aromatic side chains of amino acids Y97, F98, and F102 of the F3 zinc finger of F2F3. (c) The roles of NS1 amino acids F103 and M106 in forming the tetrameric structure. Amino acids F103 and M106 (green surfaces) of one NS1 ED interact with both the F2F3 (blue) and F2F3′ (yellow) molecules. The M106 side-chain (green) of this NS1 ED also interacts with the M106′ side-chain (red) of the second NS1 ED chain.

regulation of the function of the NS1 protein of influenza A virus), indicate that the C-terminal region of the NS1 protein, which differs between virus strains (Figure 7.1a), is responsible for at least some of the strain-specific differences in NS1 protein function. Conversely, the 2009 H1N1 pandemic virus strongly inhibits IRF3 activation, but its NS1 protein does not efficiently block 3′ processing of IFN pre-mRNAs because its CPSF30 binding site is blocked by other amino acids [39]. Mutational restoration of CPSF30 binding did not improve virus replication. Because these two mechanisms impact other functions in addi-

tion to the IFN response, there may be other reasons why only one of these mechanisms suffices for efficient virus replication.

Inhibition of the activity of two antiviral proteins: PKR and 2′-5′-oligoadenylate synthetase (OAS)

Besides inhibiting IFN induction and IFN-mediated gene expression, the NS1 protein also inhibits the antiviral activity of at least two IFN-inducible proteins, PKR and OAS (Table 7.1). The protein kinase PKR is constitutively expressed in mammalian cells and its levels are further increased by IFN treatment [40]. When PKR is functionally activated by binding dsRNA, it phosphorylates the alpha subunit of the eIF2 translation initiation factor, resulting in the inhibition of viral and cellular protein synthesis and virus replication [41]. Hence, it is crucial for many viruses, including influenza virus, to block PKR activation. It was initially proposed that the NS1 protein inhibits PKR activation via the sequestering of dsRNA by its N-terminal RNA binding domain [42,43]. However, it was shown that binding of NS1 to dsRNA is not required for NS1-mediated PKR inhibition. Thus, PKR was not activated in cells infected with a Ud virus that expresses a NS1 protein lacking dsRNA binding activity (i.e., containing a R38A mutation) [44]. The NS1 protein inhibits PKR activation by direct binding to PKR [45,46]. *In vitro* binding assays showed that the NS1 protein binds to the N-terminal 230-amino acid region of PKR, resulting in inhibition of PKR activation [46]. These binding assays showed that the 123–127 amino acid region of the NS1 protein is required for PKR binding. The same NS1 sequence is required for inhibiting PKR activation during influenza virus infection: recombinant Ud viruses expressing NS1 proteins with A substitutions at either 123 and 124, or at 126 and 127 do not block PKR activation and eIF2α phosphorylation [45]. These experiments attributed the inhibition of PKR activation solely to the action of the NS1 protein. In agreement with this, an influenza virus that does not express the NS1 protein regains a significant amount of its replication and virulence in PKR knockout mice [47]. In contrast, others have provided evidence that a host factor activated during viral infection, p58IPK, has an important role in inhibiting PKR activation in influenza A virus infected cells [48,49].

OAS is an IFN-induced protein that is activated by dsRNA to produce polyA chains with 2′-5-phosphodiester bonds [50]. These polyA chains bind to and activate a constitutive enzyme, RNase L, which then cleaves viral and cellular single-stranded RNAs, thereby inhibiting virus replication. In addition, there is evidence that some of these RNA cleavage products bind to, and activate RIG-I, and thus enhance the activation of IFN transcription [50]. The primary role of NS1 dsRNA binding activity is the inhibition of the activation of the OAS/RNase L pathway [44]. This role was established using a Ud virus encoding a NS1 protein with a R38A mutation.

This mutation eliminates at least two functions of the NS1 protein: dsRNA binding and the NLS1 [44]. However, nuclear localization of the Ud NS1 protein was not affected by the R38A mutation, due to the presence of a second NLS, NLS2. The R38A mutation resulted in a large (1000-fold) attenuation of virus replication during multiple cycle growth. Activation of the OAS/RNase L pathway accounted for most, but not all of this attenuation [44]. The underlying defect responsible for the residual attenuation is not known, but it is not due to an increase in IFN production because no such increase was detected in Ud R38A-infected cells [44]. By contrast, the R38A mutation in combination with K41 appears to increase IFN induction by other influenza virus strains, specially the mouse-adapted H1N1 PR8 strain [25]. This may be attributable to the loss of NS1 binding to TRIM25 due to these two mutations and therefore lack of inhibition of RIG-I activation.

Induction of the PI3 K by the NS1 protein

PI3K proteins belong to a family of cellular enzymes that phosphorylate phosphatidylinositol to generate second messenger molecules that regulate several biologic processes involved in cell proliferation, apoptosis, intracellular trafficking, cytoskeletal rearrangements, and migration, among others [51]. Influenza A viruses activate the PI3K signaling pathway to promote viral infection at two stages of their replication cycle. During viral entry, virion attachment transiently activates PI3K to promote virus endocytosis. Later on during infection, and coincident with viral protein expression, PI3K is once more activated [52]. This second wave of PI3K activation is mediated by the NS1 protein (Table 7.1) [53–55]. The NS1 ED binds to the p85β regulatory subunit of PI3K (Figure 7.3), resulting in repositioning of the N-terminal domain of p85β which in turns relieves p85β-mediated inhibition of the p110 catalytic subunit of PI3K [56,57]. Similarly to NS1–CPSF30 interactions, NS1–p85β interactions appear to involve the monomeric form of the NS1 ED [57]. The highly conserved tyrosine at position 89 (Y89) and proline at position 164 (P164) of NS1 make critical contacts at the interface between NS1 and p85β [57]. A Y89F mutation in NS1 abrogates the NS1–p85β interaction and inhibits PI3K activation [56,57]. The functional consequences of NS1-mediated PI3K activation during influenza

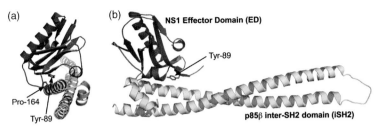

Figure 7.3. Crystal structure of the NS1–p85beta iSH2 complex. (a) Back, and (b) side cartoon representations of the four-helix bundle formed at the complex interface between three helices of the p85beta iSH2 domain and one helix of the NS1 effector domain. The p85beta iSH2 domain is shown in gold, and the NS1 effector domain is shown in red. Residues of NS1 that have been experimentally implicated in binding p85beta are highlighted. Figure courtesy of Ben Hale.

virus infection are still unclear. Active PI3K has been involved in many different functional outcomes, one of them being activation of the downstream kinase Akt [51]. Akt activation is in most instances a pro-survival signal, and therefore NS1-mediated induction of the PI3K/Akt may contribute to a delay of apoptosis of virus infected cells, contributing to enhaced virus replication [53].

The biologic consequences of the NS1 Y89F mutation is virus strain specific [58]. While this mutation prevents the second wave of PI3K/Akt activation in all Ud, PR8, and WSN influenza A virus infected cells, the mutation results in attenuated replication in tissue culture in the case of Ud and PR8 viruses [52,58,59], but not in the case of WSN virus [58]. The Y99F mutant PR8 virus [58,59], but not the Y98F mutant WSN virus [58], is attenuated in mice. These differences in phenotype correlated with the main site of activation of PI3K during wild-type viral infection, at the plasma membrane in the case of PR8 virus, and at the nuclear and perinuclear regions in the case of WSN [58].

Roles of the C-terminal motifs of the NS1 protein

The NS1 proteins of recent (after 1989) H3N2 viruses, such as A/WY/3/2003, end in the amino acid sequence ARSKV (Figure 7.1a). This sequence resembles the N-terminal sequence at the tail of histone H3, ARTKQ. Both the histone tail and the NS1 C-terminal sequence are modified at the K residue by cellular methylases and acetylases involved in chromatin remodeling [60]. As a consequence, the histone-like sequence in the NS1 acts as a histone mimic, enabling the NS1 protein to access chromatin remodeling components. Specifically, the H3N2 NS1 interacts through its histone-like tail with the human PAF1 transcription elongation complex, preventing elongation of transcription of host genes regulated by PAF1–chromatin interactions (Table 7.1) [60]. As PAF1 regulated genes include those involved in the IFN-mediated antiviral response, this epigenetic function of NS1 inhibits antiviral gene expression [60]. Thus, human H3N2 viruses have recently gained a novel NS1 inhibitory function by virtue of its NS1 C-terminal tail, which highlights the functional plasticity of the NS1 protein.

Large-scale sequence analyses of influenza viruses revealed that the NS1 proteins encoded by avian influenza viruses have a conserved C-terminal ESEV amino acid motif, whereas the NS1 proteins of human influenza viruses have a different C-terminal motif, most often RSKV when the 7 amino-acid C-terminal extension is absent (Figure 7.1a) [3]. Both of these motifs bind cellular proteins that contain a PDZ domain. Because most pathogenic H5N1 viruses possess the ESEV motif, it was postulated that this motif is a virulence determinant, specifically by targeting cellular proteins that contain particular types of PDZ domains. In fact, the ESEV domain, but not the RSKV domain, was shown to bind to several host proteins that are antiapoptotic and/or regulate cell polarity establishment [61,62]. Two studies, using either the mouse-adapted H1N1 WSN strain or a H7N1 avian virus, found that the ESEV sequence contributed to virulence in mice [63,64]. However, in

121

contrast, the NS1 protein of the highly pathogenic H5N1 A/VN/1203/04 virus has a C-terminal deletion and lacks the ESEV terminus, and the addition of a ESEV terminus did not increase virulence in mice [65].

Other NS1 functions

Viral RNA synthesis

Several studies have provided evidence for a NS1–polymerase interaction and for a role of the NS1 protein in viral RNA synthesis. For example, the Ud virus expressing a NS1 protein with A substitutions at 123 and 124 not only binds PKR and inhibits its activation, but also deregulates the normal time course of viral RNA synthesis that occurs in wt virus infected cells [45]. Gene expression in influenza A virus infected cells has been shown to be divided into an early and late phase. During the early phase the NS and NP vRNAs are selectively replicated and transcribed, whereas during the late phase all vRNAs, including the NS and NP vRNAs, are replicated and transcribed at a high rate [66,67]. In the mutant virus infected cells late, as well as early vRNAs, viral mRNAs and proteins are synthesized at high levels at very early times after infection, resulting in the enhancement of virus replication [45]. The deregulation of viral RNA synthesis also occurred in PKR–/– mouse cells, demonstrating that it is independent of PKR. This is one example where the same sequence in the NS1 protein mediates disparate functions, which may also be the case for other NS1 sequences. Similar NS1-dependent effects on viral RNA synthesis have been observed with other influenza A viruses. Work with A/VN/1203/04 and PR8 viruses that express NS1 proteins containing C-terminal truncations indicate that the NS1 protein is required for optimal transcription of late influenza virus genes, such as HA and M, but only minimally for transcription of early virus genes, such as NP [68].

Further evidence for a NS1–polymerase interaction came from the demonstration that the NS1–CPSF30 complex in infected cells is part of a macromolecular complex that contains the proteins of the virus polymerase complex that catalyzes viral RNA replication (PB1, PB2, PA, NP) [37]. Subsequent work showed that the NS1 protein probably interacts with the NP component of the viral polymerase complex

(Table 7.1) [69]. However, the mechanism by which the NS1 protein regulates the time course of viral RNA synthesis in infected cells has not yet been determined.

Viral protein synthesis

Translation of cellular mRNAs is strongly inhibited in influenza virus infected cells, and viral mRNAs are selectively translated. The NS1 protein-mediated inhibition of the production of newly synthesized cellular mRNAs (described above) probably has a role in this process, but the NS1 protein may also have a direct effect on the selective translation of viral mRNAs. For example, it was reported that the NS1 protein binds to the common viral 5′ untranslated region (UTR) of viral mRNAs [70] and also interacts with the eIF4GI and PABP1 translation factors (Table 7.1) [71,72]. Consequently, the NS1 protein may recruit these translation factors to the 5′ ends of viral mRNAs, thereby favoring the translation of viral mRNAs.

Other cellular partners

In this chapter, we have focused on specific NS1–cellular proteins interactions that have been investigated in detail both biochemically and functionally. The NS1 protein has also been reported to bind to several other host proteins, with potentially interesting biologic consequences. Because of space constrains, we only briefly describe some of these interactions in the text below. For example, in addition to the well-characterized NS1–CPSF30 interaction resulting in inhibition of cell mRNA processing, it has also been reported that the NS1 protein inhibits host gene expression by binding to, and sequestering, a complex composed of NXF1/TAP, p15/NXT, Rae1/mrnp41, and E1B-AP5 cellular proteins, which are critical components of the mRNA export machinery [73].

It has also been reported that the NS1 ED contains a Src homology type 3 (SH3) binding domain, which binds SH3 domain-containing proteins, such as Src [74], and enhances the NS1 interaction with PI3K [75]. Other cellular factors reported to interact with NS1 are RNA helicase A, Staufen, hnRNP-F, p53, hsp90, Akt, CRK/CRKL, and several others identified by the yeast-two-hybrid system [76]. Additional experimentation is needed to understand the significance of these reported interactions during viral infection.

Unique function of the NS1 protein of influenza B virus (B/NS1): Binding IFN-induced ISG15

A protein that is strongly induced by IFNα/β is ISG15, which is comprised of two ubiquitin-like (Ubl) domains connected by a short five amino acid linker [77]. The C-terminal Ubl domain contains a LRLRGG sequence at its C-terminus which is conjugated to target proteins by the sequential action of three enzymes that are also induced by IFNα/β. The E1 enzyme Ube1L activates ISG15 [78], which is then transferred to the E2 conjugating enzyme UbcH8 [79,80]. Herc5, the major ISG15 E3 ligase in humans [81,82], then conjugates ISG15 to target proteins. The first evidence for an antiviral function for ISG15 and/or its conjugation was the finding that the NS1 protein of influenza B virus (B/NS1) binds ISG15, preventing ISG15 conjugation [78], suggesting that ISG15 and/or its conjugation inhibits influenza B virus replication. The NS1 protein of influenza A virus (A/NS1) does not bind ISG15. Subsequent research showed that ISG15 conjugation inhibits influenza A virus replication [83,84], and experiments using ISG15 and Ube1L −/− mice established that ISG15 conjugation inhibits the replication of influenza A and several other viruses, including Sindbis virus and herpes simplex 1 virus [84].

The ISG15 and Ube1L knockout mice were also more susceptible to influenza B virus infection than wild-type mice [84]. However, it was not clear why the B/NS1 protein was unable to protect influenza B virus from the antiviral effects of ISG15 and/or its conjugation in wild-type mice. This issue was resolved by the demonstration that the B/NS1 protein does not bind mouse ISG15 [85,86] and in fact binds only human and nonhuman primate ISG15 proteins [85]. Surprisingly, the short five amino acid linker plays a large part in this species-specific binding [85]. The linker of human and nonhuman primate ISG15, which has a sequence that differs from other mammalian ISG15 proteins, is absolutely required for binding the B/NS1 protein. This is the first example of an influenza B protein that exhibits human (and nonhuman primate)-specific properties and hence provides one possible explanation for the restriction of influenza B virus to humans.

The B/NS1 sequence required for binding ISG15 is comprised of its RBD (amino acids 1–93) and linker region (amino acids 94–103), denoted as the N-terminal region (NTR) [78]. X-ray crystallography showed that one NTR binds two ISG15 molecules (Figure 7.4a). Each of the ISG15 molecules binds to a surface site on the B/NS1 NTR dimer composed of regions from both chains: amino acids in the RBD from one NTR chain and amino acids in the linker from the other NTR chain. The dsRNA binding site and the NLS are not occluded by ISG15 binding. Mutagenesis experiments established that both parts of the ISG15 binding site on the NTR chains are required for binding ISG15 and also for the inhibition of ISG15 conjugation as assayed in transfection experiments [78]. In addition, the crystal structure showed that a strong contact region of the B/NS1 NTR on ISG15 includes amino acids in the ISG15 linker that are specific for human and nonhuman primate ISG15 molecules (Figure 7.4b) [78], explaining the species-specificity of B/NS1 binding of ISG15. The B/NS1 NTR also interacts with amino acids in the N-terminal Ubl domain, but makes essentially no contacts with the C-terminal Ubl domain, indicating that the latter domain would be expected to be accessible to conjugating enzymes [87]. Nonetheless, B/NS1 or its NTR inhibit IFN-induced ISG15 conjugation in transfection assays [78,86]. Because the C-terminal Ubl domain of ISG15 appears to be accessible to conjugating enzymes when it is bound to the B/NS1-NTR, it is not clear how B/NS1 binding of ISG15 inhibits its conjugation.

Regulation of the function of the NS1 protein of influenza A virus

The NS1 protein undergoes at least three post-translational modifications: phosphorylation, ISG15 modification, and SUMO modification. These modifications have been reported to affect the NS1 protein and virus replication. Experiments with the H3N1 Ud virus showed that the NS1 protein is phosphorylated at both serines (Ss) and a threonine (T), specifically S42, S48, and T215 [88]. The role of these phosphorylations was evaluated by substituting other amino acids at these positions. In the case of T215, the only amino acid substitution that reduced virus replication was a A-for-T substitution [88,89], whereas all other substitutions (E to mimic constitutive phosphorylation; P to mimic the avian P-215 signature; or N) did

(a)

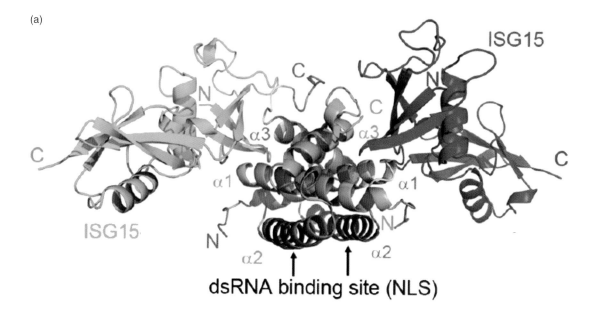

(b)

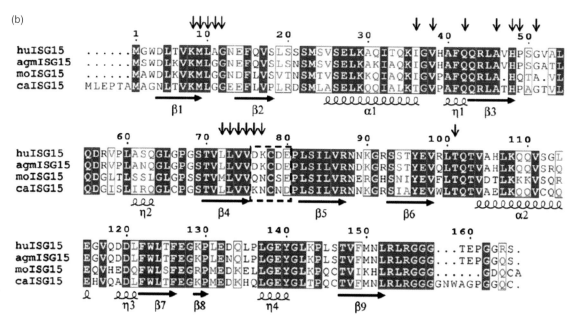

Figure 7.4. Structure of the complex of B/NS1 NTR with ISG15. (a) Each B/NS1 homodimer binds two ISG15 molecules. Each ISG15 binding site has contributions from both chains in the B/NS1 dimer. (b) The amino acids in human ISG15 that interact with B/NS1 NTR. The arrows indicate the amino acids contacting B/NS1 NTR. ISG15 amino acids 76–80 (bracketed) constitute the linker between the two Ubl domains. Two of these linker amino acids (D76 and K77), which are unique to human (hu) and nonhuman primate (agm, African green monkey) ISG15 molecules, interact with B/NS1 NTR. The linkers of mouse (mo) and canine (ca) do not have these two amino acids at positions 76 and 77. Secondary structure of ISG15 is shown below the sequence.

not affect virus replication [88]. These results indicated that attenuation resulting from the T-to-A substitution at position 215 is attributable to a deleterious structural change in the NS1 protein that is not caused by other amino acid substitutions, and that phosphorylation of T215 does not affect virus replication. At position 48 neither a S-to-A substitution, nor a S-to-D substitution affected virus replication, indicating that S48 phosphorylation does not have a role in virus replication [88]. In fact, S at position 48 in the NS1 proteins of H3N2 viruses changed to N in the mid-1980s, and the 2009 H1N1 pandemic virus has N at this position (Figure 7.1a). In contrast, at position 42, a S-to-D, but not a S-to-A substitution caused attenuation [88]. This attenuation is attributable to the loss of dsRNA-binding activity caused by the S-to-D substitution at position 42. S42 is directly involved in dsRNA binding by forming hydrogen bonds with 2′-OH groups of the dsRNA [10]. Consequently, replacing S42 with the negatively charged D amino acid not only eliminates this hydrogen bonding but also repels the negatively charged dsRNA. Hence, analogous to the R38A mutation [44], S42 phosphorylation may be expected to lead to the activation of OAS. However, because it is not known when S42 phosphorylation occurs during infection and what fraction of the NS1 protein is phosphorylated, the timing and extent of activation of the 2′-5′ OAS/RNaseL pathway by S42 phosphorylation during infection is also not known. Activated PKCα phosphorylates S42 of the Ud NS1 protein [88]. Interestingly, phosphorylation of S42, or any other S or T, of the NS1 protein of the 2009 H1N1 virus was not detected [88].

The A/NS1 protein is the primary influenza A virus target of IFN-induced ISG15 conjugation [90,91]. Transfection assays identified multiple Ks in the NS1 protein that could be ISG15 modified [90,91]. However, in infected cells IFN-induced ISG15 conjugation occurs largely on K41 in the RBD [91]. It is not known how K41 is selected over the other potential sites for ISG15 modification. K41 participates in two crucial functions: binding of dsRNA [6,10]; and binding of importin α and hence the NLS function of the RBD [5]. Surprisingly, the NS1 binding sites for dsRNA and importin α are not totally overlapping, enabling both molecules to bind to the RBD at the same time. ISG15 modification of K41 disrupted the association of the RBD with importin α, whereas

dsRNA binding activity was retained [91]. A K41R mutation in the WSN NS1 protein, which lacks NLS2, eliminated ISG15 modification of amino acid 41 and provided approximately a 10-fold protection against the antiviral action of IFN-β [91], comparable to the protection provided by overall elimination of ISG15 conjugation [83]. This result indicated that ISG15 modification of K41 of the NS1 protein inhibits influenza A virus replication in IFN-β-treated cells despite the fact that only a small fraction (~5%) of the steady state amount of the NS1 protein contains an ISG15-modified K41 amino acid. Similarly, ISG15 conjugation of filamin B also inhibits its function, despite the fact that only a small amount of this protein is ISG15 modified [92]. Interestingly, K41 is replaced by R in the NS1 proteins of H3N2 influenza A viruses isolated after 1986, suggesting that these viruses have undergone selection to counter ISG15 modification of their NS1 proteins.

The NS1 protein is also modified by another ubiquitin-like protein, SUMO [93,94]. Two Ks in the C-terminal region of NS1, K219 and K221, were identified as the sites of sumoylation [94]. Transfection assays indicated that sumoylation of these two Ks enhanced the stability of the NS1 protein. In addition, a WSN virus that expressed a NS1 protein with E rather than K at these two positions replicated somewhat slower than the wild-type virus, consistent with some enhancement of virus replication resulting from sumoylation of these two Ks.

The NS1 protein undoubtedly carries out its functions in different locations in the cell, some in the nucleus (e.g., CPSF30 binding, histone mimicry) and some in the cytoplasm (e.g., interactions with the RIG-I pathway, PKR binding, activating PI3K). It is not known where dsRNA binding occurs. Consequently, the NLSs and NES in the NS1 protein have important roles in NS1 function in infected cells. In addition, these different functions apparently involve differences in the ED–ED interaction via the helix–helix interface. This ED–ED interaction is quite weak, and is disrupted when the NS1 protein interacts with cellular protein targets, for example, with CPSF30 (Figure 7.2) and most likely with the p85β subunit of PI3 kinase (Figure 7.3). Conversely, ED–ED interactions via the W187 amino acid enhance dsRNA binding [11,13]. One interpretation of this result is that that these enhancing ED–ED interactions are intermolecular rather than intramolecular, and thus

125

provide molecular interactions between neighboring NS1 proteins on relatively long dsRNAs [11]. In other words, these ED–ED interactions may mediate cooperative dsRNA binding by the NS1 protein. In this model, the CPSF30 binding pocket is buried because NS1–NS1 interactions are mediated by the same ED interface. Consequently, this model predicts that the NS1 proteins bound to dsRNA cannot bind CPSF30. Future experiments will determine whether this model is valid.

Impact of the NS1 protein of influenza A virus in virulence, host tropism, and immune responses

Considering that the NS1 protein modulates host antiviral responses and promotes replication, it is not surprising that NS1 has a pivotal role in viral pathogenesis. Deletion of the NS1 gene from the viral genome results in a highly debilitated virus unable to efficiently replicate in immunocompetent hosts, but replicates and causes disease in IFN-deficient hosts, underscoring the importance of NS1 in inhibition of the antiviral IFN-mediated response during influenza virus infection [1]. Moreover, the NS1 protein, by virtue of its inhibition of innate immune signaling and cell gene expression, prevents optimal activation of infected antigen presenting cells. Specifically, dendritic cells infected with NS1-deficient influenza viruses, but not with wild-type viruses, are rapidly activated: they secrete proinflammatory cytokines, upregulate chemokine receptors and co-stimulatory molecules, and efficiently induce activation of T cells [95].

Strain-specific variations in the NS1 protein have been shown to result in differences in virulence. For instance, the NS1 protein of the pandemic 1918 H1N1 virus strain, which caused extremely high morbidity and mortality in humans, mediates increased virulence in nonhuman primates [96]. This phenotype correlated with specific changes in host gene expression both *in vivo* and in primary human epithelial cells in tissue culture. Notably, the 1918 NS1 protein mediated a more profound downregulation of genes associated with innate antiviral immunity and with lipid metabolism than a NS1 protein from a modern seasonal human H1N1 virus [97]. The specific

sequence features and molecular basis responsible for these differences are still unknown.

Because the NS1 protein interacts with multiple cellular factors, the ability of an animal strain of influenza virus to gain the ability to efficiently infect and transmit to humans, thereby initiating an influenza pandemic, may require specific changes in the NS1 protein to enable it to interact optimally with human proteins that may differ from the proteins of the original host. Consistent with this notion, sequence analysis of the NS1 genes from virus strains infecting different hosts (birds, pigs, horses, dogs, and humans), has revealed specific NS1 sequence variant features associated with specific hosts [98]. Moreover, adaptation of human influenza viruses to mice is known to result in adaptive NS1 changes [99]. However, our understanding of NS1 changes associated with host tropism is still very limited.

NS1 protein as an antiviral target

The multifunctional NS1 protein is an attractive target for the development of new influenza virus antivirals. Influenza A viruses that do not express the NS1 protein or express truncated forms of the NS1 protein are attenuated [2], demonstrating that a functional NS1 protein is essential for virus replication. In addition, as already described above, point mutations in the NS1 protein that disrupt critical interactions with cellular protein targets are attenuated.

One approach for identifying small molecule inhibitors of the NS1 protein has been to use a cell-based screen for chemical compounds that inhibit a NS1 function, specifically the ability of the H1N1 PR8 virus to block the activation of the IFN-β promoter [100]. Unexpectedly, one compound that was identified by this screen, denoted as ASN2, does not target the NS1 protein, but instead targets a region of the PB1 polymerase protein, resulting in the reduced expression of the mRNAs for the NS1 protein and the NEP/NS2 protein [100]. The expression of the mRNAs for the M1 and M2 mRNAs was also reduced, whereas the expression of other viral mRNAs was not affected. The molecular basis for the selective suppression of the production of these mRNAs is not known. The ASN2 compound inhibited the replication of an array of influenza A virus strains, and protected mice against a lethal infection by the WSN virus strain. An important caveat, however, is that a point mutation in the PB1 protein confers resistance to ASN2 [100], so that viruses resistant to ASN2 may readily arise.

Another approach consists in finding small molecules that revert the NS1-mediated inhibition of host gene expression in a cell-based assay [101]. This strategy has identified two classes of compounds that counteract this NS1 inhibition and inhibit virus replication. The first class consists of naphthalimides that induce expression of the host protein REDD1 which is involved in inhibition of the mTORC1 pathway [101]. As this pathway is needed for optimal replication of not only influenza A viruses, but also many other viruses, these compounds have broad antiviral activity [101]. Hence, these compounds are not specific inhibitors of the influenza virus NS1 protein. The second class consists of inhibitors of the cellular enzyme dihydroorotate dehydrogenase (DHODH), which is involved in pyrimidine synthesis [102]. Reduction of the pyrimidine pool by DHODH inhibitors promote export of cellular mRNAs in the presence of viral antagonists of this function, such as the NS1 protein of influenza A virus and the M protein of vesicular stomatitis virus [102]. Moreover, DHODH inhibition also interferes with viral RNA synthesis, which requires a high pool of pyrimidines [103]. Nevertheless, it remains to be determined whether such inhibitors are able to decrease viral replication *in vivo* without significant toxicity.

A third approach has been to screen for compounds that bind to specific regions of the NS1 protein, and to determine whether these compounds inhibit virus replication [104]. One group used a yeast screen to identify compounds that bind at some, albeit undetermined, position in the NS1 protein [105]. One of these compounds was then subjected to chemical modifications that led to compounds with increased antiviral activity [106]. Other groups are screening for compounds that bind *in vitro* to either the dsRNA-binding site in the RBD or the CPSF30-binding site in the ED [104]. The goal of this second approach is to obtain X-ray crystal or NMR structures of small molecules in complex with the NS1 protein, so that structure-based optimization of these small molecules can be undertaken.

NS1-modified viruses as potential live attenuated vaccines

Because the loss of NS1 function increases activation of antigen presenting cells, NS1-deleted influenza viruses appear to be potent inducers of immune responses in different animal models [107]. This property, together with the high levels of attenuation of NS1-deleted viruses *in vivo*, indicated that NS1-modified influenza viruses may serve as efficient live-attenuated vaccines against influenza virus. Nonhuman primates vaccinated with a human influenza H1N1 virus encoding a large carboxy-terminal deletion in its NS1 protein developed more efficacious protective immune responses against wild-type influenza virus challenge than those vaccinated with a conventional inactivated influenza virus vaccine [108]. Vaccination of pigs with NS1-modified swine influenza virus provided protection against challenge with homologous and antigenically drifted swine influenza virus strains [109]. Importantly, vaccination of healthy volunteers with an influenza virus lacking the NS1 gene proved to be safe while inducing neutralizing antibodies [110]. While these studies support the possible use of NS1-modified viruses as influenza virus vaccines, the optimal NS1 modification resulting in a safely attenuated and highly immunogenic influenza virus vaccine strain remains to be determined.

Conclusions

The NS1 protein of influenza A virus has been the focus of many studies, which have revealed several functions of this small viral protein. However, controversies about some of these functions remain, and the present authors realize that some investigators may not agree with all the statements made in this chapter. In addition, there are large gaps in the understanding of this multifunctional protein, and it is anticipated that future research will uncover surprising new functions. One of the complications is that the same sequence, or overlapping sequences of the NS1 protein may mediate more than one function, reflecting the fact that the NS1 protein in infected cells carries out different functions in different sites in the cell. In addition, evidence is accumulating that NS1 functions vary to some extent between virus strains, further complicating research. Finally, very little is currently known about the NS1 protein of influenza B virus (B/NS1), whose ED likely mediates different functions than the ED of the NS1 protein of influenza A virus (A/NS1).

References

1. García-Sastre A, Egorov A, Matassov D, Brandt S, Levy DE, Durbin JE, et al. Influenza A virus lacking the NS1 gene replicates in interferon-deficient systems. Virology. 1998;252:324–30.

2. Hale BG, Randall RE, Ortin J, Jackson D. The multifunctional NS1 protein of influenza A viruses. J Gen Virol. 2008;89:2359–76.

3. Obenauer JC, Denson J, Mehta PK, Su X, Mukatira S, Finkelstein DB, et al. Large-scale sequence analysis of avian influenza isolates. Science. 2006;311:1576–80.

4. Greenspan D, Palese P, Krystal M. Two nuclear location signals in the influenza virus NS1 nonstructural protein. J Virol. 1988;62:3020–6.

5. Melén K, Kinnunen L, Fagerlund R, Ikonen N, Twu KY, Krug RM, et al. Nuclear and nucleolar targeting of influenza A virus NS1 protein: striking differences between different virus subtypes. J Virol. 2007;81: 5995–6006.

6. Wang W, Riedel K, Lynch P, Chien CY, Montelione GT, Krug RM. RNA binding by the novel helical domain of the influenza virus NS1 protein requires its dimer structure and a small number of specific basic amino acids. RNA. 1999;5:195–205.

7. Li Y, Yamakita Y, Krug RM. Regulation of a nuclear export signal by an adjacent inhibitory sequence: The effector domain of the influenza virus NS1 protein. Proc Natl Acad Sci U S A. 1998;95:4864–9.

8. Chien CY, Tejero R, Huang Y, Zimmerman DE, Rios CB, Krug RM, et al. A novel RNA-binding motif in influenza A virus non-structural protein 1. Nat Struct Biol. 1997;4:891–5.

9. Liu J, Lynch PA, Chien CY, Montelione GT, Krug RM, Berman HM. Crystal structure of the unique RNA-binding domain of the influenza virus NS1 protein. Nat Struct Biol. 1997;4:896–9.

10. Cheng A, Wong SM, Yuan YA. Structural basis for dsRNA recognition by NS1 protein of influenza A virus. Cell Res. 2009;19:187–95.

11. Aramini JM, Ma LC, Zhou L, Schauder CM, Hamilton K, Amer BR, et al. Dimer interface of the effector domain of non-structural protein 1 from influenza A virus: an interface with multiple functions. J Biol Chem. 2011;286:26050–60.

12. Hale BG, Barclay WS, Randall RE, Russell RJ. Structure of an avian influenza A virus NS1 protein effector domain. Virology. 2008;378:1–5.

13. Kerry PS, Ayllon J, Taylor MA, Hass C, Lewis A, García-Sastre A, et al. A transient homotypic interaction model for the influenza A virus NS1 protein effector domain. PLoS ONE. 2011;6:e17946.

14. Xia S, Monzingo AF, Robertus JD. Structure of NS1A effector domain from the influenza A/Udorn/72 virus. Acta Crystallogr D Biol Crystallogr. 2009;65: 11–7.

15. Takeuchi O, Akira S. Innate immunity to virus infection. Immunol Rev. 2009;227:75–86.

16. Mibayashi M, Martinez-Sobrido L, Loo YM, Cardenas WB, Gale M Jr, García-Sastre A. Inhibition of retinoic acid-inducible gene I-mediated induction of beta interferon by the NS1 protein of influenza A virus. J Virol. 2007;81:514–24.

17. Guo Z, Chen LM, Zeng H, Gomez JA, Plowden J, Fujita T, et al. NS1 protein of influenza A virus inhibits the function of intracytoplasmic pathogen sensor, RIG-I. Am J Respir Cell Mol Biol. 2007;36:263–9.

18. Opitz B, Rejaibi A, Dauber B, Eckhard J, Vinzing M, Schmeck B, et al. IFNbeta induction by influenza A virus is mediated by RIG-I which is regulated by the viral NS1 protein. Cell Microbiol. 2007;9:930–8.

19. Pichlmair A, Schulz O, Tan CP, Naslund TI, Liljestrom P, Weber F, et al. RIG-I-mediated antiviral responses to single-stranded RNA bearing 5'-phosphates. Science. 2006;314:997–1001.

20. Myong S, Cui S, Cornish PV, Kirchhofer A, Gack MU, Jung JU, et al. Cytosolic viral sensor RIG-I is a 5'-triphosphate-dependent translocase on double-stranded RNA. Science. 2009;323:1070–4.

21. Gack MU, Shin YC, Joo CH, Urano T, Liang C, Sun L, et al. TRIM25 RING-finger E3 ubiquitin ligase is essential for RIG-I-mediated antiviral activity. Nature. 2007;446:916–20.

22. Oshiumi H, Miyashita M, Inoue N, Okabe M, Matsumoto M, Seya T. The ubiquitin ligase Riplet is essential for RIG-I-dependent innate immune responses to RNA virus infection. Cell Host Microbe. 2010;8: 496–509.

23. Zeng W, Sun L, Jiang X, Chen X, Hou F, Adhikari A, et al. Reconstitution of the RIG-I pathway reveals a signaling role of unanchored polyubiquitin chains in innate immunity. Cell. 2010;141:315–30.

24. Chien CY, Xu Y, Xiao R, Aramini JM, Sahasrabudhe PV, Krug RM, et al. Biophysical characterization of the complex between double-stranded RNA and the N-terminal domain of the NS1 protein from influenza A virus: evidence for a novel RNA-binding mode. Biochemistry. 2004;43:1950–62.

25. Gack MU, Albrecht RA, Urano T, Inn KS, Huang IC, Carnero E, et al. Influenza A virus NS1 targets the ubiquitin ligase TRIM25 to evade recognition by the host viral RNA sensor RIG-I. Cell Host Microbe. 2009;5:439–49.

26. Kuo RL, Zhao C, Malur M, Krug RM. Influenza A virus strains that circulate in humans differ in the ability of their NS1 proteins to block the activation of IRF3 and interferon-beta transcription. Virology. 2010;408:146–58.

27. Colgan DF, Manley JL. Mechanism and regulation of mRNA polyadenylation. Genes Dev. 1997;11:2755–66.

28. Wahle E, Keller W. The biochemistry of polyadenylation. Trends Biochem Sci. 1996;21:247–50.

29. Nemeroff ME, Barabino SM, Li Y, Keller W, Krug RM. Influenza virus NS1 protein interacts with the cellular 30 kDa subunit of CPSF and inhibits 3' end formation of cellular pre-mRNAs. Mol Cell. 1998;1:991–1000.

30. Das K, Ma LC, Xiao R, Radvansky B, Aramini J, Zhao L, et al. Structural basis for suppression of a host antiviral response by influenza A virus. Proc Natl Acad Sci U S A. 2008;105:13093–8.

31. Noah DL, Twu KY, Krug RM. Cellular antiviral responses against influenza A virus are countered at the posttranscriptional level by the viral NS1A protein via its binding to a cellular protein required for the 3' end processing of cellular pre-mRNAS. Virology. 2003;307:386–95.

32. Twu KY, Noah DL, Rao P, Kuo RL, Krug RM. The CPSF30 binding site on the NS1A protein of influenza A virus is a potential antiviral target. J Virol. 2006;80:3957–65.

33. Robertson JS, Schubert M, Lazzarini RA. Polyadenylation sites for influenza virus mRNA. J Virol. 1981;38:157–63.

34. Barabino SM, Hubner W, Jenny A, Minvielle-Sebastia L, Keller W. The 30-kD subunit of mammalian cleavage and polyadenylation specificity factor and its yeast homolog are RNA-binding zinc finger proteins. Genes Dev. 1997;11:1703–16.

35. Kochs G, García-Sastre A, Martinez-Sobrido L. Multiple anti-interferon actions of the influenza A virus NS1 protein. J Virol. 2007;81:7011–21.

36. Twu KY, Kuo RL, Marklund J, Krug RM. The H5N1 influenza virus NS genes selected after 1998 enhance virus replication in mammalian cells. J Virol. 2007;81:8112–21.

37. Kuo RL, Krug RM. Influenza A virus polymerase is an integral component of the CPSF30-NS1A protein complex in infected cells. J Virol. 2009;83:1611–6.

38. Spesock A, Malur M, Hossain MJ, Chen LM, Njaa BL, Davis CT, et al. The virulence of 1997 H5N1 influenza viruses in the mouse model is increased by correcting a defect in their NS1 proteins. J Virol. 2011;85:7048–58.

39. Hale BG, Steel J, Medina RA, Manicassamy B, Ye J, Hickman D, et al. Inefficient control of host gene expression by the 2009 pandemic H1N1 influenza A virus NS1 protein. J Virol. 2010;84:6909–22.

40. Hovanessian AG. The double stranded RNA-activated protein kinase induced by interferon: dsRNA-PK. J Interferon Res. 1989;9:641–7.

41. Gale MJ, Katze MG. Molecular mechanisms of interferon resistance mediated by viral-directed inhibition of PKR, the interferon-induced protein kinase. Pharmacol Ther. 1998;78:29–46.

42. Hatada E, Fukuda R. Binding of influenza A virus NS1 protein to dsRNA in vitro. J Gen Virol. 1992;73:3325–9.

43. Lu Y, Wambach M, Katze MG, Krug RM. Binding of the influenza virus NS1 protein to double-stranded RNA inhibits the activation of the protein kinase that phosphorylates the elF-2 translation initiation factor. Virology. 1995;214:222–8.

44. Min JY, Krug RM. The primary function of RNA binding by the influenza A virus NS1 protein in infected cells: Inhibiting the 2'-5' oligo (A) synthetase/RNase L pathway. Proc Natl Acad Sci U S A. 2006;103:7100–5.

45. Min JY, Li S, Sen GC, Krug RM. A site on the influenza A virus NS1 protein mediates both inhibition of PKR activation and temporal regulation of viral RNA synthesis. Virology. 2007;363:236–43.

46. Li S, Min JY, Krug RM, Sen GC. Binding of the influenza A virus NS1 protein to PKR mediates the inhibition of its activation by either PACT or double-stranded RNA. Virology. 2006;349:13–21.

47. Bergmann M, García-Sastre A, Carnero E, Pehamberger H, Wolff K, Palese P, et al. Influenza virus NS1 protein counteracts PKR-mediated inhibition of replication. J Virol. 2000;74:6203–6.

48. Goodman AG, Smith JA, Balachandran S, Perwitasari O, Proll SC, Thomas MJ, et al. The cellular protein P58IPK regulates influenza virus mRNA translation and replication through a PKR-mediated mechanism. J Virol. 2007;81:2221–30.

49. Melville MW, Tan SL, Wambach M, Song J, Morimoto RI, Katze MG. The cellular inhibitor of the PKR protein kinase, P58(IPK), is an influenza virus-activated co-chaperone that modulates heat shock protein 70 activity. J Biol Chem. 1999;274:3797–803.

50. Chakrabarti A, Jha BK, Silverman RH. New insights into the role of RNase L in innate immunity. J Interferon Cytokine Res. 2011;31:49–57.

51. Engelman JA, Luo J, Cantley LC. The evolution of phosphatidylinositol 3-kinases as regulators of growth and metabolism. Nat Rev Genet. 2006;7:606–19.

52. Ayllon J, García-Sastre A, Hale BG. Influenza A viruses and PI3K: Are there time, place, and manner restrictions? Virulence. 2012;3.

53. Ehrhardt C, Wolff T, Pleschka S, Planz O, Beermann W, Bode JG, et al. Influenza A virus NS1 protein activates the PI3K/Akt pathway to mediate antiapoptotic signaling responses. J Virol. 2007;81:3058–67.

54. Hale BG, Jackson D, Chen YH, Lamb RA, Randall RE. Influenza A virus NS1 protein binds p85beta and activates phosphatidylinositol-3-kinase signaling. Proc Natl Acad Sci U S A. 2006;103:14194–9.

55. Shin YK, Liu Q, Tikoo SK, Babiuk LA, Zhou Y. Influenza A virus NS1 protein activates the phosphatidylinositol 3-kinase (PI3K)/Akt pathway by direct interaction with the p85 subunit of PI3K. J Gen Virol. 2007;88:13–8.

56. Hale BG, Batty IH, Downes CP, Randall RE. Binding of influenza A virus NS1 protein to the inter-SH2 domain of p85 suggests a novel mechanism for phosphoinositide 3-kinase activation. J Biol Chem. 2008;283:1372–80.

57. Hale BG, Kerry PS, Jackson D, Precious BL, Gray A, Killip MJ, et al. Structural insights into phosphoinositide 3-kinase activation by the influenza A virus NS1 protein. Proc Natl Acad Sci U S A. 2010;107:1954–9.

58. Ayllon J, Hale BG, García-Sastre A. Strain-specific contribution of NS1-activated phosphoinositide 3-kinase signaling to influenza A virus replication and virulence. J Virol. 2012;86:5366–70.

59. Hrincius ER, Hennecke AK, Gensler L, Nordhoff C, Anhlan D, Vogel P, et al. A Single Point Mutation (Y89F) within the Non-Structural Protein 1 of Influenza A Viruses Limits Epithelial Cell Tropism and Virulence in Mice. Am J Pathol. 2012;180:2361–74.

60. Marazzi I, Ho JS, Kim J, Manicassamy B, Dewell S, Albrecht RA, et al. Suppression of the antiviral response by an influenza histone mimic. Nature. 2012;483:428–33.

61. Javier RT, Rice AP. Emerging theme: cellular PDZ proteins as common targets of pathogenic viruses. J Virol. 2011;85:11544–56.

62. Liu H, Golebiewski L, Dow EC, Krug RM, Javier RT, Rice AP. The ESEV PDZ-binding motif of the avian influenza A virus NS1 protein protects infected cells from apoptosis by directly targeting Scribble. J Virol. 2010;84:11164–74.

63. Jackson D, Hossain MJ, Hickman D, Perez DR, Lamb RA. A new influenza virus virulence determinant: the NS1 protein four C-terminal residues modulate pathogenicity. Proc Natl Acad Sci U S A. 2008;105:4381–6.

64. Soubies SM, Volmer C, Croville G, Loupias J, Peralta B, Costes P, et al. Species-specific contribution of the four C-terminal amino acids of influenza A virus NS1 protein to virulence. J Virol. 2010;84:6733–47.

65. Zielecki F, Semmler I, Kalthoff D, Voss D, Mauel S, Gruber AD, et al. Virulence determinants of avian H5N1 influenza A virus in mammalian and avian hosts: role of the C-terminal ESEV motif in the viral NS1 protein. J Virol. 2010;84:10708–18.

66. Shapiro GI, Gurney T Jr, Krug RM. Influenza virus gene expression: control mechanisms at early and late times of infection and nuclear-cytoplasmic transport of virus-specific RNAs. J Virol. 1987;61:764–73.

67. Skehel JJ. Early polypeptide synthesis in influenza virus-infected cells. Virology. 1973;56:394–9.

68. Maamary J, Pica N, Belicha-Villanueva A, Chou YY, Krammer F, Gao Q, et al. Attenuated influenza virus construct with enhanced hemagglutinin protein expression. J Virol. 2012;86:5782–90.

69. Robb NC, Chase G, Bier K, Vreede FT, Shaw PC, Naffakh N, et al. The influenza A virus NS1 protein interacts with the nucleoprotein of viral ribonucleoprotein complexes. J Virol. 2011;85:5228–31.

70. Park YW, Katze MG. Translational control by influenza virus. Identification of cis-acting sequences and trans-acting factors which may regulate selective viral mRNA translation. J Biol Chem. 1995;270:28433–9.

71. Aragón T, de La Luna S, Novoa I, Carrasco L, Ortín J, Nieto A. Eukaryotic translation initiation factor 4GI is a cellular target for NS1 protein, a translational activator of influenza virus. Mol Cell Biol. 2000;20:6259–68.

72. Burgui I, Aragon T, Ortin J, Nieto A. PABP1 and eIF4GI associate with influenza virus NS1 protein in viral mRNA translation initiation complexes. J Gen Virol. 2003;84:3263–74.

73. Satterly N, Tsai PL, van Deursen J, Nussenzveig DR, Wang Y, Faria PA, et al. Influenza virus targets the mRNA export machinery and the nuclear pore complex. Proc Natl Acad Sci U S A. 2007;104:1853–8.

74. Bavagnoli L, Dundon WG, Garbelli A, Zecchin B, Milani A, Parakkal G, et al. The PDZ-ligand and Src-homology type 3 domains of epidemic avian influenza virus NS1 protein modulate human Src kinase activity during viral infection. PLoS ONE. 2011;6:e27789.

75. Shin YK, Li Y, Liu Q, Anderson DH, Babiuk LA, Zhou Y. SH3 binding motif 1 in influenza A virus NS1 protein is essential for PI3K/Akt signaling pathway activation. J Virol. 2007;81:12730–9.

76. Shapira SD, Gat-Viks I, Shum BO, Dricot A, de Grace MM, Wu L, et al. A physical and regulatory map of

host-influenza interactions reveals pathways in H1N1 infection. Cell. 2009;139:1255–67.

77. Narasimhan J, Wang M, Fu Z, Klein JM, Haas AL, Kim JJ. Crystal structure of the interferon-induced ubiquitin-like protein ISG15. J Biol Chem. 2005;280:27356–65.

78. Yuan W, Krug RM. Influenza B virus NS1 protein inhibits conjugation of the interferon (IFN)-induced ubiquitin-like ISG15 protein. EMBO J. 2001;20:362–71.

79. Kim KI, Giannakopoulos NV, Virgin HW, Zhang DE. Interferon-inducible ubiquitin E2, Ubc8, is a conjugating enzyme for protein ISGylation. Mol Cell Biol. 2004;24:9592–600.

80. Zhao C, Beaudenon SL, Kelley ML, Waddell MB, Yuan W, Schulman BA, et al. The UbcH8 ubiquitin E2 enzyme is also the E2 enzyme for ISG15, an IFN-alpha/beta-induced ubiquitin-like protein. Proc Natl Acad Sci U S A. 2004;101:7578–82.

81. Dastur A, Beaudenon S, Kelley M, Krug RM, Huibregtse JM. Herc5, an interferon-induced HECT E3 enzyme, is required for conjugation of ISG15 in human cells. J Biol Chem. 2006;281:4334–8.

82. Wong JJ, Pung YF, Sze NS, Chin KC. HERC5 is an IFN-induced HECT-type E3 protein ligase that mediates type I IFN-induced ISGylation of protein targets. Proc Natl Acad Sci U S A. 2006;103:10735–40.

83. Hsiang TY, Zhao C, Krug RM. Interferon-induced ISG15 conjugation inhibits influenza A virus gene expression and replication in human cells. J Virol. 2009;83:5971–7.

84. Lenschow DJ, Lai C, Frias-Staheli N, Giannakopoulos NV, Lutz A, Wolff T, et al. IFN-stimulated gene 15 functions as a critical antiviral molecule against influenza, herpes, and Sindbis viruses. Proc Natl Acad Sci U S A. 2007;104:1371–6.

85. Sridharan H, Zhao C, Krug RM. Species specificity of the NS1 protein of influenza B virus: NS1 binds only human and non-human primate ubiquitin-like ISG15 proteins. J Biol Chem. 2010;285:7852–6.

86. Versteeg GA, Hale BG, van Boheemen S, Wolff T, Lenschow DJ, García-Sastre A. Species-specific antagonism of host ISGylation by the influenza B virus NS1 protein. J Virol. 2010;84:5423–30.

87. Chang YG, Yan XZ, Xie YY, Gao XC, Song AX, Zhang DE, et al. Different roles for two ubiquitin-like domains of ISG15 in protein modification. J Biol Chem. 2008;283:13370–7.

88. Hsiang TY, Zhou L, Krug RM. Roles of the phosphorylation of specific serines and threonines in the NS1 protein of human influenza A viruses. J Virol. 2012;86:10370–6.

89. Hale BG, Knebel A, Botting CH, Galloway CS, Precious BL, Jackson D, et al. CDK/ERK-mediated phosphorylation of the human influenza A virus NS1 protein at threonine-215. Virology. 2009;383:6–11.

90. Tang Y, Zhong G, Zhu L, Liu X, Shan Y, Feng H, et al. Herc5 attenuates influenza A virus by catalyzing ISGylation of viral NS1 protein. J Immunol. 2010;184:5777–90.

91. Zhao C, Hsiang TY, Kuo RL, Krug RM. ISG15 conjugation system targets the viral NS1 protein in influenza A virus-infected cells. Proc Natl Acad Sci U S A. 2010;107:2253–8.

92. Jeon YJ, Choi JS, Lee JY, Yu KR, Kim SM, Ka SH, et al. ISG15 modification of filamin B negatively regulates the type I interferon-induced JNK signalling pathway. EMBO Rep. 2009;10:374–80.

93. Pal S, Rosas JM, Rosas-Acosta G. Identification of the non-structural influenza A viral protein NS1A as a bona fide target of the Small Ubiquitin-like MOdifier by the use of dicistronic expression constructs. J Virol Methods. 2010;163:498–504.

94. Xu K, Klenk C, Liu B, Keiner B, Cheng J, Zheng BJ, et al. Modification of nonstructural protein 1 of influenza A virus by SUMO1. J Virol. 2011;85:1086–98.

95. Haye K, Burmakina S, Moran T, García-Sastre A, Fernandez-Sesma A. The NS1 protein of a human influenza virus inhibits type I interferon production and the induction of antiviral responses in primary human dendritic and respiratory epithelial cells. J Virol. 2009;83:6849–62.

96. Baskin CR, Bielefeldt-Ohmann H, Tumpey TM, Sabourin PJ, Long JP, García-Sastre A, et al. Early and sustained innate immune response defines pathology and death in nonhuman primates infected by highly pathogenic influenza virus. Proc Natl Acad Sci U S A. 2009;106:3455–60.

97. Billharz R, Zeng H, Proll SC, Korth MJ, Lederer S, Albrecht R, et al. The NS1 protein of the 1918 pandemic influenza virus blocks host interferon and lipid metabolism pathways. J Virol. 2009;83:10557–70.

98. Noronha JM, Liu M, Squires RB, Pickett BE, Hale BG, Air GM, et al. Influenza virus sequence feature variant type analysis: evidence of a role for NS1 in influenza virus host range restriction. J Virol. 2012;86:5857–66.

99. Forbes NE, Ping J, Dankar SK, Jia JJ, Selman M, Keleta L, et al. Multifunctional adaptive NS1 mutations are selected upon human influenza virus evolution in the mouse. PLoS ONE. 2012;7:e31839.

100. Ortigoza MB, Dibben O, Maamary J, Martinez-Gil L, Leyva-Grado VH, Abreu P Jr, et al. A novel small molecule inhibitor of influenza A viruses that targets

polymerase function and indirectly induces interferon. PLoS Pathog. 2012;8:e1002668.

101. Mata MA, Satterly N, Versteeg GA, Frantz D, Wei S, Williams N, et al. Chemical inhibition of RNA viruses reveals REDD1 as a host defense factor. Nat Chem Biol. 2011;7:712–9.

102. Zhang L, Das P, Schmolke M, Manicassamy B, Wang Y, Deng X, et al. Inhibition of pyrimidine synthesis reverses viral virulence factor-mediated block of mRNA nuclear export. J Cell Biol. 2012;196: 315–26.

103. Hoffmann HH, Kunz A, Simon VA, Palese P, Shaw ML. Broad-spectrum antiviral that interferes with de novo pyrimidine biosynthesis. Proc Natl Acad Sci U S A. 2011;108:5777–82.

104. Krug RM, Aramini JM. Emerging antiviral targets for influenza A virus. Trends Pharmacol Sci. 2009;30: 269–77.

105. Walkiewicz MP, Basu D, Jablonski JJ, Geysen HM, Engel DA. Novel inhibitor of influenza non-structural protein 1 blocks multi-cycle replication in an RNase L-dependent manner. J Gen Virol. 2011;92:60–70.

106. Jablonski JJ, Basu D, Engel DA, Geysen HM. Design, synthesis, and evaluation of novel small molecule inhibitors of the influenza virus protein NS1. Bioorg Med Chem. 2012;20:487–97.

107. Richt JA, García-Sastre A. Attenuated influenza virus vaccines with modified NS1 proteins. Curr Top Microbiol Immunol. 2009;333:177–95.

108. Baskin CR, Bielefeldt-Ohmann H, García-Sastre A, Tumpey TM, Van Hoeven N, Carter VS, et al. Functional genomic and serological analysis of the protective immune response resulting from vaccination of macaques with an NS1-truncated influenza virus. J Virol. 2007;81:11817–27.

109. Richt JA, Lekcharoensuk P, Lager KM, Vincent AL, Loiacono CM, Janke BH, et al. Vaccination of pigs against swine influenza viruses by using an NS1-truncated modified live-virus vaccine. J Virol. 2006;80: 11009–18.

110. Wacheck V, Egorov A, Groiss F, Pfeiffer A, Fuereder T, Hoeflmayer D, et al. A novel type of influenza vaccine: safety and immunogenicity of replication-deficient influenza virus created by deletion of the interferon antagonist NS1. J Infect Dis. 2010;201: 354–62.

8

Structure and function of the influenza virus replication machinery and PB1-F2

Andrew Mehle[1] and Jonathan A McCullers[2]

[1]Medical Microbiology and Immunology, University of Wisconsin Madison, Madison, WI, USA

[2]St. Jude Children's Research Hospital, Memphis, TN, USA

Influenza A virus is a negative-stranded RNA viruses composed of eight separate genomic fragments. Four of these segments, and over half of the nucleotides in the viral genome, encode proteins essential for gene expression and genome replication. These processes are performed by the influenza polymerase, a heterotrimer composed of the proteins PB1, PB2, and PA, and the viral nucleoprotein (NP). The polymerase assembles with the genomic RNA and NP to form a higher order ribonucleoprotein (RNP) complex that mediates transcription and replication. The polymerase *pb1* gene encodes proteins in addition to full-length PB1, notably the N-terminal truncation N40 which initiates at an internal methionine and PB1-F2 which is expressed from an internal open reading frame.

A spate of recent structural studies has brought into focus the global architecture of the viral RNPs and the first atomic level understanding of domains and proteins within the replication machinery. These findings have answered fundamental questions regarding influenza polymerase function, raised additional questions regarding the interaction of the polymerase with host proteins, and set the stage for the rationale development of antiviral compounds. This chapter highlights these recent advances and how the structures inform the function of the influenza replication machinery and PB1-F2. The biochemical activity of the influenza polymerase and its role during viral replication are described in detail in Chapter 4 (along with appropriate references) and are briefly summarized here.

The viral polymerase is ~250 kD. PB1 is the physical and catalytic core of the polymerase and binds independently to PB2 and PA to form the holoenzyme. PB1 possesses the hallmark residues that define an RNA-dependent RNA polymerase and its active site. PB1 also contains binding sites for NP and viral genomic RNAs to facilitate assembly of RNPs. PB2 binds to PB1 and NP, assisting in assembly of the RNP, and binds to m^{7}G cap at the 5′ end of host mRNAs during viral transcription. The role of PA is best defined during transcription. PA binds to PB1 and possess an endonucleolytic activity that is essential for viral transcription. PB2 and PA also appear to interact directly in cells, although this interaction is very weak compared with the binding of either subunit to PB1. All three subunits are required for both replication and transcription. Thus, as a whole, the polymerase possesses at least five distinct activities: (i) polymerase activity that is primer-dependent (transcription) and -independent (replication); (ii) endonuclease activity; (iii) cap-binding activity, (iv) sequence- and structure-specific binding of the genome termini; and (v) NP binding.

The eight viral genes are packaged into virions as RNPs (see Chapter 4), thus the viral genome, polymerase, and NP are pre-assembled and competent for transcription and replication prior to infection. Following infection, vRNPs migrate to the nucleus where the polymerase mediates initial rounds of transcription and the first steps of replication. Transcription proceeds via a "cap-snatching" mechanism; short host-derived m7G-capped RNAs are used as primers for synthesis of viral mRNAs that possess a 5′ cap and a 3′ polyA tail. PB1 binds to the 5′ end of the minus-sense genomic viral RNA (vRNA) and activates cap binding by the PB2 subunit. PB2 recognizes and binds the m7G cap from host mRNAs using a cap-binding domain in the middle of the protein. Subsequently, PB1 binds the 3′ end of vRNA and stimulates the endonucleolytic activity in the PA subunit. This leads to the cleavage of host transcripts 9–17 nucleotides downstream from the m7G cap that are then used to prime synthesis of viral mRNA. However, cleavage is not always dependent on the binding of the 3′ end of vRNA by PB1 and the efficiency of initiation is affected by sequence context of the cleavage site, showing a preference for primers ending with a CA dinucleotide. The terminal nucleotide of the capped primer is thought to base pair with the template vRNA and the PB1 subunit catalyzes nucleotide addition. Transcription continues to a conserved polyuridine stretch at the 5′ end of all vRNAs where iterative slippage and copying of the template produces a polyA tail.

Genome replication is performed by the same machinery responsible for transcription. Replication begins with vRNA templates copied to plus-sense (cRNA) intermediates, which are subsequently used as templates for synthesis of new vRNA. As in transcription, PB1 binds both the 5′ and 3′ ends of vRNA and catalyzes extension. However, cRNA synthesis differs from transcription in that it is primer-independent and bypasses the polyadenylation signal at the 5′ of the vRNA to produce full-length copies. Production of full-length cRNA also requires free NP which associates with nascent RNA and polymerase to form cRNPs. cRNPs then produce new vRNAs in a similar fashion. Following replication, vRNA segments can serve as templates for synthesis of mRNAs or can be packaged as vRNPs into newly budding virions.

Architecture of the vRNP

Original ultrastructural analysis was performed by electron microscopy of virions and vRNPs extracted from virions. These micrographs identified flexible,

rod-shaped vRNPs with helical characteristics [1]. The vRNPs extracted from virions are of different lengths, corresponding to the different sizes of the viral genes (~900–2300 nt) [2] and are closed at one end where the polymerase was localized by immunogold staining [3]. As both the 5′ and 3′ end of the genome are bound by the polymerase, they are also localized to this closed end. The opposite end contains a small loop formed by NP and RNA. The genome begins at the closed end of the loop, transits the length of the rod following a helical trajectory to the loop where it turns 180° and returns down the rod towards the polymerase. These data created a model of vRNP structure that contains a regular double-stranded helical arrangement with major and minor groove spacing between antiparallel strands of NP oligomers bound to vRNA [2].

Major advancements in understanding the structure of influenza virus vRNPs have been obtained from electron microscopy (EM) and cryo-EM reconstructions (Figure 8.1a) [4,5]. vRNPs were formed and purified with an artificial influenza-like gene to yield complexes containing ~9 NP, the trimeric polymerase, and a 248 nt model RNA. The vRNPs show a ring-like structure formed by the multimeric NP. The polymerase projects from the outside in the plane of the ring. Individual NP protomers are readily discerned with large head and body domains that form a "groove" on the exterior of the ring corresponding to the same domains in the crystal structure of NP [6,7]. Only limited contacts between NPs are detected in the oligomer. The NP ring is broken where it makes two discrete contacts with the polymerase. The two contacts between the back of the polymerase and NP are consistent with the biochemical identification of two discrete NP binding sites in PB1 and PB2 [8,9]. While this ring-like model using a minimal RNA has proven useful in understanding the general layout of the vRNP, EM data show that vRNPs formed with the longer bona fide viral RNAs assume a double-helical conformation [2]. This higher level of organization implies the presence of additional NP–NP interactions that are required to assume the helical hairpin structures.

The polymerase shows a compact, multi-lobed structure (Figure 8.1a) [4,5,10,11]. This differs dramatically from the head-to-tail assignment of binding sites between the polymerase subunits determined by biochemical and structural analyses (Figure 8.2) [12–

(a)

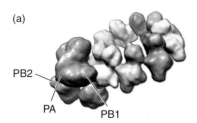

(b)

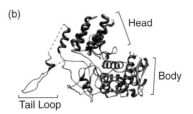

Figure 8.1. Structures of the influenza virus replication machinery. (a) Cryo-EM reconstruction of a model vRNP [5]. The polymerase is shown in purple attached to nine individual NP subunits forming a ring. The C-terminal region of PA, the N-terminal region of PB2 and the C-terminus of PB1 are marked as determined by antibody binding and epitope tagging [4]. Resolution is 12 Å for the symmetrized portion of the NP ring and 18 Å for the polymerase and adjacent NPs. Coordinates were kindly provided by Drs. J. Ortín and J. Martín-Benito. (b) Structure of influenza virus NP [6] (PDB accession 2IQH). The head, body, and tail loop are labeled. RNA binding is thought to occur in the basic groove between the head and body domains. Oligomerization involves insertion of the tail loop into a pocket on the neighboring NP protomer [6,7].

14]. Mapping of the individual subunits using either monoclonal antibodies or a large epitope tag indicated that the C-terminal half of PA is located in the middle of the polymerase on the face distal to the NP ring, whereas the N-terminal ~100 amino acids of PB2 and the C-terminus of PB1 are located on opposite sides of the structure. These positions are approximations as the N-terminus of PB2 binds directly to the C-terminus of PB1, even though these regions have been mapped to opposite sides in the EM reconstruction [4,14].

Evolving structural models continue to increase the resolution and detail of the vRNP reconstructions, with current models at 12 Å resolution for the NP ring and 18 Å for the polymerase and adjacent NPs [5]. This resolution precludes the localization of the model vRNA. It is also possible that the vRNA exhibits a large degree of flexibility, which would make structural determination by image averaging challenging. Early experiments showed that RNA in vRNPs purified from virions is sensitive to RNase digestion suggesting it is located on the outside of the structure, corresponding to the exterior of the NP ring [1,2]. The atomic structure of NP provides further support for this model (Figure 8.1b).

The structures of the influenza NP protein from an H1N1 (A/WSN/1933) and an H5N1 isolate (A/Hong Kong/483/1997) were determined (Figure 8.1b) [6,7]. The proteins crystallized as homotrimers in the absence of RNA to yield roughly crescent-shaped subunits with large head and body domains and a small "tail loop" that projects away from the body of the protein. The secondary structure is composed almost exclusively of α-helices. To date, the structure is unique amongst nucleoproteins from single-stranded RNA viruses (e.g., respiratory syncytial virus, vesicular stomatitis virus, rabies virus, Rift Valley fever virus). The head and body domains contain non-contiguous regions of the polypeptide chain that traverses between the domains three times. The two domains form a highly basic grove on the exterior of the trimer that is proposed to be the RNA binding site. The groove is lined by 16 arginines and lysines, 11 of which are highly conserved in influenza A, B, and C [6]. Mutational analysis demonstrated a critical role for several of these residues in RNA binding, most notably the cluster containing R74, R75, R174, R175, and R221 [7]. The crystal structure of NP can be docked into the cryo-EM reconstruction to create a quasi-atomic model that again places the RNA-binding groove on the outside of the ring in agreement with the biochemistry [5].

The NP structures also elucidate mechanisms for homo-oligomerization. The primary contact is made by the tail loop, amino acids 402–428. The tail loop assumes an extended conformation from the core of the protein and inserts into a hydrophobic pocket in the neighboring molecule. The tail loop makes extensive contacts between molecules by forming an intermolecular β-sheet, hydrophobic interactions, and salt bridges. Removal of the tail loop or disruption of the salt bridge between R416 in the tail loop and E339

135

in the hydrophobic pocket of the adjacent NP prevents oligomerization and impairs RNP assembly and function [5,6]. Intermolecular contacts independent of the tail loop were also observed, although their function has not been tested yet. The tail loop is connected to the core of the protein via a highly flexible linker. The positioning of the tail loop differs between the two crystal structures and further adjustments must be made in the tail loop angle to create the quasi-atomic model [5–7]. Thus, a degree of conformational plasticity at the NP–NP interface might be necessary to accommodate the various structures assumed by the vRNP during genome synthesis, vRNP assembly, and ultimately packing into virions.

Conformational flexibility extends to the viral polymerase as well. The polymerase subunits are imported into the nucleus of infected cells where they assemble to form new polymerase molecules (see Chapter 4). The trimeric polymerase assembles separately before binding to genomic RNA and NP to form the RNP complexes. EM reconstructions of the unbound polymerase shows a hollow globular conformation with a small "horn" projecting from the surface [11]. The molecule displays a clear opening to an interior cavity. Whereas free polymerase is in an open conformation, structural models of RNA-bound polymerase and those in vRNPs show a more compact overall shape [4,5,10]. In addition to the two contacts now observed between the bound polymerase and the NP ring, the cavity observed in the unbound structure is collapsed and filled with density, possibly vRNA [10,11]. Movements on the other side of the molecule indicate that a large mass containing the N-terminus of PB2 is repositioned from the bulky central domain to a projection adjacent the top of the polymerase. The host protein Hsp90, a protein folding chaperone, has recently been shown to aid incorporation of PB2 into the polymerase trimer and possibly facilitates these rearrangements [15]. PB2 mutants have been identified that form the free polymerase trimer but fail to assemble into the vRNP complex, raising the possibility that these mutants cannot undergo the conformational transition illustrated by the EM reconstructions [16,17].

Whether these conformational differences will be as dramatic in high resolution structures as they appear in these initial models remains to be determined. Additionally, the assignment of subunits on to the reconstructred polymerase is likely to be refined as the quality of models and localizations increases. Together, these studies have provided a model for the overall architecture of the replication machinery and highlighted the conformational rearrangements the polymerase and NP undergo during assembly into vRNPs. See note at end of chapter. Biochemical studies suggest each of these steps is tightly regulated, and they are almost certainly influenced by host factors.

Atomic structure of the influenza polymerase

A high resolution structure of the polymerase holoenzyme has not been determined to date, due in large part to the difficulty in recombinantly expressing and purifying sufficient quantities of the trimeric complex. Nonetheless, several strategies have been used to overcome this limitation and determine the structures of isolated domains; structures encompassing almost all of PA and a large portion of PB2 have been determined whereas limited structural information exists only for the extreme termini of PB1.

PA

The PA subunit contains two large soluble domains separated by a naturally occurring tryptic cleavage site downstream of R256 [18]. The structures of both domains have been determined (Figure 8.2) [12,13,19,20]. The N-terminal domain contains an α/β architecture where five mixed β-strands form a gently twisting sheet surrounded by seven α-helices. Helices 2–5 build a negative cavity on one side of the protein with β-strand 3 at the base. The cavity is lined by highly conserved residues and contains coordinated divalent metals, either 2 Mn^{2+} [19] or one Mg^{2+} ion [20]. It was readily apparent that this cavity represented an endonuclease active site and was shown to be the endonuclease involved in cap-snatching by the polymerase [20]. Based on sequence and structural similarity, the endonuclease has been proposed to be member of the PD-(D/E)xK nuclease superfamily [19]. Phosphodiester hydrolysis begins with the deprotonation of an attacking nucleophile by a base in the active site; the nucleophile is often water for metal-dependent nucleases. The geometry of the PA active site coupled with enzymatic analysis of mutants implicates K134 as the catalytic base.

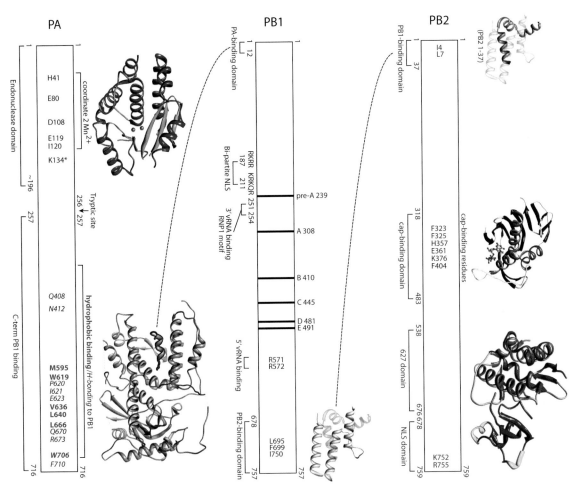

Figure 8.2. Domains, structures, and critical residues of the influenza virus polymerase. The overall domain structure of the three polymerase subunits PB1, PB2, and PA is diagrammed and inter-subunit contacts are indicated by dashed lines. The signature domains defining an RNA-dependent RNA polymerase are shown in PB1 as thick black lines [49]. See the text for details on critical residues and their proposed function. Structures are depicted using the indicated PDB accession: PA endonuclease domain [19,20], 2W69; PA C-terminus with PB1 N-terminal peptide (in blue) [12,13], 3CM8; PB1(blue)–PB2(orange) interface [14], 3A1G; PB2 cap-binding domain with m^{7}GTP cap analog [27], 2VQZ; and the PB2 627 and NLS domains [28,29], 2VY6.

The isolated endonuclease domain displays nonspecific activity cleaving single-stranded RNA, single-stranded DNA, and single-stranded circular DNA, with a preference for unstructured single-stranded RNA. This activity and that of the intact trimeric polymerase is strictly metal dependent [19,21,22]. However, the exact metal, Mn^{2+} or Mg^{2+}, is disputed [19–23]. Mn^{2+} was observed in one crystal structure,

Mg^{2+} in the other, although in both cases the metals were present at high levels in the crystallization buffers. Mn^{2+} is coordinated by amino acid side-chains at two sites in PA: site Mn1 is composed of E80, D108, and two water molecules and site Mn2 contains H41, D108, E199, and I120. The coordinating residues are highly conserved across influenza virus A, B, and C, and mutation of these sites impairs endonuclease activity [21]. Structures with Mg^{2+} show coordination only in the first metal-binding site. Co-crystal structures containing the endonuclease and nucleoside monophosphates in the presence of Mg^{2+} again show a metal ion in the first binding site and a water in the second position [23]. These structures reveal nucleotide bound as a product of the cleavage reaction with a well-ordered 5′ phosphate near the catalytic center and a distal nucleoside binding site. Mn^{2+} stimulates endonuclease activity to a greater extent than Mg^{2+}, binds with ~500-fold higher affinity, occupies both metal coordination sites, and provides the largest increase in thermal stability for the endonuclease domain [19,21,22]. Moreover, structures of the endonuclease domain from the polymerase of two other cap-snatching viruses, La Crosse virus and lymphocytic choriomenengitis virus, show a strikingly similar topology and a preference for Mn^{2+} [24,25]. Yet, Mg^{2+} is present in cells at a much higher concentration and is capable of supporting endonuclease activity of the isolated domain and the polymerase, raising the possibility that both metals may have a role in catalysis in the infected cell [20,22,23].

The C-terminal domain of PA interacts with the extreme N-terminus of PB1, and a detailed binding interface between the two proteins was elucidated in the structure [12,13,26]. The C-terminus assumes a "dragon head" shape with PB1 bound tightly by α-helices in the "jaws" of the domain through a series of hydrophobic contacts, hydrogen bonds, and van der Waals interactions. Key residues are highlighted in Figure 8.2. The PB1 peptide forms a short helix from residues 5–11 with the core motif $L_7L_8F_9L_{10}$ most important for binding; mutations in the LLFL motif abrogate binding to PA, reduce polymerase activity, and severely impair virus replication [26]. Similarly, mutation of the key contact sites in PA disrupts binding and the synthesis of vRNA, cRNA, and mRNA [12,13]. Much of the binding to PB1 involves main chain interactions, yet there is little tolerance for sequence variation in this region. As one might expect, these residues are absolutely conserved amongst influenza A strains. The back of the head contains a positively charged groove encompassing several conserved basic residues. The groove might be involved in RNA binding, although aside from binding to PB1 and possibly other host factors the function of this rather large domain remains unclear.

Finally, while the N-terminus of this domain is located near the jaw, it is a long unstructured region, suggesting that it may function as a flexible linker to the endonuclease domain at the opposite end of PA.

PB2

The function of PB2 is best characterized during viral transcription where it recognizes the host mRNAs used during cap-snatching via their m^7G cap. The PB2 cap-binding domain was identified from a clever screen for soluble PB2 fragments termed ESPRIT and was subsequently crystalized in the presence of the m^7GTP cap analog (Figure 8.2) [27]. The cap-binding domain is derived from the central region of PB2 spanning residues ~318–483. The domain assumes an α–β fold. Two separate β-sheets cradle three α-helices and the m^7GTP residue. An additional region distinct from the cap-binding site contains another α-helix and a C-terminal moiety of short β-strands. The cap-binding pocket is localized to the intersection of the two β-sheets and the base of two α-helices. Cap binding is dominated by π–π interactions between the guanine base, F404 and H357, which stack as an aromatic sandwich with the base in the middle. E361 and K376 specifically recognize the guanine base via hydrogen bonds. F323 also contributes by stacking on the ribose. Mutation of these critical residues disrupts cap-binding and in many cases selectively impairs cap-dependent mRNA production, but not cap-independent synthesis of genomic RNA [27]. The acidic phosphate group on the nucleotide is accommodated by H357, K339, R355, H432, and N429. Despite showing no sequence similarity, the cap-binding pocket in PB2 shares a remarkably similar geometry to that of other viral and cellular cap-binding proteins.

ESPRIT screening also identified soluble domains at the C-terminus of PB2 including the nuclear localization signal (NLS) and the 627 domain (Figure 8.2) [28,29]. The PB2 NLS is located in the domain containing residues 678–759. Nuclear magnetic resonance (NMR) imaging revealed a compact α–β structure with three antiparallel β-strands supporting an amphipathic α-helix [28]. The NLS was subsequently co-crystallized with importin α5, one of several importin α receptors utilized by PB2 to gain entry to the nucleus (see Chapter 4). Upon binding to its nuclear import receptor, the extreme C-terminus of PB2 assumes an extended conformation positioning a classical bipartite NLS into a super-helical groove on importin α5. The PB2 NLS motif 736-RKRX$_{12}$KRIR-755 directs the transport of heterologous fusion proteins into the nucleus and, when mutated, disrupts binding of PB2 to importin α5 and subsequent nuclear import [28,29].

In the absence of its nuclear import receptor, the C-terminal domain of PB2 packs against the 627 domain which is located immediately upstream in the polypeptide chain. A conformational rearrangement is likely to occur between these domains to accommodate binding of the NLS by importin α. The 627 domain is a unique combination of a six helix cluster with five β-strands curling around the back (Figure 8.2) [29–31]. The domain is named after amino acid 627, a key determinant of host range and pathogenicity that regulates polymerase activity in a species-specific fashion. Most avian influenza isolates encode a glutamic acid at this position and function poorly in human cells, whereas most pre-2009 human isolates encode a lysine which conveys enhanced polymerase activity and virus replication [16,17,32]. A shift occurred with the outbreak of the 2009 H1N1 pandemic virus. PB2 from these viruses and their descendants retained the avian-signature E627 but acquired the SR polymorphism which place an arginine at residue 591. The SR polymorphism functions in concert with other changes in these polymerases to selectively enhance polymerase activity in mammalian host [31,33]. The structure shows that residue 627 lies on the front of the domain in a loop that connects the helix cluster to the β-strands on the back. The loop forms a so-called φ-structure as it encircles the α-helix from residues 589–605, approximating the shape of the φ symbol. Residues in the φ loop are solvent exposed with their side-chains pointing away from the body of the protein. Structures containing either E627 or K627 have both been solved and are superimposable, thus adaptive changes at 627 do not result in any large-scale rearrangement [29]. The structure of the 627 domain from a pandemic 2009 H1N1 virus with the SR polymorphism and E627 has also been determined and it too displays a nearly identical conformation [31]. The most notable difference is that R591 in the 2009 H1N1 protein appears to fill a small cleft that is present in the other structures.

To further illustrate the high degree of similarity, there are currently five 627 domain structures from human H1N1 and H3N2 viruses with K627, a human H1N1 mutant with E627, a 2009 pandemic H1N1 virus with the SR polymorphism and E627, and a human H5N1 virus containing K627. Pairwise comparisons of the cores show that the RMSD of the α-C varies no more than 0.63 Å. However, a dramatic difference is apparent when the surface electrostatics are considered. The lysine-containing 627 domain presents a large basic face centered on residue 627 and the φ-loop, which is significantly disrupted by the avian-signature E627. The structures and additional functional experiments revealed that PB2 requires a large basic face in the 627 domain for efficient polymerase activity in human cells [17,29,31,33]. It has been suggested to be involved in interactions with proteins or possibly RNA, and it is known to have a role in vRNP assembly, yet the exact functions of this domain and its surface are still unknown [16,17,29,30].

The structure of the PB1–PB2 interface was solved and confirmed that the extreme N-terminus of PB2 binds to the very C-terminus of PB1 (Figure 8.2) [14]. The interface is a series of interleaved α-helices, three each from PB1 and PB2, which buries ~1400 Å^2. It is predominantly characterized by hydrogen bonding and salt bridges between the proteins. The hydrophobic residues PB2 I4 and L7 are completely buried at the interface and mutations at these sites prevent polymerase assembly and activity. The PB1 residues L695, F699, and I750 are essential for stable binding to PB2, but are not absolutely required for polymerase activity. Thus, while PB1 and PB2 are over 750 amino acids in length, the minimal site of interaction consists of rather small regions located at the termini.

Role of PB1-F2

Composition and structure

Gene segment 2 of influenza A viruses has multiple AUG sites of initiation, from which three polypeptides can be produced [34]. PB1 is initiated in canonical fashion from AUG1. N40 is a shortened version of PB1 produced from the fifth AUG in the same frame as PB1 through reinitiation after aborted initiation at the third AUG. PB1-F2 is a small peptide produced in the +1 reading frame from the fourth AUG through leaky ribosomal scanning. The context in which each of the first five AUGs are presented in an individual virus affects regulation of the three products, leading to incompletely understood relationships in expression between the proteins [34]. Research on the function(s) of these proteins is complicated *in vitro* and *in vivo* by this regulation; deletion of the AUG start site for one protein or expression of a gene product from plasmids instead of in the context of the full virus can alter expression of the other proteins, likely impacting function and thus pathogenesis.

Depending on the virus strain, PB1-F2 can be up to 90 amino acids in length, but sequence analyses suggest that numerous truncated forms exist in nature. The proposed secondary structure of PB1-F2 predicts two major domains, a disordered, "spaghetti strand" N-terminal domain, and a cationic, hydrophobic C-terminal domain with three closely approximated α-helix regions (comprising amino acids 37–48, 53–64, 68–83) [35]. The latter two are most likely to form helices in a membrane environment. PB1-F2 proteins can cause pore formation when inserted into membranes, resulting in detectable conduct of ions through the resulting impermanent channels. The significance of this finding in terms of pathogenesis is not clear. However, the third predicted α-helix contains a mitochondrial targeting sequence, which has given rise to speculation that pore formation, ion channel activity, or protein–protein interactions in the mitochondrial membrane contribute to pathogenesis through disruption of mitochondria and subsequent cell death [36].

Functions

At least three broad functions have been proposed for PB1-F2. Upon its discovery, PB1-F2 was shown to cause cell death, presumably mediated by targeting to mitochondria and either direct membrane disruption or interaction with other proteins involved in apoptosis [36]. Although this phenomenon does contribute to morbidity *in vivo* in mouse models, it appears to be confined to a limited set of H1N1 viruses from the early twentieth century [37]. The required C-terminal motif is not found in modern, circulating animal or human influenza virus strains. Thus, it is unclear whether this function is of relevance to current seasonal or future pandemic disease.

In addition to its demonstrated ability to oligomerize in membranes, PB1-F2 may interact directly with other proteins expressed from gene segment 2 and modify their functions. It has been proposed that binding of PB1 and delay of its exit from the nucleus could enhance replication. Several laboratories have demonstrated *in vitro* differences in replication after deletion or alteration of PB1-F2, suggesting that PB1–PB1-F2 interactions or differential regulation of the three gene segment 2 proteins could impact viral growth and thus virulence. However, little support for this hypothesis has been found *in vivo* to this point, as viral titers in mice and pathogenesis of these altered strains are not typically affected by loss of PB1-F2 [38].

In *in vivo* models of disease, the effects of PB1-F2 appear to be largely mediated through interactions with the immune system. The PB1-F2 proteins from certain influenza virus strains clearly potentiate inflammatory responses to either the virus itself, co-infecting bacteria, or both [39]. This is manifest as enhanced influx of leukocytes such as neutrophils and macrophages into the lungs and airways, accompanied by increases in proinflammatory cytokines. In the setting of secondary bacterial pneumonia following influenza, this has a profound effect on the pathogenesis of serious infections by further enhancing inflammation and increasing bacterial outgrowth in the lungs. The mechanism is unclear at present, but may involve interferon antagonism through interference with the retinoic acid-inducible gene I (RIG-I)/mitochondrial antiviral signaling protein (MAVS) complex [40]. Following PB1-F2 expression *in vitro* or *in vivo*, this interaction with RIG-I/MAVS prevents activation of interferon regulatory factor (IRF)-3, with the result that interferon (IFN)-β induction in response to the virus is inhibited, more infiltration of immune cells into the lungs occurs, and morbidity increases. Thus, PB1-F2 appears to be a multifunction peptide with anti-interferon activity similar to the nonstructural protein NS-1. Whether this interferon inhibitory activity is also involved in the enhanced response to bacteria following influenza or a separate function is involved is unclear, as is the generalizability of the anti-interferon activity to clinically relevant strains.

Evolution and adaptation

The polymerase acquires an array of adaptive mutations as it moves from host to host. Some of these mutations, such as the change at PB2 amino acid 627, have direct bearing on polymerase activity, virus replication, host range, and pathogenicity (see above). Like PB2 amino acid 627, most are located on the surface of the various protein domains, raising the possibility that these changes might be involved in recognizing host proteins in a species-specific fashion [29]. The mechanisms of adaptation for most of the changes described to date, even the well-studied PB2 amino acid 627, remain elusive, but the structures described here provide some insight. The most concrete example involves the D701N adaptive mutation in PB2. PB2 N701 is a rare polymorphism in human viruses associated with increased polymerase activity and virulence in mice [41]. The PB2 D701N mutation is predicted to disrupt a salt bridge and destabilize the compact conformation of the unbound NLS [28]. The destabilized NLS selectively demonstrates enhanced binding to the human but not avian import receptor importin α1 resulting in increased nuclear localization and polymerase activity [42]. Thus, this change might accelerate the adaptation of PB2 to a new host by enhancing binding to essential cellular co-factors. The structure of the PB2 627 domain also provided a model for the ability of the 2009 H1N1 polymerase to overcome species barriers [29,31,33]. 2009 H1N1 viruses encode the normally restrictive PB2 E627 along with the newly emerged SR polymorphism at

the upstream residues 590–591. Within the structure of the 627 domain the SR polymorphism is located at the end of the α-helix encircled by the φ-loop, juxtapositioning R591 and E627. Based on predictions of surface electrostatics, R591 has been suggested to partially neutralize the charge of E627 [33]. Additionally, R591 induces a very minor change in the topology by filling a cleft [31]. The SR polymorphism might therefore partially recreate the basic face in the 627 domain required for function in human cells, but again the exact role of this surface needs to be determined.

Polymorphisms in PB1-F2 might influence viral tropism and pathogenicity as well. All influenza viruses infecting humans are zoonotic reassortants comprised of gene segments that derive ultimately from an avian reservoir. Nearly all avian PB1-F2 sequences are full length and contain a C-terminal sequence predicted to contribute to inflammation [43]. Analysis of lineages after introduction of these strains into humans or pigs show evidence of permanent truncation during adaptation in mammalian hosts (Figure 8.3). This occurred in the H1N1 lineage derived from 1918 in the late 1940s in humans, but numerous examples of truncation of multiple subtypes after individual introductions into pigs exist. Further functional analysis of H3N2 subtype viruses indicated a loss of the PB1-F2 protein's contribution

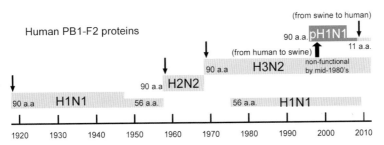

Figure 8.3. PB1-F2 expression during evolution of influenza A viruses in various species. The characteristics of PB1-F2 proteins expressed by viruses circulating in humans during the last century are pictured. Box heights and inset text indicate length of the circulating PB1-F2 proteins in relation to time. Downward arrows indicate new pandemic strains. The darker shaded box represents the nonhuman PB1-F2 protein. Human PB1-F2s tended to become truncated or lose functionality through mutation over time during adaptation. The upward arrow represents the acquisition by a swine H1N1 strain of a nonfunctional, full-length PB1-F2 from a human H3N2 strain; this protein was later truncated prior to emergence in a human pandemic strain in 2009. Avian PB1-F2 proteins are almost all full length and proinflammatory by sequence (not pictured). Swine PB1-F2 proteins are highly variable in length and sequence. Reprinted from McAuley and McCullers [50] with permission.

to pathogenicity during adaptation without truncation in the decades that it has circulated after introduction into humans in 1968 [43]. The 2009 H1N1 pandemic strain contained a gene segment 2 derived from a human H3N2 virus that had undergone a truncation event during circulation in pigs, prior to passing back into humans. Thus, the H1N1 and H3N2 seasonal influenza A virus strains as well as the currently circulating H1N1 pandemic lineage strain all have a nonfunctional PB1-F2 [37,43]. Lack of this virulence factor has been implicated in the relatively mild virulence of these strains in recent years coupled with the relatively low rate of secondary bacterial complications compared with historic pandemic viruses. However, surveys of PB1-F2 protein sequences in swine reservoirs suggest that great diversity of PB1-F2 length and sequence exists, suggesting that another swine-derived pandemic strain might contain an active PB1-F2 and thus be more pathogenic. Because most H5N1 subtype strains express an active, inflammatory PB1-F2, it remains a pandemic threat in this context as well.

The observation that nearly all PB1-F2 sequences derived from avian influenza viruses are full length implies that this protein has some functional utility in infection of birds, perhaps related to the viral life cycle in its natural host niche, the gut. Conversely, loss of function during adaptation in mammalian lungs implies it is disposable in humans and pigs. Limited study in mallard ducks suggests that PB1-F2 is important for disease severity and systemic spread of H5N1 subtype viruses in this host [44]. However, the reasons for its conservation remain unexplored.

Our current understanding of the role of PB1-F2 in pathogenesis is that PB1-F2 containing gene segments which are recent émigrés from the avian reservoir can contribute significantly to pathogenesis through interactions with the immune system. This virulence is lost over time as novel viruses adapt to mammalian lungs. Although in select backgrounds (e.g., the 1918 pandemic strain and highly pathogenic H5N1 subtype viruses) PB1-F2 contributes directly to virulence [39,44], its ability to enhance bacterial superinfections may be more important in most instances. In this context, pandemic surveillance and planning must take the length and specific C-terminal sequence of PB1-F2 into account in prioritization of viruses for study and vaccine production. Although it seems unlikely to be a key factor in disease caused by current seasonal influenza strains, its immune effects may be a major contributor to future pandemics. As a dispensable protein during infection in mammals it probably is not a good vaccine target, but inhibition of its effects either through antiviral approaches or immunomodulation might be a viable strategy to reduce pandemic morbidity and mortality.

Perspectives

Significant progress has been made in our understanding of the structure and function of the influenza polymerase gene products and replication machinery. Biochemical and structural studies have established robust models for polymerase-mediated cap-snatching and replication. Conspicuously absent is an atomic-resolution structure of the polymerase holoenzyme, which has so far resisted determination despite attempts by multiple groups. Nonetheless, continued advancement of the cryo-EM and EM reconstructions and crystallographic approaches have the potential to overcome the current obstacles. Perhaps one of the most important consequences is that the structures provide a solid foundation for the rational development of much-needed antiviral compounds. Peptides derived from the N-terminus of PB1 block polymerase assembly, and the structure of this interaction site is facilitating the derivatization of high affinity binders with potent activity [45]. The endonuclease domain of PA has also been a frequent target of antiviral compounds. The inhibitor 2, 4-dioxo-4-phenylbutanoic acid (DPBA) blocks activity of the isolated endonuclease domain and the intact polymerase, markedly reducing viral replication [19,46]. Co-crystal structures of the La Crosse virus endonuclease domain with DPBA confirms that the inhibitor disrupts function by coordinating the two Mn^{2+} ions in the active site [25]. This structure likely has direct parallels to the mode of inhibition for the influenza virus endonuclease domain, allowing systematic structure–affinity relationship analysis and refinement for more potent and specific compounds. Finally, the entire RNP is a potential target for antiviral compounds. The compound "nucleozin" was discovered to target NP and cause its aggregation, reducing replication and pathogenicity of some viral strains [47]. The structure of a nucleozin derivative complexed to NP shows a remarkable mode of action where the compound binds a pocket split between different NP monomers liganding them in a nonfunctional body-to-body orientation [48]. Thus, these initial studies extend the conclusions drawn from the structural and biochemical data to provide compelling results that, it is hoped, will spur the advancement of antiviral therapies targeting the influenza virus replication machinery.

Note added in proof

While this chapter was in press, the reconstructions of native RNPs with genome-length RNA were published. They reveal a double-helical conformation composed of NP strands with opposite polarity and also suggest differential modes of polymerase function during replication and transcription [51,52].

Acknowledgments

Drs. Mehle and McCullers declare no conflicts of interest. Dr. Mehle is a Shaw Scientist and his effort is supported by an NIH Pathway to Independence award R00GM088484. Dr. McCullers' effort is supported in part by the American Lebanese Syrian Associated Charities (ALSAC).

References

1. Pons MW, Schulze IT, Hirst GK. Isolation and characterization of the ribonucleoprotein of influenza virus. Virology. 1969;39(2):250–9.

2. Compans RW, Content J, Duesberg PH. Structure of the ribonucleoprotein of influenza virus. J Virol. 1972;10(4):795–800.

3. Murti KG, Webster RG, Jones IM. Localization of RNA polymerases on influenza viral ribonucleoproteins by immunogold labeling. Virology. 1988;164(2):562–6.

4. Area E, Martin-Benito J, Gastaminza P, Torreira E, Valpuesta JM, Carrascosa JL, et al. 3D structure of the influenza virus polymerase complex: localization of subunit domains. Proc Natl Acad Sci U S A. 2004;101(1):308–13.

5. Coloma R, Valpuesta JM, Arranz R, Carrascosa JL, Ortin J, Martin-Benito J. The structure of a biologically active influenza virus ribonucleoprotein complex. PLoS Pathog. 2009;5(6):e1000491.

6. Ye Q, Krug RM, Tao YJ. The mechanism by which influenza A virus nucleoprotein forms oligomers and binds RNA. Nature. 2006;444(7122):1078–82.

7. Ng AK, Zhang H, Tan K, Li Z, Liu JH, Chan PK, et al. Structure of the influenza virus A H5N1 nucleoprotein: implications for RNA binding, oligomerization, and vaccine design. FASEB J. 2008;22(10):3638–47.

8. Biswas SK, Boutz PL, Nayak DP. Influenza virus nucleoprotein interacts with influenza virus polymerase proteins. J Virol. 1998;72(7):5493–501.

9. Medcalf L, Poole E, Elton D, Digard P. Temperature-sensitive lesions in two influenza A viruses defective for replicative transcription disrupt RNA binding by the nucleoprotein. J Virol. 1999;73(9):7349–56.

10. Resa-Infante P, Recuero-Checa MA, Zamarreno N, Llorca O, Ortin J. Structural and functional characterization of an influenza virus RNA polymerase-genomic RNA complex. J Virol. 2010;84(20):10477–87.

11. Torreira E, Schoehn G, Fernandez Y, Jorba N, Ruigrok RW, Cusack S, et al. Three-dimensional model for the isolated recombinant influenza virus polymerase heterotrimer. Nucleic Acids Res. 2007;35(11):3774–83.

12. He X, Zhou J, Bartlam M, Zhang R, Ma J, Lou Z, et al. Crystal structure of the polymerase PA(C)-PB1(N) complex from an avian influenza H5N1 virus. Nature. 2008;454(7208):1123–6.

13. Obayashi E, Yoshida H, Kawai F, Shibayama N, Kawaguchi A, Nagata K, et al. The structural basis for an essential subunit interaction in influenza virus RNA polymerase. Nature. 2008;454(7208):1127–31.

14. Sugiyama K, Obayashi E, Kawaguchi A, Suzuki Y, Tame JRH, Nagata K, et al. Structural insight into the essential PB1-PB2 subunit contact of the influenza virus RNA polymerase. EMBO J. 2009;28(12):1803–11.

15. Naito T, Momose F, Kawaguchi A, Nagata K. Involvement of Hsp90 in assembly and nuclear import of influenza virus RNA polymerase subunits. J Virol. 2007;81(3):1339–49.

16. Labadie K, Dos Santos Afonso E, Rameix-Welti MA, van der Werf S, Naffakh N. Host-range determinants on the PB2 protein of influenza A viruses control the interaction between the viral polymerase and nucleoprotein in human cells. Virology. 2007;362(2):271–82.

17. Mehle A, Doudna JA. An inhibitory activity in human cells restricts the function of an avian-like influenza virus polymerase. Cell Host Microbe. 2008;4(2):111–22.

18. Hara K, Schmidt FI, Crow M, Brownlee GG. Amino acid residues in the N-terminal region of the PA subunit of influenza A virus RNA polymerase play a critical role in protein stability, endonuclease activity, cap binding, and virion RNA promoter binding. J Virol. 2006;80(16):7789–98.

19. Dias A, Bouvier D, Crepin T, McCarthy AA, Hart DJ, Baudin F, et al. The cap-snatching endonuclease of influenza virus polymerase resides in the PA subunit. Nature. 2009;458(7240):914–8.

20. Yuan P, Bartlam M, Lou Z, Chen S, Zhou J, He X, et al. Crystal structure of an avian influenza polymerase PA(N) reveals an endonuclease active site. Nature. 2009;458(7240):909–13.

21. Crepin T, Dias A, Palencia A, Swale C, Cusack S, Ruigrok RW. Mutational and metal binding analysis of the endonuclease domain of the influenza virus polymerase PA subunit. J Virol. 2010;84(18):9096–104.

22. Doan L, Handa B, Roberts NA, Klumpp K. Metal ion catalysis of RNA cleavage by the influenza virus endonuclease. Biochemistry. 1999;38(17):5612–9.

23. Zhao C, Lou Z, Guo Y, Ma M, Chen Y, Liang S, et al. Nucleoside monophosphate complex structures of the endonuclease domain from the influenza virus polymerase PA subunit reveal the substrate binding site inside the catalytic center. J Virol. 2009;83(18):9024–30.

24. Morin B, Coutard B, Lelke M, Ferron F, Kerber R, Jamal S, et al. The N-terminal domain of the arenavirus L protein is an RNA endonuclease essential in mRNA transcription. PLoS Pathog. 2010;6(9):e1001038.

25. Reguera J, Weber F, Cusack S. Bunyaviridae RNA polymerases (L-protein) have an N-terminal, influenza-like endonuclease domain, essential for viral cap-dependent transcription. PLoS Pathog. 2010;6(9): e1001101.

26. Perez DR, Donis RO. Functional analysis of PA binding by influenza A virus PB1: effects on polymerase activity and viral infectivity. J Virol. 2001;75(17):8127–36.

27. Guilligay D, Tarendeau F, Resa-Infante P, Coloma R, Crepin T, Sehr P, et al. The structural basis for cap binding by influenza virus polymerase subunit PB2. Nat Struct Mol Biol. 2008;15(5):500–6.

28. Tarendeau F, Boudet J, Guilligay D, Mas PJ, Bougault CM, Boulo S, et al. Structure and nuclear import function of the C-terminal domain of influenza virus polymerase PB2 subunit. Nat Struct Mol Biol. 2007;14(3):229–33.

29. Tarendeau F, Crepin T, Guilligay D, Ruigrok RW, Cusack S, Hart DJ. Host determinant residue lysine 627 lies on the surface of a discrete, folded domain of influenza virus polymerase PB2 subunit. PLoS Pathog. 2008;4(8):e1000136.

30. Kuzuhara T, Kise D, Yoshida H, Horita T, Murazaki Y, Nishimura A, et al. Structural basis of the influenza A virus RNA polymerase PB2 RNA-binding domain containing the pathogenicity-determinant lysine 627 residue. J Biol Chem. 2009;284(11):6855–60.

31. Yamada S, Hatta M, Staker BL, Watanabe S, Imai M, Shinya K, et al. Biological and structural characteriza-

tion of a host-adapting amino acid in influenza virus. PLoS Pathog. 2010;6(8).

32. Subbarao EK, London W, Murphy BR. A single amino acid in the PB2 gene of influenza A virus is a determinant of host range. J Virol. 1993;67(4):1761–4.

33. Mehle A, Doudna JA. Adaptive strategies of the influenza virus polymerase for replication in humans. Proc Natl Acad Sci U S A. 2009;106(50):21312–6.

34. Wise HM, Barbezange C, Jagger BW, Dalton RM, Gog JR, Curran MD, et al. Overlapping signals for translational regulation and packaging of influenza A virus segment 2. Nucleic Acids Res. 2011;39(17):7775–90.

35. Bruns K, Studtrucker N, Sharma A, Fossen T, Mitzner D, Eissmann A, et al. Structural characterization and oligomerization of PB1-F2, a proapoptotic influenza A virus protein. J Biol Chem. 2007;282(1):353–63.

36. Chen W, Calvo PA, Malide D, Gibbs J, Schubert U, Bacik I, et al. A novel influenza A virus mitochondrial protein that induces cell death. Nat Med. 2001;7(12):1306–12.

37. McAuley JL, Chipuk JE, Boyd KL, Van De Velde N, Green DR, McCullers JA. PB1-F2 proteins from H5N1 and 20 century pandemic influenza viruses cause immunopathology. PLoS Pathog. 2010;6(7):e1001014.

38. McAuley JL, Zhang K, McCullers JA. The effects of influenza A virus PB1-F2 protein on polymerase activity are strain specific and do not impact pathogenesis. J Virol. 2010;84(1):558–64.

39. McAuley JL, Hornung F, Boyd KL, Smith AM, McKeon R, Bennink J, et al. Expression of the 1918 influenza A virus PB1-F2 enhances the pathogenesis of viral and secondary bacterial pneumonia. Cell Host Microbe. 2007;2(4):240–9.

40. Varga ZT, Ramos I, Hai R, Schmolke M, Garcia-Sastre A, Fernandez-Sesma A, et al. The influenza virus protein PB1-F2 inhibits the induction of type i interferon at the level of the MAVS adaptor protein. PLoS Pathog. 2011;7(6):e1002067.

41. Gabriel G, Dauber B, Wolff T, Planz O, Klenk HD, Stech J. The viral polymerase mediates adaptation of an avian influenza virus to a mammalian host. Proc Natl Acad Sci U S A. 2005;102(51):18590–5.

42. Gabriel G, Herwig A, Klenk HD. Interaction of polymerase subunit PB2 and NP with importin alpha1 is a determinant of host range of influenza A virus. PLoS Pathog. 2008;4(2):e11.

43. Alymova IV, Green AM, van de Velde N, McAuley JL, Boyd KL, Ghoneim HE, et al. Immunopathogenic and antibacterial effects of H3N2 influenza A virus PB1-F2 map to amino acid residues 62, 75, 79, and 82. J Virol. 2011;85(23):12324–33.

44. Schmolke M, Manicassamy B, Pena L, Sutton T, Hai R, Varga ZT, et al. Differential contribution of PB1-F2 to

the virulence of highly pathogenic H5N1 influenza A virus in mammalian and avian species. PLoS Pathog. 2011;7(8):e1002186.

45. Wunderlich K, Juozapaitis M, Ranadheera C, Kessler U, Martin A, Eisel J, et al. Identification of high-affinity PB1-derived peptides with enhanced affinity to the PA protein of influenza A virus polymerase. Antimicrob Agents Chemother. 2011;55(2):696–702.

46. Tomassini J, Selnick H, Davies ME, Armstrong ME, Baldwin J, Bourgeois M, et al. Inhibition of cap (m7GpppXm)-dependent endonuclease of influenza virus by 4-substituted 2,4-dioxobutanoic acid compounds. Antimicrob Agents Chemother. 1994;38(12):2827–37.

47. Kao RY, Yang D, Lau LS, Tsui WH, Hu L, Dai J, et al. Identification of influenza A nucleoprotein as an antiviral target. Nat Biotechnol. 2010;28(6):600–5.

48. Gerritz SW, Cianci C, Kim S, Pearce BC, Deminie C, Discotto L, et al. Inhibition of influenza virus replication via small molecules that induce the formation of higher-order nucleoprotein oligomers. Proc Natl Acad Sci U S A. 2011;108(37):15366–71.

49. Biswas SK, Nayak DP. Mutational analysis of the conserved motifs of influenza A virus polymerase basic protein 1. J Virol. 1994;68(3):1819–26.

50. McAuley JL, McCullers JA. Bacterial super-infections: the other side of influenza pathogenesis. Influenza Other Respir Viruses. 2011;5(Suppl. 1):2–53.

51. Arranz R, Coloma R, Chichon FJ, Conesa JJ, Carrascosa JL, Valpuesta JM, et al. Negative stained electron microscopy reconstruction of the viral polymerase of influenza A virus ribonucleoprotein isolated from virions. Conformation 1. Science. 2012;338: 1634–1637.

52. Moeller A, Kirchdoerfer RN, Potter CS, Carragher B, Wilson IA. Organization of the influenza virus replication machinery. Science. 2012;338:1631–1634.

The genome and its manipulation: Recovery of the 1918 virus and vaccine virus generation

Gabriele Neumann[1] and Yoshihiro Kawaoka[1,2,3,4]

[1]Influenza Research Institute, Department of Pathobiological Sciences, School of Veterinary Medicine, University of Wisconsin-Madison, Madison, WI, USA

[2]Department of Special Pathogens, International Research Center for Infectious Diseases, Institute of Medical Science, University of Tokyo, Tokyo, Japan

[3]Division of Virology, Department of Microbiology and Immunology, Institute of Medical Science, University of Tokyo, Tokyo, Japan

[4]ERATO Infection-Induced Host Responses Project, Saitama, Japan

Reverse genetics encompasses techniques for the artificial generation of wild-type and mutant influenza viruses [1,2]. These techniques have, for example, allowed the recreation and experimental testing of the pandemic 1918 influenza virus [3,4], and the development of novel influenza vaccines; these two topics are discussed in detail below.

The pandemic 1918 virus – an elusive killer virus is identified

In 1918, the world was not only plagued by the countless casualties on the battlefields of World War I, but also by a yet greater disaster that claimed even more lives and did not spare civilians. In the spring of 1918, a respiratory disease emerged that soon traveled with American soldiers to Europe; this first wave was highly infectious but claimed few lives. In contrast to other parts of the world, the outbreak was extensively reported in the uncensored Spanish press, which may be why the pandemic of 1918 is also known as "Spanish" influenza. From August through November 1918, a second wave of considerably higher mortality spread around the world. Most infections were characterized by a sudden onset of symptoms including high fever and severe headache. The infection appeared to be limited to the respiratory tract with no evidence of systemic spread. A sizeable number of deaths was likely caused by secondary bacterial pneumonia [5–7], which may be attributed to the lack of antibiotics in this era.

In 1918, influenza viruses had not yet been identified and therefore no virus samples were stored that would help unlock the secrets of this deadly disease. In the 1950s, researchers tried to isolate the pandemic virus from corpses preserved in the permafrost of Alaska but failed. However, in the late 1990s, a successful attempt was made by Taubenberger and colleagues: RNA was recovered from formalin-fixed, paraffin-embedded lung tissue samples of two soldiers who had succumbed to the pandemic 1918 virus [8,9], and from an Inuit whose body was exhumed from a mass grave in the permafrost of Alaska [9]. Amplification of the extracted RNA by using reverse transcription polymerase chain reaction (RT-PCR) yielded the sequences of all eight vRNAs [8–14]. Phylogenetic analyses confirmed earlier seroarcheologic findings that the pandemic virus was an influenza A virus of the H1N1 subtype. Further sequence analysis

Textbook of Influenza, Second Edition. Edited by Robert G. Webster, Arnold S. Monto, Thomas J. Braciale, and Robert A. Lamb.

suggested that the pandemic 1918 virus shared an ancestor with avian viruses. Reassortant viruses were then generated that possessed single or multiple pandemic 1918 vRNA segments in the background of contemporary human H1N1 viruses [3,14–16]. With the reconstruction of all eight vRNA segments, the pandemic 1918 virus was eventually rebuilt [3,4]. The generation of wild-type and reassortant pandemic 1918 viruses now opened the door to study the viral and cellular determinants that contributed to the high pathogenicity of this virus.

Virulence and pathogenicity of pandemic 1918 virus infections

The recreated pandemic 1918 virus is highly pathogenic in mice, ferrets, and nonhuman primates [3,4,17–20]. In all three animal models, the virus replicated to high titers in the lungs of infected animals but did not cause systemic infection, just as it had in humans infected in 1918. Cynomolgus macaques (*Macaca fascicularis*) infected with 7×10^6 plaque-forming units (pfu) of the pandemic 1918 virus had to be euthanized on day 8 post-infection because of the severity of their diseases symptoms [4], whereas highly pathogenic avian H5N1 influenza viruses do not uniformly kill nonhuman primates. Ferrets infected with pandemic 1918 virus also developed disease symptoms [17,18] and most of the infected animals succumbed to their infection [17]. By contrast, the 1918 pandemic virus is of low pathogenicity in pigs, which may have a critical role in the genesis of new pandemic viruses; however, their role in the generation of the pandemic 1918 virus remains elusive. In addition, the pandemic 1918 virus is of low pathogenicity in chickens and mallard ducks, in keeping with its lack of sequence motifs that confer high pathogenicity in chickens.

A recent report summarized autopsy findings from 68 human cases of pandemic 1918 virus infection [7]. The major pathologic findings were bronchitis, bronchiolitis, primary viral pneumonia with diffuse alveolar damage, often in combination with acute pulmonary hemorrhage or edema, and hyaline membrane formation. The alveolar airspaces were filled with inflammatory cells, but also desquamated epithelial cells, edema fluid, erythrocytes, and fibrin. Viral antigen was detected in bronchiolar epithelial cells, type I and II pneumocytes, and in alveolar epithelial cells and macrophages. Similar pathologic findings were made in animals infected with the reconstituted pandemic 1918 virus. In infected macaques, the 1918 virus replicated to high titers in the upper and lower respiratory tract [4], in contrast to contemporary human H1N1 viruses, which are mainly isolated from the upper respiratory tract. The lungs of animals infected with the pandemic 1918 virus showed alveolar damage with edema and hemorrhage. Virus antigen was detected in alveolar cells and bronchiolar epithelial cells. In ferrets, bronchiolitis, alveolitis, and lung hemorrhagic lesions were observed [17,18]. Viral antigen was detected in peribronchial glands, alveolar epithelial cells, and macrophages [17,18]. Similarly, lung damage with edema, as well as rapid infiltration of neutrophils and macrophages, was found in mice infected with the pandemic 1918 virus [3,19,21,22].

Overall, the pathologic findings observed with pandemic 1918 virus infections are similar to those in patients infected with highly pathogenic H5N1 influenza viruses, or in severe cases of infection with pandemic (H1N1) 2009 virus. Collectively, these infections are characterized by virus replication in the lower and upper respiratory tract, diffuse alveolar damage with rapid infiltration of neutrophils and macrophages, high levels of proinflammatory cytokines, and – for pandemic 1918 and pandemic (H1N1) 2009 virus infections – secondary bacterial coinfections.

Host responses to infection with pandemic 1918 virus

Several studies including transcriptomics and proteomics analyses have assessed the host responses in mice or nonhuman primates to infection with the pandemic 1918 virus or with viruses possessing the pandemic 1918 virus hemagglutinin (HA) and neuraminidase (NA) genes in the background of contemporary human H1N1 influenza viruses. Hallmarks of infection with these viruses included the induction of high levels of genes involved in innate immune responses, T-cell and macrophage activation, apoptosis, and tissue damage [19,23–27]. In particular, proinflammatory cytokines and chemokines such as interleukin-6 (IL-6), monocyte chemoattractant

147

protein 1 MCP-1, or macrophage inflammatory protein 1α (MIP-1α) were upregulated [19,21–25,27]. Interestingly, fewer interferon α (IFNα)-induced genes were activated upon pandemic 1918 virus infection compared with infection with a human H1N1 control virus. This finding may suggest a reduced sensitivity to type I IFN responses. At the proteomics level, a virus possessing the pandemic 1918 HA and NA genes combined with the remaining genes of a contemporary human influenza virus triggered the upregulation of proteins that have a role in innate and adaptive immunity as well as the upregulation of proteins involved in protein synthesis and metabolic processes, such as oxidative phosphorylation [28]. In mice lacking the IL-1 receptor (IL1RKO), many more genes were differentially expressed upon infection with the pandemic 1918 virus compared with wild-type mice or mice lacking the tumor necrosis factor (TNF) receptor-1 (TNFRKO), suggesting that IL-1 receptor signaling may have an important role in host transcriptional responses to this infection [29]. In addition, in IL1RKO mice, gene expression of TNF-α and other chemokines was increased compared with TNFRKO and wild-type mice. Together with the observed differences in pathogenicity, these data suggest that IL-1 receptor signaling induces protective pathways upon pandemic 1918 virus infection, whereas signaling through the TNF-α receptor increases the severity of infection.

Proinflammatory cytokines and chemokines are also upregulated in individuals and animals infected with highly pathogenic avian H5N1 or pandemic 2009 H1N1 viruses. However, differences exist in the innate immune responses to infection with the pandemic 1918 virus compared with infection with highly pathogenic avian H5N1 viruses [26,27].

The influenza viral NS1 protein is an IFN antagonist and as such affects host cell responses (see also section on viral determinants of pandemic 1918 virus pathogenicity). In one study, an A/WSN/33 (H1N1; WSN) virus bearing the pandemic 1918 virus NS segment (which encodes NS1 and the nuclear export protein, NS2; NEP) was tested in human lung epithelial (A549) cells [30,31]. While the parental WSN virus induced several IFN-stimulated genes including IRF9, ISG15, MxA, and IFITM1, these genes were not upregulated in A549 cells infected with the WSN virus possessing the pandemic 1918 NS segment. Another study tested the pandemic 1918 NS gene in

the genetic background of seasonal human A/USSR/90/77 (H1N1) virus; again, the pandemic 1918 NS1 protein was more efficient in suppressing IFN upregulation compared with the NS1 protein of the control virus [32]. Imbalanced host immune responses thus appear to be a hallmark of infections with highly pathogenic influenza viruses.

Bacterial coinfections in pandemic 1918 virus infections

A recent analysis of lung tissues from victims of the pandemic 1918 virus has provided histologic evidence of acute bacterial pneumonia in all cases studied [7]. Previous reports identified bacterial pneumonia in lung tissue samples from pandemic 1918 virus victims [5] and in antemortem cultures from patients who presented with pneumonia during the 1918 pandemic [6]. Bacterial pneumonia was also reported in an appreciable number of human infections with pandemic 2009 H1N1 virus, although it does not seem to have a major role in human infections with highly pathogenic avian H5N1 influenza viruses. The most commonly detected bacterial pathogens in coinfections with influenza viruses are *Streptococcus pneumoniae*, *Staphylococcus aureus*, and *Haemophilus influenzae*. Several reports indicate that infections with these bacteria increase the severity of influenza virus infections.

Viral determinants of pandemic 1918 virus pathogenicity

Individual pandemic 1918 viral genes have been tested in the context of a contemporary human H1N1 virus, and vice versa. These studies revealed that the pandemic 1918 HA and the polymerase proteins (PB2, PB1, PA) are critical for viral pathogenicity; in addition, the pandemic 1918 PB1-F2, NS1, and NA proteins (all discussed in detail below) also affect pathogenicity.

Hemagglutinin (HA)

The HA protein is a known determinant of viral pathogenicity. It mediates virus binding to host cells and fusion of the viral and endosomal membranes, resulting in the release of viral ribonucleoprotein complexes into the cytoplasm of infected cells. Viruses possessing the pandemic 1918 HA (or pandemic 1918 HA and NA) genes in the background of recent human viruses are considerably more pathogenic in mice and nonhuman primates than are control viruses that possess the HA, NA, or both HA and NA genes of recent human influenza viruses [3,15,16,20,23–26], causing lung damage, influx of alveolar macrophages and neutrophils, and upregulation of cytokines and chemokines genes [23–26]. These findings indicate that the pandemic 1918 HA has a critical role in the pathogenicity of this virus.

The HA protein is synthesized as a precursor that is post-translationally cleaved into HA1 and HA2 subunits. This cleavage exposes the "fusion peptide"at the N-terminus of HA2. The fusion peptide facilitates the fusion of the viral and endosomal membranes, a step that is critical for virus replication. All highly pathogenic avian influenza viruses possess a multibasic amino acid sequence at the HA cleavage site which is recognized by ubiquitous proteases, allowing systemic spread of these viruses in their hosts. By contrast, the pandemic 1918 virus HA protein, similar to that of low pathogenic viruses, possesses a single basic amino acid at the HA cleavage site. This cleavage sequence is recognized by a limited number of proteases that presumably reside in the respiratory or intestinal tract of mammalian or avian species, thus restricting virus replication to these organs. Interestingly, however, replication of the pandemic 1918 virus in Madin–Darby canine kidney (MDCK) cells does not require the addition of exogenous trypsin, a feature conferred by the pandemic 1918 NA protein [3]. Trypsin-independent HA cleavage has also been shown for the WSN virus. The WSN virus's NA protein sequesters plasminogen; the cleavage product of plasminogen, plasmin, then facilitates HA cleavage. However, a recent study found that the pandemic 1918 NA protein-dependent spread of the pandemic 1918 virus does not require plasminogen recruitment, leaving in question the mechanism of the trypsin independence of the pandemic 1918 virus.

The HA protein also mediates virus binding to sialic acid-containing receptors on host cells, a step that confers host range restriction. Avian influenza viruses bind efficiently to sialic acid (Sia) linked to galactose by an α2,3-linkage (Siaα2,3), which is expressed on epithelial cells in the intestinal tract of avian species.

In contrast, human influenza viruses have higher specificity for Siaα2,6, the predominant sialic acid on epithelial cells in the respiratory tract of humans. The ability to recognize Siaα2,6 is believed to be a critical prerequisite for a pandemic virus; in fact, the earliest isolates of the 1957 and 1968 pandemic viruses possessed HA with human-type receptor-binding specificity, although their HA genes were of avian virus origin, based on phylogenic analysis. Taubenberger and colleagues reconstituted three different 1918 HA genes [9].At amino acid position 190 (H3 numbering), which is known to determine the receptor-binding specificity of H1 HAs, all three pandemic 1918 HA proteins possessed an aspartic acid, that is the "human-type" amino acid (avian influenza viruses bear a glutamic acid residue at this position). The receptor-binding specificity of H1 HAs is also affected by the amino acid at position 225; two pandemic 1918 HA genes (A/South Carolina/1/1918 and A/Brevig Mission/1/1918) possess a "human-type" aspartic acid at this position, whereas the pandemic 1918 A/New/York/1/1918 HA encodes an "avian-type" glycine residue. Partial sequences are available for two additional isolates [33]: the A/London/1/1918 HA protein differs from that of A/Brevig Mission/1/1918 by one amino acid (a glycine-to-serine change at position 188, which is located near the HA antigenic site Sb and may affect receptor-binding specificity); and the A/London/1/1919 HA protein, the sequence of which deviates from the A/Brevig Mission/1/1918 HA sequence by two amino acids (a valine-to-isoleucine change at position 223 and an aspartic acid-to-glycine change at position 225). Subsequent receptor binding specificity tests demonstrated that the A/New York/1/1918 HA (encoding Asp190/Gly225) binds to both human- and avian-type receptors, whereas the other two pandemic 1918 HAs (encoding Asp190/Asp225) interact primarily with human-type receptors (Figure 9.1) [34–36].These experimental findings are in line with conclusions drawn from the X-ray crystallographic structure of the pandemic 1918 HA protein [37,38]. A pandemic 1918 virus that possessed two mutations in its HA (Asp190Glu and Asp225Gly) was generated by using reverse genetics. The mutant virus no longer transmitted among ferrets through respiratory droplets, although it maintained its lethal phenotype in infected animals [17,39]. Interestingly, the Asp225Gly mutation has also been found in some human pandemic 2009 H1N1 isolates and

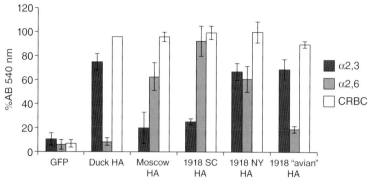

Figure 9.1. Receptor-binding specificity of pandemic 1918 HA variants. Human embryonic kidney (293T) cells were transfected with plasmids expressing green fluorescent protein (GFP; control), avian-type HA (A/duck/Ukraine/1/63 HA; Duck HA), human-type HA (A/Moscow/10/99 HA; Moscow HA), pandemic A/South Carolina/1/18 HA (1918 SC HA; encoding Asp190/Asp225), pandemic A/New York/1/18 HA (1918 NY HA; encoding Asp190/Gly225), or A/New York/1/18 HA mutated to encode Glu190/Gly225 (1918 "avian" HA). Transfected cells were incubated with chicken red blood cells (CRBC), or with desialylated CRBC subsequently resialylated with the help of Siaα2,3- or Siaα2,6-specific sialyltransferases (α2,3; α2,6). Bound CRBC were lysed and quantified by measuring hemoglobin release through absorbance at 540 nm. Bars represent averages of three separate experiments. With permission from Glaser et al. [34] with permission from the American Society for Microbiology.

appears to correlate with more severe outcome of infection in humans. Although HA receptor-binding specificity is recognized as a critical determinant of pathogenicity, the pandemic 1918 wild-type and mutant HA genes (with Siaα2,3-, Siaα2,6-, or dual Siaα2,6/Siaα2,6-specificity) all confer lethality in mice, suggesting that the pandemic 1918 virus HA gene possesses pathogenicity determinants independent of receptor-binding specificity.

In 2009, an influenza A virus of the H1N1 subtype caused the first pandemic of the twenty-first century. The infection pattern of this pandemic was similar to that of previous pandemics with low infection rates among the elderly, which typically experience high rates of infection with seasonal influenza viruses. This low infection rate among the elderly may originate from antigenic cross-reactivity between the pandemic (H1N1) 2009 virus and close descendants of the pandemic 1918 virus, due to shared antigenic epitopes between the HA proteins of the two pandemic viruses.

Replication complex

The viral replication complex comprises the three polymerase subunits (PB2, PB1, PA) and the nucleo-protein NP. This replication complex affects pathogenicity, possibly by mediating efficient virus replication which leads to high virus titers that overwhelm the host immune responses. Some individuals infected with pandemic 1918 virus died from viral pneumonia. This observation, together with the rapid progression of pandemic 1918 virus infections, suggested that the 1918 virus replicated efficiently in the lungs of infected individuals. By contrast, seasonal human influenza viruses typically do to not replicate to high titers in the lower respiratory tract of humans. This concept is supported by the finding of highly efficient pandemic 1918 virus replication in the lungs of infected ferrets and nonhuman primates [4,17,18]. Reverse genetics studies have demonstrated that the polymerase and NP genes of the pandemic 1918 virus, particularly the PB1 gene, are critical for efficient replication in mammals [3,18,20,39]. A virus possessing the pandemic 1918 virus polymerase and NP vRNAs together with the remaining four vRNAs of A/Kawasaki/173/2001 (H1N1) virus replicated in the trachea and lungs of infected ferrets to titers similar to those observed upon infection with wild-type 1918 virus [18]. Conversely, a virus bearing the A/Kawasaki/173/2001 polymerase and NP genes in combination with the pandemic 1918 HA, NA, M, and NS vRNAs replicated in the trachea, but not the lungs, of ferrets [18]. In addition, the pandemic 1918 virus and a reassortant possessing the pandemic 1918 virus replication complex caused more severe lung pathology than a contemporary human H1N1 influenza virus (Figure 9.2) [18]. Thus, the replication complex of the pandemic 1918 virus is critical for its efficient replication in the lower respiratory tract of ferrets. Further analysis revealed that the pandemic 1918 PB1 gene in the background of the A/Kawasaki/173/2001 virus conferred efficient replication in the lower respiratory tract of ferrets [18].

The pandemic 1918 virus PB2 polymerase subunit encodes a lysine residue at position 627. This amino acid is involved in host range and enhances the pathogenicity of highly pathogenic avian H5N1 viruses in mice [40]. Most human influenza viruses encode lysine at PB2-627, whereas avian influenza viruses typically possess glutamic acid at this position. Several studies have demonstrated that PB2-627K provides a replicative advantage in mammalian hosts, in particular at the lower temperature of the upper respiratory tract. In line with this finding, lysine at PB2-627K is selected during virus replication in humans, mice, and pigs, and interestingly also during virus replication in ostriches and ostrich cells. Collectively, these data indicate that PB2-627K is critical for influenza virus replication in mammalian cells. A noticeable exception are the pandemic 2009 H1N1 viruses, which possess the avian-type amino acid at PB2-627; however, the lack of a basic amino acid at this position is compensated for by a nearby basic amino acid.

One study demonstrated that the pandemic 1918 virus PB2 gene (in addition to the HA gene) is critical for respiratory droplet transmission of the pandemic virus in ferrets [39].Currently, the underlying mechanism is unknown, but the pandemic 1918 virus PB2 gene may contribute to the high replicative ability of the virus, and this may be a prerequisite for virus transmission.

NS1

The NS1 protein executes its IFN antagonism primarily by modulating the host immune responses (see section on host responses to infection with pandemic 1918 virus). The pandemic 1918 NS gene in the genetic background of the WSN virus attenuated the recombinant virus in mice [14].By contrast, more severe symptoms were observed in ferrets infected with the A/USSR/90/77 (H1N1) virus bearing the pandemic 1918 NS gene than those animals infected with control viruses encoding the A/Puerto Rico/8/34 (H1N1) or A/USSR/90/77 NS genes [32]. Both studies, however, found that the pandemic 1918 NS1 controls host immune responses very efficiently.

The carboxy-terminal four amino acids of NS1 form a PDZ domain-binding motif that is recognized by PDZ domain proteins, a large family of proteins with roles in multiple cellular processes including signaling, apoptosis, trafficking, cell polarity, and tight junction integrity. Most human influenza virus NS1 proteins encode a PDZ domain-binding motif with the sequence RSKV, whereas most avian influenza virus NS1 proteins possess an ESEV motif. The PDZ domain-binding motif found in the pandemic 1918 virus NS1 protein is KSEV, which deviates from the human- and avian-type motifs. This motif was tested in the background of the WSN virus, which possesses the RSEV motif [41]. The WSN virus encoding the pandemic 1918-like KSEV motif replicated in MDCK cells to titers similar to those obtained for the WSN virus, but caused more rapid weight loss in mice, was cleared less efficiently from the lungs of infected animals, and caused more severe alveolitis and hemorrhage [41]. The differences in virulence did not correlate with IFN expression levels [41], suggesting that the NS1 protein affects virulence through different mechanisms. Similarly, the avian influenza virus ESEV motif slightly increased the severity of disease compared with the human influenza virus RSKV motif [41]. Recent studies suggest that the PDZ domain-binding motif may affect the regulation of apoptosis or the integrity of tight junctions in virus-infected cells. Both of these processes may contribute to disease pathogenicity in infected individuals or animals.

PB1-F2

The PB1-F2 protein is expressed from the +1 reading frame of the PB1 gene. It is encoded by most avian and human influenza viruses.By contrast, most swine influenza viruses do not encode this protein due to several in-frame stop codons. PB1-F2 increases viral pathogenicity, inflammation, and the frequency and severity of bacterial coinfections in a strain-specific

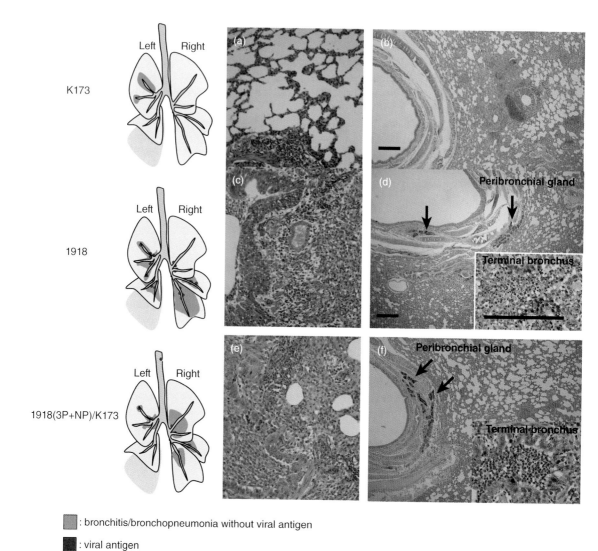

: bronchitis/bronchopneumonia without viral antigen

: viral antigen

Figure 9.2. Pathologic examination of lungs of infected ferrets. On day 3 post-infection, lung samples were collected from ferrets infected with 10^5 pfu pandemic 1918 virus, human A/Kawasaki/173/2001 (H1N1, K173) virus, or a virus possessing the polymerase and NP genes of pandemic 1918 virus together with the remaining genes from Kaw virus (1918(3P + NP)/K173 virus). Lung samples were examined for pathologic changes. (a) In lungs of ferrets infected with K173 virus, peribronchitis and bronchopneumonia were observed in some lung lobes, but (b) no viral antigen was detected. Infection with 1918 virus (c) or 1918(3P + NP)/K173 virus (e) resulted in moderate to severe peribronchitis and bronchopneumonia. Viral antigens were detected mainly in the peribronchial gland (arrows) and rarely in the terminal bronchial epithelium (d and f). (Scale bars, 100 μm.) On the left, the distribution of viral antigen and bronchitis/bronchopneumonia is shown schematically. The left lower lobes of the lungs (gray) were used for virologic examination. Reproduced with courtesy of Yoshihiro Kawaoka, Department of Pathobiological Sciences, University of Wisconsin-Madison.

manner [42–46]. It may accomplish these effects through the induction of apoptosis, interaction with and nuclear retention of PB1, or an IFN-antagonistic function mediated by obstructing the RIG-I–IPS-1 pathway.

Sequence comparison of highly pathogenic avian H5N1 PB1-F2 proteins revealed an amino acid change (Asn66Ser) that correlated with pathogenicity [46]. Interestingly, the PB1-F2 protein of the pandemic 1918 virus also encodes serine (the amino acid correlated with a high-pathogenicity phenotype) at position 66. To assess the significance of PB1-F2-Ser66, WSN viruses possessing an H5N1 PB1 segment encoding PB1-F2-Asn66 or Ser66 were generated [46]. Similarly, two pandemic 1918 viruses were generated encoding the two PB1-F2 variants. PB1-F2 proteins encoding serine at position 66 conferred higher virus titers and increased pathogenicity in mice, as compared with their counterparts encoding an asparagine residue at this position [46,47]. In particular, the dose required to kill 50% of infected mice (MLD_{50}) was ~1000-fold higher for the pandemic 1918 virus encoding PB1-F2-Asn66 than for that for the virus encoding PB1-Ser66, demonstrating the attenuating effect of the PB1-F2-Ser66Asn mutation in the background of the pandemic 1918 virus. Moreover, H5N1 and 1918 PB1-F2 proteins encoding serine at position 66 induced higher levels of cytokines in the lungs of infected mice.

In a more detailed study, transcriptomics analyses were carried out for the lungs of mice infected with WSN viruses possessing an H5N1 PB1 gene that encodes PB1-F2-Ser66 or -Asn66 [47]. One day after infection, the more pathogenic PB1-F2-Ser66 variant caused a delay in the upregulation of IFN-regulated genes as compared with the virus expressing PB1-F2-Asn66. However, on days 3 and 5 post-infection, the more pathogenic PB1-F2-Ser66 virus activated more genes related to host immune responses than did the less pathogenic PB1-F2-Asn66 virus. These findings further support the concept that PB1-F2 interferes with host immune responses and that the magnitude of this effect may be determined by the amino acid at position 66 of PB1-F2.

NA

The neuraminidase protein cleaves the α-ketosidic linkage between a terminal sialic acid and an adjacent sugar residue. This reaction removes sialic acid residues from cellular glycoconjugates and viral proteins and balances the sialic acid-binding function of HA in the binding and release of viruses. The sialidase activity of most epidemic human and swine virus NA proteins is irreversibly lost at acidic pH (pH 4.0–5.0). By contrast, the NA proteins of duck viruses and pandemic 1957 and 1968 viruses (both of the N2 subtype) remain active at pH 4.0–5.0. A recent study found that the pandemic 1918 virus NA protein also possesses low pH stability [48]. The deletion of threonine at position 435 and an asparagine-to-glycine change at position 455 are responsible for this phenotype. Viruses possessing a low pH-stable NA protein replicate more efficiently in culture cells, most likely because these low pH-stable NA proteins maintain their enzymatic function under the pH conditions in the endosome.

Generation of vaccine viruses

Reverse genetics approaches are now also employed to generate inactivated and live attenuated vaccine viruses. In classic approaches for influenza A virus vaccine generation, cells are coinfected with the selected circulating strain and human lab-adapted A/Puerto Rico/8/34 (H1N1) virus (which confers high-growth properties in embryonated chicken eggs and is therefore used routinely for the generation of inactivated vaccine viruses) or attenuated A/Ann Arbor/1/60 (H2N2) virus (for the generation of live attenuated vaccine viruses). Then, vaccine viruses are selected that possess (at least) the HA and NA segments of the circulating virus in the background of the A/Puerto Rico/8/34 or A/Ann Arbor/1/60 viruses. This selection process can be cumbersome. By providing the eight vRNAs from plasmids, reverse genetics allows one to generate any specific gene constellation without the need for subsequent selection steps.

Even more importantly, reverse genetics is now used to generate candidate vaccines to highly pathogenic avian H5N1 influenza viruses. Because of their high pathogenicity in humans, work with these viruses is restricted to biosafety level 3 containment facilities, thus generally precluding vaccine virus generation in large-scale industrial settings. In addition, highly pathogenic avian H5N1 influenza viruses kill chicken embryos, resulting in low virus yields in embryonated chicken eggs, the most commonly used system to amplify vaccine viruses (although cell culture systems are now approved in Europe for human vaccine virus production). This limitation can be overcome by replacing the multibasic HA cleavage sequence (see section on viral determinants of pandemic 1918 virus pathogenicity) with a single basic amino acid; this modification attenuates the virus so that it can be handled in biosafety level 2 containment and also yields higher virus titers in embryonated chicken embryos.

A number of H5N1 candidate vaccines have now been generated, most of which possess the attenuated H5 HA and matching NA genes in the genetic background of the A/Puerto Rico/8/34 virus. Early clinical trials indicated low immunogenicity of these vaccines, requiring high amounts of antigen or repeated immunization or both, potentially in combination with adjuvants [49,50]. Since then, many studies has been carried out to evaluate: (i) different vaccine doses in the presence or absence of different adjuvants; (ii) inactivated vaccines propagated in embryonated chicken eggs or cell culture; (iii) live attenuated vaccines; and (iv) the immunogenicity and cross-protection of vaccines directed towards different (sub)clades of H5 HAs. Overall, H5 HA appears to be of low immunogenicity in mammals. However, high doses of antigen administered once or twice, or the addition of an adjuvant, may elicit protective antibody titers. Similarly, candidate vaccines to avian influenza viruses of the H7 and H9 subtypes are now in various stages of development.

Influenza vaccines provide a wide range of protection, depending on the antigenic match between the circulating virus and the vaccine strain, the immunogenic and health status of the vaccinated individual, and other factors. Improvements are needed in vaccine virus yield, level of attenuation (for live virus vaccines), immunogenicity/efficacy, and cross-protection. Reverse genetics approaches are actively being used to test and screen mutations in viral proteins yield such improvements. In one example, an A/Puerto Rico/8/34 virus has been identified that grows to higher titers in MDCK and Vero cells (both of which are used in Europe for influenza vaccine virus growth) when compared with the A/Puerto Rico/8/34 isolate currently used for vaccine production. Testing for individual amino acid changes in the high-growth isolate revealed that mutations PB2 and NS1 affected

this virus's growth properties in MDCK cells, whereas a mutation in the HA2 subunit of its HA affected the virus yield in Vero cells.

In conclusion, the ability to manipulate influenza viruses has markedly increased our understanding of virulence determinants, and has had a major impact on influenza virus vaccine generation and production.

References

1. Fodor E, Devenish L, Engelhardt OG, Palese P, Brownlee GG, Garcia-Sastre A. Rescue of influenza A virus from recombinant DNA. J Virol. 1999;73(11): 9679–82.

2. Neumann G, Watanabe T, Ito H, Watanabe S, Goto H, Gao P, et al. Generation of influenza A viruses entirely from cloned cDNAs. Proc Natl Acad Sci U S A. 1999;96(16):9345–50.

3. Tumpey TM, Basler CF, Aguilar PV, Zeng H, Solorzano A, Swayne DE, et al. Characterization of the reconstructed 1918 Spanish influenza pandemic virus. Science. 2005;310(5745):77–80.

4. Kobasa D, Jones SM, Shinya K, Kash JC, Copps J, Ebihara H, et al. Aberrant innate immune response in lethal infection of macaques with the 1918 influenza virus. Nature. 2007;445(7125):319–23.

5. Morens DM, Taubenberger JK, Fauci AS. Predominant role of bacterial pneumonia as a cause of death in pandemic influenza: implications for pandemic influenza preparedness. J Infect Dis. 2008;198(7):962–70.

6. Chien YW, Klugman KP, Morens DM. Bacterial pathogens and death during the 1918 influenza pandemic. N Engl J Med. 2009;361(26):2582–3.

7. Sheng ZM, Chertow DS, Ambroggio X, McCall S, Przygodzki RM, Cunningham RE, et al. Autopsy series of 68 cases dying before and during the 1918 influenza pandemic peak. Proc Natl Acad Sci U S A. 2011;108 (39):16416–21.

8. Taubenberger JK, Reid AH, Krafft AE, Bijwaard KE, Fanning TG. Initial genetic characterization of the 1918 "Spanish" influenza virus. Science. 1997;275(5307): 1793–6.

9. Reid AH, Fanning TG, Hultin JV, Taubenberger JK. Origin and evolution of the 1918 "Spanish" influenza virus hemagglutinin gene. Proc Natl Acad Sci U S A. 1999;96(4):1651–6.

10. Taubenberger JK, Reid AH, Lourens RM, Wang R, Jin G, Fanning TG. Characterization of the 1918 influenza virus polymerase genes. Nature. 2005;437(7060): 889–93.

11. Reid AH, Fanning TG, Janczewski TA, Lourens RM, Taubenberger JK. Novel origin of the 1918 pandemic influenza virus nucleoprotein gene. J Virol. 2004;78 (22):12462–70.

12. Reid AH, Fanning TG, Janczewski TA, McCall S, Taubenberger JK. Characterization of the 1918 "Spanish" influenza virus matrix gene segment. J Virol. 2002;76(21):10717–23.

13. Reid AH, Fanning TG, Janczewski TA, Taubenberger JK. Characterization of the 1918 "Spanish" influenza virus neuraminidase gene. Proc Natl Acad Sci U S A. 2000;97(12):6785–90.

14. Basler CF, Reid AH, Dybing JK, Janczewski TA, Fanning TG, Zheng H, et al. Sequence of the 1918 pandemic influenza virus nonstructural gene (NS) segment and characterization of recombinant viruses bearing the 1918 NS genes. Proc Natl Acad Sci U S A. 2001;98(5): 2746–51.

15. Tumpey TM, Garcia-Sastre A, Mikulasova A, Taubenberger JK, Swayne DE, Palese P, et al. Existing antivirals are effective against influenza viruses with genes from the 1918 pandemic virus. Proc Natl Acad Sci U S A. 2002;99(21):13849–54.

16. Tumpey TM, Garcia-Sastre A, Taubenberger JK, Palese P, Swayne DE, Basler CF. Pathogenicity and immunogenicity of influenza viruses with genes from the 1918 pandemic virus. Proc Natl Acad Sci U S A. 2004;101(9): 3166–71.

17. Tumpey TM, Maines TR, Van Hoeven N, Glaser L, Solorzano A, Pappas C, et al. A two-amino acid change in the hemagglutinin of the 1918 influenza virus abolishes transmission. Science. 2007;315(5812):655–9.

18. Watanabe T, Watanabe S, Shinya K, Kim JH, Hatta M, Kawaoka Y. Viral RNA polymerase complex promotes optimal growth of 1918 virus in the lower respiratory tract of ferrets. Proc Natl Acad Sci U S A. 2009;106 (2):588–92.

19. Kash JC, Tumpey TM, Proll SC, Carter V, Perwitasari O, Thomas MJ, et al. Genomic analysis of increased host immune and cell death responses induced by 1918 influenza virus. Nature. 2006;443(7111):578–81.

20. Pappas C, Aguilar PV, Basler CF, Solorzano A, Zeng H, Perrone LA, et al. Single gene reassortants identify a critical role for PB1, HA, and NA in the high virulence of the 1918 pandemic influenza virus. Proc Natl Acad Sci U S A. 2008;105(8):3064–9.

21. Perrone LA, Plowden JK, Garcia-Sastre A, Katz JM, Tumpey TM. H5N1 and 1918 pandemic influenza virus infection results in early and excessive infiltration of macrophages and neutrophils in the lungs of mice. PLoS Pathog. 2008;4(8):e1000115.

22. Belser JA, Wadford DA, Pappas C, Gustin KM, Maines TR, Pearce MB, et al. Pathogenesis of pandemic influenza A (H1N1) and triple-reassortant swine influenza A (H1) viruses in mice. J Virol. 2010;84(9): 4194–203.

23. Kash JC, Basler CF, Garcia-Sastre A, Carter V, Billharz R, Swayne DE, et al. Global host immune response: pathogenesis and transcriptional profiling of type A influenza viruses expressing the hemagglutinin and neuraminidase genes from the 1918 pandemic virus. J Virol. 2004;78(17):9499–511.

24. Kobasa D, Takada A, Shinya K, Hatta M, Halfmann P, Theriault S, et al. Enhanced virulence of influenza A viruses with the haemagglutinin of the 1918 pandemic virus. Nature. 2004;431(7009):703–7.

25. Tumpey TM, Garcia-Sastre A, Taubenberger JK, Palese P, Swayne DE, Pantin-Jackwood MJ, et al. Pathogenicity of influenza viruses with genes from the 1918 pandemic virus: functional roles of alveolar macrophages and neutrophils in limiting virus replication and mortality in mice. J Virol. 2005;79(23):14933–44.

26. Baskin CR, Bielefeldt-Ohmann H, Tumpey TM, Sabourin PJ, Long JP, Garcia-Sastre A, et al. Early and sustained innate immune response defines pathology and death in nonhuman primates infected by highly pathogenic influenza virus. Proc Natl Acad Sci U S A. 2009;106(9):3455–60.

27. Cilloniz C, Shinya K, Peng X, Korth MJ, Proll SC, Aicher LD, et al. Lethal influenza virus infection in macaques is associated with early dysregulation of inflammatory related genes. PLoS Pathog. 2009;5(10): e1000604.

28. Brown JN, Palermo RE, Baskin CR, Gritsenko M, Sabourin PJ, Long JP, et al. Macaque proteome response to highly pathogenic avian influenza and 1918 reassortant influenza virus infections. J Virol. 2010;84(22): 12058–68.

29. Belisle SE, Tisoncik JR, Korth MJ, Carter VS, Proll SC, Swayne DE, et al. Genomic profiling of tumor necrosis factor alpha (TNF-alpha) receptor and interleukin-1 receptor knockout mice reveals a link between TNF-alpha signaling and increased severity of 1918 pandemic influenza virus infection. J Virol. 2010;84(24): 12576–88.

30. Geiss GK, Salvatore M, Tumpey TM, Carter VS, Wang X, Basler CF, et al. Cellular transcriptional profiling in influenza A virus-infected lung epithelial cells: the role of the nonstructural NS1 protein in the evasion of the host innate defense and its potential contribution to pandemic influenza. Proc Natl Acad Sci U S A. 2002; 99(16):10736–41.

31. Billharz R, Zeng H, Proll SC, Korth MJ, Lederer S, Albrecht R, et al. The NS1 protein of the 1918 pandemic influenza virus blocks host interferon and lipid metabolism pathways. J Virol. 2009;83(20):10557–70.

32. Meunier I, von Messling V. NS1-mediated delay of type I interferon induction contributes to influenza A virulence in ferrets. J Gen Virol. 2011;92(Pt 7):1635–44.

33. Reid AH, Janczewski TA, Lourens RM, Elliot AJ, Daniels RS, Berry CL, et al. 1918 influenza pandemic caused by highly conserved viruses with two receptor-binding variants. Emerg Infect Dis. 2003;9(10):1249–53.

34. Glaser L, Stevens J, Zamarin D, Wilson IA, Garcia-Sastre A, Tumpey TM, et al. A single amino acid substitution in 1918 influenza virus hemagglutinin changes receptor binding specificity. J Virol. 2005;79(17):11533–6.

35. Stevens J, Blixt O, Glaser L, Taubenberger JK, Palese P, Paulson JC, et al. Glycan microarray analysis of the hemagglutinins from modern and pandemic influenza viruses reveals different receptor specificities. J Mol Biol. 2006;355(5):1143–55.

36. Srinivasan A, Viswanathan K, Raman R, Chandrasekaran A, Raguram S, Tumpey TM, et al. Quantitative biochemical rationale for differences in transmissibility of 1918 pandemic influenza A viruses. Proc Natl Acad Sci U S A. 2008;105(8):2800–5.

37. Gamblin SJ, Haire LF, Russell RJ, Stevens DJ, Xiao B, Ha Y, et al. The structure and receptor binding properties of the 1918 influenza hemagglutinin. Science. 2004;303(5665):1838–42.

38. Stevens J, Corper AL, Basler CF, Taubenberger JK, Palese P, Wilson IA. Structure of the uncleaved human H1 hemagglutinin from the extinct 1918 influenza virus. Science. 2004;303(5665):1866–70.

39. Van Hoeven N, Pappas C, Belser JA, Maines TR, Zeng H, Garcia-Sastre A, et al. Human HA and polymerase subunit PB2 proteins confer transmission of an avian influenza virus through the air. Proc Natl Acad Sci U S A. 2009;106(9):3366–71.

40. Hatta M, Gao P, Halfmann P, Kawaoka Y. Molecular basis for high virulence of Hong Kong H5N1 influenza A viruses. Science. 2001;293(5536):1840–2.

41. Jackson D, Hossain MJ, Hickman D, Perez DR, Lamb RA. A new influenza virus virulence determinant: the NS1 protein four C-terminal residues modulate pathogenicity. Proc Natl Acad Sci U S A. 2008;105(11):4381–6.

42. Chen W, Calvo PA, Malide D, Gibbs J, Schubert U, Bacik I, et al. A novel influenza A virus mitochondrial protein that induces cell death. Nat Med. 2001;7(12):1306–12.

43. Zamarin D, Ortigoza MB, Palese P. Influenza A virus PB1-F2 protein contributes to viral pathogenesis in mice. J Virol. 2006;80(16):7976–83.

44. Zamarin D, Garcia-Sastre A, Xiao X, Wang R, Palese P. Influenza virus PB1-F2 protein induces cell death through mitochondrial ANT3 and VDAC1. PLoS Pathog. 2005;1(1):e4.

45. McAuley JL, Hornung F, Boyd KL, Smith AM, McKeon R, Bennink J, et al. Expression of the 1918 influenza A virus PB1-F2 enhances the pathogenesis of viral and secondary bacterial pneumonia. Cell Host Microbe. 2007;2(4):240–9.

46. Conenello GM, Zamarin D, Perrone LA, Tumpey T, Palese P. A single mutation in the PB1-F2 of H5N1 (HK/97) and 1918 influenza A viruses contributes to increased virulence. PLoS Pathog. 2007;3(10):1414–21.

47. Conenello GM, Tisoncik JR, Rosenzweig E, Varga ZT, Palese P, Katze MG. A single N66S mutation in the PB1-F2 protein of influenza A virus increases virulence by inhibiting the early interferon response in vivo. J Virol. 2011;85(2):652–62.

48. Takahashi T, Kurebayashi Y, Ikeya K, Mizuno T, Fukushima K, Kawamoto H, et al. The low-pH stability discovered in neuraminidase of 1918 pandemic influenza A virus enhances virus replication. PLoS ONE. 2010;5(12):e15556.

49. Treanor JJ, Campbell JD, Zangwill KM, Rowe T, Wolff M. Safety and immunogenicity of an inactivated subvirion influenza A (H5N1) vaccine. N Engl J Med. 2006;354(13):1343–51.

50. Bresson JL, Perronne C, Launay O, Gerdil C, Saville M, Wood J, et al. Safety and immunogenicity of an inactivated split-virion influenza A/Vietnam/1194/2004 (H5N1) vaccine: phase I randomised trial. Lancet. 2006;367(9523):1657–64.

10

Pathogenesis

Hans Dieter Klenk, Wolfgang Garten, and Mikhail Matrosovich

Institut für Virologie, Philipps-Universität, Marburg, Germany

Introduction

Many species are susceptible to natural and experimental influenza virus infection, and there are wide variations in disease depending on the virus and the host. Conclusions from studies obtained in a given animal may not apply to other species and are therefore to be generalized only with caution. Remarkably, however, important determinants of pathogenesis resemble each other in different hosts. It is also evident that some of the mechanisms underlying pathogenicity determine host range and transmissibility.

Pathogenesis is the result of a complex interplay between virus and host at the systemic, the cellular, and the molecular level, and it involves the interaction of all viral proteins with many host factors. In this chapter we first highlight the major disease symptoms of influenza virus infection in mammalian and avian hosts and the key mechanisms at the systemic and the cellular level. We then focus in more detail on the viral proteins that are the major determinants of pathogenicity and some of their cellular interaction partners.[1] Our understanding of these interactions is far from complete, but it is to be expected that with the elucidation of the host cell proteome and of the structures of all viral proteins we will learn more about them in the not too distant future.

[1]Whenever possible we will limit references to reviews and to articles that contain extensive citations.

Disease in mammalian and avian hosts

Mammalian influenza

Human influenza is a highly contagious disease that is transmitted by the airborne route. Virus replication normally reaches its peak 2–3 days after infection. The period of virus shedding is 5–7 days and may last as long as 2 weeks in infants and children. After an incubation time of 1–5 days, patients develop acute respiratory disease symptoms with headache, high fever, myalgia, nausea, and malaise. Severe cases are typically associated with primary influenza pneumonia or combined viral–bacterial pneumonia. Persons usually at risk for complications during a seasonal epidemic are the elderly and patients with cardiovascular diseases, metabolic disorders, or immunosuppression. In contrast, in some pandemics, notably those of 1918 and 2009, severe cases were observed predominantly in younger age groups without an underlying disease. Less frequent complications are myositis, myocarditis, and Reye's syndrome, a severe disease with brain and liver involvement and usually lethal outcome.

Human influenza viruses typically replicate in the epithelia of the conducting airways. They contain a diverse population of cell types that vary depending on the region of the airways (nose, trachea, bronchi) [1]. The two major cell types exposed on the surface of these epithelia are ciliated cells and nonciliated secretory cells.

Textbook of Influenza, Second Edition. Edited by Robert G. Webster, Arnold S. Monto, Thomas J. Braciale, and Robert A. Lamb.
© 2013 John Wiley & Sons, Ltd. Published 2013 by John Wiley & Sons, Ltd.

The secretory cells together with the cells of subepithelial glands produce mucins and other biologically active molecules which are incorporated in the airway surface liquid and mucous blanket. Ciliar beating moves the blanket up and out of the airways towards the pharynx where mucus is swallowed together with trapped foreign particles and microorganisms.

The main complication of human influenza is extension of the infection to the alveoli (often with secondary bacterial infection) resulting in pneumonia. The alveolar epithelium consists of type I and II pneumocytes [1]. The type I cells are very flat cells that constitute about 40% of the alveolar lining cells but occupy 90% of the alveolar surface. They form the structure of the alveolar wall and function as barrier between air space and blood. Type II pneumocytes cover approximately 5% of the alveolar surface. They resorb fluid from the alveolar lumen and produce lung surfactant which is important for reducing alveolar surface tension. They also serve as reserve cells which mature into type I cells in response to alveolar damage. Alveolar macrophages, terminally differentiated cells of the myeloid lineage, are also present in the alveolar space; they have an important role in clearing exogenous and endogenous particles and debris. Damage to the alveolar epithelium impairs the gas exchange function of the lung and causes severe, occasionally fatal, respiratory dysfunction [2].

The respiratory tract is the primary target of infection not only with human, but also with mammalian influenza viruses in general. Influenza in pigs is characterized by tracheobronchitis and bronchointerstitial pneumonia which is associated with fever, dry cough, and nasal discharge. Morbidity is high, but mortality is usually low. The clinical and pathophysiologic symptoms of equine influenza are similar (see Chapters 12 and 13).

Avian influenza

Avian influenza is quite different from human influenza and there are wide variations in the pathogenetic properties of avian influenza viruses in different bird species [3]. Based on the pathobiologic properties in poultry, avian influenza viruses are categorized as low pathogenic (LPAI) or highly pathogenic (HPAI) viruses. LPAI viruses cause asymptomatic infections in wild aquatic birds. When introduced into domestic poultry, infections may also be asymptomatic or associated with mild disease. LPAI viruses are shed in the feces. A common route of dissemination among aquatic birds is therefore through contaminated water. HPAI viruses which occur primarily in gallinaceous species are also shed in feces with high concentrations. However, these viruses are more readily transmitted among birds in densely populated flocks by the nasal and oral routes through contact with virus-contaminated materials. In contrast to the local LPAI virus infection of the intestinal or respiratory tract, HPAI viruses cause systemic infection. As a result, virus can be recovered from many organs of infected animals. Large hemorrhages distributed all over the body, edema, and cutaneous ischemia are major symptoms of the disease. The final stage of the infection can be characterized by the emergence of neurologic signs, such as photophobia and dullness. HPAI viruses have been found to specifically target lymphocytes and lymphoid tissues, myocytes in the heart muscle, and endothelial cells, and tropism to these cells may have an important pathogenic role in systemic virus dissemination and in the vascular leakage underlying hemorrhages and edema. HPAI virus infection has rarely been observed in domestic water fowl or wild birds in the past. However, over the last decades H5N1 viruses have evolved with the unique capacity to infect such birds with a wide spectrum of disease symptoms ranging from asymptomatic local infection to severe systemic spread and death as seen in poultry.

Avian influenza virus infections in mammalian host

LPAI viruses of subtypes H7N2, H7N3, H7N7, and H9N2 may infect humans with, generally, mild disease symptoms (for references see [4]). However, we are currently witnessing an outbreak of human pneumonia with a high case-fatality rate caused by a LPAI virus of subtype H7N9. HPAI viruses of serotypes H7 and H5 have also been transmitted to humans, and the H5N1 infections, in particular, occur with severe disease and high lethality. The primary targets in the lung are alveolar epithelial cells and alveolar macrophages. Occasionally, dissemination to other organs, such as the central nervous system and the gastrointestinal tract, has been observed. When compared with seasonal human influenza viruses, human H5N1 infections are characterized by high levels of cytokines and chemokines, which may contribute to the severity of the disease [4].

H5N1 viruses cause also severe disease in many nonhuman mammalian hosts. The primary target is also the lung, but spread to other organs is common, including brain, liver, heart, kidney, spleen, intestine, pancreas, and adrenal gland. LPAI viruses of many subtypes may infect pigs and other non-human mammals with severity of disease varying over a wide range (reviewed by [5]).

Pathogenic mechanisms

Tropism

Cell and tissue tropism that targets the virus to the respiratory tract or, in the case of avian viruses, to the intestinal tract, is a key determinant of pathogenicity. Evidence is increasing that the tropism of influenza viruses within the human respiratory tract has a major impact on the outcome of infection. The crucial role of the receptor specificity of hemagglutinin (HA) has been well established [6], but it is reasonable to assume that many other interactions between viral proteins and host factors contribute not only to species specificity, but also to cell and tissue tropism.

Spread of infection

Proteolytic activation of HA is the prime factor that determines whether infection is confined to a specific organ or whether it is disseminated throughout the organism [7,8]. Other factors regulating spread of infection are virus release from infected cells by neuraminidase (NA), the functional balance between HA and NA (see below), and the site of virus budding on polarized cells.

Virus load

An important parameter for the severity of disease is the virus load. It depends to a large extent on the replication efficiency of the viral polymerase (see below), but other factors, such as the number of infected cells and NA-mediated virus release, may also contribute.

Escape of host defense

Evasion of the immune response is not only crucial for the emergence of new virus variants and, thus, for the epidemiology of human influenza, but it also promotes the development of disease in the infected individual. Influenza viruses have developed different strategies to accomplish this involving different virus genes. Escape of adaptive immunity is based on antigenic shift and drift of the surface glycoproteins (see Chapter 18), whereas the NS1 protein has a particularly important role in pathogenesis by antagonizing innate immune responses (see Chapter 17).

Modulation of inflammatory response

Influenza viruses induce inflammation and cytokine release to various extents in infected tissues [9]. Because the inflammatory response causes virus clearance, but also tissue destruction, it may have enhancing or mitigating effects on pathogenesis. There is evidence that these effects differ depending on the virus, but the mechanisms responsible for these variations are not understood yet.

Synergism between influenza viruses and bacteria

It has long been known that coinfection with *Streptococcus pneumoniae*, *Haemophilus influenzae* and other bacteria significantly contributes to the severity of disease caused by influenza viruses. In fact, bacterial coinfection is believed to have played a critical part during the 1918 pandemic [10].

Damage of virus-infected cells allowing bacterial invasion of the respiratory epithelium has often been proposed as an explanation for the synergism. An enhanced susceptibility to bacterial super-infections may also result from the ability of the virus to impair functions of neutrophils which are essential for containment of bacteria. Deactivation of neutrophils does not require internalization of virus particles and is mediated by the HA-dependent polyvalent virus binding to the sialic acid-containing receptors on the surface of neutrophils (for references, see [11]). The viral NA activity can also have a role in promoting bacterial coinfections by desialylating the surface of airway epithelium and exposing cryptic oligosaccharide receptors used by bacteria for adhesion [12]. Furthermore, it has been suggested that the capacity of influenza viruses to promote bacterial coinfection is linked to the proinflammatory motif of PB1-F2.

Whereas in all of these instances viral infection has paved the way for bacterial infections, there is also evidence for bacterial support of virus replication. Thus, it has been shown that various bacteria, including *Staphylococcus aureus*, secrete proteases that activate HAs at monobasic cleavage sites and promote the development of pneumonia in mice after combined viral–bacterial infection [13].

Hemagglutinin determines tropism and spread of infection

HA initiates infection by binding to cell receptors and by inducing membrane fusion. The receptor specificity of HA is an important determinant not only of host range and transmissibility, but also of pathogenicity. Fusion activity depends on proteolytic cleavage of HA, and cleavage activation has a prime role in virus pathogenicity.

Receptor specificity

The receptor determinant of influenza viruses is sialic acid, mostly *N*-acetyl-neuraminic acid (Neu5Ac). In natural glycoconjugates, sialic acids are α2-3- or α2-6-linked to galactose (Gal), α2-6-linked to *N*-acetyl-glucosamine (GlcNAc) and *N*-acetyl-galactosamine (GalNAc), and α2-8-linked to the second Neu5Ac residue. Influenza viruses generally do not bind to α2-8-linked Neu5Ac moieties and can recognize only α2-3- or α2-6-linked sialic acid epitopes (Neu5Acα2-3/6Gal and Neu5Acα2-6GalNAc/GlcNAc) (for references see [6]). There are differences in the receptor-binding specificity of human and avian influenza viruses (for references see Chapter 8). Human influenza viruses preferentially bind to sialic acid with an α2-6-linkage (Neu5Acα2-6Gal). This preference correlates with abundant expression of Neu5Acα2-6Gal moieties on epithelial cells in the human trachea. In contrast, avian influenza viruses preferentially recognize the Neu5Acα2-3Gal motif that is matched by Neu5Acα2-3Gal sequences on epithelial cells in the intestinal tract of waterfowl. The receptor-binding specificity of human and avian influenza viruses suggests that avian influenza viruses need to acquire the ability to recognize human-type receptors to cause a pandemic. Thus, the receptor specificity of HA is a determinant of host range.

There is increasing evidence that receptor specificity also has an important role in pathogenesis.

Studies on human and avian virus infection in differentiated cultures of human airway epithelial cells (HAE) indicated that some cells in the human airway epithelium express sufficient amounts of receptors to allow infection with avian viruses and that receptor specificity determines the viral cell tropism in the epithelium. Early in infection of HAE cultures, human viruses preferentially infect nonciliated cells containing Neu5Acα2-6Gal receptors, whereas avian viruses mainly infect ciliated cells displaying Neu5Acα2-3Gal receptors (Figure 10.1) (for references see [6]).

More recently, analyses of sialic acid expression in fixed histologic sections of human lung tissues using linkage-specific lectins indicated that the concentrations of Neu5Acα2-6Gal and Neu5Acα2-3Gal motifs vary depending on the region of the respiratory tract. Whereas nasal and tracheobronchial epithelial cells mainly express 6-linked sialic acids, there is a decrease of these receptors and a concomitant increase of Neu5Acα2-3Gal receptors in the lower respiratory tract with about equal amounts of both receptor types in the bronchiolar and alveolar tissues [14].

Abundant expression of Neu5Acα2-6Gal and paucity of Neu5Acα2-3Gal moieties in human nasal and tracheobronchial cells seems to be one of the critical factors preventing human-to-human transmission of avian influenza viruses, as efficient replication of the virus in these tissues is required for its efficient airborne transmission via sneezing and coughing. However, the presence of avian-type receptors in the terminal bronchioles and alveoli will allow replication of the avian viruses deep in the lung and, thus, increase their pathogenicity in humans. Although formal proof for this theory is still missing, it is supported by indirect experimental evidence. For example HPAI H5N1 viruses with Neu5Acα2-3Gal receptor specificity efficiently bind to human alveolar epithelial cells and macrophages in *in vitro* binding assays [15] and they cause severe pneumonia with viral replication in pneumocytes and diffuse alveolar damage in humans.

Furthermore, enhanced binding to Neu5Acα2-3Gal receptors resulting from a D222G mutation in the hemagglutinin has been observed with virus isolates obtained from severe cases during the H1N1 2009 pandemic (for references see [16]). The same mutation was also found in fatal cases from the 1918 influenza pandemic. Taken together, these observations indicate that the receptor specificity of the

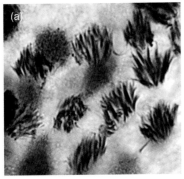
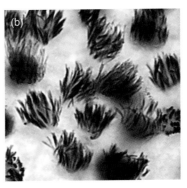
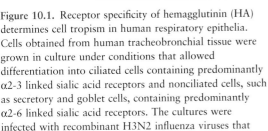

Figure 10.1. Receptor specificity of hemagglutinin (HA) determines cell tropism in human respiratory epithelia. Cells obtained from human tracheobronchial tissue were grown in culture under conditions that allowed differentiation into ciliated cells containing predominantly α2-3 linked sialic acid receptors and nonciliated cells, such as secretory and goblet cells, containing predominantly α2-6 linked sialic acid receptors. The cultures were infected with recombinant H3N2 influenza viruses that differed only by two amino acids in the receptor-binding site of HA resulting in specificity for either α2-3 linked or α2-6 linked sialic acid receptors [60]. The cultures were fixed 7h post infection and double-immunostained for virus antigen (brown) and cilia of ciliated cells (gray). The results show that the virus with specificity for α2-6 linked receptors infects predominantly nonciliated cells (a), whereas the virus with α2-3 specificity infects ciliated cells (b).

hemagglutinin is an important pathogenicity determinant of influenza viruses in humans.

Although most avian viruses recognize terminal 2-3-linked sialylgalactosyl moieties they vary in their specificity for the next sugar residues of the receptor [6]. For example, duck viruses preferentially bind to type I and III sequences (Neu5Ac2-3Gal1-3GalNac/GlcNAc) and do not tolerate the presence of a fucose (Fuc) substituent. The typical feature of H5 and H7 viruses adapted to gallinaceous land-based birds (chicken, quail, turkey) is strong virus binding to sulfated and fucosylated type II sequences, such as Neu5Acα2-3Galβ1-4(Fucα1-3)(6-O-HS0$_3$)GlcNAc (Su–SLe^x). These sequences are expressed on endothelial cells and leukocytes in mammals, with their levels increasing significantly during inflammation. Interestingly, HPAI viruses have a strong tropism to endothelia in chicken embryos [17] and to primary human pulmonary microvascular endothelial cells [18]. The distinctive receptor-mediated endotheliotropism may very likely be an important determinant for the systemic infection in birds [8,17] and for the severe lesions in the human lung caused by these viruses.

Fusion activation

Cleavage of HA is necessary for fusion activity and therefore for the infectivity of the virus. The cleavage site is located in a circular loop projecting away from the surface of the precursor HA0 (see Chapter 5). The activating enzymes are provided by the host. Proteolytic activation of HA is a prime determinant of pathogenicity, in particular with avian influenza viruses that display large variations in cleavability [19,20].

HA of mammalian influenza viruses and of LPAI viruses is activated at a monobasic cleavage site by proteases that are present only in respiratory or intestinal epithelia. Infection is therefore restricted to these organs (Figure 10.2). Initially, trypsin and a number of trypsin-like proteases, such as plasmin, blood clotting factor Xa, and tryptase Clara have been found to activate HA with a monobasic cleavage site *in vitro* (for references see [7,8]). However, it is unlikely that they activate these viruses in their natural setting. More recently, the serine proteases HAT, TMPRSS2 [21], and TMPRSS4 [22] from

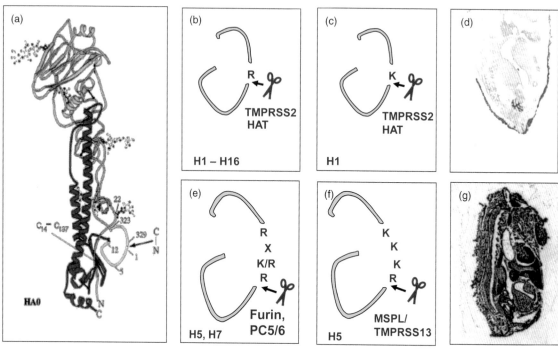

Figure 10.2. Proteolytic activation of HA determines spread of infection. The precursor HA0 is cleaved at a loop containing the cleavage site (yellow) into fragments HA1 (blue) and HA2 (red) (for details and references see Chapter 5) (a). LPAI and mammalian viruses have a monobasic cleavage site which is usually arginine (b), or in a few cases lysine (c). Viruses with a monobasic cleavage site are activated in the human respiratory tract by proteases TMPRSS2 and HAT (b, c). Infection with LPAI viruses is localized in the cloaca and the chorioallantoic membrane of chicken embryos (d). HPAI viruses are activated at multibasic cleavage sites by furin and PC5/PC6 (e), or in a few cases by MSPL/TMPRSS13 (f). Since these proteases are ubiquitous, HPAI viruses cause systemic infection in chicken embryos (g). Viral mRNA was detected by *in-situ* hybridization in chicken embryos infected with LPAI virus A/chick/Germany/N/49 (H10N7) (d) and HPAI virus A/FPV/Rostock/34 (H7N1) (g) Adapted from Garten and Klenk [7] with permission of S. Karger AG; for further references see text.

human airway epithelium have been found to activate human influenza A viruses as well as LPAI viruses. Interestingly, these enzymes are membrane-bound by an amino-terminal hydrophobic anchor (type I membrane proteins). TMPRSS2 is localized on intracellular membranes and activates newly synthesized HA during exocytosis, whereas HAT activates budding virus as well as incoming virus at the plasma membrane (Figure 10.3) [23]. These enzymes are autocatalytically activated and they are normally responsible for regulation of sodium homeostasis and other physiologic functions of the epithelia. Bacterial proteases may also activate HAs of restricted cleavability and promote the development of pneumonia in mice after combined viral–bacterial infection [13].

HPAI viruses are activated by a different cleavage mechanism. Their HAs are activated at multibasic cleavage sites by furin, a member of the proprotein convertase family of eukaryotic subtilisin-like serine endoproteases. The ubiquity of this enzyme accounts for the systemic infection typical for these viruses (Figure 10.2). Furin is a type I membrane protein of the constitutive secretory pathway. It is partially released at the plasma membrane as soluble enzyme and partially retrieved into the trans-Golgi network where it accumulates and colocalizes with HA.

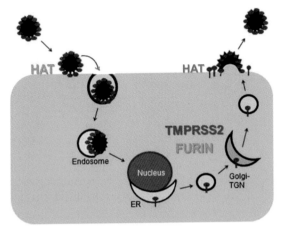

Figure 10.3. Cellular compartmentation of HA activating proteases. HA is activated by host proteases that have different substrate specificities and are located in different compartments of the cell. Furin activates newly synthesized HAs with multibasic cleavage sites when passing through the trans-Golgi network (TGN). HAs with monobasic cleavage sites are activated either during exocytosis by TMPRSS2 also located in the TGN or on virus budding from the plasma membrane by HAT. Virus particles containing uncleaved HA can also be activated by HAT when entering cells.

Furin has a broad substrate spectrum of biologically important proteins, including nerve growth factor, insulin receptor, anthrax and shigella toxins, and many others [7]. There are other proprotein convertases that resemble furin in structure and substrate specificity. One of them, PC5/6, also activates HAs with multibasic cleavage sites. The HAs of most HPAI viruses have the consensus sequences R-X-K/R-R or R-X-X-R at the cleavage site, motifs that are both recognized by furin. Among the few exceptions to these rules are HAs that contain the unusual tetrapeptide K-K-K-R. These HAs are cleaved by the serine protease TMPRSS13 (for references see [16]).

A multibasic cleavage site is not the only requirement for high cleavability. Another important determinant is a carbohydrate side-chain close to the cleavage site that interferes with protease accessibility. Loss of this carbohydrate resulted in enhanced HA cleavability and pathogenicity. However, masking of the cleavage site by this oligosaccharide was also overcome when the number of basic amino acids was increased (for references see [7]). Taken together, these observations indicate that the high cleavability of the HPAI virus HA depends on the multibasic amino acid motif, an extended cleavage site loop, and the absence of a masking carbohydrate.

HPAI viruses are derived from LPAI viruses by acquisition of a multibasic cleavage site (Table 10.1). This has first been observed in laboratory studies involving sequential cell culture passages of strains A/seal/Massachusetts/1/80 (H7N7) and A/turkey/Oregon/71 (H7N3). In the latter case, the acquisition of the furin recognition motif resulted from recombination of the HA gene with 28S ribosomal RNA. The HA gene may not only recombine with cellular RNA, but also with other viral gene segments, as has been observed when new HPAI viruses emerging in the field have been analyzed. Thus, comparison of A/chicken/Chile/02 (H7N3) isolates revealed that the HA genes of the highly pathogenic strains had an insertion of 30 nucleotides at the cleavage site which was presumably derived from the nucleoprotein gene of the unrelated A/gull/Maryland/704/77 (H13N6) virus. Recombination between HA and matrix protein genes of the same virus generated the highly pathogenic A/chicken/BC/04 (H7N3) viruses. Polymerase slippage has been suggested as an alternative strategy by which a multibasic cleavage site is generated. However, there are other examples where the mechanism of insertion is not understood (for references see [7]).

It is also not clear why the acquisition of a multibasic cleavage site and therefore the generation of HPAI viruses occur in nature apparently only with subtypes H5 and H7. High cleavability was observed when multibasic cleavage sites have been inserted into HAs of other subtypes by recombinant DNA technology [24], and some viruses containing such HAs were highly pathogenic for chickens [25]. Thus, it appears that confinement of naturally occurring HPAI viruses to subtypes H5 and H7 cannot be attributed to structural restrictions of the HA protein, but that the constraints are more likely at the RNA level.

There is evidence that proteolytic activation of HA has also a pathogenetic function with mammalian viruses, but here this role is not as clear as it is with avian viruses. Thus, equine H7N7 viruses have an HA with a multibasic cleavage site, yet do not differ significantly in their relatively moderate pathogenicity

Table 10.1. HPAI viruses are derived from LPAI viruses by acquisition of a multibasic HA cleavage site. Cleavage sites of pairs of LPAI and HPAI viruses are shown that have been isolated during the same outbreak or have been obtained *in vitro* by serial cell culture passage in the absence of trypsin. Sequence comparison reveals insertions which enlarge the loop at the cleavage site and generate multibasic motifs recognized by furin and PC6 (for references see [7,16]).

Virus isolates	Pathogenicity	Cleavage site	
		HA1	HA2
Turkey/Ore/71 (H7N3)	Low	PENPKT——————————R↓GLF	
Turkey/Ore/TC1 (H7N3)	High	PENPKTSLSPLYPGRTTDLHVRTAR↓GLF	
Chicken/Chi/176822/02 (H7N3)	Low	PEKPKT——————————R↓GLF	
Chicken/Chi/4957/02 (H7N3)	High	PEKPKT——————CSPLSRCRKTR↓GLF	
Chicken/CN/6/04 (H7N3)	Low	PENPKT——————————R↓GLF	
Chicken/BC/NS1337-1/04 (H7N3)	High	PENPKQ——————AYQKRMTR↓GLF	
Chicken/Mex/31381-7/94 (H5N2)	Low	PQPET——————————R↓GLF	
Chicken/Que/4588-19/95 (H5N2)	High	PQ——————————RKPKTR↓GLF	
Turkey/Ita/99 (H7N1)	Low	PEIPKG——————————R↓GLF	
Turkey/Ita/99 (H7N1)	High	PEIPKG——————————SRVRR↓GLF	
Seal/Mass/1/80 (H7N7)	Low	PENPKT——————————R↓GLF	
Seal/Mass/SC32 (H7N7)	High	PENPKT——————————RGRR↓GLF	

from equine H3N8 viruses displaying a monobasic cleavage site (see Chapter 13). It has been reported that HA of the 1918 H1N1 pandemic virus, although lacking a multibasic cleavage site, displays high cleavability and this feature may contribute to the pathogenicity of the virus. It has also been speculated that NA may be involved in cleavage, but the precise activation mechanisms is not clear [26]. H5N1 infection studies demonstrated that the multibasic cleavage site is a virulence factor of this virus in mammals, but that its contribution to pathogenicity varied with different animal species, underscoring the role of host genetic differences in the susceptibility of mammals to H5N1 infections [27].

In contrast to natural evolution where HPAI viruses generally appear to be derived from LPAI viruses, recombinant viruses with reduced pathogenicity can be generated by *in vitro* mutation at the cleavage site. Thus, replacement of the multibasic cleavage site of a highly pathogenic H5N1 virus by a single arginine resulted in an attenuated virus that can be used for mass production of an inactivated pandemic vaccine. Protease activation mutants that are cleaved by elastase, an activating enzyme not occurring in a natural setting, are even less pathogenic and have the potential to be used as live vaccines (for references see [7]).

Several protease inhibitors have been developed that interfere with HA activation and virus replication [23,28]. Because these compounds target cellular enzymes they will not elicit the generation of drug-resistant viruses. This should be a major advantage when compared with conventional influenza antivirals, such as neuraminidase inhibitors.

Pathogenicity is a multifactorial trait: receptor specificity, N-glycosylation and fusion activity of HA determine lung pathogenicity in mice

Experimental infection of mice is a common model for studying influenza virus pathogenicity. Nonadapted viruses usually produce asymptomatic infection in mice, although they can replicate in the respiratory tract with high titers. Serial passage results in the selection of adaptive mutants which can cause lethal viral pneumonia resembling severe human infection. Extensive genetic and phenotypic analyses of mouse-adapted human viruses indicated that three characteristics of HA are critical for the high virulence in the mouse lung.

One of these features is receptor specificity. Mice mainly express Neu5Acα2-3Gal receptors in all regions of the respiratory tract. Therefore, adaptation of human influenza viruses to mice typically results in the acquisition/enhancement of Neu5Acα2-3Gal binding. By contrast, mouse adaptation of avian viruses can occur without significant changes in receptor specificity.

Another common type of mouse-adaptation mutations is the loss of N-linked high-mannose glycans from the globular heads of HA and NA (for references see [29]). These glycans mediate binding of surfactant protein D (SP-D) and mannose-binding lectin (MBL), collagenous Ca^{2+}-dependent multimeric lectins (collectins) present in respiratory secretions and blood, respectively. SP-D and MBL neutralize the virus by several mechanisms, including steric hindrance of the receptor-binding site of HA, inhibition of the enzymatic activity of NA, aggregation of virions, and activation of complement-dependent pathways. Virus variants with reduced HA glycosylation obtained by mouse passages or generated by reverse genetics were less sensitive to inhibition by collectins *in vitro* and more virulent in mice than their fully glycosylated counterparts. Furthermore, the HAs of the influenza viruses that caused the pandemics in 1918, 1957, 1968, and 2009 had only a few N-glycosylation sites on the globular head, which is a typical feature of HA of avian and avian-origin swine viruses. HA glycosylation of these viruses increased during post-pandemic circulation in humans resulting in more collectin binding sites. Consequently, recombinant influenza viruses with the HAs of pandemic viruses showed lower binding to SP-D and significantly higher pathogenicity for mice than isogenic viruses with the HA of seasonal human viruses [30]. These findings indicate that reduced glycosylation and increased resistance to collectins might contribute to enhanced pathogenicity of pandemic and zoonotic influenza viruses in humans.

Finally, there is evidence that HA stability has an important role in pneumotropism and, thus, in the pathogenicity for mice. Membrane fusion involves an irreversible conformational transition of HA that depends on pH and temperature (see Chapter 5). To prevent premature inactivation of HA and to ensure efficient fusion a pH optimum and an optimal transition temperature are critical for infectivity. It is therefore reasonable to assume that pH and temperature optima differ with viruses targeting the upper and the lower respiratory tract. This concept is supported by the observation that pneumotropic mouse viruses that were derived from human viruses replicating predominantly in the upper airways displayed adaptive mutations in HA2 that decreased the pH optimum substantially [31].

Interestingly, transmissibility of influenza viruses appears to be determined by similar factors. Studies in which H5N1 viruses have been adapted to ferrets demonstrated that mutational changes in receptor specificity, glycosylation, and stability of HA resulted in a virus that could infect the animals through the air [32,33].

Neuraminidase promotes virus release and destroys decoy receptors

The major function of NA is mitigation of unfavorable interactions of HA with receptors. At the early stages of infection NA destroys decoy receptors on mucins, cilia, and cellular glycocalix that interfere with virus access to functional receptors on the plasma membrane of target cells. At the late stages of the viral life cycle, NA removes sialic acids from virus progeny and infected cells and thus prevents virus aggregation and promotes its detachment and spread (for references see [34]). Because HA and NA have opposite activities, a balance between their interactions with sialic acid-containing receptors and inhibitors in host target tissues is essential for efficient virus replication. This balance can be disturbed by various mechanisms, such as reassortment, virus transmission to a new host, antigenic drift, and therapeutic inhibition of NA. The resulting decrease in the viral fitness is usually overcome by restoration of the functional balance owing to compensatory mutations in HA, NA, or both proteins. Thus, the ability of NA to ensure efficient viral growth in host tissues has an important role in pathogenesis.

Polymerase determines replication rates

To mediate replication and transcription of the viral genome, the polymerase has to enter the nucleus of the host cell. The efficiency of the polymerase depends therefore at least in part on its ability to cross the nuclear envelope. There is now increasing evidence that this barrier has not only an important role in host restriction, but that it also modulates pathogenicity and transmissibility of the virus.

The structure of the viral polymerase complex is still poorly understood, but there has been remarkable progress in the structural elucidation of its individual subunits as reviewed in Chapter 8 of this book and elsewhere [35]. To summarize these data briefly, large parts of PA – the amino terminal domain (aa 1–197) and the carboxy-terminal domain (aa257–716) – have been crystallized. The carboxy-terminal domain of PA contains the PB1 binding site, whereas the amino-terminal domain is the cap-snatching endonuclease. The PB2 domains with known structure include an amino-terminal peptide (aa 1–35) that interacts with the carboxy-terminal end of PB1, the cap-binding domain (aa 320–483), a domain involved in host interaction carrying the adaptive mutation site 627 (aa 538–678), followed by the carboxy-terminal NLS domain (aa 678–759) that contains the classic bipartite nuclear localization sequence R736-K-R-X_{12}-K-R-I-R755. PB1, the central scaffold for trimer assembly, is the RNA-dependent RNA polymerase. Short amino-terminal (aa 1–15) and carboxy-terminal (aa 685–757) sequences interacting with PA and PB2, respectively, are the only parts of PB1 currently known at atomic resolution.

Specific mutations in the polymerase subunits, particularly in PB2, are involved in the adaptation of avian viruses to mammalian hosts. Some of these adaptive mutations, which have been found to enhance polymerase activity and replication rates in mammalian cells, are also responsible for increased pathogenicity in the new host (for references see [36]). The most prominent of these mutation sites is located at position 627 of PB2 which is usually glutamic acid in avian and lysine in mammalian strains. Being first

recognized as a determinant of host range [37], it was later identified as a major pathogenicity determinant of HPAI viruses in mammalian hosts [38]. When an avian influenza virus infects a mouse or a human the E627K mutation occurs very rapidly. Thus, the mammalian signature has been found in numerous human H5N1 isolates [39]. Another important determinant of host range and pathogenicity is amino acid 701 of PB2 which is aspartic acid with avian and asparagine with mammalian viruses. There is evidence that mutations D701N and E627K promote airborne transmission in guinea pigs and that 701N can compensate for the lack of 627K. Another compensatory mutation has been observed in PB2 of the 2009 pandemic H1N1 virus, where the exchange Q591R accounts for the absence of 627K (for references see [16]).

Adaptive mutations in viral proteins are expected to optimize interactions with host-specific proteins or to adjust to other physiologic constraints, that is to the low temperature in the mammalian upper respiratory tract as suggested for PB2 mutation E627K [36]. Recently, several studies have employed gene silencing techniques in search of host factors involved in influenza virus replication [40,41]. Each of these studies has identified numerous such factors including proteins mediating nuclear-cytoplasmic transport. The underlying molecular mechanisms are still poorly understood, except for the interaction of PB2 with importin α, a component of the classic nuclear import pathway acting as an adaptor that recognizes cargo proteins with a nuclear localization signal. Mutation D701N observed after mouse adaptation of an avian influenza virus enhanced binding of PB2 to importin α in mammalian cells. Likewise, importin α binding of NP was enhanced by mutation N319K in this protein [42]. These observations were in agreement with another study showing that mutation D701N facilitates exposure of the nuclear localization signal at the carboxy-terminus of PB2 [43]. Facilitated recruitment by importin α resulted in increased nuclear transport of PB2 and NP and enhanced transcription and replication activities in mammalian cells [42]. Furthermore, there is a switch in the specificity for importin α isoforms upon interspecies transmission. PB2 and NP of avian viruses prefer importin α3, whereas importin α7 preference is observed with mammalian viruses [44]. The mechanism by which E627K exerts its effect on pathogenicity is less well understood. There is evidence that it also depends on interaction with importin α, yet in a mode not involving nuclear transport [45].

NS1 modulates host responses

As reviewed in Chapter 7 of this volume and elsewhere [46], NS1 is a multifunctional protein with a high degree of structural variability. It modulates different steps in the viral life cycle, such as viral RNA replication and viral protein synthesis. Furthermore, and above all, it inhibits the innate immune response of the host by blocking retinoic acid-inducible gene I (RIG-I)-mediated interferon production as well as the synthesis and the antiviral effects of interferon-stimulated proteins, such as double-stranded RNA (dsRNA)-dependent protein kinase R (PKR), 2'5'-oligoadenylate synthetase (OAS), and the Mx proteins. By all of these regulatory mechanisms NS1 can also affect pathogenesis.

Modulation of the IFN response

The N-terminal part of NS1 comprising amino acids 1–73 encompasses the RNA-binding domain. Alanine substitution of basic amino acids at positions 38 and 41 believed to be involved in RNA binding and, thus, in the inhibition of the RIG-I-signaling pathway resulted in increased interferon production and virus attenuation indicating that interferon antagonism and pathogenicity depend on the RNA-binding capacity of NS1. Interestingly, pathogenicity can also be modulated in a manner not dependent on RNA binding when an adjacent amino acid is mutated (for references see [46]). Taken together, these observations indicate that the N-terminal domain has an important role in the interferon antagonism of NS1 and, thus, in pathogenicity, and that this function depends, at least partly, on its RNA binding ability.

The effector domain (amino acid 74 to the C-terminus) of NS1 also interferes with the interferon response. This domain binds and sequesters CPSF30, a cellular protein that is required for the processing of mRNA, including interferon mRNA. The CPSF30 binding site of NS1 displays a motif with a consensus sequence at amino acids 103 and 106, and mutations at these positions have been shown to alter pathogenicity [47]. CPSF30 binding has also been modulated by other mutations in the effector domain,

and these mutations affect pathogenicity, too. The C-terminal end has been implicated to enhance the interferon antagonistic properties by stabilizing the dimeric structure of NS1, another prerequisite for RNA binding. Consequently, C-terminal truncation of NS1 resulted in attenuation of influenza viruses [46].

NS1 may also interfere by other mechanisms with the innate immune response. Hypercytokinemia is a typical feature of fatal human infections with highly pathogenic avian H5N1 viruses [39], and it has been shown that NS1 of these viruses induces high levels of proinflammatory cytokines and complete resistance to the antiviral effects of interferon [46]. The overproduction of proinflammatory cytokines appears to be paralleled by a concomitant decrease of anti-inflammatory cytokines, such as interleukin-10 (IL-10) [48]. Similarly, an imbalanced innate immune response has been observed after infection with the 1918 influenza virus [9]. Thus, atypical modulation of the host immune response by NS1 may be a feature shared by highly pathogenic influenza viruses. However, there is also evidence that excessive viral replication rates may outrun a timely antiviral host response [49]. Thus, the high pathogenicity of these viruses may not only result from specific NS1 properties, but may also reflect the fact that they take advantage of the lag phase between the onset of infection and the induction of the antiviral defense system.

Modulation of signaling cascades

Carbohydrate receptors at the cell surface and HA activating proteases are not the only host factors utilized by influenza viruses. In fact, they take advantage of many signaling pathways of the cell to optimize their replication and thereby often redirect or alter these regulatory systems.

Many proteins involved in signaling cascades communicate via PDZ domains. These domains specifically recognize and bind to short C-terminal peptide motifs of 4–5 amino acids, the PDZ domain ligands (PL). The NS1 proteins of avian influenza viruses have a PL with the sequence ESEV or EPEV at positions 227–230 [50]. These authors also showed that NS1 of avian viruses as well as that of the 1918 virus that has an avian-like PL motif, too, are able to bind to up to 30 human PDZ domain-containing proteins, whereas this was not the case with human

NS1 proteins in which the PL sequence was RSKV. The introduction of avian or 1918 PL sequences into the NS1 protein of WSN virus increased pathogenicity in mice as indicated by a loss of body weight, severe alveolitis, and reduced survival [51]. The specific signaling cascades targeted and disrupted by these NS1 proteins and their role in pathogenesis still have to be identified. However, it appears that viral proteins with PL motifs commonly target cellular proteins controlling tight junction formation, cell polarity, and apoptosis, and that the perturbation of such functions is a strategy used by viruses to enhance replication, dissemination within, and transmission between hosts [52].

Modulation of apoptosis

Many types of cells infected with influenza viruses have been found to undergo apoptosis, a form of programmed cell death. Two main apoptotic pathways have been observed: the extrinsic pathway mediated by transmembrane receptors of the TNF receptor superfamily that bind TNFα, TRAIL, and FasL as major ligands; and the intrinsic pathway involving mitochondria and non-receptor-mediated stimuli (for references see [53]). When cells were infected with an attenuated virus lacking NS1, activation by caspases, central components of the apoptotic machinery, and other parameters of apoptosis were enhanced as compared with wild-type virus [54]. However, NS1 expressed from a vector in the absence of the other viral proteins was found to enhance apoptosis [55]. Thus, it appears that NS1 has proapoptotic and antiapoptotic properties, and there is evidence that NS1 exerts its antiapoptotic effects early and its proapoptotic effects late in infection.

NS1 is involved in several mechanisms that might explain its antiapoptotic properties. Thus, NS1 activates the phosphatidylinositol-3-kinase (PI3K) pathway which inhibits proapoptotic factors, such as caspases 3 and 9. Furthermore, the NS1 proteins of the 1918 virus and of avian viruses carry an SH3 domain binding motif at positions 212–216 that interacts with CRK and CRKL adaptor proteins. This interaction may competitively limit apoptotic responses triggered by mitogenic activated protein kinases (MAPK) which also bind to CRK. The serine/threonine kinase PKR that activates the extrinsic apoptosis pathway is also a binding partner of NS1 [53].

Thus, suppression of PKR by NS1 also reduces programmed cell death in influenza virus infected cells.

Taken together, it appears that, in the course of infection, NS1 regulates apoptosis in opposite directions. Reduced apoptosis early in infection would promote genome replication and synthesis of viral proteins, while enhanced apoptosis late in the replication cycle may increase release of progeny virus and promote clearance of cells that can no longer be used for virus growth.

PB1-F2 and PA-X – other modulators of host responses

There is increasing evidence that PB1-F2, an accessory protein encoded by the second viral RNA segment, also has an important role in pathogenesis. PB1-F2 has been shown to interact in vitro with mitochondrial proteins and induce apoptosis through permeabilization of the mitochondrial outer membrane and release of mediator proteins [56]. It also affects polymerase activity and replication efficiency with some strains. In vivo studies have revealed an immunomodulatory function of PB1-F2 exerted either by enhancing inflammatory responses [57] or by interferon antagonism [53]. The viruses causing the pandemics of 1918 (H1N1), 1957 (H2N2), and 1968 (H3N2) as well as the highly pathogenic avian H5N1 strains contain PB1-F2 proteins that enhance lung inflammation via an elevation of cytokines in bronchoalveolar lavage fluid and a significant influx of neutrophils and macrophages, and the enhanced inflammatory responses contributed also to the morbidity and pathogenicity of these viruses in mice. With the pandemic H3N2 virus the proinflammatory activity appears to be mediated by four specific amino acids in PB1-F2, and this motif is also responsible for an enhanced susceptibility to bacterial coinfection. Seasonal strains derived from the pandemic viruses lost the proinflammatory potential as a result of PB1-F2 truncations in the H1 lineage or mutations in the H3 lineage [58]. Thus, it appears that loss of the proinflammatory potential of PB1-F2 contributes to the relatively diminished frequency of severe infections in post-pandemic periods.

Very recently, another accessory influenza A protein termed PA-X has been discovered. PA-X is a fusion protein comprising the N-terminal endonuclease domain of the PA protein and a short C-terminal domain encoded by an overlapping open reading frame in segment 3 of the viral genome that is accessed by ribosomal frame shifting. By virtue of its endonuclease activity PA-X is believed to be involved in the shut-off of host gene expression, and there is evidence from studies in a mouse model that PA-X decreases pathogenicity by controlling the kinetics of inflammatory, apoptotic, and T-lymphocyte signaling pathways. These observations support the notion that immunopathology has an important role in influenza virus infection [59].

Acknowledgments

We thank Sabine Fischbach for expert secretarial help. We acknowledge recent financial support of our own work by the Deutsche Forschungsgemeinschaft (SFB 593), the Bundesministerium fuer Bildung und Forschung (FluResearchNet), the von Behring-Roentgen-Stiftung, the LOEWE Program of the State of Hessen (Universities of Giessen and Marburg Lung Center), the Wellcome Trust grant WT085572MF, and the European Commission FP7 projects FLUPOL, FLUPHARM, FLUPIG and PREDEMICS.

References

1. Tomashefski JF, Farver CF. Anatomy and histology of the lung. In: Tomashefski JF, editor. Dail and Hammar's Pulmonary Pathology, 3rd ed. New York: Springer; 2008. p. 20–48.
2. Kuiken T, Taubenberger JK. Pathology of human influenza revisited. Vaccine. 2008;26(Suppl. 4):D59–66.
3. Pantin-Jackwood MJ, Swayne DE. Pathogenesis and pathobiology of avian influenza virus infection in birds. Rev Sci Tech. 2009;28:113–36.
4. Peiris M. Avian influenza viruses in humans. Rev Sci Tech. 2009;28:161–73.
5. Reperant LA, Rimmelzwaan GF, Kuiken T. Avian influenza viruses in mammals. Rev Sci Tech. 2009;28: 137–59.
6. Matrosovich MN, Gambaryan AS, Klenk HD. Receptor specificity of influenza viruses and its alteration during interspecies transmission. In: Klenk HD, Matrosovich M, Stech J, editors. Avian Influenza. Basel: Karger; 2008. p. 134–55.
7. Garten W, Klenk HD. Cleavage activation of the influenza virus hemagglutinin and its role in pathogenesis.
8. Steinhauer DA. Role of hemagglutinin cleavage for the pathogenicity of influenza virus. Virology. 1999;258: 1–20.
9. Kash JC, Tumpey TM, Proll SC, Carter V, Perwitasari O, Thomas MJ, et al. Genomic analysis of increased host immune and cell death responses induced by 1918 influenza virus. Nature. 2006;443:578–81.
10. Morens DM, Taubenberger JK, Fauci AS. Predominant role of bacterial pneumonia as a cause of death in pandemic influenza: implications for pandemic influenza preparedness. J Infect Dis. 2008;198:962–70.
11. Matrosovich MN, Klenk HD, Kawaoka Y. Receptor specificity, host range and pathogenicity of influenza viruses. In: Kawaoka Y, editor. Influenza Virology: Current Topics. Wymondham, England: Caister Academic Press; 2006. p. 95–137.
12. McCullers JA. Insights into the interaction between influenza virus and pneumococcus. Clin Microbiol Rev. 2006;19:571–82.
13. Tashiro M, Ciborowski P, Klenk HD, Pulverer G, Rott R. Role of Staphylococcus protease in the development of influenza pneumonia. Nature. 1987;325:536–7.
14. Shinya K, Ebina M, Yamada S, Ono M, Kasai N, Kawaoka Y. Avian flu: influenza virus receptors in the human airway. Nature. 2006;440:435–6.
15. van Riel D, Munster VJ, de Wit E, Rimmelzwaan GF, Fouchier RA, Osterhaus AD, et al. Human and avian influenza viruses target different cells in the lower respiratory tract of humans and other mammals. Am J Pathol. 2007;171:1215–23.
16. Klenk HD, Garten W, Matrosovich M. Molecular mechanisms of interspecies transmission and pathogenicity of influenza viruses: lessons from the 2009 pandemic. Bioessays. 2011;33:180–8.
17. Klenk HD. Infection of the endothelium by influenza viruses. Thromb Haemost. 2005;94:262–5.
18. Ocana-Macchi M, Bel M, Guzylack-Piriou L, Ruggli N, Liniger M, McCullough KC, et al. Hemagglutinin-dependent tropism of H5N1 avian influenza virus for human endothelial cells. J Virol. 2009;83:12947–55.
19. Horimoto T, Kawaoka Y. Reverse genetics provides direct evidence for a correlation of hemagglutinin cleavability and virulence of an avian influenza A virus. J Virol. 1994;68:3120–8.
20. Klenk HD, Rott R. The molecular biology of influenza virus pathogenicity. Adv Virus Res. 1988;34:247–81.
21. Boettcher E, Matrosovich T, Beyerle M, Klenk HD, Garten W, Matrosovich M. Proteolytic activation of influenza viruses by serine proteases TMPRSS2 and HAT from human airway epithelium. J Virol. 2006;80: 9896–8.

22. Bertram S, Glowacka I, Steffen I, Kuhl A, Pohlmann S. Novel insights into proteolytic cleavage of influenza virus hemagglutinin. Rev Med Virol. 2010;20: 298–310.

23. Boettcher-Friebertshäuser E, Freuer C, Sieloff F, Eickmann M, Uhlendorff J, Steinmetzer T, et al. Cleavage of influenza virus hemagglutinin by airway proteases TMPRSS2 and HAT differs in subcellular localization and susceptibility to protease inhibitors. J Virol. 2010; 84:5605–14.

24. Ohuchi R, Ohuchi M, Garten W, Klenk HD. Human influenza virus hemagglutinin with high sensitivity to proteolytic activation. J Virol. 1991;65:3530–7.

25. Veits J, Weber S, Stech O, Breithaupt A, Graber M, Gohrbandt S, et al. Avian influenza virus hemagglutinins H2, H4, H8, and H14 support a highly pathogenic phenotype. Proc Natl Acad Sci U S A. 2012;109: 2579–84.

26. Tumpey TM, Basler CF, Aguilar PV, Zeng H, Solorzano A, Swayne DE, et al. Characterization of the reconstructed 1918 Spanish influenza pandemic virus. Science. 2005;310:77–80.

27. Suguitan AL Jr, Matsuoka Y, Lau YF, Santos CP, Vogel L, Cheng LI, et al. The multibasic cleavage site of the hemagglutinin of highly pathogenic A/Vietnam/ 1203/2004 (H5N1) avian influenza virus acts as a virulence factor in a host-specific manner in mammals. J Virol. 2012;86:2706–14.

28. Zhirnov OP, Klenk HD, Wright PF. Aprotinin and similar protease inhibitors as drugs against influenza. Antiviral Res. 2011;92:27–36.

29. Ward AC. Virulence of influenza A virus for mouse lung. Virus Genes. 1997;14:187–94.

30. Qi L, Kash JC, Dugan VG, Jagger BW, Lau YF, Sheng ZM, et al. The ability of pandemic influenza virus hemagglutinins to induce lower respiratory pathology is associated with decreased surfactant protein D binding. Virology. 2011;412:426–34.

31. Ping J, Keleta L, Forbes NE, Dankar S, Stecho W, Tyler S, et al. Genomic and protein structural maps of adaptive evolution of human influenza A virus to increased virulence in the mouse. PLoS ONE. 2011;6:e21740.

32. Herfst S, Schrauwen EJ, Linster M, Chutinimitkul S, de Wit E, Munster VJ, et al. Airborne transmission of influenza A/H5N1 virus between ferrets. Science. 2012; 336:1534–41.

33. Imai M, Watanabe T, Hatta M, Das SC, Ozawa M, Shinya K, et al. Experimental adaptation of an influenza H5 HA confers respiratory droplet transmission to a reassortant H5 HA/H1N1 virus in ferrets. Nature. 2012;486:420–8.

34. Wagner R, Matrosovich M, Klenk HD. Functional balance between haemagglutinin and neuraminidase in influenza virus infections. Rev Med Virol. 2002;12:159–66.

35. Boivin S, Cusack S, Ruigrok RW, Hart DJ. Influenza A virus polymerase: structural insights into replication and host adaptation mechanisms. J Biol Chem. 2010;285:28411–7.

36. Naffakh N, Tomoiu A, Rameix-Welti MA, van der Werf S. Host restriction of avian influenza viruses at the level of the ribonucleoproteins. Annu Rev Microbiol. 2008; 62:403–24.

37. Subbarao EK, London W, Murphy BR. A single amino acid in the PB2 gene of influenza A virus is a determinant of host range. J Virol. 1993;67:1761–4.

38. Hatta M, Gao P, Halfmann P, Kawaoka Y. Molecular basis for high virulence of Hong Kong H5N1 influenza A viruses. Science. 2001;293:1840–2.

39. de Jong MD, Simmons CP, Thanh TT, Hien VM, Smith GJ, Chau TN, et al. Fatal outcome of human influenza A (H5N1) is associated with high viral load and hypercytokinemia. Nat Med. 2006;12:1203–7.

40. Karlas A, Machuy N, Shin Y, Pleissner KP, Artarini A, Heuer D, et al. Genome-wide RNAi screen identifies human host factors crucial for influenza virus replication. Nature. 2010;463:818–22.

41. Koenig R, Stertz S, Zhou Y, Inoue A, Hoffmann HH, Bhattacharyya S, et al. Human host factors required for influenza virus replication. Nature. 2010;463:813–7.

42. Gabriel G, Herwig A, Klenk HD. Interaction of polymerase subunit PB2 and NP with importin alpha1 is a determinant of host range of influenza A virus. PLoS Pathog. 2008;4:e11.

43. Tarendeau F, Boudet J, Guilligay D, Mas PJ, Bougault CM, Boulo S, et al. Structure and nuclear import function of the C-terminal domain of influenza virus polymerase PB2 subunit. Nat Struct Mol Biol. 2007;14:229–33.

44. Gabriel G, Klingel K, Otte A, Thiele S, Hudjetz B, Arman-Kalcek G, et al. Differential use of importin-alpha isoforms governs cell tropism and host adaptation of influenza virus. Nat Commun. 2011;2:156.

45. Resa-Infante P, Jorba N, Zamarreno N, Fernandez Y, Juarez S, Ortin J. The host-dependent interaction of alpha-importins with influenza PB2 polymerase subunit is required for virus RNA replication. PLoS ONE. 2008;3:e3904.

46. Hale BG, Randall RE, Ortin J, Jackson D. The multifunctional NS1 protein of influenza A viruses. J Gen Virol. 2008;89:2359–76.

47. Spesock A, Malur M, Hossain MJ, Chen LM, Njaa BL, Davis CT, et al. The virulence of 1997 H5N1 influenza viruses in the mouse model is increased by correcting a defect in their NS1 proteins. J Virol. 2011;85: 7048–58.

48. Lipatov AS, Webby RJ, Govorkova EA, Krauss S, Webster RG. Efficacy of H5 influenza vaccines produced by reverse genetics in a lethal mouse model. J Infect Dis. 2005;191:1216–20.

49. Haller O, Kochs G, Staeheli P. Influenza a virus virulence and innate immunity: recent insights from new mouse models. In: Klenk HD, Matrosovich MN, Stech J, editors. Avian Influenza. Basel: Karger; 2008. p. 195–209.

50. Obenauer JC, Denson J, Mehta PK, Su X, Mukatira S, Finkelstein DB, et al. Large-scale sequence analysis of avian influenza isolates. Science. 2006;311:1576–80.

51. Jackson D, Hossain MJ, Hickman D, Perez DR, Lamb RA. A new influenza virus virulence determinant: the NS1 protein four C-terminal residues modulate pathogenicity. Proc Natl Acad Sci U S A. 2008;105: 4381–6.

52. Javier RT, Rice AP. Emerging theme: cellular PDZ proteins as common targets of pathogenic viruses. J Virol. 2011;85:11544–56.

53. Herold S, Ludwig S, Pleschka S, Wolff T. Apoptosis signaling in influenza virus propagation, innate host defense, and lung injury. J Leukoc Biol. 2012;92:75–82. doi: 10.1189/jlb.1011530.

54. Zhirnov OP, Konakova TE, Wolff T, Klenk HD. NS1 protein of influenza A virus down-regulates apoptosis. J Virol. 2002;76:1617–25.

55. Schultz-Cherry S, Dybdahl-Sissoko N, Neumann G, Kawaoka Y, Hinshaw VS. Influenza virus NS1 protein induces apoptosis in cultured cells. J Virol. 2001;75: 7875–81.

56. Chen W, Calvo PA, Malide D, Gibbs J, Schubert U, Bacik I, et al. A novel influenza A virus mitochondrial protein that induces cell death. Nat Med. 2001;7: 1306–12.

57. McAuley JL, Hornung F, Boyd KL, Smith AM, McKeon R, Bennink J, et al. Expression of the 1918 influenza A virus PB1-F2 enhances the pathogenesis of viral and secondary bacterial pneumonia. Cell Host Microbe. 2007;2:240–9.

58. McAuley JL, Chipuk JE, Boyd KL, Van De Velde N, Green DR, McCullers JA. PB1-F2 proteins from H5N1 and 20 century pandemic influenza viruses cause immunopathology. PLoS Pathog. 2010;6:e1001014.

59. Jagger BW, Wise HM, Kash JC, Walters KA, Wills NM, Xiao YL, et al. An overlapping protein-coding region in influenza A virus segment 3 modulates the host response. Science. 2012;337:199–204.

60. Matrosovich M, Matrosovich T, Uhlendorff J, Garten W, Klenk HD. Avian-virus-like receptor specificity of the hemagglutinin impedes influenza virus replication in cultures of human airway epithelium. Virology. 2007; 361:384–90.

PART 3

Evolution and ecology of influenza viruses

Section Editor: Robert G. Webster

Ecology and evolution of influenza viruses in wild and domestic birds

Ron A.M. Fouchier[1] and Yi Guan[2]

[1]Department of Viroscience, Erasmus MC, Rotterdam, The Netherlands
[2]Center of Influenza Research, School of Public Health, University of Hong Kong, Hong Kong, China

Introduction

Recognition of the influenza ecosystem

Influenza has been recognized as a disease of humans for many centuries. Fowl plague, now referred to as highly pathogenic avian influenza (HPAI), was one of the first diseases known to be caused by a virus. That these apparently distinct diseases share a common cause was only recognized in 1955. However, the first influenza virus was isolated neither from humans nor birds but from pigs. In the early 1930s, Richard Shope published a series of manuscripts describing the isolation and characterization of swine influenza viruses. A few years later, the first human influenza virus was isolated. The realization that the progenitors of all these animal and human viruses were circulating in wild bird populations did not occur until the 1990s.

Aquatic birds as the natural reservoir of influenza A viruses

Influenza A viruses are classified on the basis of two glycoproteins, hemagglutinin (HA) and neuraminidase (NA), expressed on the surface of the virus particles [1]. In wild birds and poultry throughout the world, influenza A viruses representing 16 HA and 9 NA antigenic subtypes have been detected [2] and can be found in numerous combinations, which are referred to as virus subtypes (e.g., H1N1, H16N3). The seventeenth subtype of HA and tenth subtype of NA, reported in 2012, are the only subtypes not yet detected in wild birds [3]. Influenza viruses can infect and cause disease in a wide range of host species, including humans, pigs, horses, mink, dogs, cats, and marine mammals, yet avian species were the original hosts of all these mammalian influenza A viruses (Figure 11.1).

Interspecies transmission of avian influenza viruses

All influenza A viruses in terrestrial poultry and mammals were directly or indirectly derived from viruses originally resident in aquatic birds [1]. Generally, interspecies transmission occurs more frequently from aquatic birds to terrestrial poultry than from birds to mammals. However, results from recent surveillance studies suggest that introductions of avian influenza viruses to mammals are not rare events. Since the HPAI Asian H5N1 and low pathogenic avian influenza (LPAI) H9N2 virus lineages became endemic in many countries in Asia and Africa, sporadic human infections by these avian viruses have occurred. Avian-origin H1N1 and H3N8 lineages have been established in European pigs since 1979 and in horses since 1963, respectively. Phylogenetic

Textbook of Influenza, Second Edition. Edited by Robert G. Webster, Arnold S. Monto, Thomas J. Braciale, and Robert A. Lamb.
© 2013 John Wiley & Sons, Ltd. Published 2013 by John Wiley & Sons, Ltd.

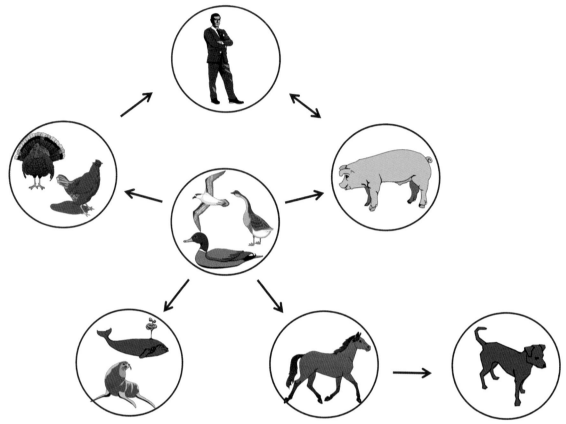

Figure 11.1. The main hosts of influenza A virus, with wild aquatic birds as the natural viral reservoir.

analyses revealed that all the human pandemic influenza viruses of the twentieth century had gene segments of contemporary avian origin when they emerged, suggesting that interspecies transmission of avian influenza viruses was directly involved in the genesis of human pandemic viruses.

Natural reservoirs

Recognition of influenza viruses in wild birds worldwide

The earliest influenza surveillance studies in wild birds used classic methods in virology, such as isolating virus from embryonated chicken eggs inoculated with fecal samples or cloacal swabs. Those landmark studies of wild ducks and shorebirds in North America were the first to reveal the high prevalence of avian influenza viruses in species such as mallards and turnstones [4–6]. Since then, it has been recognized that many wild bird species may harbor influenza viruses. Birds of wetlands and aquatic environments, such as the Anseriformes (particularly ducks, geese, and swans) and Charadriiformes (particularly gulls, terns, and waders), which are distributed globally, except for the most arid regions, constitute the major natural LPAI virus reservoir species [1,7].

The implementation of high-throughput molecular diagnostic methods around the end of the twentieth century has allowed the intensity of surveillance studies to increase substantially [8], making avian influenza viruses one of the most extensively studied wildlife disease agents at the beginning of the twenty-first century. LPAI viruses have now been isolated from well over 100 wild bird species [7]. Despite their prevalence in the bird reservoir and poultry, relatively few influenza virus subtypes have been detected in mammalian species.

Wild birds: anseriformes

Numerous surveillance studies of wild ducks in the Northern Hemisphere have revealed a high prevalence of LPAI viruses, primarily in juvenile birds, with a peak in early fall prior to and at the start of southbound migration. In North America, virus prevalence has been estimated to be ~60% in ducks sampled at marshalling sites close to the Canadian breeding areas in early fall, 0.4–2% at the wintering grounds in the southern United States, and ~0.25% during spring migration [1]. Similar patterns have been observed in northern Europe. However, virus prevalence during the spring migration of up to 6.5% has been reported in Europe [9]. Surveillance of the nesting grounds of ducks in Alaska and Siberia before winter migration revealed the presence of LPAI viruses in 2.5–8% of birds. These patterns of prevalence raise the possibility that LPAI viruses can persist in ducks all year and that high virus prevalence is driven by young individuals when they congregate in large numbers. However, this does not exclude the possibility that additional host species or preservation of infectious influenza viruses in frozen lakes over the winter have important roles in the perpetuation of avian influenza viruses.

Subtypes H1–H16 of HA and N1–N9 of NA have been detected in LPAI viruses in ducks, although some subtypes are detected more frequently than others (e.g., H3, H4, and H6 versus H2 or H9) and H13 and H16 seem mainly restricted to gulls. The general prevalence of influenza viruses and the specific distribution of subtypes vary among different surveillance studies depending on species, time, and place. In long-term studies in Canada, cyclic patterns of influenza virus subtypes were reported, with peaks in virus isolation of an HA subtype followed 1–2 years later by reduced rates of isolation of this subtype [6]. This observation is of particular interest but awaits confirmation in other long-term surveillance studies.

Dabbling ducks of the Anas genus, with mallards (Anas platyrhynchos) being the most extensively studied species, appear to be infected with influenza viruses more frequently than are other birds [6,7,9]. Dabbling ducks feed primarily on surface waters and may switch breeding grounds between years (abmigration), partially because of mate choice. This behavior could provide an opportunity for LPAI viruses to be transmitted between different host subpopulations. Consecutive or simultaneous infections with different subtypes of influenza A viruses are common in dabbling ducks, suggesting that only partial homo- and heterosubtypic immunity is induced by infection of the birds with an influenza A virus [10].

Experimental infection studies to assess the influence of prior infection with influenza A virus on reinfections showed that although mallards were reinfected with influenza A viruses, the duration of virus shedding was markedly reduced upon reinfection. This reduction was most pronounced when subsequent infection occurred with a virus of the same HA subtype. The duration of infection was estimated from field studies to be approximately 10 days [10], which is in agreement with the shedding duration of 7–17 days observed in experimental infections [11,12]. The transient nature of these infections and the relatively short shedding time suggest that the spatial dynamics of influenza A viruses are mainly explained by circulation within bird flocks or by relay transmission between staging areas where the birds congregate.

Until recently, the prevalence of LPAI viruses in wild ducks in the Southern Hemisphere and potential transmission between the hemispheres were largely unknown. There is little connectivity between northern and southern Anatidae species, and most species stay all year on each breeding continent. Anatidae of Oceania are mainly resident and do not perform regular seasonal migrations. As a consequence, there appears to be sufficient geographic separation for the LPAI viruses of Oceania to form more or less distinct virus lineages [13]. Although surveillance data for South America and Africa are still limited, most data suggest that LPAI viruses of ducks in the northern and southern latitudes can be linked.

As opposed to the endemicity of avian influenza viruses in dabbling ducks, the prevalence of avian influenza viruses in other Anseriformes species suggests that avian influenza virus infections behave epidemically in those species. In geese and swans in northern Europe, avian influenza viruses are only detected after the arrival of the birds at their wintering grounds, where they come into contact with reservoir species such as the ubiquitous mallards [9]. This observation suggests that frequent spill-over from the endemic host (able to sustain long-term continuous circulation of the avian influenza virus) occurs to more transient hosts (able to sustain circulation of the influenza virus only for a limited period of time). Although variation in time and space may occur, the overall picture is that among the Anseriformes, virus prevalence in dabbling ducks is higher than that in other ducks, geese, and swans.

Wild birds: charadriiformes

The first recorded isolation of influenza virus from a wild bird was from a common tern (*Sterna hirundo*) in 1961 [14]. This HPAI H5N3 virus was responsible for an outbreak in South Africa during which at least 1300 of these birds died. This event remains unusual because this outbreak in wild birds could not be linked with outbreaks in poultry. The most frequently detected LPAI virus subtypes in gulls are H13 and H16, virus subtypes generally not found in Anseriformes [2,9]. The genes of gull H13 and H16 viruses are genetically distinct from those of influenza viruses from Anseriformes hosts, suggesting that gull H13 and H16 viruses have been separated for sufficient time to allow genetic differentiation [2]. This conclusion concurs with the observation that gull influenza viruses do not readily infect ducks upon experimental inoculation [1]. Although other influenza virus subtypes are also occasionally detected in terns and gulls [7], it is plausible that these viruses are not endemic in these birds, only in Anseriformes. A recent study in Argentina demonstrated the presence of an H13 LPAI virus in gulls in South America that was genetically distinct from viruses circulating in gulls elsewhere, potentially as the result of geographic isolation [15].

Influenza viruses can be detected in a small proportion of gulls, with the highest virus prevalence reported in late summer and early fall. Most gull species breed in colonies, with adults and juveniles crowded in a small space, creating good opportunities for virus spread. This situation contrasts with that in dabbling ducks, which do not breed in dense colonies, and epizootics could be more easily initiated when birds congregate in large numbers during molt, migration, or wintering.

Waders in the Charadriidae and Scolopacidae families are adapted to either marine or freshwater wetland areas and often live side-by-side with ducks. Long-term influenza virus surveillance studies are still sparse, but data from North America suggest a distinct role of these birds in the perpetuation of certain virus subtypes. Influenza viruses of subtypes H1–H12 have been isolated from birds migrating through the eastern United States, with higher prevalence rates of certain HA subtypes (H1, H3, H7, H9–H12) and a larger variety of HA–NA combinations than from ducks in Canada, suggesting that waders maintain a wider spectrum of viruses. Moreover, compared with the seasonal prevalence of influenza viruses in ducks, that in waders seems to be reversed, with higher virus prevalence rates (~14%) during spring migration [6]. This observation has led to the hypothesis that different families of wetland birds are involved in perpetuation of LPAI virus and suggests a role for waders, which may carry the virus north to the ducks' breeding grounds in spring.

However, genetic analyses have not revealed striking differences between influenza viruses from ducks and waders in the Americas, suggesting that these viral gene pools are not separated [16,17]. The results of a large multi-year surveillance study of Charadriiformes in the Americas [18] suggest that LPAI virus infections among shorebirds may be localized, species-specific, and highly variable with respect to virus subtypes. It is thus plausible that the Delaware Bay area, where many initial shorebird studies were performed, has provided data that may not be translated directly to shorebirds in other parts of the world; studies in waders elsewhere have produced results dissimilar to those of Delaware Bay. Because many wader species of the Northern Hemisphere are long-distance, intercontinental migrants, they have the potential to distribute LPAI viruses around the globe. Although it is clear that waders are permissive to LPAI viruses, to what extent they contribute to LPAI virus epidemiology remains less clear and requires further study.

Wild birds: other species

Avian influenza viruses infect many other bird species [7], but it is unclear whether the virus is endemic in these species or whether the virus is a transient pathogen. Species in which avian influenza viruses are endemic share the same habitat, at least part of the year, with species in which influenza viruses are detected occasionally. A comparative analysis of influenza wild bird surveillance data indicated that feeding in surface waters was an indicator of avian influenza prevalence [19]. In most bird species, influenza A virus prevalence is lower than that in dabbling ducks, but studies that sample throughout the full annual cycle are limited, and it is possible that peak prevalence has been missed because of its seasonal nature or location. In addition, avian influenza virus surveillance efforts have typically been focused on species that are easily caught or are present in accessible areas at high concentrations. Therefore, the current status of our knowledge may only partly reflect the true ecology of avian influenza viruses with respect to host reservoir species.

Perpetuation, replication, and transmission in the wild bird populations

In wild birds, LPAI viruses are thought to preferentially infect cells lining the intestinal tract [20]. As a result, virus can be excreted in high concentrations in bird feces. Influenza viruses can remain infectious in lake water for prolonged periods: up to 4 days at 22°C and more than 30 days at 0°C [20]. The relatively high virus prevalence in birds living in aquatic environments may, in part, be due to this relative stability in surface waters, facilitating efficient transmission via a fecal–oral route [1,5]. Preservation of LPAI virus viability in frozen surface waters has been suggested to contribute to LPAI virus epidemiology, by enabling the virus to infect birds after their return to the breeding grounds in spring. Whether and to what extent the conservation of LPAI viruses in frozen surface waters contributes to LPAI virus epidemiology still remain largely unknown.

Although it has long been known that significant LPAI virus replication can be observed in the respiratory tract of wild birds [11], this notion has received renewed attention due, in part, to studies on HPAI viruses. Although transmission via the fecal–oral route may be the primary mode of LPAI virus transmission in many bird species, transmission via respiratory secretions may also occur and may be relevant

for particular bird species, for instance, land-based birds. In addition, fecal–cloacal transmission (via "cloacal drinking") has been postulated to represent a third potential route of transmission. More studies are needed to identify the most efficient routes of transmission in different wild bird families.

In mallards, the frequency of avian influenza detection in cloacal samples is twice as high as that in oropharyngeal samples, and the amount of virus in cloacal samples is higher [8,21]. In contrast, in white-fronted geese (Anser albifrons albifrons) the detection frequency is higher in oropharyngeal samples than in cloacal samples, and a comparable amount of virus is shed via both routes [22]. Thus, the site of replication and route of transmission may be species-specific, and transmission via the respiratory route may be relevant for bird species in which fecal–oral transmission would prove difficult.

In general, avian influenza viruses replicate in birds without inducing apparent signs of disease [11,12,23]. In naturally infected mallards, pathologic consequences of avian influenza virus infection were found to be minimal [24]. A longitudinal study in migratory mallards in Sweden indicated that avian influenza virus infection may reduce the body mass of mallards [10]. It is unclear whether the low body mass of infected mallards is a direct effect of the infection or whether birds in poor physical condition are more susceptible to acquiring an infection [10]. A study on the effect of natural avian influenza virus infection on free-living Bewick's swans (Cygnus columbianus bewickii) showed that infected swans fuelled and fed at reduced rates, displayed delayed migration, and traveled shorter distances than did uninfected Bewick's swans [25]. Although the direct effect of LPAI virus infections on the health of wild birds is limited, such virus infections may have effects of ecologic significance.

Influenza in domestic birds

Recognition of influenza viruses in domestic birds worldwide

Most of the influenza activity recognized in domestic birds was associated with disease outbreaks of both high and low pathogenicity viruses. The H9, H6, and

H3 subtypes are commonly seen as low pathogenic viruses in terrestrial poultry, and some strains have become established and been prevalent over the long term in poultry. Only the H5 and H7 subtypes of influenza viruses have caused major highly pathogenic outbreaks in poultry. Field surveillance and laboratory animal studies suggest that all HPAI H5 or H7 viruses were derived from their LPAI counterpart strains in aquatic birds by a series of passages in poultry [26,27].

Surveillance in China of apparently healthy domestic ducks showed that they host most subtypes of influenza viruses (H1–H11 and N1–N9). The most frequent subtypes were H3, H4, and H6. Viruses could be detected year-round and even from the pool water where ducks were raised [28]. The distribution of subtypes has changed since 2003 when the Asian H5N1 HPAI viruses became endemic throughout south and east Asia, with about 30% of duck influenza viruses being of this subtype. This finding suggests that domestic ducks in China may have become the major reservoir host species for the H5N1 HPAI virus and the source of its endemicity.

Domestic geese also harbor most influenza virus subtypes, but isolation rates are much lower than those in domestic ducks, except for HPAI H5N1. The other, more frequent, subtypes were H3, H4, and H6. Domestic geese were the original species from which the Asian HPAI H5N1 virus was isolated.

Interaction between wild and domestic birds

Migratory ducks usually travel on pathways that include inland lakes (such as Poyang and Dongting lakes in China), where large numbers of domestic waterfowl are farmed along the shore. Consequently, the migrating birds will share the same water body as the domestic birds. Parallel surveillance of migratory ducks and neighboring (or sentinel) domestic ducks found similar viruses in both sets of birds, with isolation rates in sentinel domestic ducks being 5–10 times that of the migratory ducks [29]. This finding emphasizes the effect of population density on the prevalence of influenza viruses in the host. Similar findings were obtained from surveillance in South Korea.

Frequent transmissions of viruses between migratory and domestic ducks occur. Phylogenetic analyses show that most influenza viruses prevalent in migratory and domestic ducks are characteristic of the gene

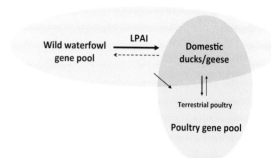

Figure 11.2. The interaction of the influenza virus gene pools in waterfowl (blue) and poultry (yellow). The H1–H16 and N1–N9 subtypes of avian influenza viruses are maintained in wild waterfowl and pass to domestic aquatic birds. Viruses in domestic aquatic birds become part of the poultry virus gene pool and circulate at much higher densities because of industrial farming practices. Transmission of viruses from these farmed birds, or wild birds, can then lead to the emergence and establishment of viruses in terrestrial poultry. Terrestrial poultry viruses transmit less frequently to domestic aquatic birds and their viruses may return to wild birds.

pool and match other viruses found in their migratory flyways or geographic regions. Thus, domestic ducks and geese also serve as natural reservoirs for the influenza virus and facilitate transmission to other domestic poultry (Figure 11.2). Whether distinct domestic avian virus lineages could be transmitted back to migratory birds is still controversial. However, the detection of Asian H5N1 HPAI viruses in many species of wild birds highlights the frequency of wild birds being exposed to viruses of domestic bird origin. The rapid expansion of the geographic distribution of H5N1 viruses gives further support to the hypothesis that virus transmission from domestic to migratory birds occurs [30].

Terrestrial poultry

Chickens are the most common domestic poultry species, and large farm populations are found worldwide. In some geographic regions, the H9N2 and H6 subtypes of influenza viruses have become established and prevalent [31,32]. Other subtypes have occasionally been isolated from chickens, but these have failed to become established or cause major outbreaks. The chicken is also the major poultry type that could facilitate the genesis of highly pathogenic H5 or H7 subtype viruses. Viruses of the H9N2 lineage in chickens have contributed to the multiple genetic reassortant variants of the Asian H5N1 lineage that have caused major outbreak and transmission waves in many countries [33].

Turkeys are intensively farmed in the United States and Europe, and influenza outbreaks have been observed since the early 1960s. This species appears to be one of the most permissive influenza host species. Most subtypes of viruses (H1–H11) have been isolated from it, although H5, H7, and H9 seem to be detected most frequently. Consistently, influenza outbreaks in turkeys were associated with farms situated on migratory waterfowl flyways until preventative measures were taken. H9N2 viruses were isolated from turkeys as early as 1966 in the United States but have become prevalent in Israel more recently. H7 outbreaks have occurred in the United States, with viruses isolated from 1971 to 2005, and a highly pathogenic H7N1 outbreak occurred in Italy in 1999. Turkeys are also sensitive to some mammalian-adapted viruses, such as the 2009 H1N1 pandemic virus.

Influenza activity has been detected in other terrestrial poultry species, such as quail, chukar, Guinea fowl, partridge, and pheasant (collectively called minor poultry). These birds have small population sizes in comparison to that of chickens, but with increased populations since the 1990s. The first influenza viruses isolated from diseased quail were H9N2 viruses in 1988 and 1992 in Hong Kong [33]. Surveillance in southern China revealed that G1-like H9N2 viruses and W312-like H6N1 viruses were prevalent over the long term in minor poultry. In laboratory experiments, quail and partridges appear to be permissive to most subtypes of aquatic bird influenza viruses [34]. Thus, quails have been proposed to act as a "mixing vessel" between aquatic and terrestrial birds to facilitate the genesis and emergence of the viruses prevalent in chickens.

Prevalence and perpetuation in poultry

Maintenance in domestic ducks and geese

The long history of farming vast numbers of domestic ducks and geese across China and South-East Asia has contributed to establishing an influenza gene pool. Influenza viruses can be isolated year round in domestic birds, with seasonal and spatial variations, and at higher rates than in migratory birds. Several ecologic factors favor the maintenance of influenza viruses in domestic birds. Ponds and rice fields become ideal places to spread viruses within and across the bird populations [28] as ducks and geese shed viruses into the water to form "virus soups." Many of the large duck farms in China are located on major lakes that are also aggregation sites for overwintering migratory birds. These large water bodies provide ample opportunities for virus exchange among ducks from different populations and between domestic and migratory birds. The extent of interchange between viruses of domestic and migratory aquatic birds is not yet known.

Current farming practices in China have shortened the development period of ducks to 45–60 days. Ducks could possibly shed influenza viruses for up to 22 days, a significant portion of their lifespan. As flock numbers are maintained, ducks of different age groups are always present in farms, creating an effectively unlimited pool of immunologically naïve hosts to allow these viruses to persist in the duck population. Almost every city and town in China and South-East Asia has live-poultry markets where domestic ducks and geese from different regions come into close contact and can spread viruses within markets and back to farms.

Establishment and development in terrestrial poultry

Influenza viruses in terrestrial poultry were initially introduced from migratory birds. Mixed species backyard poultry farms may be the infectious source for some Asian countries. However, the change to industrial scale, high-density terrestrial poultry farms has allowed LPAI viruses to become established in these birds. Only a few subtypes of LPAI viruses, such as H9N2 and H6N1, are known to persist over the long-term in terrestrial poultry. The H9N2 virus has established multiple lineages in chickens and minor poultry in Asia since the mid-1990s, coincident with the start of large-scale farming in these regions [33]. In Taiwan, a region with a relatively isolated influenza ecosystem and high-density poultry farming, an H6N1 virus has been prevalent in chickens for more than three decades [35]. The endemic H9N2 and H6N1 viruses in terrestrial poultry cause very limited disease symptoms. Co-circulation of two different subtypes of influenza viruses in the same species facilitates genetic reassortment events that generate novel variants, as observed with the H9N2 and H5N1 virus lineages in southern China.

After H9N2 and H6N1 viruses became established in terrestrial poultry, these viruses changed their replication site from the intestine to the trachea. Many more virus isolates were obtained from tracheal swabs and the birds' drinking water than from cloacal swabs. Virus transmission among the population occurred mainly through close contact or drinking water.

When H5 and H7 subtype viruses are introduced into terrestrial poultry, they may eventually evolve into HPAI viruses if they are prevalent in these poultry for some time. The HPAI H5 and H7 viruses have not become established in terrestrial poultry because their high pathogenicity either destroys the bird population or they are subject to control measures (see below). Improved techniques now make rapid diagnosis and early detection of virus introductions possible, allowing interventions to prevent further spread of the virus and to reduce the chance of viruses changing their pathogenicity. Such early detection and intervention may be the reasons that viruses have not become established in poultry in Western countries even though several disease outbreaks have occurred.

Genesis and development of highly pathogenic H5 and H7 influenza viruses

The HA protein of the influenza A virus is initially synthesized as a single polypeptide precursor (HA0) and then cleaved into HA1 and HA2 subunits by proteases. The cleaved protein mediates binding of the virus to host cells, followed by fusion with endosomal membranes [1]. Influenza viruses of subtypes H5 and H7, but not those of other HA subtypes, have become highly pathogenic following introduction in poultry and may cause outbreaks of HPAI. The switch from an LPAI virus phenotype, common in wild birds and poultry, to the HPAI virus phenotype is achieved by the introduction of basic amino acid residues into the HA0 cleavage site, which facilitates systemic virus replication. HPAI isolates have been obtained primarily from commercially raised poultry.

Since the 1990s, HPAI outbreaks have occurred frequently. Although most of these HPAI outbreaks were controlled relatively quickly, HPAI H5N1 viruses have continued to circulate in poultry in the Eastern Hemisphere since 1997. The introduction of HPAI H5N1 viruses to wild birds and the subsequent spread of the virus throughout Asia, the Middle East, Africa, and Europe has focused attention on the role of wild birds in the geographic spread of HPAI H5N1 viruses [36]. Large-scale, wild-bird surveillance programs were implemented in many parts of the world to determine the role of wild birds in the spread of HPAI H5N1 viruses and to serve as a sentinel system to detect the introduction of HPAI H5N1 viruses into new geographic areas.

HPAI H5N1 virus

H5N1 outbreaks in domestic birds

Unlike most HPAI outbreaks, which occur in chickens, the initial outbreak of the Asian H5N1 virus occurred in domestic geese in Guangdong, China in 1996. This HPAI H5N1 virus did not receive attention until one of its genetic variants, the HK/97-like virus, caused a major outbreak in live-poultry markets and 18 human infections, with six fatalities, in Hong Kong in 1997. This incident suggested that the HPAI H5N1 viruses could have pandemic potential, which made the world seriously consider pandemic preparedness plans and systematic influenza surveillance to monitor the activity and evolution of this virus.

After the Hong Kong "bird flu" incident, the HK/97-like H5N1 virus disappeared in the field although its primary precursor virus (Goose/GD-like) continued to circulate in geese, causing only limited clinical symptoms. In July 2000, the H5N1 virus was detected in domestic ducks in southern China, with novel reassortant H5N1 variants replacing the Goose/GD-like virus in the field by December 2000. These novel reassortant H5N1 variants caused the second major outbreak in poultry in Hong Kong. In 2002, further reassortant variants of H5N1 viruses caused a series of outbreaks in the poultry farms and markets of Hong Kong. H5N1 activity was detected throughout the year except for the summer months.

In late 2003 and early 2004, H5N1 genotype Z viruses spread to eight countries in East and South-

East Asia, causing the first H5N1 dissemination wave and more than 30 human infections. After this event, H5N1 viruses became endemic in the poultry of Vietnam and Indonesia. In April 2005, an HPAI H5N1 outbreak was observed at Qinghai Lake, China [30]. Subsequently, the virus was transmitted widely, forming the second dissemination wave (see below). This occurrence raised the possibility that the HPAI H5N1 virus might be being transmitted over long distances via bird migration.

Surveillance in poultry markets in several provinces of southern China since 2001 has revealed that the virus was present in apparently health birds, mainly domestic ducks and geese. In late 2005, H5N1 genotype V (Fujian-like, or clade 2.3.4) viruses became predominant and were transmitted to Vietnam and Malaysia in the third dissemination wave [37]. Since these events, the H5N1 virus has developed into a panzootic in poultry in the Eastern Hemisphere and persistently caused sporadic human infections in several countries. The development of the Asian H5N1 virus lineage is summarized in Figure 11.3.

H5N1 in wild birds

After the 1997 HPAI outbreak in Hong Kong, the H5N1 HPAI virus reappeared in 2002 in waterfowl at two parks in Hong Kong and was detected in other captive and wild birds. It resurfaced again in 2003 and has devastated the poultry industry in large parts of South-East Asia since 2004. In 2005, the first reported outbreak in wild migratory birds occurred in April–June at Qinghai Lake, China. This HPAI H5N1 virus outbreak in wild birds affected large numbers of birds such as bar-headed geese (*Anser indicus*) and brown-headed gulls (*Larus brunnicephallus*) [30]. After the HPAI H5N1 virus outbreak in wild birds, the virus rapidly spread westwards across Asia, Europe, the Middle East, and Africa. Several countries have reported finding infected wild birds, predominantly mute swans (*Cygnus olor*), whooper swans (*Cygnus cygnus*), and tufted ducks (*Aythya fuligula*), although small numbers of cases in other species (raptors, gulls, and herons) have been reported as well [7].

Although numerous wild birds have become infected, whether they have an active role in the geographic spread of the disease has been much debated. It has been argued that infected birds would be too severely affected to continue migration and thus would be unlikely to spread the H5N1 virus. Although this may be true for some wild birds, several bird species survive experimental infections and shed the H5N1 virus without apparent disease signs [38,39]. In addition, wild birds may be partially immune owing to previous exposures to LPAI influenza viruses. Finally, several studies suggest that HPAI viruses may become less pathogenic to ducks upon experimental infection while retaining high pathogenicity for chickens [38–40]. Outbreaks in Europe, where infected wild birds were found in countries that did not experience outbreaks among poultry, indicate that wild birds can indeed carry the virus to previously unaffected areas.

Despite intensive surveillance programs, HPAI H5N1 viruses have predominantly been found in dead wild birds. Only in limited cases were HPAI H5N1 viruses detected in apparently healthy birds. This observation raises the question of whether these infections have indeed become endemic in wild bird populations or whether the HPAI H5N1 virus is being reintroduced repeatedly by poultry or human activities. Recent studies reported a high prevalence of HPAI H5N1 in China, suggesting that HPAI H5N1 circulates endemically there.

H5N1 in mammals

The HPAI H5N1 viruses originally caused sporadic human infections during the Hong Kong "bird flu" incident. Since their dissemination, sporadic infections in mammalian hosts have occurred. Occasional infections have been observed in tigers, leopards, domestic cats, dogs, and pigs. All the H5N1 reassortant variants have had the ability to cause human infections, but these remain sporadic and the ability of the virus to transmit from human-to-human is limited. Recent work has suggested that only a few amino acid substitutions may be required to make the virus become transmissible via aerosols in the ferret model.

Both in the context of a wholly avian H5N1 virus and in the context of a reassortant with seven genes of the 2009 pandemic H1N1 virus and the H5 hemagglutinin, two substitutions in the receptor binding site, the loss of a glycosylation site at the tip of HA, and a change further away from the globular head

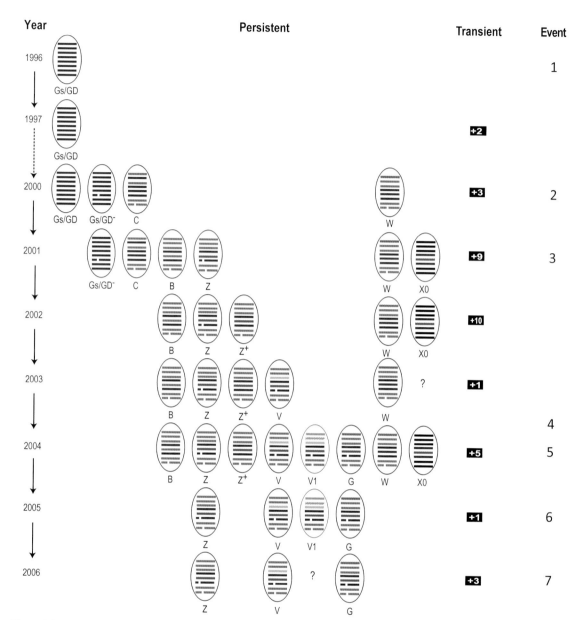

Figure 11.3. Genotypes and development of H5N1 influenza viruses in southern China (1996–2006). The numbers of transient genotypes are given in boxed text. Development events: (1) the emergence of the prototype Goose/GD-like virus in domestic geese (red) in Guangdong; (2) the interspecies transmission and reassortment of H5N1 in domestic ducks; (3) the emergence of multiple reassortant genotypes, only their HA and NA genes remained Goose/GD-like (red) and all internal genes had different origins (other colors); (4) predominance and dissemination of genotype Z viruses to South-East Asia (Wave 1); (5) endemicity of multiple sublineages in China and South-East Asia; (6) dissemination of clade 2.2 virus to Europe, south Asia and Africa via migratory birds after the Qinghai Lake outbreak (Wave 2); (7) dissemination of clade 2.3.4 virus (Fujian-like virus, genotype V) to South-East Asia (Wave 3). Reproduced from Duan et al. [50] with permission from Elsevier.

were sufficient to yield airborne virus. In these studies, a change in the receptor specificity towards α-2,6-linked sialic acids and an increase in the stability of HA were crucial for the change in the transmission phenotype [41,42]. These data indicate that H5N1 viruses have the ability to be transmitted via aerosols or respiratory droplets between mammals, and thus pose a significant pandemic threat.

Interspecies transmission

Interspecies transmission from aquatic birds to terrestrial poultry

Interspecies transmission of many subtypes of viruses from aquatic birds to terrestrial poultry has been frequently reported in most surveillance work. However, most of these cases were isolated events with no subsequent disease outbreak or corresponding virus circulation being observed, so the possibility that laboratory or environmental contamination occurred cannot be excluded. The turkey is probably the most susceptible poultry species; more than 10 subtypes of aquatic bird-origin influenza viruses have been detected in this bird. However, none of these viruses became established or prevalent over the long term.

To date, only H9 and H6 subtype viruses have become prevalent in terrestrial poultry, especially chickens. Since the mid-1990s, multiple lineages of H9N2 influenza viruses from aquatic birds have been established in chickens and minor poultry in Asia. The G1-like H9N2 viruses are prevalent in chickens in many Middle Eastern and southern Asian countries and in minor poultry in China. Ck-Bei-like H9N2 viruses have been prevalent in chickens in China since 1994, while the Korean-like H9N2 viruses were only prevalent in chickens in southern Korea during this time [33].

The H6N1 viruses that have circulated in chickens in Taiwan for more than three decades originated from an aquatic bird virus, and the H6N1 virus of minor poultry in China resulted from reassortment between a G1-like H9N2 virus and an avian H6 virus. The H6 virus that caused a disease outbreak in chickens in California was an intercontinental transmission of a Eurasian gene pool avian virus [43].

Interspecies transmission to humans and other mammals

Long-term prevalence of H9N2 and H6 LPAI viruses in terrestrial poultry led to a change in their tissue tropism. The viruses gradually adapted from replicating in the intestine to replicating in the trachea, which may change the transmission pattern from "fecal–oral" to aerosol.

Wherever viral etiologic diagnoses were conducted, sporadic H9N2 human infections were detected from patients with flu-like illness. Human serologic surveys have revealed that seroconversion rates in H9N2 endemic regions range from 1.0–1.8%, suggesting that interspecies transmission from birds to humans are not rare [44,45]. A similar situation has been observed in swine. However, there is no evidence to suggest that mammal-to-mammal transmission of H9N2 viruses has occurred.

Evolution of influenza A virus in different hosts

Evolution of influenza viruses in aquatic birds and the formation of Eurasian and American influenza gene pools

Genetically, LPAI viruses can be divided into two lineages: Eurasian and American. This division is probably the result of long-term ecologic and geographic separation of wild birds, and hence the viruses, of the Eastern and Western Hemispheres. For each of the eight gene segments of LPAI viruses, a distinction between Eurasian and American lineages can be made [16,17]. However, bird populations of North America and Eurasia are not completely separated; several waterfowl and shorebird species cross between hemispheres during migration or have overlapping breeding ranges. As a consequence, LPAI viruses carrying a mix of genes from the American and Eurasian lineages have been isolated, indicating that allopatric speciation is only partial [16,46]. Detection of LPAI viruses with genes of the American lineage in Eurasia and vice versa is still a relatively rare phenomenon; thus, the partial geographic isolation of LPAI virus hosts seems sufficient to facilitate divergent evolution of separate gene pools [16,17]. Recent studies in Australia and South America have revealed genetic lineages of influenza A virus in wild birds that are distinguishable from the lineages of Eurasia and North America [13]. It is likely that novel signals of temporal, spatial, and host-related variation in LPAI virus evolution will become evident after high-throughput sequencing of these viruses.

The evolution of LPAI viruses in wild birds is relatively slow compared with their evolution in mammals [1] but certainly is not negligible. Within both the American and Eurasian genetic lineages, multiple sublineages of viral genes co-circulate, but there are generally no consistent temporal or spatial correlations [16,17].

Genetic data from duck and shorebird LPAI virus isolates from the Americas suggest an active interplay between these host species. Although certain HA subtypes are reported to be more prevalent in either shorebirds or ducks in North America [6], this does not seem to have resulted in differences in the genetic composition of LPAI viruses obtained from these two reservoirs. This situation contrasts with that of the LPAI viruses of the H13 and H16 subtypes, which are predominantly isolated from gulls and terns and have evolved into a separate genetic lineage of LPAI viruses: the gull lineage.

Reassortment

The segmented nature of the influenza virus genome enables evolution by a process known as genetic reassortment, the mixing of genes from two or more influenza viruses. Studies in wild birds indicate that genetic "sublineages" do not persist but frequently reassort with other viruses [17]. As a result, LPAI viruses of a particular subtype do not necessarily have the same genetic make-up, even within a single year or a single host species. The high prevalence of LPAI virus in some wild bird species and the detection of concomitant infections in single birds [17,47] support the notion that reassortment occurs frequently in nature. An analysis of full virus genomes revealed a high proportion of mixed subtype infections and high rates of genome reassortment, leading to the conclusion that LPAI viruses have transient "genome constellations" [17].

Evolution of influenza viruses in domestic birds

Most influenza viruses from domestic ducks and geese behave similarly to the rest of the influenza viruses. That is they have limited amino acid substitutions, undergo frequent reassortment with segments from different subtypes of viruses, and do not form the lineages seen in viruses of aberrant hosts. After introduction into terrestrial poultry, the surface and internal genes of influenza viruses underwent significant changes. The driving forces may have included adaptation to a new host, reassortment events, and host immune pressure. Molecular traits such as NA stalk deletions and NS1 truncations are commonly observed.

H6 viruses in domestic ducks of coastal regions in southern China have formed distinct viral lineages. These lineages have characteristics of adaptation to aberrant hosts; such as deletions in the NA stalk region, truncations in the *NS1* gene, and an increase in the number of viruses that were isolated from tracheal samples [48]. The large numbers of birds kept in high densities and the rapid turnover of birds which provides continuous naïve hosts for the virus may have facilitated these lineages forming.

Evolution of the HPAI H5N1 virus

The genesis and development of the H5N1 Asian viruses is associated with several uncommon evolutionary patterns. These viruses are mainly maintained in domestic ducks and geese and co-circulate with different subtypes of influenza viruses, creating many opportunities for genetic reassortment. Thus, this virus lineage has become the only HPAI lineage to generate many reassortant variants, particularly from 2000 to 2002. The results of dating the emergence of the different reassortants or genotypes suggest that these variants were generated in three waves. Each of these reassortment events led to new dominant variants, new outbreaks in terrestrial poultry, and the expansion of the geographic distribution of the virus (see above). After becoming endemic in poultry in a region, the H5N1 viruses developed into locally distinct sublineages. These sublineages have significant genetic and antigenic differences. In China, multiple sublineages co-circulated in different provinces from 2003 to 2006 [36]. All the genetic variants of the Asian H5N1 lineage that were recognized by 2012 were originally identified in China. The virus has become endemic only in regions that have domestic ducks or have vaccination programs.

Conclusions and outlook

Despite the relatively intense surveillance studies that have been performed for many years in North America and Eurasia, our understanding of the global distribution of LPAI viruses in wild bird populations is limited. Serologic evidence indicates that LPAI viruses occasionally circulate in Antarctica [49], and it is reasonable to assume that LPAI viruses are distributed globally wherever competent host species are present. Some subtypes may be rare or may not be detected annually in surveillance studies. Simply because of the limitations of available methods, studies are currently biased toward species that are easy to sample during migration or wintering.

To understand the global patterns of LPAI viruses in wild birds, it will be crucial to integrate virus and host ecology with long-term surveillance studies to provide more insight into the year-round perpetuation of LPAI viruses in wild birds. Possible intercontinental contacts among ducks and shorebirds in areas where migrating birds from the northern and southern latitudes mix are of particular interest. We need to know whether LPAI viruses are perpetuated in ducks alone and whether the interface between ducks and shorebirds, which seems to occur in North America, also occurs on other continents.

By using high-throughput sequencing technology, it should be possible to gain more insight into the genetic variability and evolution of LPAI viruses in wild birds and to integrate this information with epidemiology and virus-host ecology. Transmission routes remain largely unknown for many wild bird species. Similarly, the effect of immunity induced by exposure to LPAI virus on subsequent reinfections of wild birds remains an important area for further research. Increased interest in avian influenza provides an opportunity to increase our knowledge not only of HPAI viruses, but also of LPAI viruses in wild birds.

The influenza viruses prevalent in domestic birds might be the main sources of the viruses that infect humans and other domesticated mammalian species because these hosts all share the same ecosystem and have a much higher likelihood of interacting with each other than with wild birds. The long-term endemicity of H9N2 viruses in Asia and H5N1 viruses in Asia and Africa poses a persistent pandemic threat to humans. Surveillance of influenza viruses in wild and domestic birds and the interface of these hosts with other host species is necessary to understand and mitigate these threats.

References

1. Webster RG, Bean WJ, Gorman OT, Chambers TM, Kawaoka Y. Evolution and ecology of influenza A viruses. Microbiol Rev. 1992;56(1):152–79.
2. Fouchier RA, Munster V, Wallensten A, Bestebroer TM, Herfst S, Smith D, et al. Characterization of a novel influenza A virus hemagglutinin subtype (H16) obtained from black-headed gulls. J Virol. 2005;79(5):2814–22.
3. Tong S, Li Y, Rivailler P, Conrardy C, Castillo DA, Chen LM, et al. A distinct lineage of influenza A virus from bats. Proc Natl Acad Sci U S A. 2012;109(11):4269–74.
4. Slemons RD, Johnson DC, Osborn JS, Hayes F. Type-A influenza viruses isolated from wild free-flying ducks in California. Avian Dis. 1974;18(1):119–24.
5. Webster RG, Morita M, Pridgen C, Tumova B. Ortho- and paramyxoviruses from migrating feral ducks: characterization of a new group of influenza A viruses. J Gen Virol. 1976;32(2):217–25.
6. Krauss S, Walker D, Pryor SP, Niles L, Chenghong L, Hinshaw VS, et al. Influenza A viruses of migrating wild aquatic birds in North America. Vector Borne Zoonotic Dis. 2004;4(3):177–89.
7. Olsen B, Munster VJ, Wallensten A, Waldenstrom J, Osterhaus AD, Fouchier RA. Global patterns of influenza a virus in wild birds. Science. 2006;312(5772):384–8.
8. Munster VJ, Baas C, Lexmond P, Bestebroer TM, Guldemeester J, Beyer WE, et al. Practical considerations for high-throughput influenza A virus surveillance studies of wild birds by use of molecular diagnostic tests. J Clin Microbiol. 2009;47(3):666–73.
9. Munster VJ, Baas C, Lexmond P, Waldenstrom J, Wallensten A, Fransson T, et al. Spatial, temporal, and species variation in prevalence of influenza A viruses in wild migratory birds. PLoS Pathog. 2007;3(5):e61.
10. Latorre-Margalef N, Gunnarsson G, Munster VJ, Fouchier RA, Osterhaus AD, Elmberg J, et al. Effects of influenza A virus infection on migrating mallard ducks. Proc Biol Sci. 2009;276(1659):1029–36.
11. Kida H, Yanagawa R, Matsuoka Y. Duck influenza lacking evidence of disease signs and immune response. Infect Immun. 1980;30(2):547–53.
12. Fereidouni SR, Grund C, Hauslaigner R, Lange E, Wilking H, Harder TC, et al. Dynamics of specific antibody responses induced in mallards after infection by or immunization with low pathogenicity avian influenza viruses. Avian Dis. 2010;54(1):79–85.

13. Hansbro PM, Warner S, Tracey JP, Arzey KE, Selleck P, O'Riley K, et al. Surveillance and analysis of avian influenza viruses, Australia. Emerg Infect Dis. 2010; 16(12):1896–904.

14. Becker WB. The isolation and classification of Tern virus: influenza A-Tern South Africa – 1961. J Hyg (Lond). 1966;64(3):309–20.

15. Pereda AJ, Uhart M, Perez AA, Zaccagnini ME, La Sala L, Decarre J, et al. Avian influenza virus isolated in wild waterfowl in Argentina: evidence of a potentially unique phylogenetic lineage in South America. Virology. 2008; 378(2):363–70.

16. Krauss S, Obert CA, Franks J, Walker D, Jones K, Seiler P, et al. Influenza in migratory birds and evidence of limited intercontinental virus exchange. PLoS Pathog. 2007;3(11):e167.

17. Dugan VG, Chen R, Spiro DJ, Sengamalay N, Zaborsky J, Ghedin E, et al. The evolutionary genetics and emergence of avian influenza viruses in wild birds. PLoS Pathog. 2008;4(5):e1000076.

18. Hanson BA, Luttrell MP, Goekjian VH, Niles L, Swayne DE, Senne DA, et al. Is the occurrence of avian influenza virus in Charadriiformes species and location dependent? J Wildl Dis. 2008;44(2):351–61.

19. Garamszegi LZ, Moller AP. Prevalence of avian influenza and host ecology. Proc Biol Sci. 2007;274(1621): 2003–12.

20. Webster RG, Yakhno M, Hinshaw VS, Bean WJ, Murti KG. Intestinal influenza: replication and characterization of influenza viruses in ducks. Virology. 1978;84 (2):268–78.

21. Ellstrom P, Latorre-Margalef N, Griekspoor P, Waldenstrom J, Olofsson J, Wahlgren J, et al. Sampling for low-pathogenic avian influenza A virus in wild Mallard ducks: oropharyngeal versus cloacal swabbing. Vaccine. 2008;26(35):4414–6.

22. Kleijn D, Munster VJ, Ebbinge BS, Jonkers DA, Muskens GJ, Van Randen Y, et al. Dynamics and ecological consequences of avian influenza virus infection in greater white-fronted geese in their winter staging areas. Proc Biol Sci. 2010;277(1690):2041–8.

23. Jourdain E, Gunnarsson G, Wahlgren J, Latorre-Margalef N, Brojer C, Sahlin S, et al. Influenza virus in a natural host, the mallard: experimental infection data. PLoS ONE. 2010;5(1):e8935.

24. Daoust PY, Kibenge FS, Fouchier RA, van de Bildt MW, van Riel D, Kuiken T. Replication of low pathogenic avian influenza virus in naturally infected Mallard ducks (Anas platyrhynchos) causes no morphologic lesions. J Wildl Dis. 2011;47(2):401–9.

25. van Gils JA, Munster VJ, Radersma R, Liefhebber D, Fouchier RA, Klaassen M. Hampered foraging and migratory performance in swans infected with low-pathogenic avian influenza A virus. PLoS ONE. 2007; 2(1):e184.

26. Horimoto T, Rivera E, Pearson J, Senne D, Krauss S, Kawaoka Y, et al. Origin and molecular changes associated with emergence of a highly pathogenic H5N2 influenza virus in Mexico. Virology. 1995;213(1):223–30.

27. Ito T, Goto H, Yamamoto E, Tanaka H, Takeuchi M, Kuwayama M, et al. Generation of a highly pathogenic avian influenza A virus from an avirulent field isolate by passaging in chickens. J Virol. 2001;75(9):4439–43.

28. Shortridge KF. Pandemic influenza: a zoonosis? Semin Respir Infect. 1992;7(1):11–25.

29. Duan L, Zhu H, Wang J, Huang K, Cheung CL, Peiris JS, et al. Influenza virus surveillance in migratory ducks and sentinel ducks at Poyang Lake, China. Influenza Other Respir Viruses. 2011;5(Suppl. 1):65–8.

30. Chen H, Smith GJ, Zhang SY, Qin K, Wang J, Li KS, et al. Avian flu: H5N1 virus outbreak in migratory waterfowl. Nature. 2005;436(7048):191–2.

31. Xu KM, Smith GJ, Bahl J, Duan L, Tai H, Vijaykrishna D, et al. The genesis and evolution of H9N2 influenza viruses in poultry from southern China, 2000 to 2005. J Virol. 2007;81(19):10389–401.

32. Cheung CL, Vijaykrishna D, Smith GJ, Fan XH, Zhang JX, Bahl J, et al. Establishment of influenza A virus (H6N1) in minor poultry species in southern China. J Virol. 2007;81(19):10402–12.

33. Guan Y, Shortridge KF, Krauss S, Webster RG. Molecular characterization of H9N2 influenza viruses: were they the donors of the "internal" genes of H5N1 viruses in Hong Kong? Proc Natl Acad Sci U S A. 1999;96 (16):9363–7.

34. Perez DR, Lim W, Seiler JP, Yi G, Peiris M, Shortridge KF, et al. Role of quail in the interspecies transmission of H9 influenza A viruses: molecular changes on HA that correspond to adaptation from ducks to chickens. J Virol. 2003;77(5):3148–56.

35. Lee MS, Chang PC, Shien JH, Cheng MC, Chen CL, Shieh HK. Genetic and pathogenic characterization of H6N1 avian influenza viruses isolated in Taiwan between 1972 and 2005. Avian Dis. 2006;50(4): 561–71.

36. Guan Y, Smith GJ, Webby R, Webster RG. Molecular epidemiology of H5N1 avian influenza. Rev Sci Tech. 2009;28(1):39–47.

37. Smith GJ, Fan XH, Wang J, Li KS, Qin K, Zhang JX, et al. Emergence and predominance of an H5N1 influenza variant in China. Proc Natl Acad Sci U S A. 2006;103(45):16936–41.

38. Hulse-Post DJ, Sturm-Ramirez KM, Humberd J, Seiler P, Govorkova EA, Krauss S, et al. Role of domestic ducks in the propagation and biological evolution of

highly pathogenic H5N1 influenza viruses in Asia. Proc Natl Acad Sci U S A. 2005;102(30):10682–7.

39. Chen H, Smith GJ, Li KS, Wang J, Fan XH, Rayner JM, et al. Establishment of multiple sublineages of H5N1 influenza virus in Asia: implications for pandemic control. Proc Natl Acad Sci U S A. 2006;103(8): 2845–50.

40. Sturm-Ramirez KD, Hulse-Post J, Govorkova EA, Humberd J, Seiler P, Puthavathana P, et al. Are ducks contributing to the endemicity of highly pathogenic H5N1 influenza virus in Asia? J Virol. 2005;79(17): 11269–79.

41. Imai M, Watanabe T, Hatta M, Das SC, Ozawa M, Shinya K, et al. Experimental adaptation of an influenza H5 HA confers respiratory droplet transmission to a reassortant H5 HA/H1N1 virus in ferrets. Nature. 2012; 486(7403):420–8

42. Herfst S, Schrauwen EJ, Linster M, Chutinimitkul S, de Wit E, Munster VJ, et al. Airborne transmission of influenza A/H5N1 virus between ferrets. Science. 2012; 336(6088):1534–41.

43. Webby RJ, Woolcock PR, Krauss SL, Walker DB, Chin PS, Shortridge KF, et al. Multiple genotypes of non-pathogenic H6N2 influenza viruses isolated from chickens in California. Avian Dis. 2003;47(3 Suppl.): 905–10.

44. Chen Y, Zheng Q, Yang K, Zeng F, Lau SY, Wu WL, et al. Serological survey of antibodies to influenza A viruses in a group of people without a history of influenza vaccination. Clin Microbiol Infect. 2011;17(9):1347–9.

45. Jia N, de Vlas SJ, Liu YX, Zhang JS, Zhan L, Dang RL, et al. Serological reports of human infections of H7 and H9 avian influenza viruses in northern China. J Clin Virol. 2009;44(3):225–9.

46. Makarova NV, Kaverin NV, Krauss S, Senne D, Webster RG. Transmission of Eurasian avian H2 influenza virus to shorebirds in North America. J Gen Virol. 1999;80(Pt 12):3167–71.

47. Sharp GB, Kawaoka Y, Jones DJ, Bean WJ, Pryor SP, Hinshaw V, et al. Coinfection of wild ducks by influenza A viruses: distribution patterns and biological significance. J Virol. 1997;71(8):6128–35.

48. Huang K, Zhu H, Fan X, Wang J, Cheung CL, Duan L, et al. Establishment and lineage replacement of H6 influenza viruses in domestic ducks in southern China. J Virol. 2012;86(11):6075–83.

49. Austin FJ, Webster RG. Evidence of ortho- and paramyxoviruses in fauna from Antarctica. J Wildl Dis. 1993;29(4):568–71.

50. Duan L, Bahl J, Smith GJ, Wang J, Zhang LJ, Zhang JX, et al. The development and genetic diversity of H5N1 influenza virus in China, 1996–2006. Virology 2008;380:243–54.

12 Influenza in swine

Richard Webby[1] and Juergen Richt[2]

[1]Department of Infectious Diseases, St. Jude Children's Research Hospital, Memphis, TN, USA
[2]College of Veterinary Medicine, Kansas State University, KS, USA

Influenza as a swine disease

Influenza is an endemic contagious disease of swine in many regions of the world. The viruses are detected year-round, although seasonal peaks occur in temperate regions. In uncomplicated cases the disease course is typically mild and self-limiting, usually lasting 3–7 days. Swine influenza viruses typically infect the epithelium of the respiratory tract, leading to its disruption and subsequent bronchiole attenuation and interstitial pneumonia, although there are strain-to-strain variations in severity [1]. Clinical signs of swine influenza are similar to the signs and symptoms observed in humans, including fever, depression, anorexia, coughing, dyspnea, respiratory distress, nasal discharge, and weakness. At the herd level, uncomplicated influenza typically results in morbidity approaching 100%, with a low mortality rate of less than 1% [2]. More severe disease can occur when swine influenza viruses act in concert with other respiratory pathogens, such as *Mycoplasma hyopneumoniae*, *Actinobacillus pleuropneumoniae*, *Pasteurella multocida*, *Bordetella bronchiseptica*, *Haemophilus parasuis*, porcine reproductive and respiratory syndrome virus, and porcine circovirus type 2, which together form the porcine respiratory diseases complex.

Molecular epidemiology of swine influenza viruses

The molecular epidemiology of influenza viruses in swine can superficially appear remarkably similar to that in humans, in that H1N1, H1N2, and H3N2 subtype viruses are those that circulate or have previously circulated. However, the similarity stops there. In humans, these virus lineages are monophyletic and circulate globally within a given timeframe with evolution occuring when new variants emerge to displace previous variants along the branch of a phylogenetic tree. In contrast, H1 and H3 influenza viruses were introduced into swine on multiple occasions, pools of viruses differ according to geographic region, and the introduction of new viruses does not necessarily result in displacement of existing endemic strains (at least not within the timeframe seen in humans). In addition, while mutations are introduced into the viral genomes at a similar rate in both hosts, human and swine influenza viruses are under different selective pressure for changes in their antigenic sites [3]. Swine influenza viruses undergo much slower and more gradual antigenic evolution. Many of the differences between the characteristics of influenza viruses in human and swine hosts are explained most parsimoniously by the absence of substantial and prolonged

Textbook of Influenza, Second Edition. Edited by Robert G. Webster, Arnold S. Monto, Thomas J. Braciale, and Robert A. Lamb.
© 2013 John Wiley & Sons, Ltd. Published 2013 by John Wiley & Sons, Ltd.

herd immunity in swine. In the swine population, naïve animals are continually introduced, the lifespan is short, and there are relatively few multiple repeat exposures to influenza virus. Swine also experience much less intercontinental movement which contributes to the geospatial uniqueness of swine influenza viruses.

The available literature on swine influenza viruses includes a few detailed longitudinal studies (or groups of studies) from some regions of the world while offering numerous stand-alone publications describing well-known or unique viruses isolated from individual outbreaks in different countries. While there is

interest and merit in reviewing all such reports, this chapter concentrates on the major lineages of viruses in areas representing the largest and most complete datasets (South-East Asia, Europe, and North America) to make the best use of the available space and present the evolution of swine influenza viruses over time. While there is some regional overlap of viruses and events, the molecular epidemiology and the timing of these events is remarkably unique to each region. Highlighting this geographic variation is the timing of interspecies transmission of human viruses to swine as depicted in Figure 12.1 and as discussed below.

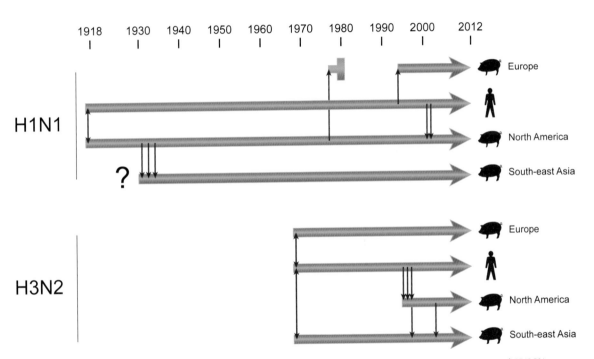

Figure 12.1. Impact of human H1N1 and H3N2 influenza viruses and/or HA and NA genes on swine influenza in Europe, South-East Asia, and North America. **H1N1.** The 1918 Spanish H1N1 influenza virus entered humans and North American swine around the same time (classical-swine H1N1). At undetermined times during the 1900s the virus spread on multiple occasions from North American swine to Asian swine and around 1976 from North American swine to European swine. Further transmission of more recent lineages of human H1 virus HA genes to swine occurred in Europe (reassortant H1N2) in the mid 1990s and at least twice in North American in

the early 2000s (triple reassortant H1N1 and H1N2). **H3N2.** The 1968 H3N2 pandemic virus entered humans and swine in Europe and Asia at approximately the same time (A/Port Chalmers/1/1973 – A/Victoria/3/1975 lineages). During the mid-1990s human virus HA and/or NA genes transmitted from humans to swine in North America on at least three occasions (triple reassortant H3N2). One of these viruses later transmitted from swine in North America to swine in Asia. In 1997, A/Sydney/5/97-like human viruses transmitted to swine in Asia.

Molecular epidemiology in North America

The first influenza virus ever detected was isolated from a pig in North America in 1930. This virus, the classical-swine H1N1 virus, was subsequently found to be derived from the same, or similar, lineage as the 1918 human "Spanish flu" pandemic virus. This finding was consistent with anecdotal reports from the 1918 period that pigs and people developed respiratory illness simultaneously. Taken together, this indicates that the classical-swine H1N1 virus became established in North American swine at approximately the same time as the 1918 pandemic [4]. This virus was subsequently predominant in the North American swine for about 70 years until the mid-1990s when the triple reassortant H3N2 viruses emerged. The limited genetic and antigenic data suggest that the early H1N1 viruses were not under strong selective pressure and were a comparatively homogenous population. H3N2 viruses had been found in North American swine, but rarely and apparently as the result of reverse zoonotic infection with contemporary human viruses. There is no evidence that H3N2 viruses circulated to any extent before 1995, despite isolated findings in the United States and Canada [5]. Due to the rather benign nature of the classical-swine H1N1 viruses there was little industrial or academic interest in swine influenza and, until the H3N2 viruses emerged, systematic molecular data on swine influenza viruses were limited to studies in slaughterhouses [6].

Perhaps the most notable epidemiologic event in North American swine influenza occurred toward the end of 1998, when the H3N2 triple reassortant swine influenza viruses were initially detected in outbreaks of swine respiratory disease in Texas, Minnesota, and Iowa (it was retrospectively shown that these viruses had caused outbreaks earlier that year) [5,7]. These triple reassortant viruses contained gene segments from classical-swine H1N1 viruses (NP, M, NS), human H3N2 viruses (PB1, HA, NA), and avian viruses (PB2, PA). The PB2 and PA genes of the triple reassortants, although also of avian origin, were phylogenetically distinct from their counterparts in the Eurasian-avian H1N1 swine viruses (Figure 12.2). The nearly simultaneous detection of similar viruses in three states suggested that they were already widespread, and serologic data showed that by 1999 these viruses had clearly become endemic [8]. Hemagglutinin-based phylogenetic analyses of these viruses showed that they were related to human viruses of the 1995 era, suggesting that viruses with at least the surface glycoproteins of the 1998 triple reassortants had likely been circulating in pigs for a number of years before detection. Regardless of the series of events that generated the triple reassortants (i.e., did the avian virus genes enter the swine virus population before the human-virus genes or vice versa, or perhaps at the same time?), it is clear that their impact was substantial. Not only was that impact measurable in a number of practical ways, such as increased economic impact leading to higher vaccination rates and diagnostic interest, but there was also a subsequent and dramatic change in the genetic make-up of circulating viruses. What had once been a stable viral reservoir of classical-swine H1N1 virus for almost 70 years was now dynamic and diverse.

Soon after detection of the first H3N2 triple reassortant, a plethora of newly generated reassortants were detected. Evidence showed reassortment not only between triple reassortant and classical-swine H1N1 lineage viruses [9–11], but also between triple reassortant and additional H3N2 human-lineage viruses [8], triple reassortant and H1N1 human-lineage viruses [12], and even triple reassortant and H2N3 avian-lineage viruses [13]. Some of the identified reassortants were transient, some circulated for a period of time, and at least three have continued to circulate. The common feature of all of these reassortment events was retention of the avian/human-virus polymerase components, and viruses with the so-called triple reassortant internal gene (TRIG) cassette have now displaced the classical-swine viruses, which no longer circulate. Using a Bayesian phylogeographic analysis, Nelson et al. [14] showed that the spatial dissemination of one lineage of H1 virus closely followed the long-distance transportation of swine from the Southern States into the corn-rich Midwestern States. The authors concluded that the practice of transporting massive numbers of swine into this area for fattening provided a permissive environment for reassortment.

A number of wholly avian viruses have been isolated from swine in North America, primarily in Canada, but none appeared to have become established [15,16]. The 2009 human pandemic H1N1 virus has further complicated our understanding of North American swine influenza viruses. The pan-

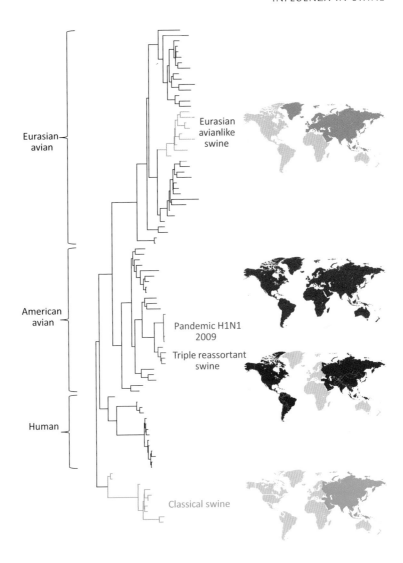

Figure 12.2. Phylogenetic tree showing the origin (major genetic clades shown in black) and relationships of the PB2 genes of the major swine influenza virus lineages (shown in color). Also shown are the continents where these major swine influenza virus lineages have been recently identified.

demic virus was not found in North American swine before the pandemic but was detected on multiple subsequent occasions. Although the initial reports of isolation likely reflected human-to-swine transmission events, the virus has undoubtedly been maintained since then by swine-to-swine transmission. As observed after the entrance of the triple reassortant viruses in the late 1990s (and as observed in other parts of the world with the pandemic virus), next-generation reassortants were subsequently observed in swine in the United States [17,18]. These next-generation reassortants contain combinations of gene segments from triple reassortant and pandemic viruses. The fact that one such next-generation virus was isolated from humans throughout 2011 and 2012 [19] ensures the intense ongoing interest of both public and veterinary health sectors in influenza in North American swine. Although the future endemicity of the pandemic virus (and its reassortant derivatives) in swine is uncertain, current evidence suggests the likely long-term maintenance of at least some of this additional viral diversity.

Molecular epidemiology in Europe

The classical-swine H1N1 viruses were first detected in pigs in North American in 1930 at approximately the time of the 1918 pandemic. However, the classical-swine H1N1 virus was not detected in Europe until 1976, likely as the result of importation of animals from the United States [20]. If classical H1N1 influenza viruses were established in swine in Europe before this time, their presence went undetected. The introduction of influenza virus into the European swine population was first detected not long after the human H3N2 pandemic of 1968. Early variants of the human H3N2 viruses were detected in Asian and European swine but, for reasons not understood, apparently not in North America. Although it is difficult to determine how many times H3N2 viruses were introduced into European swine, the lineage that became endemic was most related to human viruses of the A/Port Chalmers/1/1973 and A/Victoria/3/1975 H3N2 lineages. No other lineages of influenza virus except the H3N2 and classical H1N1 subtypes were detected in European swine until 1979, when a distinct wholly avian H1N1 virus was isolated [21]. This virus, referred to as Eurasian avian-like H1N1, appeared very well adapted to the swine host and displaced the classical-swine H1N1 virus surprisingly quickly [3]. Perhaps because of the short period of co-circulation or the incompatibility of gene segments, no evidence of reassortment between the classical-swine and Eurasian avian-like H1N1 viruses was found. In contrast, the dominant H3N2 viruses, rather than being displaced by the Eurasian avian-like H1N1 viruses, quickly incorporated the H1N1 internal gene combination. In one study, all 11 characterized H3N2 viruses isolated between 1992 and 1995 had internal genes derived from the Eurasian avian-like H1N1 virus [22]. In 1994, a new reassortant identified in the United Kingdom contained the Eurasian avian-like H1N1 internal genes, the N2 of the H3N2 virus, and an H1 from a contemporary human seasonal virus [23]. This virus subsequently spread to continental Europe, where it co-circulates with the reassortant H3N2 and Eurasian avian-like H1N1 viruses.

Despite the co-circulation of the three lineages, they differ geographically in their prevalence and dominance. More than 50% of swine in Belgium, Germany, Italy, and Spain are reported to have immunity to most of the endemic strains, while other countries, such as the Czech Republic and Poland, are primarily affected by the European avian-like H1N1 (seroprevalence rates ≥12%) [24]. The authors of these studies postulated that the epidemiologic disparities between countries might be partly linked to the density of farmed swine, with a greater prevalence related to higher density. Pandemic H1N1 2009 viruses were detected in European swine after their detection in humans. Within 12 months of the isolation of the virus in humans, nine European countries had reported detection of the pandemic virus in swine to the World Organization for Animal Health.

Molecular epidemiology in South-East Asia

The epidemiology of swine influenza viruses in South-East Asia is complex, as it combines the emergence of specific lineages in this area and the introduction of the major North American and European lineages, presumably via importation of animals. The large number of swine in South-East Asia, particularly China, also provides ample opportunity for virus spread and evolution. Although the 2009 pandemic has renewed interest in swine influenza virus surveillance in the region, including Thailand and Vietnam, most information comes from studies in Hong Kong, Japan, South Korea, and Taiwan. Swine influenza virus in South-East Asia was reported to have likely coincided with the 1918 influenza pandemic, as simultaneous illness in swine and in humans was described [25]. The first influenza virus to be isolated in South-East Asia, in the mid-1970s, was of the classical-swine H1N1 lineage [26]. Interestingly, large-scale sequence analyses of classical H1N1 viruses isolated from Hong Kong slaughterhouses over a prolonged period demonstrated that these viruses did not form a monophyletic group. Instead, they were interspersed with North American influenza viruses, indicating that they may have been introduced multiple times [27]. Classical-swine H1N1 viruses have also been isolated in other South-East Asian countries, including Mainland China, Japan, South Korea, and Thailand. These data strongly suggest that, as in North America (but not as in Europe), the 1918 human pandemic led to a stable swine lineage of H1N1 virus, although this conclusion cannot be confirmed. What is clearer is that, as in Europe but not in North America, the early human pandemic H3N2 viruses did enter South-East Asia and become endemic in pigs.

H3N2 influenza virus was first isolated in the region from Taiwanese swine in the late 1960s, contemporaneously with disease in humans [28]. It is difficult to estimate accurately when stable H3N2 lineages were established in the region's swine, but repeated isolation of early A/Port Chalmers/1/1973-like and A/Victoria/3/1975-like H3N2 viruses in China, Thailand, and Japan show that it was likely not long after the pandemic. Unique to Asia is the fact that a second, wholly human, H3N2 virus appears to have become established in pigs. These A/Sydney/5/1997-like H3N2 viruses were first detected in Hong Kong slaughterhouses in 1998 and co-circulated with the A/Port Chalmers/1/1973 and A/Victoria/3/1975 H3N2 lineages [29]. It is worthy of note that viruses with the triple reassortant backbone but with A/Sydney/5/1997-like HA and NA genes were detected in the United States, although they were apparently not maintained for extended periods. Somewhat surprisingly, H3N2 viruses were continuously isolated in Hong Kong from before 1998–2005 but have since not been abundant, although they remain in other countries in the region in various forms [30].

The first imported European swine influenza virus that gained a foothold in swine in South-East Asia was detected in Hong Kong slaughterhouses in 2001. This virus, the European avian-like H1N1 virus, was genetically similar to its counterparts in Europe, strongly suggesting intercontinental transport of swine as its source. As recently noted, the introduction of this lineage of virus into southern China (the source of swine for the Hong Kong slaughterhouse) shows a temporal relation to the reduced rate of isolation of the classical-swine H1N1 lineage viruses, analogous to events observed in Europe [26]. The lack of sustained, systematic surveillance in other parts of South-East Asia makes it unclear whether the classical swine viruses are being displaced over a geographic region greater than southern China. The second detected import of a modern swine influenza virus into South-East Asia occurred in South Korea in 2003. This import was an H3N2 triple reassortant virus from North America [31]. Unlike the European

avian-like H1N1 viruses, which appear to have been introduced only once into South-East Asia, the North American triple reassortant was found to have been introduced multiple times [32].

With classical H1N1, human-like H3N2, triple reassortant H3N2, and European avian-like H1N1 viruses circulating simultaneously in South-East Asia, the detection of multiple reassortant viruses was to be expected. Reassortants representing all of these major lineages have been widely described [30]. The 2009 pandemic H1N1 virus was also detected in multiple South-East Asian countries soon after its establishment in humans. By the end of 2009, China, Indonesia, Japan, Korea, Taiwan, and Thailand had all reported detection of the virus. As seen in other regions of the world, detection of the pandemic virus in swine was rapidly followed by reports of reassortant viruses containing gene segments from pandemic and endemic swine viruses [33,34].

Cross-species transmission of swine influenza viruses

Like most influenza viruses, swine influenza viruses are limited primarily to their host reservoir. However, swine influenza viruses may sporadically breach their host range barrier, leading to self-limiting replication in a new host population. Swine influenza viruses have been identified in a number of hosts, including humans, turkeys, and ducks. Of these, turkeys appear to be most susceptible to infection. There are numerous reports of swine-to-turkey interspecies transmission events, which may reflect an intrinsic susceptibility of turkeys to swine influenza viruses or simply increased exposure. Turkeys in the United States and Europe have been infected with H3 and/or H1 viruses, and some sectors of the turkey industry have resorted to vaccination to minimize the virus's impact. Canada has also reported infection of turkeys with swine influenza viruses. Although typically not a lethal disease in turkeys, swine influenza virus infection can cause reduced egg production and associated economic losses.

There have been sporadic reports of infection of ducks with swine influenza viruses, although in at least one case the ducks were swabbed in the vicinity of a swine farm, and environmental contamination cannot be ruled out. Experimentally, swine influenza viruses have been shown to replicate in (and in some cases to be transmissible in) mice, quail, and ferrets. Perhaps the best-documented recipient of swine influenza virus spillover is the human host. Both serologic and virologic confirmation of swine-to-human transmission has been reported, and all of the major global lineages of swine influenza viruses have been detected in humans. In a thorough review of the literature up to early 2006, Myers et al. [35] identified 50 reports of confirmed swine-to-human influenza virus transmission events. Fourteen percent of these infections were lethal [35]. The infections were typically self-limiting, with the exception of one outbreak among military personnel at Fort Dix, United States, in 1976. In this outbreak there was evidence of substantial human-to-human spread of a classical-swine H1N1 virus, and as many as 230 soldiers were infected [36]. The other major exception to the usual self-limiting nature of swine influenza virus infection in humans is the 2009 pandemic H1N1 virus, which, although not detected in its pandemic form in swine before appearing in humans, was most likely of swine origin.

The exact mechanisms underlying the usual failure of swine influenza virus to spread in humans are not clear, but at least two major factors are likely involved. The first is that, although both swine and human-adapted viruses recognize the sialic acid receptor in the α2-6 conformation, there is a HA-mediated host range barrier. This barrier is most clearly demonstrated by experimental infection of swine with human influenza viruses, as in a study by Landolt et al. [37]. In this study, swine were inoculated intranasally with a human-origin H3N2 virus. Although the virus replicated, as measured by viral titers in nasal swabs, its replication kinetics were slower, and its nasal swab titers were lower, than those of a swine-adapted virus [37]. This effect was reversed by replacing the human-virus HA and NA genes with the corresponding genes from the swine virus by reverse genetics [38]. In follow-up studies, these investigators found differences between the binding of human and swine-adapted viruses to sialic acids on host cells; they hypothesized that this difference was the primary determinant of the less efficient replication of human viruses in swine [39]. Extrapolation of these data suggest that there are important fundamental differences in either the host-receptor avidity of human and

swine influenza viruses or in the exact α2-6 sialic acid conformations that they bind.

A second factor that is likely to limit swine influenza virus spread in humans is the extent of pre-existing population immunity. Many major swine influenza virus lineages have HA proteins (the major target of neutralizing antibodies) ancestrally related to those of human viruses; therefore, portions of the human population have cross-reactive immunity to them. As human influenza viruses evolve antigenically at a faster rate in a human population than in a swine population, however, this cross-protection is progressively lost. The end result is age-dependent susceptibility to swine influenza virus infection. The epidemiology of the 2009 H1N1 pandemic is well explained by this phenomenon. Much of the elderly population had been exposed to viruses antigenically similar to the 2009 pandemic strain and were largely unaffected by it, while the young and those with underlying conditions experienced more severe disease. It is likely that similar cross-reactive responses may limit the spread of current H1N1 and H3N2 swine viruses in the human population

Swine as intermediate hosts

In 1985, Scholtissek et al. [40] formally proposed, on the basis of observational and experimental evidence, that swine might be the mixing vessel for the generation of human pandemic influenza viruses. The "mixing vessel" theory holds that simultaneous infection of swine with avian-adapted and mammalian-adapted viruses creates an environment where reassortant viruses can be generated. Such human–avian virus reassortants were responsible for the 1957 and 1968 pandemics. An important piece of the experimental evidence came from laboratory infection of swine with avian influenza viruses of a range of HA subtypes, from H4 to H13, to document their susceptibility to these viruses [41]. The results showed that at least one virus of each HA subtype was capable of prolonged replication in swine. These studies have subsequently been interpreted as indicating that swine are susceptible to a wide range of avian influenza viruses. The caveats concerning this study were that very high doses of virus inoculum were used and that other host species were not tested to determine whether the broad range of avian influenza virus susceptibility is unique to swine under these conditions. A second major contribution to the mixing vessel hypothesis came from work designed to identify the mechanism responsible for the dual susceptibility of swine to avian and mammalian viruses. The study found that the cells of the swine respiratory tract contain receptors preferred by both human (α-2-6-linked sialic acid) and avian (α-2-3-linked sialic acid) influenza viruses [42].

Although it is now clear that swine are not unique in possessing both forms of the receptor and that certain avian and even human hosts have both [43,44], there is ample evidence that swine can indeed foster the generation of reassortant viruses. An example was shown in 2006 when H2N3 influenza viruses were isolated from two pig facilities in the United States state of Missouri [13]. These viruses were of particular concern to public health because of the known pandemic potential of H2 viruses. The 1957 pandemic had been caused by a virus of the H2N2 subtype, and as the virus did not circulate in humans after the emergence of the 1968 H3N2 pandemic virus, anyone born after 1968 would have little neutralizing H2 immunity. The swine H2N3 virus was isolated from barns in geographic proximity, but they did not share any common staff or animal supply chains, raising concern about how far the viruses might have spread. Retrospectively, the viruses did not appear to have spread beyond these two premises, and there was no evidence of spread to humans in contact with the animals. Sequencing of the two isolated viruses showed that they were reassortants comprising avian virus-like HA, NA, and PA genes with their remaining segments derived from the endemic triple reassortant viruses, consistent with the swine mixing vessel theory. Use of water from a nearby pond that was frequented by waterfowl was the likely source of the contamination of swine with the avian virus genes. Similar practices were identified as likely sources of avian viruses isolated at Canadian pig farms in prior years. In these cases, H4N6, H3N3, and H1N1 viruses had been isolated from single barns, and no evidence of reassortment with endemic viruses was detected [15,16]. The sequences of the H2N3 viruses revealed genetic signatures of mammalian adaptation. Specifically, they had a leucine at position 226 of the HA. This mutation is linked to better binding to the α-2-6 receptor, is not found in aquatic bird viruses, and was detected in the 1957

pandemic H2N2 viruses. These findings support not only the fact that avian viruses can infect swine, but also that replication of these viruses in swine can select for α-2-6 sialic acid binding properties which was also previously suggested by Ito et al. [42].

The fact that swine can support reassortment of viruses from different host reservoirs and that replication in pigs can promote adaptation of viruses to the mammalian receptor conformation, means there is great interest in the ability of swine to act as maintenance hosts for other avian viruses sporadically isolated from humans. Such viruses include not only H9N2 viruses, but also the highly pathogenic H7 and H5 viruses. The only evidence of swine infection with H7 viruses was associated with a poultry outbreak of H7N7 virus in the Netherlands in 2003. This virus was transmitted to humans involved in the slaughter of birds, and in some cases to their family members [45]. Although no virus was isolated, there was serologic evidence for H7 infection of pigs, but only at farms where poultry were positive for the virus. These findings suggested infection via environmental contaminants, without substantial further onward transmission.

The available data on the replication of highly pathogenic H5N1 viruses in swine are unclear. Isolation of H5N1 virus from swine has been reported in Indonesia and China, countries where the virus is, or has been, widespread in poultry. There is no solid evidence of sustained pig-to-pig transmission of H5N1 viruses, and infection via environmental contamination cannot be completely ruled out. Attempts to experimentally model H5N1 infection of swine have suggested that sustained transmission is unlikely. Two studies have experimentally infected swine with H5N1 viruses of different clades [46,47]. Both studies used a large virus inoculum, and inoculated pigs shed virus poorly if at all. Although H5N1 viruses have been isolated from swine in field conditions, these experimental data suggest that swine are poorly susceptible and do not appear to be major contributors to the epidemiology of H5N1 viruses.

Data on the other avian virus subtype of concern, H9N2, are also not conclusive. During systematic slaughterhouse surveillance for influenza viruses in Hong Kong from 1998 to 2010, H9N2 viruses were isolated from swine but were a minority of the total influenza virus burden (2 of 672 viruses) [29]. Studies of H9N2 viruses isolated from pigs in Mainland

China identified as many as 10 different genotypes between 1998 and 2007 [48], but it remains unclear how many of these viruses were maintained in swine and how many were transient infections from poultry.

Although the 2009 pandemic H1N1 virus is addressed in detail in other chapters of this textbook, a brief examination of its genesis may provide clues to viral factors that can contribute to the transformation of a swine influenza virus to a human pathogen. The pandemic virus was a reassortant derived from the Eurasian avian-like H1N1 and triple reassortant H1 viruses; its NA and M gene segments were derived from the former and the remaining gene segments from the latter. Although the direct precursors of the virus are not known, the 2009 pandemic viruses are readily transmissible in ferrets, whereas viruses of the parental lineages are typically not. While the precise underlying mechanisms remain uncertain, it is clear that the specific combination of gene segments is crucial to the pandemic virus's transmissibility [49,50]. In addition, it is likely that key changes in at least the viral HA are required to generate the transmissible phenotype. Perhaps the main take-home message here is that a reassortant swine virus was generated that apparently had biologic properties not seen in either parental virus lineage. Considering the rather prolific nature of reassortment in swine, as described above, this fact raises some concern.

Challenges to the control of swine influenza

Swine influenza viruses continue to present a danger to veterinary and public health; however, control of the virus and the resulting disease are subject to multiple challenges, not the least of which is that influenza is rarely lethal in swine. Infected swine may take longer to reach slaughter weight and pregnant gilts might deliver stillborn piglets, both crucial economic factors that prompt intervention in hog-dense production systems. In contrast, in developing regions of the world veterinary funds must be used for other more economically devastating viral diseases (e.g., foot and mouth disease and classical and African swine fever viruses), and control of swine influenza is not a high priority. Similarly, surveillance is lacking in many regions, and therefore the burden of influ-

enza in swine populations in these areas is unknown. Even in developed countries, where pigs are reared in large numbers and reduction in time to market weight imposes a significant financial burden, control of the disease is challenging because of the diversity of circulating viruses. In regions of the world where swine are vaccinated for influenza, the primary formulation is inactivated whole virus with oil-in-water adjuvants. There is experimental evidence that these vaccines are effective and can produce broad reactive responses. However, these responses are not broad enough to cover the full diversity of circulating viruses, and the timing of vaccination to coincide with the decline of maternal immunity can limit vaccine use to swine of certain ages. Compounding these issues is the fact that in most of the developed world, where influenza vaccines are used, the veterinary regulatory authorities do not allow rapid updates in vaccine composition. Updating an influenza virus strain in a vaccine for agricultural use can require complete vaccine reregistration, at substantial financial and time costs. While the search for more cross-reactive and "universal" vaccines for humans has taken on high priority, such approaches are in fact more urgently needed in swine. They are unlikely to materialize, however, because of the relative lack of economic incentive for development of these newer swine vaccines.

Challenges in swine influenza surveillance

The complex nature of the global molecular epidemiology of swine influenza viruses and the infrequent yet repetitive incursions of these viruses into the human host place a heavy burden on surveillance data. For a number of reasons, influenza virus surveillance in swine lags behind that in humans and even in poultry populations. An important reason is that swine influenza is not a reportable disease in most countries. Thus, there is no requirement to report its presence, and there is often a valid reason not to. For example, although the World Organization for Animal Health (OIE) clearly and publicly stated that the pandemic H1N1 virus in swine did not warrant the interruption of international trade of pork products, trade was in fact interrupted in a number of cases, and pork sales dropped because of consumer perception that eating pork was dangerous. Under these circumstances, industry had valid concerns about openly reporting illness and submitting samples.

Perhaps one of the greatest lessons learned from the 2009 pandemic is that communication of scientific information to consumers is crucial. The use of the term "swine flu" during the early stages of the pandemic had a lasting effect on pork consumption. Despite the best attempts of various national and international agencies to change this nomenclature, it persisted in the media and even in scientific venues. Because of this concern and because of the close down and culling of infected animals on a farm in Canada after the first reverse zoonotic transmission of the pandemic virus (an unfortunate response, from a public and veterinary health perspective), levels of swine surveillance data for many areas plummeted after the pandemic.

Three methods are typically used for swine influenza virus surveillance: sampling of animals with signs of respiratory illness, sampling of slaughtered swine, and active collection of samples at the farm level. Each of these methods has it pros and cons, and the perfect system would incorporate aspects of all three. Sampling of diseased swine (piggybacking on disease diagnostics) yields by far the highest percentage of positive samples, as sampling can be targeted to animals with respiratory illness. This method also offers more rapid identification of pathogens, which is important for animal health status, as samples are often collected and screened within a shorter timeframe. The disadvantages of this form of sample collection are sampling bias (as asymptomatic pigs are not sampled), over-representation of samples from commercial-type systems, and the absence of information about prevalence. This form of sampling is most productive in the more industrialized regions of the world, where sophisticated veterinary diagnostic systems can rapidly identify the pathogens and where these services are used routinely.

Slaughterhouse surveillance has also proved to be a fruitful source of information about circulating influenza viruses. This method is simplest, in that large numbers of samples can easily be collected, and it can be less politically sensitive than on-farm surveillance. A disadvantage of this type of surveillance is that rates of isolation are typically low (approximately 2–5% in published reports) for a number of reasons, not the least of which is that slaughter age is likely not the most susceptible age. It may also be

misleading to use slaughterhouse virologic data to estimate prevalence, as some amplification of infection can occur if animals are penned together for periods before slaughter. Theoretically, due to health requirements for animals to enter the human food chain, this method of sample collection should also bias sampling toward asymptomatic animals.

The third method (sampling animals at the farm level) is the most difficult to perform but is potentially the most informative. This method can be used to sample animals of all age and health status. Farm surveillance is not only the most labor-intensive virologic surveillance method, but also the most politically challenging, as entry to farms is required and samples can be linked to individual premises. Nevertheless, the ability to sample both diseased and healthy animals and to obtain true prevalence data make this surveillance method desirable where resources are available and where it is politically feasible.

Knowledge gaps

Both the H5N1 outbreaks and the 2009 pandemic generated a much-needed boost in the funding of and interest in swine influenza research. However, there are a number of key issues that remain to be addressed. From an epidemiologic point of view, the circulating swine influenza viruses are still poorly defined in some regions of the world. Not surprisingly, these regions also often have less than optimal data on influenza viruses in other hosts. The types of swine influenza viruses in much of South America, Africa, and parts of Asia remain undocumented, as does their prevalence in the various swine production systems employed.

From the public health perspective, a number of other fundamental questions remain; the answers to these questions will allow full utilization of the global surveillance data being collected. A priority in this area is delineation of the molecular changes that are required to allow a swine-adapted virus to become a full-fledged human pathogen capable of community spread. Are there molecular signatures that should be watched for? Do some lineages of virus have a greater capacity for these changes, or can they even become human pathogens without changes?

From a veterinary health perspective these questions can be reversed. They are then about the changes necessary for successful establishment of human viruses or virus segments in swine. H3N2 viruses and segments of the early 1970s and mid-1990s human lineages became established in swine, yet those between these years apparently did not: was this a result of virologic or epidemiologic factors? A major factor limiting swine influenza virus spread and establishment in humans is the nature of the human population's pre-existing immunity. Before 2009, the subtype similarities described in the human and swine virus populations did not suggest that swine influenza viruses posed a significant threat to human health. However, the 2009 pandemic showed that substantial age-dependent population immunity was not sufficient to limit virus spread. Therefore, we must make it a priority to determine the point at which the human population may become more susceptible to establishment of the older H3N2 swine influenza virus lineages; while H5, H7, and H9 viruses remain a theoretical threat to human health, H1 and H3 viruses have already demonstrated their potential.

As a scientific discipline, we also have much to learn from swine influenza viruses about basic viral properties. The apparent promiscuity of swine influenza virus reassortment provides a real-world basis for understanding the mechanisms that control this fundamental influenza virus evolutionary process. Unraveling the immune mechanisms behind the absence of the typical proinflammatory response to highly pathogenic H5N1 virus infection in swine could also provide key leads for understanding the basis of H5N1-induced immunopathology. All in all, a substantial amount of work still remains.

Acknowledgments

This work was supported by the National Institute of Allergy and Infectious Diseases (NIAID), Centers of Excellence for Influenza Research and Surveillance (CEIRS) under Contract No. HHSN266200700005C.

References

1. Thacker EL, Thacker BJ, Janke BH. Interaction between Mycoplasma hyopneumoniae and swine influenza virus. J Clin Microbiol. 2001;39(7):2525–30.

2. Vincent AL, Ma W, Lager KM, Janke BH, Richt JA. Swine influenza viruses a North American perspective. Adv Virus Res. 2008;72:127–54.

3. Brown IH. The epidemiology and evolution of influenza viruses in pigs. Vet Microbiol. 2000;74(1–2):29–46.

4. Smith GJ, Bahl J, Vijaykrishna D, Zhang J, Poon LL, Chen H, et al. Dating the emergence of pandemic influenza viruses. Proc Natl Acad Sci U S A. 2009;106 (28):11709–12.

5. Karasin AI, Schutten MM, Cooper LA, Smith CB, Subbarao K, Anderson GA, et al. Genetic characterization of H3N2 influenza viruses isolated from pigs in North America, 1977–1999: evidence for wholly human and reassortant virus genotypes. Virus Res. 2000;68(1):71–85.

6. Olsen CW, Carey S, Hinshaw L, Karasin AI. Virologic and serologic surveillance for human, swine and avian influenza virus infections among pigs in the north-central United States. Arch Virol. 2000;145(7):1399–419.

7. Zhou NN, Senne DA, Landgraf JS, Swenson SL, Erickson G, Rossow K, et al. Genetic reassortment of avian, swine, and human influenza A viruses in american pigs. J Virol. 1999;73(10):8851–6.

8. Webby RJ, Swenson SL, Krauss SL, Gerrish PJ, Goyal SM, Webster RG. Evolution of swine H3N2 influenza viruses in the United States. J Virol. 2000;74(18):8243–51.

9. Karasin AI, Olsen CW, Anderson GA. Genetic characterization of an H1N2 influenza virus isolated from a pig in Indiana. J Clin Microbiol. 2000;38(6):2453–6.

10. Ma W, Gramer M, Rossow K, Yoon KJ. Isolation and genetic characterization of new reassortant H3N1 swine influenza virus from pigs in the midwestern United States. J Virol. 2006;80(10):5092–6.

11. Webby RJ, Rossow K, Erickson G, Sims Y, Webster R. Multiple lineages of antigenically and genetically diverse influenza A virus co-circulate in the United States swine population. Virus Res. 2004;103(1–2):67–73.

12. Vincent AL, Ma W, Lager KM, Gramer MR, Richt JA, Janke BH. Characterization of a newly emerged genetic cluster of H1N1 and H1N2 swine influenza virus in the United States. Virus Genes. 2009;39(2):176–85.

13. Ma W, Vincent AL, Gramer MR, Brockwell CB, Lager KM, Janke BH, et al. Identification of H2N3 influenza A viruses from swine in the United States. Proc Natl Acad Sci U S A. 2007;104(52):20949–54.

14. Nelson MI, Lemey P, Tan Y, Vincent A, Lam TT, Detmer S, et al. Spatial dynamics of human-origin H1 influenza A virus in North American swine. PLoS Pathog. 2011;7(6):e1002077.

15. Karasin AI, Olsen CW, Brown IH, Carman S, Stalker M, Josephson G. H4N6 influenza virus isolated from pigs in Ontario. Can Vet J. 2000;41(12):938–9.

16. Karasin AI, West K, Carman S, Olsen CW. Characterization of avian H3N3 and H1N1 influenza A viruses isolated from pigs in Canada. J Clin Microbiol. 2004; 42(9):4349–54.

17. Ducatez MF, Hause B, Stigger-Rosser E, Darnell D, Corzo C, Juleen K, et al. Multiple reassortment between pandemic (H1N1) 2009 and endemic influenza viruses in pigs, United States. Emerg Infect Dis. 2011;17(9): 1624–9.

18. Liu Q, Ma J, Liu H, Qi W, Anderson J, Henry SC, et al. Emergence of novel reassortant H3N2 swine influenza viruses with the 2009 pandemic H1N1 genes in the United States. Arch Virol. 2012;157(3):555–62.

19. Lindstrom S, Garten R, Balish A, Shu B, Emery S, Berman L, et al. Human infections with novel reassortant influenza A(H3N2)v viruses, United States, 2011. Emerg Infect Dis. 2012;18(5):834–7.

20. Nardelli L, Pascucci S, Gualandi GL, Loda P. Outbreaks of classical swine influenza in Italy in 1976. Zentralbl Veterinarmed B. 1978;25(10):853–7.

21. Pansaert M, Ottis K, Vandeputte J, Kaplan MM, Bachmann PA. Evidence of natural transmission of influenza A virus from wild ducks to swine and its potential importance for man. Bull WHO. 1981;59:75–8.

22. Campitelli L, Donatelli I, Foni E, Castrucci MR, Fabiani C, Kawaoka Y, et al. Continued evolution of H1N1 and H3N2 influenza viruses in pigs in Italy. Virology. 1997;232(2):310–8.

23. Brown IH, Chakraverty P, Harris PA, Alexander DJ. Disease outbreaks in pigs in Great Britain due to an influenza A virus of H1N2 subtype. Vet Rec. 1995;136 (13):328–9.

24. Van RK, Brown IH, Durrwald R, Foni E, Labarque G, Lenihan P, et al. Seroprevalence of H1N1, H3N2 and H1N2 influenza viruses in pigs in seven European countries in 2002–2003. Influenza Other Respir Viruses. 2008;2(3):99–105.

25. Kilbourne ED. Influenza pandemics of the 20th century. Emerg Infect Dis. 2006;12(1):9–14.

26. Zhu H, Webby R, Lam TT, Smith DK, Peiris JS, Guan Y. History of swine influenza viruses in Asia. Curr Top Microbiol Immunol. 2011 Sep 23; DOI: 10.1007/82_2011_179.

27. Vijaykrishna D, Smith GJ, Pybus OG, Zhu H, Bhatt S, Poon LL, et al. Long-term evolution and transmission dynamics of swine influenza A virus. Nature. 2011;473 (7348):519–22.

28. Kundin WD. Hong Kong A-2 influenza virus infection among swine during a human epidemic in Taiwan. Nature. 1970;228(274):857.

29. Peiris JS, Guan Y, Markwell D, Ghose P, Webster RG, Shortridge KF. Cocirculation of avian H9N2 and contemporary "human" H3N2 influenza A viruses in pigs

30. Choi YK, Pascua PN, Song MS. Swine influenza viruses: an Asian perspective. Curr Top Microbiol Immunol. 2012 Jan 21; DOI: 10.1007/82_2011_195.

31. Song DS, Lee JY, Oh JS, Lyoo KS, Yoon KJ, Park YH, et al. Isolation of H3N2 swine influenza virus in South Korea. J Vet Diagn Invest. 2003;15(1):30–4.

32. Pascua PN, Song MS, Lee JH, Choi HW, Han JH, Kim JH, et al. Seroprevalence and genetic evolutions of swine influenza viruses under vaccination pressure in Korean swine herds. Virus Res. 2008;138(1–2):43–9.

33. Kitikoon P, Sreta D, Na Ayudhya SN, Wongphatcharachai M, Lapkuntod J, Prakairungnamthip D, et al. Brief report: molecular characterization of a novel reassorted pandemic H1N1 2009 in Thai pigs. Virus Genes. 2011;43(1):1–5.

34. Vijaykrishna D, Poon LL, Zhu HC, Ma SK, Li OT, Cheung CL, et al. Reassortment of pandemic H1N1/2009 influenza A virus in swine. Science. 2010;328 (5985):1529.

35. Myers KP, Olsen CW, Gray GC. Cases of swine influenza in humans: a review of the literature. Clin Infect Dis. 2007;44(8):1084–8.

36. Gaydos JC, Hodder RA, Top FH Jr, Allen RG, Soden VJ, Nowosiwsky T, et al. Swine influenza A at Fort Dix, New Jersey (January-February 1976). II. Transmission and morbidity in units with cases. J Infect Dis. 1977;136(Suppl.):S363–8.

37. Landolt GA, Karasin AI, Phillips L, Olsen CW. Comparison of the pathogenesis of two genetically different H3N2 influenza A viruses in pigs. J Clin Microbiol. 2003;41(5):1936–41.

38. Landolt GA, Karasin AI, Schutten MM, Olsen CW. Restricted infectivity of a human-Lineage H3N2 influenza A virus in pigs is hemagglutinin and neuraminidase gene dependent. J Clin Microbiol. 2006;44(2):297–301.

39. Bateman AC, Busch MG, Karasin AI, Olsen CW. Infectivity phenotypes of H3N2 influenza A viruses in primary swine respiratory epithelial cells are controlled by sialic acid binding. Influenza Other Respi Viruses. 2012;6:424–33.

40. Scholtissek C, Burger H, Kistner O, Shortridge KF. The nucleoprotein as a possible major factor in determining host specificity of influenza H3N2 viruses. Virology. 1985;147(2):287–94.

41. Kida H, Ito T, Yasuda J, Shimizu Y, Itakura C, Shortridge KF, et al. Potential for transmission of avian influenza viruses to pigs. J Gen Virol. 1994;75(Pt 9):2183–8.

42. Ito T, Couceiro JN, Kelm S, Baum LG, Krauss S, Castrucci MR, et al. Molecular basis for the generation

in pigs of influenza A viruses with pandemic potential. J Virol. 1998;72(9):7367–73.

43. Kimble B, Nieto GR, Perez DR. Characterization of influenza virus sialic acid receptors in minor poultry species. Virol J. 2010;7:365.

44. Shinya K, Ebina M, Yamada S, Ono M, Kasai N, Kawaoka Y. Avian flu: influenza virus receptors in the human airway. Nature. 2006;440(7083):435–6.

45. Fouchier RA, Schneeberger PM, Rozendaal FW, Broekman JM, Kemink SA, Munster V, et al. Avian influenza A virus (H7N7) associated with human conjunctivitis and a fatal case of acute respiratory distress syndrome. Proc Natl Acad Sci U S A. 2004;101(5):1356–61.

46. Choi YK, Nguyen TD, Ozaki H, Webby RJ, Puthavathana P, Buranathal C, et al. Studies of H5N1 influenza virus infection of pigs by using viruses isolated in vietnam and Thailand in 2004. J Virol. 2005;79(16): 10821–5.

47. Lipatov AS, Kwon YK, Sarmento LV, Lager KM, Spackman E, Suarez DL, et al. Domestic pigs have low susceptibility to H5N1 highly pathogenic avian influenza viruses. PLoS Pathog. 2008;4(7):e1000102.

48. Yu H, Hua RH, Wei TC, Zhou YJ, Tian ZJ, Li GX, et al. Isolation and genetic characterization of avian origin H9N2 influenza viruses from pigs in China. Vet Microbiol. 2008;131(1–2):82–92.

49. Lakdawala SS, Lamirande EW, Suguitan AL Jr, Wang W, Santos CP, Vogel L, et al. Eurasian-origin gene segments contribute to the transmissibility, aerosol release, and morphology of the 2009 pandemic H1N1 influenza virus. PLoS Pathog. 2011;7(12):e1002443.

50. Yen HL, Liang CH, Wu CY, Forrest HL, Ferguson A, Choy KT, et al. Hemagglutinin-neuraminidase balance confers respiratory-droplet transmissibility of the pandemic H1N1 influenza virus in ferrets. Proc Natl Acad Sci U S A. 2011;108(34):14264–9.

13 Equine/Canine/Feline/Seal influenza

Thomas M. Chambers[1], Edward J. Dubovi[2] and Ruben O. Donis[3]

[1]Department of Veterinary Science, Maxwell H. Gluck Equine Research Center, University of Kentucky, Lexington, KY, USA

[2]Animal Health Diagnostic Center, College of Veterinary Medicine, Cornell University, Ithaca, NY, USA

[3]Influenza Division, Centers for Disease Control and Prevention, Atlanta, GA, USA

Equine influenza

Equine influenza virus (EIV), causative agent of equine influenza (EI), is one of the most common respiratory pathogens of horses. Other equidae including donkeys and zebras are also susceptible. Among countries with significant horse populations only New Zealand and Iceland are thought to have remained continuously EI-free throughout history. A few countries including Australia, Japan, and South Africa have experienced major EI epizootics but subsequently succeeded in eradicating EIV from their horse populations through intensive vaccination and strict quarantine. EIV circulate widely in Eurasia, North America, and South America. EI is considered enzootic in the United States and the United Kingdom, and repeated outbreaks have occurred in diverse regions including mainland Europe, Africa, India, China, Mongolia, and Argentina (reviewed in [1]).

Unlike influenza in humans, EI outbreaks do not follow predictable seasonal patterns. In countries with large populations and movement of horses, EI is likely to be diagnosed in connection with sales or race meets for which horses, particularly young horses, are brought together from different national or international sources, regardless of season. The large EI epizootics in Japan (1971 and 2007), South Africa (1986 and 2003), Hong Kong (1992), and Australia (2007) were all triggered by importation of infected horses into regions where the disease had been absent, facilitated by breakdowns in quarantine regimes. As with human influenza, the spread of EIV is facilitated by the short incubation period, typically 1–3 days, coupled with frequent occurrence of subclinical infections especially in vaccinated animals.

History

Morens and Taubenberger [2] recently reviewed the history of EI-like disease prior to the virologic era. Outbreaks of equine respiratory disease resembling EI were noted as early as 1299 AD and recurred frequently over the centuries since. It is uncertain that these were actually influenza, as other equine diseases such as equine herpesvirus infection can produce some of the same clinical signs typical of influenza. As discussed below, these outbreaks were frequently recorded as being associated in both time and place with human influenza-like outbreaks; especially those happening in spring or fall rather than winter. Indeed, a mild human influenza-like epidemic in the United States in the early 1870s was popularly known as the "epizooty" because it seemed to be linked to human–horse contact during the course of an explosive equine panzootic. That panzootic had a morbidity rate of nearly 100% and mortality rate of 2%, and as Morens and Taubenberger relate, "the 1872 panzootic literally shut down the United States for several

Textbook of Influenza, Second Edition. Edited by Robert G. Webster, Arnold S. Monto, Thomas J. Braciale, and Robert A. Lamb.
© 2013 John Wiley & Sons, Ltd. Published 2013 by John Wiley & Sons, Ltd.

weeks, preventing travel, transportation, mail delivery, and delivery of goods and provisions." They note further equine epizootics through 1915–1916.

In the modern virologic era, EIV have been identified as influenza A viruses and two subtypes are recognized: equine-1 (H7N7) and equine-2 (H3N8) (Figure 13.1). Influenza B and C viruses have never been found in horses. The first serologic association of influenza virus with equine respiratory disease was from an outbreak in 1955, and the first strain of EIV, influenza

A/equine/Prague/56 (equine-1), was isolated from an outbreak in Czechoslovakia in 1956 [3]. Similar strains soon appeared elsewhere in Europe, and were first isolated in 1963 in both the United Kingdom and United States. This virus was shown to be antigenically similar to subtype H7 fowl plague strains, and serologic studies indicated equine-1 virus had already been circulating for at least a few years prior to 1956.

In 1963 a new EIV strain of subtype H3N8 appeared, with prototype influenza A/equine/Miami/

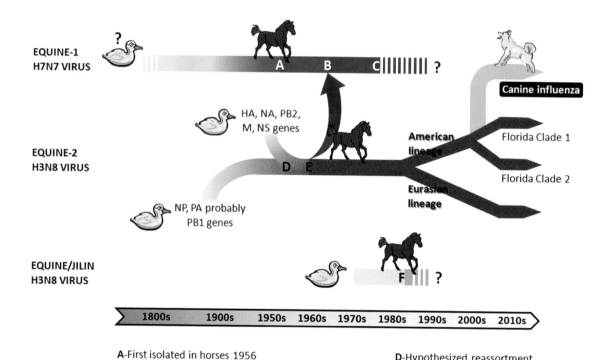

A-First isolated in horses 1956

B-Internal gene segments replaced by equine-2 1964-1973

C-Last confirmed isolate 1979

D-Hypothesized reassortment

E-First isolated in horses 1963

F-Isolated in horses 1989-90

Figure 13.1. Timelines of known (solid) and hypothetical (hatched) genetic histories of equine influenza virus. Timeline is not to scale. Host species of known or hypothetical influenza virus strains are shown by pictograms: avian, equine, or canine. Letters refer to key events as described beneath. The origin of the equine-1 lineage is primitive and its origin, presumably from avian influenza virus ancestors, is uncertain. An arrow (B) indicates that between 1964 and 1973, reassortment between viruses of the equine-1 and equine-2 lineages occurred. This resulted in one-way introduction of five equine-2 genes (PB1, PB2, PA, NP, NS) into equine-1 viruses while its corresponding ancestral genes were lost. It

is thought to be extinct (C) but this remains uncertain, as shown by a hatched terminus. The equine-2 lineage now consists of multiple co-circulating sublineages or clades defined by HA sequence and antigenic relationships, as shown by multiple parallel arrows. The equine/Jilin lineage arose suddenly from an avian influenza parent virus (F); did not trigger a panzootic and disappeared after 2 years. The origin of the only known lineage of canine influenza from equine-2 influenza is shown (blue), at latest 2003 and no earlier than late 1990s, and has persisted through this writing (2012). Other introductions of influenza into canines have occurred but, so far as is known, did not persist.

63 (equine-2) [4]. This strain differed from Prague/56-type strains in that it spread at a faster rate, generally caused more severe clinical signs especially in foals, and initially occurred in both juvenile and adult horses. The equine-2 EI panzootic may have originated in South America but was first observed in southern Florida in early February 1963, and by mid-May it had disseminated across the United States. It reached Europe in 1965, facilitated by international transport of horses and by quarantine practices ineffective for influenza control.

The 1963 emergence of subtype H3 EIV, followed in 1968 by the human pandemic with serologically cross-reactive H3 influenza, raised the possibility that equine and human H3 influenza viruses might be related. Further, seroarchaeologic studies indicate that an H3N8 virus previously circulated in humans starting with a pandemic in 1890, and on this basis it was suggested that equine-2 influenza viruses may have been a source of genes for novel or re-emerging human influenza viruses [5]. Against this, sequencing studies and phylogenetic analyses show that the equine H3 HA is only distantly related to H3 HA of humans or any other species. The human H3 HA lineage clearly originated around 1965 either directly or indirectly from an avian ancestor; whereas the equine-2 H3 HA lineage was calculated to have diverged from an avian ancestor around 1952 [6]. Thus, equine-2 EIV was not a progenitor of human H3 influenza virus.

Equine-1 and equine-2 virus subtypes co-circulated in horses from 1963 to at least 1979. In some outbreaks viruses of both subtypes were isolated. Equine-1 viruses have not been isolated in North or South America or western Europe since 1979, and so are now considered to be extinct. Subsequent reports of equine-1 virus outbreaks have come from India and Egypt, but these have so far been unconfirmed by international reference laboratories. Serologic evidence for exposure of unvaccinated horses to equine-1 virus was reported from various countries. However, serologic evidence alone, in the absence of a virus isolate, remains suspect because equine serum α_2-macroglobulin is a nonspecific inhibitor of hemagglutination using chicken or guinea pig erythrocytes [7], yielding false positive reactions in the standard hemagglutination inhibition (HAI) test for influenza antibodies. Owing to the absence of any confirmed isolations for 20 years, in 1999 the OIE Expert Surveillance Panel for equine influenza recommended that there was no longer any justification for continued inclusion of equine-1 virus strains in vaccines. Nonetheless, surveillance programs for equine influenza must continue to watch for possible re-emergence of that subtype from hidden reservoirs.

In 1989 a novel strain of influenza virus appeared in horses. This virus, influenza A/equine/Jilin/89 virus, arose in Jilin and Heilonjiang provinces in north-east China where it caused a massive outbreak, infecting over 20 000 horses with approximately 400 deaths [8]. Jilin/89 virus is subtype H3N8, but not a member of the equine-2 EIV lineage. Genetic analysis revealed that it was most similar in all gene segments to H3N8 influenza viruses of avian species [8]. The virus has not been reisolated since 1990. Serologic evidence from 1993–1994 indicated it might still be circulating, but this is believed to be a result of "original antigenic sin" brought about by a later epizootic of conventional equine-2 influenza. If the avian-like virus had persisted in horses it was possible for it to have reassorted with conventional equine-2 influenza virus, but such has not been detected. The Jilin/89 outbreak lends credence to the theoretical avian genetic ancestry for equine-1 and equine-2 EIV.

Pathology

EIV infects and replicates in the ciliated epithelium of the upper respiratory tract. These cells are killed by apoptosis, resulting in breakdown of the mucociliary escalator and increased susceptibility to secondary opportunistic infections. Primary influenza in horses is characterized by dry hacking cough, pyrexia, and nasal discharge which is initially serous and becomes mucopurulent after 1 or 2 days (reviewed in [9]). In experimental challenges featuring high virus inocula the incubation period between exposure and presentation of signs is typically 2 days. In the field it may be longer, although EI is known to cause fast-spreading outbreaks. A stochastic model yielded a transmission rate for EI in an unvaccinated population as 1.85/day, and the reproduction number as 10.18 [10]. Morbidity rates as high as 98% have been reported. Virus shedding, as detected by egg or cell culture based assays, generally persists for 5–7 days and does not correlate with disease severity: horses can be subclinically infected, or recovered from clinical signs within 1–2 days, while continuing to shed detectable levels of virus for 1–5 days thereafter. There is evidence (P.D. Kirkland, Elizabeth Macarthur Agricultural Institute, New South Wales, Australia, personal communication) that EIV-infected horses frequently harbor viral RNA detectable by polymerase chain reaction (PCR) for up to 15 days post-exposure, and in some cases for >30 days. The equine-1 (H7N7) subtype, despite an HA characteristic of high-pathogenicity avian influenza (HPAI) virus, was no more virulent in EIV-naïve adult horses than the equine-2 (H3N8) subtype, if as much. Strain differences in pathogenicity of equine-2 viruses have been observed, but these are relatively subtle: increased coughing, magnitude and duration of pyrexia, and expression of proinflammatory cytokines including type 1 interferon (IFN) and interleukin-6 (IL-6) [1,11]. Neurologic signs and nonsuppurative encephalitis, although rare, have been reported. Influenza is potentially fatal in equine neonates, particularly in cases of failure of passive transfer of colostrum, or when the dam is infectious at time of birth. Antibiotic therapy is frequently used to control secondary bacterial infections, which can produce life-threatening bronchopneumonia. Antiviral agents (rimantadine, oseltamivir) have been studied and are experimentally efficacious (although rimantadine was shown to be impractical in horses) but there are no reports of their use in the field.

Virus characterization

Antigenic drift reduces the effectiveness of vaccination with outdated strains; thus, with the apparent extinction of equine-1 EIV, most surveillance attention has focused upon the H3 HA of the equine-2 EIV isolated from field outbreaks. Virus characterization by HA sequencing and comparative antigenicity has revealed a succession of virus strains evolving with increasing complexity. These are ordered as follows:
1. Pre-divergence strains: prior to ca. 1989, H3N8 EIV evolved apparently in a single lineage albeit with a few unexplained outliers [12].
2. In 1987–1989, EIV H3 HA evolved into two diverging, antigenically distinct branches, termed the American and Eurasian lineages, which initially circulated in different parts of the world but did not co-circulate until the American lineage penetrated to Europe in 1992. Eurasian lineage penetration into the

Americas, so far as is known, was limited to a single outbreak in 1990 [13].
3. In 2000–2002, sublineages of the American lineage were identified, the South American, Kentucky, and Florida sublineages. In 2003, the Florida sublineage evolved into two distinct clades: Florida clades 1 and 2 [14].

This revised nomenclature abandons the geographic distinctions, perhaps advantageously as since 2003 the majority of documented outbreaks worldwide have been caused by Florida-sublineage strains. But phylogenetic–geographic correlations have not disappeared. In recent years Florida clade 2 strains have predominated in Europe but been largely absent from the United States. Another, more fine-grained classification scheme has been published [15] featuring 12 clades of which Florida clades 1 and 2 are the most recent. A mathematical model of phylodynamic evolution of EIV accounts for the spread of the American lineage to Europe – but not the reverse – by positing more effective quarantine restrictions by the United States than Europe [16]. Perhaps so, but horse import restrictions between Europe and the United States were nearly as minimal in either direction, so it seems unlikely that regulatory practices posed a one-way barrier to international transmission of EIV.

The rate of antigenic drift in the HA1 subunit of EIV H3 HA is about 1.8×10^{-3} nucleotide and 1.4×10^{-3} amino acid substitutions per site per year, about one-third as fast as in human H3 HA (4.6×10^{-3} nucleotide and 6.0×10^{-3} amino acid substitutions per site per year) [6,13,17]; thus, vaccine strain updating is less frequently needed than in human influenza vaccines. Recently, the technique of antigenic cartography has been applied to EIV (Figure 13.2) [18]. This analytic method facilitates high-resolution quantitative antigenic comparison of large numbers of virus strains using large numbers of reference antisera. The findings support the antigenic divergence of the Eurasian lineage and Florida clades 1 and 2 (called clade 3 subsets in [18]), with only two key amino acid positions: strains in the Florida clade 1 cluster (red) have 159S and 189N, D, Q, or E; the Florida clade 2 cluster (blue) have 159N and 189N, D, Q, or E; the Eurasian cluster (green) have 159N and 189K. Two phylogenetically Eurasian lineage strains that antigenically map to the Florida clade 2 cluster have 189E, while one Florida clade 1 strain

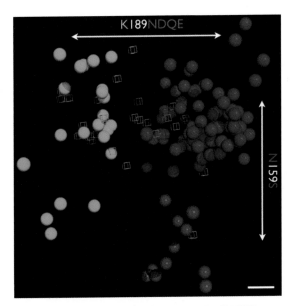

Figure 13.2. Antigenic map of equine-2 (H3N8) EIV, 1968–2007, showing the amino acid substitutions that were found to define the antigenic properties of the three clusters. The relative positions of isolates (colored spheres) and antisera (gray cubes) were calculated so that distances between isolates and antisera in the map correspond with minimal error to comparative titers in the hemagglutination inhibition (HAI) assay. The scale bar represents 1 unit of antigenic distance, or a twofold dilution of antiserum in the HAI assay. As only relative positions of antigens are determined, orientation of the map within the axes is free. Isolate colors represent distinct antigenic clusters: blue, early American lineage and Florida clade 2 strains; green, Eurasian lineage strains; red, Florida clade 1 strains. A few virus isolates are phylogenetically in one lineage but antigenically in another (see text). Reprinted from N.S. Lewis et al. [18]; Copyright © 2011, American Society for Microbiology. All Rights Reserved.

and two old American-lineage strains that antigenically map to the Eurasian cluster have 189K. For two of the three clusters there was no discernible antigenic drift within the cluster over time, signifying the unimportance of other amino acid changes: genetic evolution was relatively continuous but antigenic evolution was punctuated.

These findings were instrumental in the 2010 *Office International des Epizooties*/World Health Organiza-

tion recommendation that EIV vaccines for the international market should contain both clade 1 and 2 viruses of the Florida sublineage; whereas the Eurasian lineage, though still persisting, has been unimportant in recent years. Experimental and field studies have shown that even vaccines with imperfectly matched virus strains can provide protection if titers are sufficiently high. But modeling of experimental challenge data using challenge viruses homologous and heterologous to vaccines indicate heightened risk of infection, slightly heightened chance and duration of virus shedding, although no difference in the latent period preceding virus shedding. Consequently, even though these individual differences may be small, they combine to give greater risk of transmission and initiation of an outbreak in a horse population resulting from vaccine strain–challenge strain mismatches [19].

Occasionally, EIV strains are isolated that are genetically anachronistic, resembling strains several years older. Recent examples have been found in Germany and France, but the most prominent examples were isolated around 1987 from Argentina, Brazil, and India, which most closely resemble the equine-2 prototype, Miami/63 [17]. This evolutionary stasis or "frozen evolution" has not been convincingly explained as a natural phenomenon. If anachronistic strains persist in hidden reservoirs in nature, they pose the threat of re-emergence as circulating strains and vaccines increasingly lose their resemblance.

Suzuki et al. [20] explored the receptor binding characteristics of equine-1 and equine-2 viruses. They showed that sialic acid α2-3 galactose was the predominant moiety in equine tracheal epithelium, as in avians but unlike humans in which sialic acid α2-6 galactose predominates. Further, in equine trachea 97% of sialic acid was of the N-glycolyl type, rather than the N-acetyl type prevalent in human trachea. Similarly, in ganglioside binding assays both subtypes of EIV reacted preferentially with sialic acid α2-3 galactose and about equally strongly with both N-acetyl and N-glycolyl forms. This receptor preference was confirmed by measurement of virus shedding in the equine experimental challenge model, using a set of mutant EIV differing in HA receptor specificity. Receptor preference provides one rationale for the failure of the known EIV strains to cause outbreaks in humans, whereas they succeeded in canines.

The N8 NA of equine-2 EIV has not been studied to the same extent as the corresponding H3 HA, but it has had a similarly complex evolution. It falls into four subgroups within the N8 spectrum, one of which – represented only by the equine/Jilin/89 isolates – is shared with avian influenza viruses. The phylogenetic tree of equine N8 NA has a similar structure to equine H3 HA, featuring clades corresponding to the American and Eurasian lineages and Florida clades 1 and 2 [15]. The estimated nucleotide substitution rate of 1.7×10^{-3} per site per year is nearly as high as HA, and indeed the number of amino acid substitutions along the main trunk of this phylogenetic tree from 1963 through 2008 is 50 compared to 48 for the equivalent HA tree, indicating that equine immunologic selective pressures are similar on both viral surface antigens. The estimated date of origin of the equine N8 NA lineage was variously estimated as 1951 to 1955, similar to the 1952 estimate for HA. This suggests that equine-2 HA and NA evolved together and possibly were introduced together into EIV but, as with HA, the equine-2 NA lineage apparently had already diverged from identified avian N8 NA lineages long before. NA of equine-1 virus forms a distinct subgroup of the N7 spectrum, not shared with avian influenza N7 NA, and known to be shared only with a single swine H1N7 isolate. Nothing is known about antigenic–genetic variation within this subgroup.

Phylogenetic analysis of the genes encoding the "internal" virus proteins (PB1, PB2, PA, NP, M1/2, NS1/NEP) reveal reassortment between the equine-1 and equine-2 subtypes of EIV [21]. The prototype equine-1 virus, influenza A/equine/Prague/56, is remarkable in that its "internal" genes are primitive and are the closest known to the presumptive common ancestor between type A and type B influenza viruses estimated to have arisen around 1800 [22]. The "internal" genes of the equine-2 subtype are phylogenetically diverse in origin. NP and PA genes appear to be the first to have diverged from avian ancestors, perhaps in the late nineteenth century, which recalls the suggestion by Morens and Taubenberger [23] that the 1872 North American equine influenza epizootic was associated with an explosive highly lethal epizootic of poultry disease which might have been HPAI. PB1 diverged more recently, and the PB2, M, and NS genes clearly diverged relatively recently, around 1952, which coincides with the divergence of HA and

NA [22]. The general clade structure of HA and NA is similarly replicated with minor topologic differences in all the internal genes and most particularly PA whose main trunk lineage accumulated nearly as many amino acid substitutions as HA and NA [15]. In the period 1964–1973, while the equine-1 and equine-2 subtypes co-circulated, reassortment between them yielded viruses possessing H7 HA, N7 NA, and M genes from the equine-1 progenitor and the polymerase, NP, and NS genes from the equine-2 progenitor [21]. The phylodynamic analysis of Murcia et al. [15] suggests this happened more than once. All equine-1 H7N7 virus isolates since 1973 derive from these reassortments and, except for M, the internal genes of the prototype Prague/56 strain disappeared. The functional segregation of M gene with HA, probably associated with M2 ion channel activity, has been noted for HPAI also [21].

Also of interest is a C-terminal truncation of NS1 evident in most but not all EIV isolated since 2002, resulting from introduction of a stop codon at amino acid position 220 [14]. The truncation eliminates 12 amino acids from the C-terminus, including a putative PDZ domain ligand hypothesized to be a virulence determinant for avian influenza viruses in human cells [24]. The effect of this on virulence of EIV is uncertain, as no EIV have a high-pathogenicity phenotype in equids.

Equine-1 EIV, however, do have a high-pathogenicity phenotype in Balb/c mice [25]. This subtype features the HPAI genotype of multiple basic amino acids at the HA1/HA2 connecting peptide (R-K-K-R for Prague/56 HA) and replicate in cell culture with efficient cleavage of HA in the absence of exogenous trypsin. When inoculated intranasally into mice, a variety of equine-1 EIV were lethal on first passage, that is without prior adaptation. Occasionally, virus was detected in brain as well as lung tissues. By comparison, equine-2 EIV as well as human/swine/avian H1 and H3 strains replicated in infected mouse lungs but caused no mortality or disease signs. Equine-1 virus strains lethal for mice included the prototype Prague/56 strain and also strains post-dating the 1964–1973 reassortment that replaced most internal genes with those of equine-2 virus, suggesting that mouse lethality was associated with HA, NA, or M which did not reassort. Equine-1 virus is not itself lethal in chickens; however, reassortant viruses containing equine-1 HA and five or more genes from influenza A/chicken/Pennsylvania/1370/83 (H5N2) virus were lethal in chickens with spread of virus to the brain. Equine-1 virus has been used as a model to study viral pathogenesis in mice. Repeated mouse passage increases its neurovirulence, and this has been associated with mutations in polymerase genes including in particular the PB2-E627K substitution, already implicated in virulence enhancement of HPAI in mammals [26]. It is not understood why, in comparison with mice, equine-1 EIV were not highly pathogenic in horses, in neither their original Prague/56-like configuration nor their post-1973 reassortant configuration of internal genes. Aspects of innate immunity such as a functional Mx response in horses but not Balb/c mice might be responsible.

Vaccines

Vaccination for EIV has been utilized since the late 1960s. Most vaccines for EIV have been conventional virus–adjuvant mixtures administered by intramuscular injection. These are effective at stimulating serum antibody responses, especially in post-weanling horses and, when these incorporate virus strains that are well matched with the currently circulating EIV strains, such antibody responses are effective in proportion to their magnitude (reviewed in [27]). Vaccine responses in foals <4–6 months old are affected by maternal antibody interference, and a minority of horses appear to be inherently poor responders. Also, conventional inactivated-virus vaccines using alum adjuvants – for many years the most widely used kind – induce an equine immunoglobulin G (IgG) isotype profile dominated by IgG(T), which is poorly protective, whereas natural infection induces predominantly equine IgGa and IgGb isotypes in serum as well as mucosal IgA [28]. Another important limitation is that serum antibody responses have a short half-life especially in young horses. However, post-infection clinical and virologic immunity to EIV persists up to 1 year, much longer than serum antibody responses [29], suggesting long-lasting mucosal antibody or cytotoxic T-lymphocyte responses.

The goal of triggering protective, long-lasting humoral and cellular immune responses by vaccination has made the equine fertile ground for new vaccine technologies. Vaccines using ISCOM (Immune-Stimulating COMplexes of antigens with saponins) or ISCOM-matrix (ISCOM cage-like complexes containing saponin, cholesterol and phospholipid) as adjuvants, modified-live virus (MLV) vaccines, and live recombinant canarypox-HA vaccines have all been brought to market, and DNA vaccination has been studied. The MLV licensed in the United States is a cold-adapted EIV administered intranasally. In EIV-naïve horses this vaccine induces low to undetectable serum HAI antibodies and virus shedding although reduced is not eliminated, but a single dose provides long-lasting clinical protection from experimental challenge. Similar results have been obtained from a prototype MLV whose attenuation results from truncation of viral NS1 [30], restricting its replication in interferon-competent hosts. This MLV was generated from plasmid DNA by reverse genetics, so in principle its antigenic updating should be readily accomplished by site-directed mutagenesis as needed. MLV vaccines for EIV have not been widely accepted owing to perceived risk of reversion to virulence; however, such reversion has not yet been demonstrated to occur. The canarypox-HA vaccine when tested by experimental vaccination/challenge induces long-lasting clinical protection, humoral IgGa and IgGb serum antibody responses, and also evidence for cytotoxic T lymphocyte responses based on increased IFN-γ responses post-challenge [31]. This vaccine should be equally amenable to updating. It was the only vaccine approved for use in Australia for control of their 2007 EI outbreak, most importantly because it allowed discrimination of vaccinated from infected horses by comparative serology for HA versus NA antibodies.

Experimental challenge models

Mice and hamsters have been used as small animal models for *in vivo* EIV infection studies, with virus administered by the intranasal route, and virus replication titrated in excised lungs. The equine-1 (H7N7) phenotype of mouse lethality provides a handy measuring stick for, for example, assessment of novel vaccine technologies. Equine-2 viruses replicate and induce seroconversion, though not clinical signs, in mice and hamsters, and both have been used to estimate effects of antigenic drift on EIV vaccine efficacy.

Studies of horse immune responses to EIV infection, including vaccine efficacy studies, require an equine experimental challenge model. Attempts in the

1960s to develop such a model, featuring liquid virus inoculums administered by nasal catheter, failed to induce the expected clinical signs. Mumford et al. [32] developed the method that is widely used today, in which low-passage virus is aerosolized and inhaled by horses either through a mask or while standing within an enclosure. In EIV-naïve horses this model reliably induces typical clinical signs of EI, albeit the virus dose required for full expression of clinical signs can be 10^3- to 10^4-fold greater than the minimal infectious dose. Virus shedding can be titrated from nasal swabs or washes collected repeatedly over time; serum samples are easily obtainable. The major limitation is that facility capabilities and requirement for EIV-naïve horses tend to constrain the animal numbers and hence the statistical power of individual experiments.

Infectivity of EIV for humans

EIV are thought to have originated from avian influenza virus ancestors [12]. The 1989 outbreak of avian H3N8 influenza in horses in Jilin and Heilonjiang demonstrated that equids are susceptible to introduction of avian influenza viruses [8]. However, equids were long believed to have no intermediary role in interspecies influenza transmission in nature. This view began to change in 2005 with the advent of canine influenza (see below). Recently, H3N8 EIV have also been isolated from pigs, and unpublished data from a University of Iowa sero-survey indicate that up to 10% of humans with extensive horse contact may be seropositive for EIV H3 HA (Leedom et al., personal communication), suggestive of infection without clinical disease. Experimentally, humans can be infected by EIV, as can ferrets, though not beef cattle. However, the only report describing natural infection of a human with EIV was unsupported by any virus isolate. In this author's experience, EIV researchers who conduct challenge studies in horses are often exposed to large amounts of aerosolized virus but typically exhibit no symptoms, no detectable virus shedding, and weak or absent seroconversion. The currently existing strains of EIV are not considered to be human pathogens.

EIV strains of the previous era may have been different. Morens and Taubenberger [2] published a review of historical descriptions of presumptive influenza pandemics prior to the twentieth century. Strik-ingly, they noted coincidental equine and human outbreaks of influenza-like disease as early as 1299 AD. They wrote:

> Between 1688 and 1888 . . . by our count there were 112 (of 200) years in which either significant [human] epidemics/pandemics or equine epizootics of apparent influenza were documented in Europe. Of these 112 years, combined equine epizootics and epidemics were documented in 67; equine epizootics only in 25; and epidemics only in 20 . . . Equine influenza typically appeared about 3 weeks before human influenza . . . Well before the year 1700, a strong association between human and equine influenza had been widely observed and widely accepted as a typical pattern of influenza occurrence [2].

These authors suggest elsewhere that the 1872 equine influenza panzootic was likely to have been caused by an HPAI virus [23]. The definitive causative agents of pre-twentieth century outbreaks are unknown. However, neither human biology nor equine biology have fundamentally changed since; what has changed is the role of the horse in human society. Even that change is not universal; for example, in Mongolia the ratio of horses to humans is still today about 1 : 1. Furthermore, horses, owing to racing and breeding activities, are the most frequent international air traveling mammal after humans, which would facilitate rapid spread of any newly emerging pathogen. If equines were once important in transmission of influenza viruses to humans, they can be so again.

Canine influenza

Until recently the focus of influenza studies in mammals was largely limited to humans, swine, and horses, with companion animals being considered somewhat resistant to infection. This perception changed with the emergence of the highly pathogenic avian influenza virus (H5N1) in South-East Asia. Both dogs and cats were shown to be susceptible to infection and to develop severe disease associated with the infections. At about the same time, a true canine influenza virus (CIV) was isolated from dogs in the United States. Multiple strains of influenza virus have now been identified as being able to infect dogs and in some cases induce overt disease.

Equine origin CIV (H3N8)

Early in 2004, an influenza virus was isolated from lung tissue of a greyhound that was part of a severe respiratory disease outbreak in Florida [33]. The virus was identified as a unique lineage of H3N8 influenza A virus with all eight gene segments having an equine influenza virus origin. Archival tissues identified the same virus from a case in 2003. Since then, cases of canine influenza have sporadically been identified in over a dozen states, sometimes associated with movement of dogs. Overall the seroprevalence of CIV in the United States is below 5%, but for unknown reasons the infection has remained enzootic in New York City and Colorado. Elsewhere, foxhounds in England were identified as seropositive to H3N8 but no virus was isolated. In the 2007 epizootic of H3N8 equine influenza virus in Australia, PCR and serology showed infection of dogs occurred on premises that had infected horses, but again no virus was recovered. Experimentally, equine H3N8 can be transmitted to dogs [34].

The designation of this virus as CIV is based on the fact that the canine isolates have a genome that differentiates them from the equine progenitor. At least six changes in the amino acid sequence of HA are consistently found in the CIV isolates (Table 13.1) [35]. While there has been some drift in the CIV isolates over time, the evolutionary pattern is consistently monophyletic (Figure 13.3). For CIV isolates analyzed through 2008, 19 amino acid changes are highly conserved in the CIV genome compared with EIV isolates obtained during the same time period [35]. For the CIV isolates in hand, the evidence indicates that a single successful transmission event occurred and all are derived from that event and are evolving within its unique lineage. The best guess for the emergence of CIV in the United States is in the late 1990s. There is no evidence as yet for transmission of CIV into horses, and experimental transmission studies using a CIV isolate in horses indicated that the canine virus replicated poorly in horses and was not transmitted to contact controls [36].

Pathologic descriptions associated with natural CIV infections are complicated by the presence of various other bacterial and viral agents, as CIV is generally found in situations such as shelters where dogs are in close contact. Experimentally, CIV clinical signs are

Table 13.1. Evolution of the equine-origin H3 hemagglutinin of canine influenza virus (CIV) [33,35,37].

Amino acid position[a]	Hemagglutinin								
	29	54	83	118	222	261	328	479	483
EIV (1990–2003)[b]	I[e]	N	N[f]	L[g]	W[h]	K[i]	I	G	N[j]
Emerging CIV (Florida 2003–2004)[c]	M/I[k]	K	S	L	L	K	T	G	T
Enzootic CIV (2005–2008)[d]	M/I[k]	K	S	V	L	N	T	E	T

[a]Amino acid numbering per A/Aichi/2/68 HA gene, Genbank Accession AAA43178, mature protein (without signal peptide).
[b]Amino acid residues found in all H3N8 EIVs collected between 1990 and 2003. Variations to consensus are indicated in footnotes.
[c]Amino acid residues in emerging CIVs (A/canine/Florida/242/2003 and A/canine/Florida/43/2004).
[d]Amino acid residues found in enzootic H3N8 CIV sequences (absent in Florida isolates from 2003–2004).
[e]Amino acid residues shown in IUPAC/IUB single letter codes.
[f]A few isolates have serine at position 83.
[g]One isolate has serine at position 118 (A/equine/Newmarket/1/1993).
[h]A few isolates have leucine at position 222.
[i]A few isolates have arginine or glycine at position 261.
[j]One isolate has lysine at position 483 (A/equine/Guelph/G03-0250/2003).
[k]One isolate has a mixed base isoleucine/methionine at position 29.

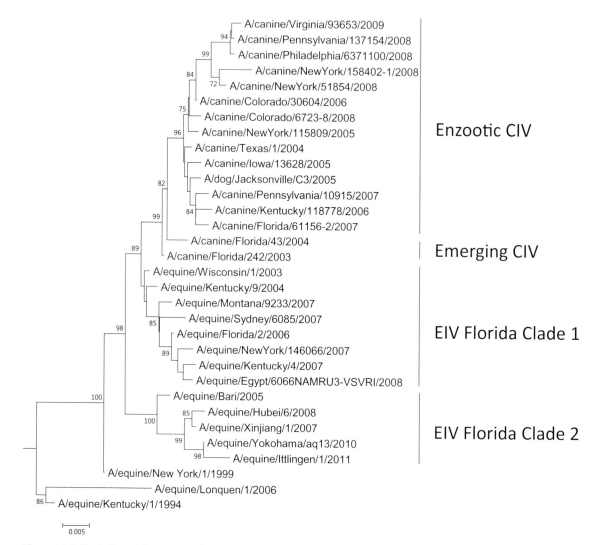

Figure 13.3. Evolution of the canine influenza virus (CIV) H3 hemagglutinin (HA) gene. The phylogenetic tree was constructed by Neighbor-Joining using MEGA software [51] and includes selected EIV H3N8 collected after 1993 as well as CIV sequences. The trees were rooted to A/equine/Miami/1/1963. The reliability of the phylogeny was assessed with 1000 bootstrap replicates. Values greater than 70% are indicated at the node of the branches. The horizontal bar denotes the unit scale of nucleotide substitutions per site for the tree branch lengths.

typical of influenza: ocular and nasal discharge, lethargy, inappetance, coughing, and a low grade fever beginning 2–3 days post infection and peaking at days 9–11. Viral titers in respiratory secretions are not impressively high (<5 logs) and peak at days 3–5 followed by rapid decline; however, virus can be readily transmitted to contact controls. Common pathologic features are tracheitis and bronchitis with necrosis and erosion of the surface epithelium and edema of the lamina propria and submucosa [37].

CIV vaccines are now commercially available and experimentally produce reductions in virus shedding and clinical signs. Vaccine effectiveness in the field has been difficult to assess.

Avian origin influenza A virus H3N2

In 2006 and 2007, epizootics of canine respiratory disease were observed in Korea [38] and China. Virus isolates belonged to the avian influenza virus lineage H3N2. Dogs developed clinical signs typical of influenza infection, and pathology noted in respiratory tissues was similar to that of H3N8 CIV. Dog-to-dog contact transmission was easily achieved. In comparison to contemporary isolates of avian H3N2, there were six amino acid changes in HA1. Additional data will be necessary to determine whether these changes are unique and consistent, signifying that a true CIV lineage of avian H3N2 derivation exists.

Avian origin influenza A virus H5N1

In 2004, a dog in Thailand died within 6 days of eating duck carcasses [39]. There was severe pulmonary edema and congestion with congestion in the liver, kidney, and spleen. Influenza virus was isolated from lung, liver, kidney, and urine samples indicating that the virus replicated in extrapulmonary tissues. Genetically, the virus was essentially the same H5N1 that was infecting birds, tigers, and humans in Thailand. Experimental infections of dogs with different H5N1 isolates confirmed the ability of the virus to initiate infections in dogs, but clinical outcomes were variable and virus was not detected in extrapulmonary tissues.

A/H1N1pdm09 virus

In 2009, clinical cases in dogs infected with human A/H1N1pdm09 virus were observed [40]. In experimental infections, clinical signs were mild and contact transmission was limited. A sero-survey in Italy in late 2009 found a small number (0.8%) of seropositive dogs.

Other

A surveillance program for canine influenza in Korea, 2007–2010, identified 49 PCR positive cases of avian-origin H3N2, but one typed as H3N1. Seven gene segments including NA were closely related to A/H1N1pdm09 virus, but HA was closely related to the avian H3 identified in dogs previously [41]. The identification of this novel virus reinforces the need for continued surveillance of companion animals for evidence of influenza A virus infections.

Feline influenza

The increased interest in the role that felines have in the epidemiology of influenza A virus infections is correlated with the increased surveillance related to the emergence of the highly pathogenic avian virus collectively referred to as H5N1 and more recently to that associated with pandemic H1N1 of 2009 (A/H1N1pdm09 virus). Unlike the canine situation, there is no evidence of a lineage of influenza virus that is unique to felines.

Studies since 1970 provided experimental evidence that felines could be infected with influenza A viruses including human H2N2 and H3N2, avian H3N2 and H7N3, avian and seal H7N7, as well as influenza B virus [42]. It was demonstrated that domestic cats could be infected and shed virus for at least 6 days, and, in addition, uninfected animals in contact with the inoculated ones became infected. Significantly, a cat became infected through exposure to a human patient shedding H3N2 virus. While successful infections were documented by reisolation of the viruses and seroconversions, no clinical signs of disease were evident.

The susceptibility of felines to influenza A viruses was "rediscovered" in association with the emergence of HPAI H5N1 virus in South-East Asia in 2003–2004. Fatal infections in exotic cats and domestic cats associated with contact of birds infected with H5N1 were reported [43]. Gross lesions in two tigers and two leopards consisted of severe pulmonary consolidations with evidence of extrapulmonary hemorrhages in multiple tissues, and, surprisingly, evidence of encephalitis in a tiger and a leopard. The H5N1 virus isolated from these cases was indistinguishable from that circulating in avians in the region. In a domestic cat, interstitial pneumonia, nonsuppurative encephalitis, and lesions in the liver were noted and influenza A antigen was detected in cerebral neurons, myocardial cells, pneumocytes, hepatic cells, splenic cells, and tubular epithelial cells of the kidney. These case reports, confirmed by experimental infections [44], associated H5N1 infections with mortalities in felines and provided evidence for systemic spread of the virus including to lung, brain, heart, kidney, liver, and adrenal glands. Infectious virus was also found in fecal samples. Contact infections opened the possibility of cat-to-cat spread, but there currently is no evidence of natural feline infections in the absence of exposure to infected birds. Also, natural H5N1 infections of cats have been detected in the absence of overt disease.

The heightened surveillance associated with the emergence of what is now known as A/H1N1pdm09 virus and the awareness that influenza viruses infect dogs led to more screening of companion animals for evidence of influenza virus infections. In a pattern similar to H5N1, feline field cases associated with A/H1N1pdm09 virus were identified [45]. These included cases suggestive of transmission to household cats from infected humans. Seroconversions were detected in sentinel cats. The pattern seen with A/H1N1pdm09 virus in experimentally infected cats resembled a milder form of H5N1 induced disease.

The degree of penetration of influenza viruses into the feline population has been assessed using different serologic tests including HAI, ELISA, and microneutralization tests. These have not been validated for feline studies and results compared among the methods correlate poorly. Sero-surveys found few positive samples prior to the emergence of pandemic H1N1, but >20% positive samples collected during the first influenza season of pandemic H1N1, strongly suggesting exposure of domestic cats to H1N1. Seroprevalence for seasonal H1N1 and seasonal H3N2 were surprisingly high as well. If the HAI test is accepted as the gold standard for influenza serology, then one is left with the conclusion that felines are more affected by influenza virus than previously thought.

Influenza in marine mammals

Compared with avian and terrestrial species, marine mammals receive relatively little virologic attention because of poor accessibility. Nonetheless, susceptibility of whales and seals to infection with influenza viruses is now well established. The earliest virus isolate appears to have been obtained in 1976 from lung tissue of a South Pacific striped whale, and characterized as subtype H1N3 [46]. Influenza viruses were isolated from the lung and hilar lymph node of a stranded pilot whale in 1984, and characterized as

subtypes H13N2 and H13N9. In 1979–1980 along the United States north-eastern seaboard, an outbreak of severe respiratory infection and high mortality (20%) in harbor seals led to isolation of an H7N7 influenza virus [47]. In 1983, another pneumonia outbreak in harbor seals in the same general area as the 1979 outbreak, but with comparatively low mortality (2–4%), produced an isolate of H4N5 influenza virus, which had possibly been introduced as early as 6 months previously [48]. Follow-up surveillance in the same region led to isolations of H4N6 viruses from stranded seals in 1991, and H3N3 viruses in 1992. Exposure to subtypes H3, H6, and H10 were revealed by serologic surveys in Japan and Antarctica. Genomic analyses based on sequencing and competitive RNA–RNA hybridization indicated that the isolated viruses consistently appeared to represent recent introductions of avian influenza viruses into marine mammals. The receptor specificity preference of the seal H7N7 and whale H13N9 isolates was for sialic acid α-2,3 galactose, similar to avian but not human influenza A viruses [49], and this correlates with the receptors present in seal and whale lungs. The seal H4N5 virus, but not the seal H7N7 virus, could experimentally replicate in the intestinal tract of ducks [48]. Serologic studies of the incidence of influenza A serum antibodies in marine mammals from different regions of the world have produced varying results, ranging from zero or low incidence in some studies to a cumulative 36% (28/77, primarily against H3) in Caspian seals sampled over an 8-year period. This suggests that influenza infection of diverse marine mammal populations occurs sporadically from avian sources and, when it occurs, sometimes but not always becomes enzootic.

Some seals in the Caspian Sea study and also in a study in Uruguay were seropositive for influenza B virus, and in 1999 influenza B virus was isolated from a juvenile harbor seal stranded along the Netherlands coast [50]. The HA1 sequence of that isolate was identical to that of the human influenza B/Argentina/4105/95 strain. Testing of 971 banked Netherlands seal sera produced the estimate that 0.5–2% of that wild seal population had experienced influenza B infection since 1995, but none were detected from before 1995. Influenza B virus was thought to be restricted to humans. The manner of its introduction into seals is unknown, but it persisted in that population at a low level for 5 years and thus seals can be an animal reservoir for influenza B viruses. Whether it still persists is unknown.

Influenza virus isolations from marine mammals have been obtained in association with epizootic respiratory disease characterized by necrotizing bronchopneumonia, mass strandings, and high mortality. To these it is tempting to ascribe a causative role for influenza, but that has not been established. Viruses were isolated from lung, hilar lymph node, and brain tissues. The seals with influenza B in the Netherlands suffered respiratory disease but this could not conclusively be attributed to influenza rather than lungworm. Seals experimentally infected with the H7N7 isolate produced mild respiratory signs, pneumonitis, and eye infections but in general were not affected as severely as animals involved in the 1979–1980 epizootic. Seals experimentally infected with the H4N5 isolate shed virus but showed no overt disease signs or lung lesions. Thus, the pathogenicity of influenza viruses in marine mammals is uncertain, because the contribution of co-infections analogous to secondary bacterial complications in humans and horses, or contribution of other environmental factors, is not understood.

Acknowledgments

Any views expressed in the Work by contributors employed by the United States government at the time of writing do not necessarily represent the views of the United States government, and the contributor's contribution to the Work is not meant to serve as an official endorsement of any statement to the extent that such statement may conflict with any official position of the United States government.

References

1. Daly JM, MacRae S, Newton JR, Wattrang E, Elton DM. Equine influenza: a review of an unpredictable virus. Vet J. 2011;189(1):7–14.
2. Morens DM, Taubenberger JK. Historical thoughts on influenza viral ecosystems, or behold a pale horse, dead dogs, failing fowl, and sick swine. Influenza Other Respir Viruses. 2010;4(6):327–37.
3. Sovinova O, Tumova B, Pouska F, Nemec J. Isolation of a virus causing respiratory disease in horses. Acta Virol. 1958;2(1):52–61.
4. Waddell GH, Teigland MB, Sigel MM. A new influenza virus associated with equine respiratory disease. J Am Vet Med Assoc. 1963;143:587–90.
5. Laver WG, Webster RG. Studies on the origin of pandemic influenza. 3. Evidence implicating duck and equine influenza viruses as possible progenitors of the Hong Kong strain of human influenza. Virology. 1973;51(2):383–91.
6. Bean WJ, Schell M, Katz J, Kawaoka Y, Naeve C, Gorman O, et al. Evolution of the H3 influenza virus hemagglutinin from human and nonhuman hosts. J Virol. 1992;66(2):1129–38.
7. Rogers GN, Pritchett TJ, Lane JL, Paulson JC. Differential sensitivity of human, avian, and equine influenza A viruses to a glycoprotein inhibitor of infection: selection of receptor specific variants. Virology. 1983;131(2):394–408.
8. Guo Y, Wang M, Kawaoka Y, Gorman O, Ito T, Saito T, et al. Characterization of a new avian-like influenza A virus from horses in China. Virology. 1992;188(1):245–55.
9. Landolt GA, Townsend HGG, Lunn DP. Equine influenza infection. In: Sellon DC, Long MT, editors. Equine Infectious Diseases. St. Louis: Saunders; 2007. p. 124–33.
10. Glass K, Wood JL, Mumford JA, Jesset D, Grenfell BT. Modelling equine influenza 1: a stochastic model of within-yard epidemics. Epidemiol Infect. 2002;128(3):491–502.
11. Wattrang E, Jessett DM, Yates P, Fuxler L, Hannant D. Experimental infection of ponies with equine influenza A2 (H3N8) virus strains of different pathogenicity elicits varying interferon and interleukin-6 responses. Viral Immunol. 2003;16(1):57–67.
12. Kawaoka Y, Bean WJ, Webster RG. Evolution of the hemagglutinin of equine H3 influenza viruses. Virology. 1989;169(2):283–92.
13. Daly JM, Lai AC, Binns MM, Chambers TM, Barrandeguy M, Mumford JA. Antigenic and genetic evolution of equine H3N8 influenza A viruses. J Gen Virol. 1996;77(Pt 4):661–71.
14. Bryant NA, Rash AS, Russell CA, Ross J, Cooke A, Bowman S, et al. Antigenic and genetic variations in European and North American equine influenza virus strains (H3N8) isolated from 2006 to 2007. Vet Microbiol. 2009;138(1–2):41–52.
15. Murcia PR, Wood JL, Holmes EC. Genome-scale evolution and phylodynamics of equine H3N8 influenza A virus. J Virol. 2011;85(11):5312–22.
16. Koelle K, Khatri P, Kamradt M, Kepler TB. A two-tiered model for simulating the ecological and evolutionary dynamics of rapidly evolving viruses, with an application to influenza. J R Soc Interface. 2010;7(50):1257–74.

17. Endo A, Pecoraro R, Sugita S, Nerome K. Evolutionary pattern of the H 3 haemagglutinin of equine influenza viruses: multiple evolutionary lineages and frozen replication. Arch Virol. 1992;123(1–2):73–87.

18. Lewis NS, Daly JM, Russell CA, Horton DL, Skepner E, Bryant NA, et al. Antigenic and genetic evolution of equine influenza A (H3N8) virus from 1968 to 2007. J Virol. 2011;85(23):12742–9.

19. Park AW, Daly JM, Lewis NS, Smith DJ, Wood JL, Grenfell BT. Quantifying the impact of immune escape on transmission dynamics of influenza. Science. 2009; 326(5953):726–8.

20. Suzuki Y, Ito T, Suzuki T, Holland RE Jr, Chambers TM, Kiso M, et al. Sialic acid species as a determinant of the host range of influenza A viruses. J Virol. 2000;74(24): 11825–31.

21. Ito T, Kawaoka Y, Ohira M, Takakuwa H, Yasuda J, Kida H, et al. Replacement of internal protein genes, with the exception of the matrix, in equine 1 viruses by equine 2 influenza virus genes during evolution in nature. J Vet Med Sci. 1999;61(8):987–9.

22. Webster RG, Bean WJ, Gorman OT, Chambers TM, Kawaoka Y. Evolution and ecology of influenza A viruses. Microbiol Rev. 1992;56(1):152–79.

23. Morens DM, Taubenberger JK. An avian outbreak associated with panzootic equine influenza in 1872: an early example of highly pathogenic avian influenza? Influenza Other Respir Viruses. 2010;4(6):373–7.

24. Obenauer JC, Denson J, Mehta PK, Su X, Mukatira S, Finkelstein DB, et al. Large-scale sequence analysis of avian influenza isolates. Science. 2006;311(5767): 1576–80.

25. Kawaoka Y. Equine H7N7 influenza A viruses are highly pathogenic in mice without adaptation: potential use as an animal model. J Virol. 1991;65(7):3891–4.

26. Shinya K, Watanabe S, Ito T, Kasai N, Kawaoka Y. Adaptation of an H7N7 equine influenza A virus in mice. J Gen Virol. 2007;88(Pt 2):547–53.

27. Paillot R, Hannant D, Kydd JH, Daly JM. Vaccination against equine influenza: quid novi? Vaccine. 2006;24 (19):4047–61.

28. Nelson KM, Schram BR, McGregor MW, Sheoran AS, Olsen CW, Lunn DP. Local and systemic isotype-specific antibody responses to equine influenza virus infection versus conventional vaccination. Vaccine. 1998;16(13): 1306–13.

29. Hannant D, Mumford JA, Jessett DM. Duration of circulating antibody and immunity following infection with equine influenza virus. Vet Rec. 1988;122(6): 125–8.

30. Quinlivan M, Zamarin D, Garcia-Sastre A, Cullinane A, Chambers T, Palese P. Attenuation of equine influenza viruses through truncations of the NS1 protein. J Virol. 2005;79(13):8431–9.

31. Paillot R, Kydd JH, Sindle T, Hannant D, Edlund Toulemonde C, Audonnet JC, et al. Antibody and IFN-gamma responses induced by a recombinant canarypox vaccine and challenge infection with equine influenza virus. Vet Immunol Immunopathol. 2006;112(3–4): 225–33.

32. Mumford JA, Hannant D, Jessett DM. Experimental infection of ponies with equine influenza (H3N8) viruses by intranasal inoculation or exposure to aerosols. Equine Vet J. 1990;22(2):93–8.

33. Crawford PC, Dubovi EJ, Castleman WL, Stephenson I, Gibbs EP, Chen L, et al. Transmission of equine influenza virus to dogs. Science. 2005;310(5747):482–5.

34. Yamanaka T, Nemoto M, Tsujimura K, Kondo T, Matsumura T. Interspecies transmission of equine influenza virus (H3N8) to dogs by close contact with experimentally infected horses. Vet Microbiol. 2009;139(3–4): 351–5.

35. Rivailler P, Perry IA, Jang Y, Davis CT, Chen LM, Dubovi EJ, et al. Evolution of canine and equine influenza (H3N8) viruses co-circulating between 2005 and 2008. Virology. 2010;408(1):71–9.

36. Quintana AM, Hussey SB, Burr EC, Pecoraro HL, Annis KM, Rao S, et al. Evaluation of infectivity of a canine lineage H3N8 influenza A virus in ponies and in primary equine respiratory epithelial cells. Am J Vet Res. 2011;72(8):1071–8.

37. Castleman WL, Powe JR, Crawford PC, Gibbs EPJ, Dubovi EJ, Donis RO, et al. Canine H3N8 Influenza Virus Infection in Dogs and Mice. Vet Pathol. 2010;47 (3):507–17.

38. Song D, Kang B, Lee C, Jung K, Ha G, Kang D, et al. Transmission of avian influenza virus (H3N2) to dogs. Emerg Infect Dis. 2008;14(5):741–6.

39. Songserm T, Amonsin A, Jam-on R, Sae-Heng N, Pariyothorn N, Payungporn S, et al. Fatal avian influenza A H5N1 in a dog. Emerg Infect Dis. 2006;12(11): 1744–7.

40. Lin D, Sun S, Du L, Ma J, Fan L, Pu J, et al. Natural and experimental infection of dogs with pandemic H1N1/2009 influenza virus. J Gen Virol. 2012;93(Pt 1):119–23.

41. Song D, Moon HJ, An DJ, Jeoung HY, Kim H, Yeom MJ, et al. A novel reassortant canine H3N1 influenza virus between pandemic H1N1 and canine H3N2 influenza viruses in Korea. J Gen Virol. 2012;93(Pt 3):551–4.

42. Paniker CK, Nair CM. Infection with A2 Hong Kong influenza virus in domestic cats. Bull World Health Organ. 1970;43(6):859–62.

43. Keawcharoen J, Oraveerakul K, Kuiken T, Fouchier RA, Amonsin A, Payungporn S, et al. Avian influenza H5N1 in tigers and leopards. Emerg Infect Dis. 2004;10 (12):2189–91.

44. Kuiken T, Rimmelzwaan G, van Riel D, van Amerongen G, Baars M, Fouchier R, et al. Avian H5N1 influenza in cats. Science. 2004;306(5694):241.

45. Sponseller BA, Strait E, Jergens A, Trujillo J, Harmon K, Koster L, et al. Influenza A pandemic (H1N1) 2009 virus infection in domestic cat. Emerg Infect Dis. 2010;16(3):534–7.

46. Lvov DK, Zdanov VM, Sazonov AA, Braude NA, Vladimirtceva EA, Agafonova LV, et al. Comparison of influenza viruses isolated from man and from whales. Bull World Health Organ. 1978;56(6):923–30.

47. Geraci JR, St Aubin DJ, Barker IK, Webster RG, Hinshaw VS, Bean WJ, et al. Mass mortality of harbor seals: pneumonia associated with influenza A virus. Science. 1982;215(4536):1129–31.

48. Hinshaw VS, Bean WJ, Webster RG, Rehg JE, Fiorelli P, Early G, et al. Are seals frequently infected with avian influenza viruses? J Virol. 1984;51(3):863–5.

49. Ito T, Kawaoka Y, Nomura A, Otsuki K. Receptor specificity of influenza A viruses from sea mammals correlates with lung sialyloligosaccharides in these animals. J Vet Med Sci. 1999;61(8):955–8.

50. Osterhaus AD, Rimmelzwaan GF, Martina BE, Bestebroer TM, Fouchier RA. Influenza B virus in seals. Science. 2000;288(5468):1051–3.

51. Kumar S, Tamura K, Nei M. MEGA3: integrated software for Molecular Evolutionary Genetics Analysis and sequence alignment. Brief Bioinform. 2004;5(2):150–63.

14 Emergence and evolution of the 1918, 1957, 1968, and 2009 pandemic virus strains

Taia T. Wang[1] and Peter Palese[2,3]

[1]Laboratory of Molecular Genetics and Immunology, Rockefeller University, New York, NY, USA

[2]Department of Microbiology, Icahn School of Medicine at Mount Sinai, New York, NY, USA

[3]Department of Medicine, Icahn School of Medicine at Mount Sinai, New York, NY, USA

Definition of pandemic influenza disease

Designation of pandemic scale human disease is classically determined by the existing prevalence and geographic spread of a specific infectious agent [1]. Because influenza viruses cause acute illness (~5–7 days) and spread is typically restricted by climate, the prevalence and regional distribution of influenza disease at any one time is highly variable [2]. Therefore, the word "pandemic," when applied to influenza viruses, is often used to describe an ongoing epidemic of unusually large proportion, or it may be used in a predictive context to identify potential pandemic strains based on antigenic novelty of the virus's hemagglutinin protein.

Risk for pandemic influenza disease is high when a circulating virus meets three criteria:
1. The virus causes human disease.
2. The virus demonstrates sustained human-to-human transmission.
3. The virus expresses a hemagglutinin that is antigenically novel for most or all of the population.

These three criteria have defined which influenza outbreaks are classified, historically, as pandemics. For example, the disease epidemic caused by the reemergence of H1N1 viruses in 1977 does not meet this classic definition because a majority of the population had pre-existing immunity against the strain (see the section on re-emergence of H1N1 viruses in 1977).

In response to the 2009 pandemic, the World Health Organization (WHO) developed updated guidelines that define six distinct phases of an influenza pandemic; each phase is associated with recommended actions that can be taken to reduce further spread of a pandemic strain, including enhancing disease surveillance, limiting travel and developing new vaccines [3].

Background

More than a dozen human influenza virus pandemics are thought to have occurred since the start of the sixteenth century [4]. The majority of these were identified from written accounts of large-scale disease epidemics that match the clinical phenotype and epidemiologic patterns commonly associated with influenza disease. There are serologic data and other documentation supporting the occurrence of a pandemic caused by an H3 subtype virus beginning in 1889 – this 1889 influenza outbreak is the first for which serologic evidence exists [5]. Viruses exist only for the four most recent pandemic strains of 1918, 1957, 1968, and 2009 (Figure 14.1a). While the three most recent pandemic viruses were isolated from

Textbook of Influenza, Second Edition. Edited by Robert G. Webster, Arnold S. Monto, Thomas J. Braciale, and Robert A. Lamb.
© 2013 John Wiley & Sons, Ltd. Published 2013 by John Wiley & Sons, Ltd.

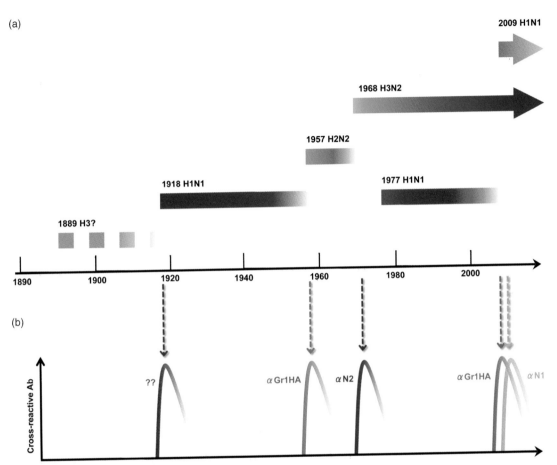

Figure 14.1. Human influenza A viruses in the human population. (a) Influenza pandemics occurred in 1889 (H3, likely), 1918 (H1), 1957 (H2), 1968 (H3), and 2009 (H1). Pandemics were followed by circulation of strains according to seasonality for the duration indicated. Color shading within bars represents antigenic drift of seasonal virus strains. The line representing circulation of the 1889 pandemic virus is broken, indicating uncertainty around the subtype and duration of circulation of this strain. (b) Representation of elevated population immunity against the stalk of group 1 hemagglutinins (Gr1HA) (group 1 hemagglutinin subtypes: H1, H2, H5, H6, H8, H9, H11, H12, H13, H16, and H17) that may have resulted in the extinction of seasonal H1N1 following the 1957 pandemic; elevated immunity against the N2 may have caused the extinction of H2N2 following the 1968 pandemic; elevated immunity against both the stalk of group 1 hemagglutinins and the N1 protein may have resulted in extinction of seasonal H1N1 following the pandemic of 2009.

humans, the 1918 virus was recreated by reverse genetics [6,7].

Of the 17 known hemagglutinin and the nine (possibly 10) known neuraminidase subtypes [8], only viruses expressing H1, H2, or H3 and N1 or N2 subtype proteins are known to have caused pandemic human disease. Other viral subtypes emerge only spo-

radically in humans and it is not known whether they are, in fact, capable of adapting to cause sustained human disease.

Immunity against influenza viruses is largely mediated by neutralizing antibodies, which are specific for the hemagglutinin protein. The antigenic similarity of two viruses and the cross protective immunity that

219

Table 14.1. Percentage identity between amino acids of HA1 proteins.

	JP/1957 (H2)	HK/1968 (H3)	CA/2009 (H1)	NJ/1976 (H1)	USSR/1977 (H1)
BM/1918*	58	35	81	89	82
JP/1957*		33			
HK/1968*			34		
CA/2009*				87	71

Reference strains: A/Brevig Mission/1/1918 (BM/1918), A/Japan/305/1957 (JP/1957), A/Hong Kong/1/1968 (HK/1968), A/New Jersey/11/1976 (NJ/1976), A/USSR/90/1977 (USSR/1977), A/California/04/2009 (CA/2009).
Sequence identity can indicate antigenic similarity: viruses with greater amino acid identity between HA1 proteins can often provide cross protective immunity. For example exposure to either the 1918 or the 1976 H1 hemagglutinin proteins provides protection against the 2009 H1 pandemic virus strain in mice [9]. In contrast, protection against the 1957 H2 or the 1968 H3 pandemic viruses was not afforded by exposure to the 1918 H1 strain; these three strains are more distinct at the levels of the HA1 amino acid sequences and protein structures. Pandemic virus strains are marked with an asterisk at left.

can be elicited by exposure to one of the viruses can be predicted, to a degree, by the percentage identity between amino acids of the hemagglutinin subunit 1 (HA1) of the expressed hemagglutinins. For example, immunity against the 2009 H1 pandemic virus can be conferred by exposure to either the 1918 or 1976 H1 viruses, which have relatively similar HA1 subunits [9]. In contrast, exposure to the 1918 virus does not provide protection against the 1957 H2 or the 1968 H3 pandemic strains, which express HA1 proteins with lower identity at the amino acid and structural levels (Table 14.1). Structural elements and antigenicity of the HA1 protein, which are not factored in when comparing amino acid sequences alone, can be assessed in the laboratory using the hemagglutination inhibition assay.

Pandemic influenza viruses, in general, cause significantly more morbidity and mortality than do seasonal strains. This is largely attributable to a lack of population immunity against pandemic strains; however, other genetic factors may also be present that increase virulence of a given strain.

Determinants of evolution and emergence of pandemic influenza virus strains

Genetic evolution of influenza viruses occurs by one of two distinct mechanisms: (i) reassortment (for-merly referred to as "recombination") of viral RNA segments, or, (ii) fixation of errors in the genome that occur during transcriptional processing. There has been no compelling evidence for homologous recombination of influenza gene segments [10].

Evolution resulting from gene segment reassortment

Reassortment of influenza virus segments to generate a novel virus occurs when a host cell is infected by more than one distinct virus strains. Co-infection of cells by mammalian and avian viruses is unusual due to preference for different binding cofactors. Avian viruses bind more readily to sialic acid connected to galactose by an $\alpha2,3$-linkage, whereas human viruses exhibit preference for $\alpha2,6$-linked sialic acid. Affinity of the viral hemagglutinin for either $\alpha2,3$- or $\alpha2,6$-linked sialic acid is an important determinant of species tropism. Swine tissue is hypothesized to be a hospitable environment for reassortment of influenza gene segments due to general expression of both $\alpha2,6$- and $\alpha2,3$-linked sialic acids, thus enabling infection of cells by both human and avian viruses. Co-infection of a host cell by two strains may result in any of 256 (2^8) novel combinations of eight RNA segments (254 with exclusion of parental combinations) [2].

Genetic reassortment can result in the production of a human virus expressing a novel hemagglutinin glycoprotein; this phenomenon is termed "antigenic shift." Such shift events were seen in association with the influenza pandemics of 1957, 1968, and 2009. The 1918 virus may also be a product of a shift event, but this is not known with certainty, as the parental strains have not yet been identified.

Evolution resulting from fixation of genomic mutations

The polymerase of influenza viruses is a low fidelity complex lacking exonuclease activity, which generates a high rate of transcriptional mutation relative to other RNA polymerases [2]. Under neutral conditions, mutations in the influenza A virus genome occur at a rate of approximately 2.0×10^{-6} mutations per site per infectious cycle [11]. Because of the rapid kinetics of influenza virus replication, mutations can readily be selected for, or against, based on a variety of extrinsic sources of selective pressure such as pre-existing host immunity, use of antiviral drugs, epistatic interaction between mutations, or change in host environment. In addition, mutations may simply become fixed because they do not result in significantly decreased viral fitness [12]. Human influenza A viruses are exposed to considerable evolutionary pressure (relative to viruses infecting other species) and undergo fixed genetic change at a rate of approximately 1×10^{-3} to 8×10^{-3} base substitutions per site per year, depending on the segment [13,14]. The rate of change in nonhuman viruses varies and is lowest in strains hosted by animals with a short lifespan, which are less likely to be infected by multiple different influenza A viruses.

The rates of evolutionary change amongst the eight influenza RNAs are highest in the HA, NA, and M,

which code for envelope proteins, and in the NS segment, which codes for the protein functioning in antagonism of the host antiviral–interferon system. The frequency of fixed missense mutations is generally highest in the HA gene due to evolutionary pressure towards the selection of antigenically novel virus strains.

Fixed structural change in the viral hemagglutinin is called "antigenic drift" and occurs over time secondary to transcriptional error in combination with immune selection. Repeated exposure of a population to influenza viruses via infection (and possibly vaccination) results in continuous remodeling of antibody specificities that drive the progressive antigenic drift of circulating viruses. Neutralizing antibodies select for mutations in antigenic sites that are within the globular head (HA1) of the hemagglutinin.

Emergence of novel virus strains

Distinct lineages of influenza A viruses have become stably adapted to either avian or mammalian species. For a novel human virus to emerge, it must transition from a nonhuman host species or undergo reassortment with a nonhuman strain, resulting in antigenic shift. Some of the determinants of viral host switch between avian and mammalian species have been identified (Table 14.2; for a review of viral fitness factors see Chapters 8–10).

Extinction of seasonal strains

When pandemic viruses emerge, existing seasonal strains often disappear from the human population (Figure 14.1a). Though this interesting phenomenon

Table 14.2. Examples of markers of pathogenicity/increased virulence in mammals.

Segment	Disease increased in mammals	Reference
1: PB2	Mutations associated with determination of host tropism	42,43
2: PB1	Expression of PB1-F2	44
4: HA	Antigenic novelty and α2,6-linked sialic acid receptor specificity	45–47
6: NA	Neuraminidase inhibitor resistance	48
8: NS	Robust interferon antagonist activity	28,49,50

has not been explained definitively, it is possible that the abrupt genesis of population immunity elicited during a pandemic results in the suppression and, ultimately, the extinction of existing seasonal viruses. The specificity of antibodies that are both capable of being boosted by the pandemic virus and of extinguishing existing seasonal strains varies depending on the specific pandemic and seasonal viruses involved. The 1957 H2N2 virus would likely have boosted population immunity against the conserved stalk of group 1 hemagglutinins, which include the H1 subtype; this might have led to the disappearance of seasonal H1N1 virus strains. The 1968 pandemic virus boosted immunity against the N2 protein, which might have caused seasonal H2N2 viruses to be eliminated. Re-emerged H1N1 viruses in 1977 would not have boosted antibodies against the hemagglutinin or neuraminidase of H3N2 viruses; therefore H3N2 and H1N1 viruses co-circulated, seasonally, until 2009. Antibodies generated during the 2009 H1N1 pandemic that targeted conserved regions of the H1 stalk and the N1 protein likely caused seasonal H1N1 viruses to disappear (Figure 14.1b) [15,16].

The 1918, 1957, 1968, and 2009 influenza virus pandemics

Development of nucleotide sequencing technology has enabled genetic analysis of the most recent pandemic strains. Analysis is limited by a paucity of available sequences from pre-1975 avian H1 and H2 subtype viruses; however, increased surveillance efforts over the last decade enabled a detailed analysis of the 2009 pandemic strain. In all cases, it is unknown how many reassortment events lead to the formation of pandemic viruses and how long the strains existed and adapted in the human reservoir prior to causing pandemic disease. See reference [17] to review methods that can be used to study the phylogenetics of influenza viruses.

The H1N1 "Spanish" influenza pandemic of 1918

The influenza pandemic of 1918 was the single most deadly pandemic on record, with an associated global mortality in excess of 50 million people [18]. Notably, this pandemic occurred in three separate waves

between 1918 and 1919. The final two waves are often associated with a mortality rate of greater than 2.5%, which is substantially higher than the rate of <1% that is typically ascribed to seasonal influenza outbreaks. While viral pneumonia caused many deaths during this pandemic, a majority of deaths occurred secondary to bacterial co-infections in the pre-antibiotic era. Epidemiologically, the 1918 pandemic was unusual for causing elevated mortality in young healthy adults in addition to persons at extremes of age; this is often referred to as the "W-shaped" mortality curve of the 1918 pandemic. After 1919, seasonal H1N1 strains circulated for nearly four decades until being replaced by H2N2 subtype viruses during the pandemic of 1957 (Figure 14.1a).

The development of reverse genetics enabled researchers to recreate the 1918 virus strain and to characterize the virus in *in vitro* and *in vivo* models of infection [6,7]. Experiments done by reassortment of the 1918 virus with seasonal H1N1 strains have specifically identified the HA, NA, and the PB1 genes as significantly increasing virulence of the 1918 strain [19]. The 1918 virus does not code for a polybasic cleavage site, which defines highly pathogenic avian influenza viruses.

Sequencing of the 1918 virus was accomplished through isolation of viral nucleic acid from preserved lung tissue taken from victims of the pandemic [20]. As sequence data from viruses predating 1918 are not yet available, the genetic origins of this pandemic strain cannot be known with certainty. Some investigators have noted that the 1918 virus shares genomic signatures with avian viruses [20–22]. Smith et al. [23] suggest that the virus is derived from a mixture of human, swine, and avian viral segments that emerged as a consequence of multiple reassortment events over several years.

In the early 1930s, the first influenza viruses were isolated from humans and from swine. These seasonal and swine H1N1 strains were found to share genes with the recreated 1918 virus; unfortunately, no sequences are currently available from other human viruses emerging prior to 1933. This paucity of data limits the utility of phylogenetic analysis of viruses emerging prior to the mid-twentieth century. At this time, we cannot unambiguously determine whether early strains with genetic similarity represent separate viral lineages that may have circulated concurrently

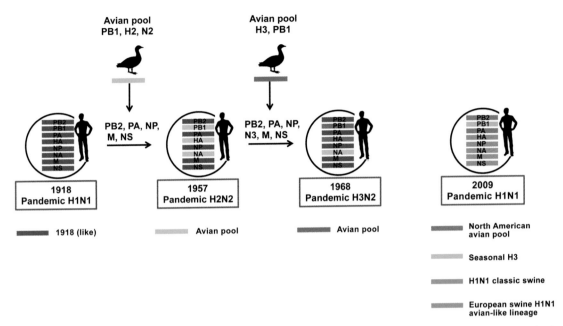

Figure 14.2. Proposed genetic origins of the 1918, 1957, 1968, and 2009 pandemic influenza virus strains. The genetic origins of the 1918 pandemic strain are not known with certainty. The 1957 and 1968 pandemic viruses incorporated genes from human seasonal viruses and avian viruses. The 2009 pandemic virus was derived from swine-adapted strains.

during the 1918 pandemic [23], or whether similar strains emerged sequentially and are, in fact, members of the same lineage (Figure 14.2).

The H2N2 "Asian" pandemic virus of 1957

In February of 1957, a virus with novel surface glycoproteins was identified in residents of southern China. Over the following months, the virus spread through Singapore, Hong Kong, and Japan, followed by the United States and the United Kingdom by October of that year. A second wave of the Asian pandemic began in January of 1958. Ultimately, this pandemic was the second most severe on record, causing approximately 70 000 excess deaths in the United States. The 1957 virus caused a similar disease phenotype to that seen in 1918; however, elevated rates of mortality in young adults did not occur.

The 1957 H2N2 virus was derived from the circulating H1N1 strain with substitution of the HA, NA, and PB1 segments for avian virus-like segments (Figure 14.2) [24,25]. Within 2 years of emergence, the pandemic H2N2 virus became a seasonal strain and circulated continuously until being replaced by H3N2 viruses during the pandemic of 1968 (Figure 14.1a).

The H3N2 "Hong Kong" pandemic virus of 1968

The third pandemic of the twentieth century began in July of 1968, with the isolation of a novel H3N2 virus from residents of Hong Kong. The virus was associated with increased disease during the 1968–1969 and 1969–1970 influenza seasons; ultimately, the 1968 pandemic was relatively mild, causing an estimated 33 000 excess deaths in the United States. It has been suggested that the lower mortality during this pandemic resulted from pre-existing antibodies against the N2 of the H2N2 seasonal strain that conferred some protection against the 1968 virus in older people [26]. Though the 1968 pandemic was relatively mild, seasonal H3N2 viruses circulating since have caused significantly more morbidity and mortality than co-circulating H1N1 strains [27].

The H3N2 pandemic virus incorporated two novel avian virus-like RNA segments, HA and PB1, in combination with six segments from the existing seasonal H2N2 virus (Figure 14.2) [28]. H3N2 viruses have circulated continuously as seasonal strains since the 1968 pandemic (Figure 14.1a).

The pandemic virus that never was: An outbreak of swine-origin H1N1 virus in 1976

In 1976 a novel swine H1N1 virus was found to be circulating amongst recruits at the Fort Dix army base in New Jersey. The virus was genetically similar to viruses that had been stably circulating in swine from the region [29]. Concern that the novel strain had potential to cause pandemic disease on the scale of that seen in 1918 prompted the US government to enact a mass-vaccination campaign; in all, 40 million people were vaccinated. Though human-to-human transmission of the novel H1N1 virus did take place, ultimately, the 1976 virus did not spread beyond the Fort Dix army base. Hundreds on the base were infected (resulting mostly in asymptomatic disease) and one fatality was attributed to the 1976 strain. Vaccination of millions of people in 1976–1977 exposed a very low rate of a previously unseen vaccine side effect – Guillain–Barré syndrome, a paralyzing autoimmune disorder which can be fatal.

Events around the emergence of the antigenically novel virus strain in 1976 revealed the degree to which influenza viruses remained a mystery. It became clear that antigenic novelty and some degree of transmissibility between humans do not determine the ability of a virus to cause widespread disease.

Reemergence of H1N1 viruses in 1977

In 1977, the H1N1 virus strain that had been in circulation just prior to the 1957 pandemic re-emerged in the human reservoir. The high degree of sequence identity between the 1950 seasonal strain and the 1977 H1N1 virus suggests that the virus may have been released back into humans from a frozen stock [30]. Because much of the population had prior exposure to the H1N1 strain, a majority of disease

occurred in those under 20 years of age. The re-emerged H1N1 virus circulated seasonally with H3N2 viruses until being replaced by the novel H1N1 pandemic virus of 2009 (Figure 14.1a).

The swine-origin H1N1 pandemic virus of 2009

In February of 2009, an antigenically novel H1N1 virus was found to be circulating in residents of La Gloria, Veracruz, Mexico. Evidence suggests that the virus may have circulated in humans for some months prior to its detection [31]. Frequent international air travel enabled the virus to spread rapidly across the globe. Whereas prior pandemic viruses crossed continents over a period of many months, the 2009 H1N1 virus spread from the initial documented cases in Mexico to 74 countries spanning every continent within 5 weeks. On 11 June 2009, the WHO declared the official start of a novel influenza pandemic.

The 2009 pandemic virus was highly transmissible, but caused relatively mild disease for a pandemic strain. The virus caused a disproportionately high rate of infection in people under the age of 65 and was remarkable for its ability to transmit during a period of warmer weather in the Northern Hemisphere where influenza viruses usually circulate according to a strict seasonal pattern. Several virulence factors of the 2009 pandemic virus have been suggested, including the M, HA, and PB2 gene segments [32–34].

The 2009 pandemic strain was derived from viruses that were stably adapted to swine hosts. It incorporated segments from two distinct virus lineages: six of the segments, PB1, PB2, PA, HA, NP, and NS were from the North American triple reassortant swine lineage while the NA and M segments were from the European avian-like swine lineage. The PB2 and PA of triple reassortant origin were derived from the North American avian lineage, the PB1 from the human H3N2 A/Sydney/5/97-like strain, and the HA, NS and NP segments were from the classical H1N1 swine lineage (Figure 14.3) [31].

H3N2 subtype viruses dominated the 2010–2011 and 2011–2012 influenza seasons, while the previously circulating seasonal H1N1 strains disappeared from the human reservoir. The disappearance of seasonal H1N1 viruses and the suppression of the novel H1N1 strain following the pandemic may have resulted from a sudden, large-scale increase in popu-

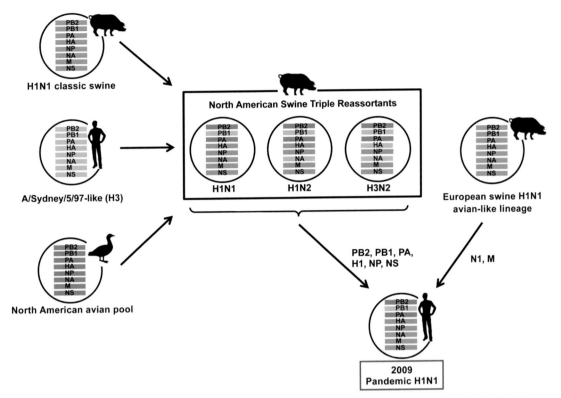

Figure 14.3. Genetic origins of the 2009 pandemic virus strain. The 2009 pandemic virus was composed completely of segments from swine-adapted virus strains. The European avian-like lineage was first isolated from swine in the 1979. In 1998, the first North American swine "triple reassortant" viruses were isolated and consisted of segments from North American avian, classical swine, and a circulating human H3N2 strain (A/Sydney/5/97-like).

lation immunity against conserved regions in the H1 stalk and the N1 protein (Figure 14.1b) [15,16].

Future influenza pandemics

Without the development of vaccines that can protect against novel virus strains, we will almost certainly see influenza pandemics in the future. How can we identify viruses with the potential to cause pandemic disease? Using established laboratory methods, we can identify antigenic novelty of the expressed hemagglutinin protein; however, this is only one requisite characteristic of a pandemic strain. The molecular correlates of influenza virus fitness in humans and determinants of stable host switch are topics of active research and discovery. Several genetic markers of viruses with increased tropism for mammalian cells have been identified, but we cannot yet reliably predict which viruses will be pathogenic, virulent, or transmissible in humans (Table 14.2). It is hypothesized that an H2 virus may cause the next influenza pandemic because humans have not been exposed to H2 protein in over 40 years.

Avian influenza viruses as potential human pathogens

Of the 17 known subtypes of hemagglutinin, all except the recently discovered H17 have been found

225

in avian populations. H5, H7, and H9 subtype avian influenza viruses are the primary subtypes that cause sporadic human infections. These subtypes are pathogenic in rare humans who are typically persons at high risk for inhaling large inoculum doses due to direct contact with infected poultry. As with infections caused by human viruses, avian viruses can cause a spectrum of clinical disease severity ranging from subclinical to fatal. Poor clinical outcome may result from higher inoculum dose, host immunodeficiency, or lack of prior exposure to influenza viruses, which can confer cross-protective immunity [35].

Viruses stably adapted to avian species can become virulent and transmissible between mammals [36–38]. Still, despite probable centuries of exposure between humans and infected mammals and birds, only H1, H2, and H3 subtypes are known to have emerged as significant human pathogens. Other influenza virus subtypes may, in fact, be incapable of causing sustained disease in humans; this is not known with certainty. To lessen the disease burden caused by influenza viruses in the future, researchers are working toward the development of a universal influenza virus vaccine [39–41]. The development of such a vaccine could prevent future influenza pandemics and could, in fact, eliminate influenza viruses from the human reservoir.

References

1. Porta M, International Epidemiological Association. A Dictionary of Epidemiology. 5th ed. Oxford; New York: Oxford University Press; 2008. xxiv, 289 p.
2. Shaw M, Palese P. Othomyxoviridae: the viruses and their replication. In: Knipe D, Howley P, editors. Fields' Virology, 6th edn. Philadelphia, PA: Lippincott Williams & Wilkins; 2011.
3. World Health Organization. Pandemic influenza preparedness and response, World Health Organization guidance document. 2009. Available from: http://www.who.int/influenza/resources/documents/pandemic_guidance_04_2009/en/index.html (last accessed 6 February 2013).
4. Beveridge WIB. Influenza: the last great plague. London: Heinemann Educational Books Ltd; 1977.
5. Dowdle WR. Influenza A virus recycling revisited. Bull World Health Organ. 1999;77(10):820–8.
6. Fodor E, Devenish L, Engelhardt OG, Palese P, Brownlee GG, Garcia-Sastre A. Rescue of influenza A virus from recombinant DNA. J Virol. 1999;73(11):9679–82.
7. Tumpey TM, Basler CF, Aquilar PV, Zengg H, Solórzano A, Swayne DE, et al. Characterization of the reconstructed 1918 Spanish influenza pandemic virus. Science. 2005;310(5745):77–80.
8. Tong S, Li Y, Conrardy C, Castillo DA, Chen LM, Recuenco S, et al. A distinct lineage of influenza A virus from bats. Proc Natl Acad Sci U S A. 2012;109(11):4269–74.
9. Manicassamy B, Medina RA, Hai R, Tsibane T, Sterts S, Nistal-Villán E, et al. Protection of mice against lethal challenge with 2009 H1N1 influenza A virus by 1918-like and classical swine H1N1 based vaccines. PLoS Pathog. 2010;6(1):e1000745.
10. Boni MF, Smith GJ, Holmes EC, Vijaykrishna D. No evidence for intra-segment recombination of 2009 H1N1 influenza virus in swine. Gene. 2012;494(2):242–5.
11. Nobusawa E, Sato K. Comparison of the mutation rates of human influenza A and B viruses. J Virol. 2006;80(7):3675–8.
12. Taubenberger JK, Kash JC. Influenza virus evolution, host adaptation, and pandemic formation. Cell Host Microbe. 2010;7(6):440–51.
13. Rambaut A, Pybus OG, Nelson MI, Viboud C, Taubenberger JK, Holmes EC. The genomic and epidemiological dynamics of human influenza A virus. Nature. 2008;453(7195):615–9.
14. Chen R, Holmes EC. Avian influenza virus exhibits rapid evolutionary dynamics. Mol Biol Evol. 2006;23(12):2336–41.
15. Palese P, Wang TT. Why do influenza virus subtypes die out? A hypothesis. MBio. 2011;2(5).
16. Pica N, Hai R, Krammer F, Wang TT, Maamary J, Eggink D, et al. Hemagglutinin stalk antibodies elicited by the 2009 pandemic influenza virus as a mechanism for the extinction of seasonal H1N1 viruses. Proc Natl Acad Sci U S A. 2012;109(7):2573–8.
17. Smith GJ, Bahl J, Vijaykrishna D. Genetic analysis. Methods Mol Biol. 2012;865:207–27.
18. Johnson NP, Mueller J. Updating the accounts: global mortality of the 1918–1920 "Spanish" influenza pandemic. Bull Hist Med. 2002;76(1):105–15.
19. Pappas C, Aquilar PV, Basler CF, Solórzano A, Zeng H, Perrone LA, et al. Single gene reassortants identify a critical role for PB1, HA, and NA in the high virulence of the 1918 pandemic influenza virus. Proc Natl Acad Sci U S A. 2008;105(8):3064–9.
20. Taubenberger JK, Reid AH, Lourens RM, Wang R, Jin G, Fanning TG. Characterization of the 1918 influenza

virus polymerase genes. Nature. 2005;437(7060): 889–93.

21. Rabadan R, Levine AJ, Robins H. Comparison of avian and human influenza A viruses reveals a mutational bias on the viral genomes. J Virol. 2006;80(23): 11887–91.

22. Webster RG, Bean WJ, Gorman OT, Chambers TM, Kawaoka Y. Evolution and ecology of influenza A viruses. Microbiol Rev. 1992;56(1):152–79.

23. Smith GJ, Bahl J, Vijaykrishna D, Zhang J, Poon LL, Chen H, et al. Dating the emergence of pandemic influenza viruses. Proc Natl Acad Sci U S A. 2009;106(28): 11709–12.

24. Scholtissek C, Rohde W, Von Hoyningen V, Rott R. On the origin of the human influenza virus subtypes H2N2 and H3N2. Virology. 1978;87(1):13–20.

25. Kawaoka Y, Krauss S, Webster RG. Avian-to-human transmission of the PB1 gene of influenza A viruses in the 1957 and 1968 pandemics. J Virol. 1989;63(11): 4603–8.

26. Schulman JL, Kilbourne ED. The antigenic relationship of the neuraminidase of Hong Kong virus to that of other human strains of influenza A virus. Bull World Health Organ. 1969;41(3):425–8.

27. Subbarao K, Swayne D, Olsen CW. Epidemiology and control of human and animal influenza. In: Kawaoka Y, editor. Influenza Virology: Current Topics. Norfolk, UK: Caister Academic Press; 2006. p. 229–80.

28. Obenauer JC, Denson J, Mehta PK, Su X, Mukatira S, Finkelstein DB, et al. Large-scale sequence analysis of avian influenza isolates. Science. 2006;311(5767):1576–80.

29. Palese P, Schulman JL. RNA pattern of "swine" influenza virus isolated from man is similar to those of other swine influenza viruses. Nature. 1976;263(5577):528–30.

30. Nakajima K, Desselberger U, Palese P. Recent human influenza A (H1N1) viruses are closely related genetically to strains isolated in 1950. Nature. 1978;274(5669): 334–9.

31. Smith GJ, Vijaykrishna D, Bahl J, Lycett SJ, Worobey M, Pybus OG, et al. Origins and evolutionary genomics of the 2009 swine-origin H1N1 influenza A epidemic. Nature. 2009;459(7250):1122–5.

32. Chou YY, Albrecht RA, Pica N, Lowen AC, Richt JA, Garcia-Sastre A, et al. The M segment of the 2009 new pandemic H1N1 influenza virus is critical for its high transmission efficiency in the guinea pig model. J Virol. 2011;85(21):11235–41.

33. Lakdawala SS, Lamirande EW, Suquitan AL Jr, Wang W, Santos CP, Vogel L, et al. Eurasian-origin gene segments contribute to the transmissibility, aerosol release, and morphology of the 2009 pandemic H1N1 influenza virus. PLoS Pathog. 2011;7(12):e1002443.

34. Zhang Y, Zhang Q, Gao Y, He X, Kong H, Jiang Y, et al. Key molecular factors in HA and PB2 contribute to the efficient transmission of the 2009 H1N1 pandemic influenza virus. J Virol. 2012;86:9666–74.

35. Palese P, Wang TT. H5N1 influenza viruses: facts, not fear. Proc Natl Acad Sci U S A. 2012;109(7):2211–3.

36. Burgos S, Burgos SA. Reports of avian influenza H5N1 in cats and dogs. Int J Poult Sci. 2007;6(12):1003–5.

37. Kuiken T, Rimmelzwaan G, van Riel D, van Amerongen G, Baars M, Fouchier R, et al. Avian H5N1 influenza in cats. Science. 2004;306(5694):241.

38. Herfst S, Schrauwen EJ, Linster M, Chutinimitkul S, de Wit E, Munster VJ, et al. Airborne transmission of influenza A/H5N1 virus between ferrets. Science. 2012;336(6088):1534–41.

39. Steel J, Lowen AC, Wang TT, Yondoloa M, Gao Q, Havye K, et al. Influenza virus vaccine based on the conserved hemagglutinin stalk domain. MBio. 2010;1(1).

40. Wang TT, Tan GS, Hai R, Pica N, Ngai L, Ekiert DC, et al. Vaccination with a synthetic peptide from the influenza virus hemagglutinin provides protection against distinct viral subtypes. Proc Natl Acad Sci U S A. 2010;107(44):18979–84.

41. Wei CJ, Boyington JC, McTamney PM, Kong WP, Pearce MB, Xu L, et al. Induction of broadly neutralizing H1N1 influenza antibodies by vaccination. Science. 2010;329(5995):1060–4.

42. Hatta M, Gao P, Halfmann P, Kawaoka Y. Molecular basis for high virulence of Hong Kong H5N1 influenza A viruses. Science. 2001;293(5536):1840–2.

43. Gabriel G, Herwig A, Klenk HD. Interaction of polymerase subunit PB2 and NP with importin alpha1 is a determinant of host range of influenza A virus. PLoS Pathog. 2008;4(2):e11.

44. Conenello GM, Zamarin D, Perrone LA, Tumpey T, Palese P. A single mutation in the PB1-F2 of H5N1 (HK/97) and 1918 influenza A viruses contributes to increased virulence. PLoS Pathog. 2007;3(10): 1414–21.

45. Schulman JL, Kilbourne ED. Independent variation in nature of hemagglutinin and neuraminidase antigens of influenza virus: distinctiveness of hemagglutinin antigen of Hong Kong-68 virus. Proc Natl Acad Sci U S A. 1969;63(2):326–33.

46. Bateman AC, Busch MG, Karasin AI, Bovin N, Olsen CW. Amino acid 226 in the hemagglutinin of H4N6 influenza virus determines binding affinity for alpha2,6-linked sialic acid and infectivity levels in primary swine and human respiratory epithelial cells. J Virol. 2008;82(16):8204–9.

47. Stevens J, Blixt O, Tumpey TM, Taubenberger JK, Paulson JC, Wilson IA. Structure and receptor specifi-

city of the hemagglutinin from an H5N1 influenza virus. Science. 2006;312(5772):404–10.

48. Le QM, Kiso M, Someya K, Sakai YT, Nquyen TH, Pham ND, et al. Avian flu: isolation of drug-resistant H5N1 virus. Nature. 2005;437(7062):1108.

49. Seo SH, Hoffmann E, Webster RG. Lethal H5N1 influenza viruses escape host anti-viral cytokine responses. Nat Med. 2002;8(9):950–4.

50. Jackson D, Hossain MJ, Hickman D, Perez DR, Lamb RA. A new influenza virus virulence determinant: the NS1 protein four C-terminal residues modulate pathogenicity. Proc Natl Acad Sci U S A. 2008;105 (11):4381–6.

PART 4

Epidemiology and surveillance

Section Editor: Arnold S. Monto

15 Influenza surveillance and laboratory diagnosis

Maria Zambon

Reference Microbiology Services, Public Health England, London, UK

Surveillance

Global virus surveillance

Every year distinct epidemics of human influenza occur during the winter seasons in both Northern and Southern Hemispheres. The rates and severity of annual epidemics vary significantly from place to place and year to year, depending on the strain and subtype circulating and the susceptibility of the population. Typically, influenza circulates in temperate zones between October to April in the Northern Hemisphere and May to September in the Southern Hemisphere, with peak epidemic periods varying according to location and climate and lasting approximately 6–12 weeks. Global virus circulation is tracked through the World Health Organization's (WHO) Global Influenza Surveillance and Response System (GISRS) [1]. Tropical regions may have prolonged low level circulation for much longer periods of time. Virus circulation and association with discrete disease epidemics is less well recognized in these regions. Historically, global influenza surveillance has focused on virologic monitoring to guide selection of vaccine strains. New WHO standards for global surveillance now focus mainly on the collection, reporting, and analysis of epidemiologic data on seasonal influenza [2]. The variability in peak activity and location emphasizes the importance of country and region-specific epidemiologic and virologic surveillance so as to optimize decisions about composition of influenza vaccines and timing of vaccination campaigns.

Clinical disease surveillance

Seasonal influenza is an acute respiratory disease in humans, with abrupt onset of fever and respiratory symptoms including cough, sore throat, coryza with associated systemic features of malaise, muscle fatigue, and headache. The spectrum of clinical infection extends from relatively mild or even asymptomatic virus shedding to severe illness, pneumonia, and death. Complications can include otitis media in children, and exacerbation of underlying cardiac and respiratory illnesses and secondary bacterial pneumonia in all ages. Unusual complications include myocarditis and encephalitis. In the developed world most influenza-associated deaths occur in the elderly, but fatal outcomes occur regularly in young adults and children with no known underlying risk factors [3, 4].

Of all common respiratory illnesses, influenza has the most dramatic effect on communities. The explosive nature of influenza outbreaks and epidemics can have a sudden impact on population morbidity and mortality within a matter of weeks. Vaccination is the major control measure. Optimizing vaccine composition to match circulating strains involves

---

Textbook of Influenza, Second Edition. Edited by Robert G. Webster, Arnold S. Monto, Thomas J. Braciale, and Robert A. Lamb.
© 2013 John Wiley & Sons, Ltd. Published 2013 by John Wiley & Sons, Ltd.

separate clinical disease and virologic surveillance. The integration of diverse and complex disease indicator information with virologic data on circulating strains demonstrates the linkage between clinically detected epidemics of influenza-like illness (ILI) and periods of virus circulation (Figure 15.1a). As recording of morbidity in various health sectors (community, primary care, hospital admissions, critical care) becomes increasingly sophisticated and better integrated with virologic surveillance data, it is becoming possible to forecast early warning of healthcare impact. Assessments of severity associated with different circulating strains and subtypes can also be refined to improve the speed of response in epidemic and pandemic periods and ensure that control measures are proportionate.

Morbidity

The impact of influenza epidemics can be demonstrated in several different ways, directly and indirectly in the community. Direct measures of healthcare utilization include family doctor consultations in primary care or hospital admissions and critical care requirements in secondary care. Indirect measures include sickness absence from school or employment and sales of medications and other symptomatic relief items (Figure 15.1b). The unpredictability of influenza epidemics limits the extrapolation of trends in disease indicators from one health sector to another, and from year to year. Outbreaks in schools or other institutions may not be reflected in hospital admission data, critical care requirements, or mortality, and vice versa. Generally, a range of indicators are used to interpret trends rather than describe absolute numbers of cases of illness.

The ability to predict the link between virus circulation in the community and requirement for secondary care is subject to considerable uncertainty, dependent on the virus strain and subtype. A comprehensive system for monitoring clinical disease and predicting healthcare utilization associated with influenza requires an assessment of:

1. Mild illness in the community not requiring medical attention. Surveillance schemes that provide this sort of information tend to focus on pre-enrolled household or family cohorts, telephone helpline calls, sales of over-the-counter medication. Population-based seroepidemiology may provide the most accurate overall denominator of asymptomatic, mild, and more severe illness.

2. Illness in the community requiring medical attention. Attendance at medical practitioner (consultation) and clinical intervention such as prescription medications may be a proxy for slightly more severe illness (Figure 15.1c).

3. Hospital admission, emergency visits, and critical care requirements are measures used to describe more severe illness episodes. These are used to reflect disease at the severe end of the spectrum, particularly in the young and the elderly.

4. Mortality statistics and cause of death reporting (Figure 15.1c).

Depending on the healthcare system, the quantitative relationship between service delivery in different sectors of healthcare can vary. Comparison of impact of influenza epidemics between countries and regions where healthcare delivery arrangements depend on diverse health infrastructure, political systems, and available funding may be extremely difficult. Having historical data sets within countries helps to establish relative impact of one epidemic over another.

Mortality

Two methodologies are used for describing and estimating influenza-related mortality [5]:

1. Methods based around individual ascertainment use death certification and laboratory diagnosis. These predominately determine patterns and risk factors for mortality. Data from these sources are used to establish vaccination policy and priority groups for interventions. Any figures of total mortality based on individual deaths are inevitably a minimum estimate as individual death recording frequently does not attribute causality [4].

2. Population-based methods use statistical techniques to estimate numbers of premature or excess deaths [6].

The total numbers of deaths generated from the two methods cannot be compared. The former are prone to underestimation, especially when identifying influenza-related deaths in older people. The latter are cruder and have to allow for confounding factors, notably other seasonal infections and climate effects. Although there are estimates of influenza mortality in individual seasons or due to pandemics globally in specific locations, these are not yet systematically applied to all countries and regions. The pattern of mortality differs considerably between pandemics and interpandemic periods, as was seen most recently in the 2009 pandemic [5].

Comparison of deaths in Europe due to the 2009 pandemic with those in the interpandemic period 1970–2008 indicates that pandemic deaths in 2009 occurred in younger and healthier persons, a common feature of pandemics where excess mortality in younger age groups is clearly seen [7]. Common methods are needed to estimate and compare influenza-related morbidity and mortality at national and regional level, and individual surveillance is required for influenza-related deaths in key groups such as pregnant women and children to support evidence-based decision making. This is particularly the case in low income countries which require good quality, local evidence to allocate scarce health system resources to deliver interventions against influenza [8].

Animal surveillance

Effective collaboration and coordination between human and animal networks is an essential requirement for: (i) the improved integration of data on animal and human viruses; (ii) the identification of unusual influenza A viruses infecting humans; (iii) the evaluation of pandemic risk; and (iv) selection of viruses for pandemic vaccines. The relationship is most obviously seen in relating the number of human cases of avian influenza in South-East Asia to the seasonality of avian influenza in wild bird populations (Figure 15.1d) and the detection of diverse viruses in humans in North America resulting from zoonotic transmission from swine [9]. Animal influenza surveillance coverage is limited, with a shortage of epidemiologic data on circulation of viruses in animal populations in most countries. Strenuous efforts are now underway to enhance virologic surveillance in animals beyond notification of disease and recognition of sporadic human infections [10].

Integrated epidemiologic and virologic surveillance

In a clinical care environment, accurate diagnosis is a key tool for individual patient management and outbreak control, leveraging intervention decisions

and infection control measures. Explosive outbreaks and sickness absence from employment are typical features of severe epidemics and pandemics, leading to an exponential surge in demand for healthcare. Maximizing the match between healthcare availability and demand requires an accurate understanding of the prevalence and severity of illness in different segments of the population, derived through surveillance indicators to ensure the most efficient health system management. The vast majority of individuals (over 98%) experiencing symptomatic influenza infection do not undergo specific influenza laboratory tests, due to cost and availability. Yet laboratory diagnosis of influenza infection for at least some cases is crucial to provide specificity to clinical disease surveillance, given the ability of influenza epidemics and pandemics to have enormous societal impact (Figure 15.1).

Influenza cannot easily be differentiated clinically from other respiratory viruses, such as respiratory syncytial virus and parainfluenza viruses, which may be co-circulating in the community. Even without the use of specific laboratory tests, the accuracy of a clinical diagnosis of influenza is much greater when physicians are made aware that influenza is circulating in the community through reports of virologic surveillance. This intelligence may lead to an accuracy of approximately 80% in clinical diagnosis alone at the height of an influenza epidemic [11]. Combined clinical and virologic surveillance from sentinel primary care facilities in the community is one of the most comprehensive and sophisticated approaches to providing a clear linkage between virus circulation and clinical illness and/or disease in the community [12]. This approach has many benefits including early warning of virus circulation and the ability to provide rapid estimates of vaccine effectiveness, but may not provide a complete picture of the health impact of influenza. The relationship between illness in the community and impact in primary care does not always directly correlate with severe illness, hospitalization, and death for a variety of reasons, including behavioral factors that govern propensity to access medical services [13, 14]. It is necessary to ensure that there is some virologic sampling associated with severe disease and hospitalization, and an integrated approach to surveillance which looks at a range of indicators.

233

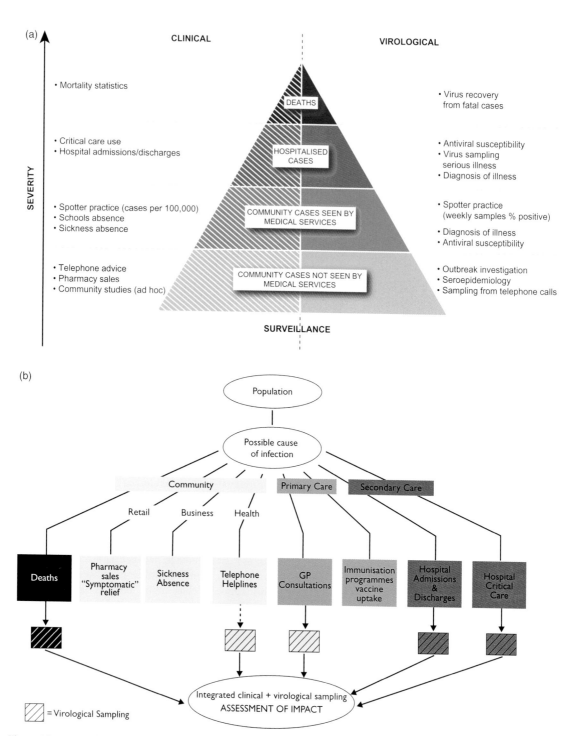

Figure 15.1. Surveillance of influenza. (a) Clinical and virologic indices used to describe severity of infection. (b) Different sources of information for surveillance of influenza. (c) Virus isolates, family doctor consultations for influenza-like illness (ILI) and death registration (all cause) England and Wales 2000–2012. (d) Relationship between highly pathogenic avian influenza outbreaks (all countries) and human H5N1 infections (all countries). Data taken from World Health Organization website, 31 July 2012 [1].

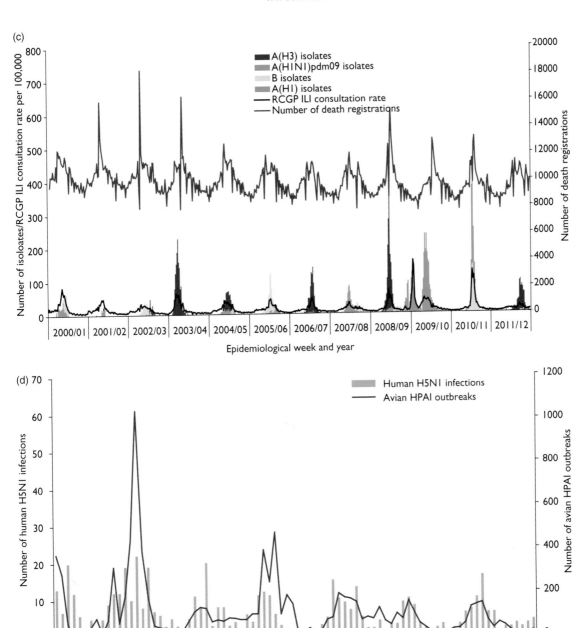

Figure 15.1. (*Continued*)

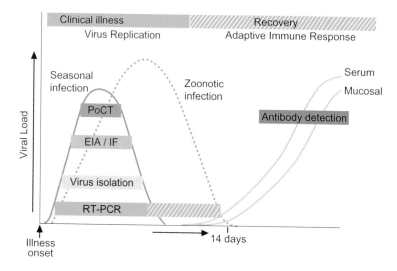

Figure 15.2. Detection of influenza during infection. Influenza detection post infection using different diagnostic tests following acute illness onset. EIA, enzyme-linked immunoassay; IF, immunofluorescence; RT-PCR, reverse transcriptase polymerase chain reaction; PoCT, point of care test.

Laboratory diagnosis

Diagnosis of acute phase illness

Specific laboratory diagnosis of seasonal influenza infection during the acute phase of illness in humans relies on the isolation of virus particles or the detection of viral components during the period of viral replication, prior to viral clearance through activation of adaptive immune response (Figure 15.2). This is usually through the analysis of respiratory tract secretions sampled by nasopharyngeal swabbing (NPS) or wash/aspirate procedures: nasopharyngeal aspirates (NPAs), nasal washes (NW), endotracheal aspirates (ETA), or bronchoalveolar lavage (BAL).

For seasonal human influenza A (H1N1, H3N2, and B) and pandemic H1N1 2009, viral shedding peaks within days of the onset of illness, and cultivable virus is readily detectable in the upper respiratory tract for up to 5–7 days, or longer in children. Non-cultivable virus nucleic acid may be detectable for several more days (Figure 15.2). Viral replication outside the respiratory tract or viremia is not generally a feature of human influenza, but recovery of viable virus from conjunctival fluid is well recognized, and viral nucleic acid may occasionally be detected outside the respiratory tract when there are unusual systemic features such as myocarditis in seasonal or zoonotic influenza A infections. In seasonal flu, viral nucleic acid is detectable at low titer in feces particu-

larly in children and immunocompromised individuals [15].

Zoonotic infections

The experiences of avian influenza A infection in humans in the last few years (H5N1, H7N7, H9N2, H7N3), unexpected presentation of some subtypes with a high case fatality and serious illness, the emergence of pandemic influenza H1N1 2009 from a swine origin [16], and sporadic zoonotic cases of swine origin influenza viruses (SOIV) in 2011–2012 [9] underlines the importance of ensuring clinical laboratory capability for rapid influenza diagnosis. This includes the ability to detect unusual subtypes of influenza associated with zoonotic transmission and the potential emergence of pandemic influenza. Physicians should remain alert to the possibility of avian influenza infection where there are risk factors involving exposure to animal reservoirs of influenza, such as birds or swine.

In zoonotic influenza A H5N1 infection, virus can be detected in respiratory tract samples, blood, and feces, indicating systemic viral replication during the acute illness phase [17]. The highest viral shedding occurs lower in the respiratory tract, reflecting the cell tropism of avian and H5 viruses [18]. Although H5N1 viral shedding may be prolonged and viral replication higher than seasonal human influenza infection (Figure 15.2), the concentration of viral protein or nucleic acid in accessible upper respiratory tract secretions is lower. Zoonotic influenza A H7 infection is associated with virus shedding in conjunctival fluid, but only in a minority of cases is virus recovered from elsewhere in the respiratory tract [19].

Initially, H5N1 illness may be indistinguishable from seasonal influenza or, in rare cases, bear no resemblance to human influenza, as has occurred in Thailand and Vietnam. H5 diagnosis is also problematic in more developed countries where H5 is not known to be endemic in birds but where there may have been unrecognized exposure by contact with poultry or wild birds, for example in Turkey and Azerbaijan in 2006 [20]. Rapid accurate diagnosis is vital for individual patient management and for control of public and animal health.

Type of clinical specimen

The type of clinical specimen collected for the diagnosis of human influenza depends largely on the diagnostic test required; the age of the patient and clinical presentation or stage of an outbreak investigation are other important considerations. Any clinical specimen intended for virus isolation and for viral genome detection should be collected as soon as possible after the onset of symptoms. Mammalian influenza A viruses replicate primarily in the epithelial cells of the respiratory tract. Sampling of the human mammalian respiratory tract for virus isolation should attempt to maximize the harvest of virally infected epithelial cells. NPW or NPA tend to have a higher cellular content but there are several acceptable respiratory tract specimens for viral genome detection, virus culture, immunofluorescence (IF), and enzyme immunoassays for viral antigen detection (see above).

The swab should be inserted deeply into the nasopharynx, rotated vigorously to collect epithelial cells, removed, and placed into viral transport medium (VTM) prior to laboratory analytical investigations. NPA are collected by placing a fine bore catheter connected to a mucous trap with vacuum suction into the nostril past the anterior nares and applying suction. After removal of the catheter from the nose, VTM or saline is suctioned through the catheter, washing cellular material into the trap. NW are collected by instilling 1–2 mL of sterile phosphate-buffered saline into the nares by using a catheter or fine bore tubing

attached to a 5-mL syringe or a bulb syringe. The saline is immediately suctioned back into the syringe, yielding a 1–2-mL sample.

Lung tissue derived from post mortem, open lung, or needle biopsy procedures can be an excellent clinical sample for virus isolation; isolation of virus from lung tissue or BAL usually indicates lower tract infection. Viral antigens or nucleic acid can be detected in formalin-fixed paraffin-embedded lung tissue by immunohistochemistry, *in situ* hybridization, or reverse transcription polymerase chain reaction (RT-PCR [21].

Although seasonal influenza causes respiratory disease, gastrointestinal illness features such as diarrhea and vomiting are regularly seen, particularly in children and immunocompromised individuals. Influenza viral RNA can be detected in fecal material and, in a very small proportion of cases, infectious virus can be recovered. The exact explanation for detection of seasonal influenza A virus in feces is not yet forthcoming as receptor availability and limited replication in intestinal cells do not suggest extensive local replication. Notwithstanding these observations, fecal samples are not a particularly useful diagnostic sample and there is little clinical predictive value from the detection of viral RNA in stools [15].

Avian influenza viruses replicate in both the respiratory and intestinal tracts and virus is shed in the feces of feral birds and ducks [22], but may also be shed in the respiratory tract of domestic chickens. Fecal transmission is thought to be a major route of transmission from and between birds and between birds and humans. Cloacal swabs are the sample of choice for avian influenza isolation from wild birds, although tracheal secretions may also be a useful sample source if domestic poultry are infected with avian influenza A viruses.

Following zoonotic transmission of nonhuman subtypes of influenza A to humans, viral receptors and replication competence will affect the tropism of the virus and the tissues and body fluids in which the virus may be detected, as has been demonstrated for H5N1 and H7 viruses. In this situation, a broad range of tissues may yield infectious virus recovery and a different spectrum of illness, as has been reviewed [23]. In contrast to seasonal influenza virus infection, feces may be a useful sample for virus recovery as viral loads are much higher.

Transport

Transport conditions should be optimized to maintain viral infectivity and ensure maximal recovery. Specimens should be transported immediately at 4°C or frozen at −70°C. The infectivity of enveloped viruses is generally rapidly destroyed at room temperature, although influenza is moderately stable compared with other respiratory viral pathogens, for example respiratory syncytial virus (RSV). Although the highest virus yields are in samples taken within 24–48 hours of onset of illness, influenza viruses can be recovered even after several days from respiratory specimens sent by post. The VTM used can be critical in ensuring good virus recovery. Ideally, VTM should include a balanced salt solution at neutral pH with protein stabilizers such as gelatine or bovine serum albumin (BSA), and antibiotics to reduce or inhibit growth of commensal or pathogenic bacteria.

Alternative approaches to sampling and transport of biologic material containing influenza viruses includes the use of dried clinical samples using various storage matrices [24]. As diagnosis shifts increasingly towards genetic analysis, there are several advantages to this approach which is likely to improve the ability to ship and store material from remote locations or where a cold chain cannot be assured. Such methodology is tried and tested for other RNA viruses such as HIV and hepatitis C virus and allows recovery of viral genomic material suitable for RT-PCR and sequencing, but will not provide recovery of infectious virus. Dried swab materials have been used for the virologic detection of influenza in the community in public health surveillance networks with good results [25].

Types of laboratory tests

There are an ever increasing number of laboratory tests available for the diagnosis of influenza, to detect the presence of viral footprints: antigens, encoded enzymes, nucleic acid, infected cells, or infectious particles in respiratory secretions. Serologic tests rely on the detection of the adaptive (antibody) immune response to influenza infection, and tend to be applied retrospectively once virus replication is reduced or terminated. The application of different tests and testing strategies depends on the information required, the speed with which the information is needed, the

sample provided, and the stage of illness (Figure 15.2, Table 15.1).

The WHO global surveillance programs which track the evolution of human influenza virus deliver an array of detailed virologic information, crucial for vaccine formulation decisions [26]. Such programs remain critically dependent on cultured virus isolates provided from clinical laboratories following sampling of cases during acute illness in community or hospital settings. Pinpointing the emergence of antigenic variants of human influenza requires virus amplification in cell culture or embryonated eggs to obtain virus particles in adequate concentrations (approximately 10^7–10^8 particles per mL of culture fluid) to provide sufficient viral hemagglutinin (HA) protein for analysis. Innovations, including the use of engineered mammalian cell lines, such as MDCK cells expressing enhanced levels of 2,6-sialic acid virus receptor [27], may enhance sensitivity for detection of human viruses, but have not reduced the time taken for the virus to grow. Virus culture may take up to 7 days. Virus isolation as a diagnostic methodology is therefore not useful for immediate patient clinical management due to the time taken to grow the virus. However, there are important clinical and public health advantages that accrue from more rapid laboratory confirmation of subtype-specific diagnosis during the acute phase of illness.

Influenza diagnostics to guide patient management

Current practice dictates that a suitable clinical sample is transported to the laboratory for processing, analysis, interpretation, and reporting. Depending on the setting, this will introduce delays in clinical decision making if treatment or infection control is dependent on the results of laboratory testing. Although virus culture and viral genome detection using nucleic acid amplification techniques (NAAT), such as real time RT-PCR, are the gold standards of laboratory tests for influenza, these require specialized facilities and equipment, highly trained laboratory staff, and workflow processes that depend on batched analysis. The application of these technologies tends to require a complex infrastructure environment present in a minority of secondary care facilities.

The use of simple but rapid diagnostic techniques such as antigen detection or direct IF is much more

Table 15.1. Influenza diagnostic investigations.

Method	Sample	Time	Throughput	Skill	Equipment	Setting	Advantages	Disadvantages
RT-PCR	Any respiratory tract sample	4–6 h	High depending on automation 50–100 per day	High specialized	Highly specialized	Secondary care	Sensitive	High skill (complex) laboratory infrastructure
Rapid PoCT	As per manufacturer	15–60 min	1–20 depending on batch size	Low skill minimal lab requirement	Nil or minimum	Community Primary care Pharmacies ER Any clinical environment	Rapid specific	Low sensitivity Poor negative predictive value
IF	NPS NW BAL ETT	4–6 h	Low 1–20 No automation	Highly skilled	Specialized equipment of infrastructure required	Secondary care	Rapid	Poor specificity and sensitivity
EIA antigen Detection	NPS NW BAL ETT	2–4 h	High depending on automation 100+	Medium generic ELISA skills	Specialized equipment	Secondary care	Simple Automatable	Poor sensitivity
Virus Culture	Any respiratory tract sample	3–7 d	Medium	Highly specialized	Highly specialized equipment and infrastructure	Secondary or tertiary care	Gold standard	Labour intensive Specialized Complex Laboratory infrastructure
Serology (HAI or MN)	Serum	Requires paired sera 14 d apart	High 100 +	Highly specialized	Infrastructure required	Tertiary Highly specialized	Gold standard	Retrospective

BAL, bronchoalveolar aspirate; ER, emergency room; ETT, endotracheal aspirate; HAI, hemagglutination inhibitor; MN, microneutralization; NPS, nasopharyngeal swab; NW, nasal wash; PoCT, point of care test; RT-PCR, reverse transcriptase polymerase chain reaction.

appropriate close to acute hospital facilities, where speed of diagnosis is necessary to support early antiviral therapy and local infection control measures. In this situation, antigenic information is less important. Sensitivity of these tests must be high to avoid false negative results, and the amount of specialized equipment and operator skill should be minimized to allow handling of large numbers of specimens and rapid processing. Whilst diagnosis using IF can be obtained within a few hours, the sensitivity and specificity are low, and still requires specialist operator skill and equipment. It is a reasonably low cost diagnostic service to provide, but is increasingly being replaced by more rapid point of care tests (PoCT), which have similar levels of sensitivity, improved specificity, and require a low skill level but do not require highly specialized equipment (Table 15.1).

Point of care diagnostics

Rapid PoCT for influenza were developed alongside neuraminidase inhibitor (NI) drugs for treatment of human influenza in the 1990s to assist individual patient management so that sampling and analysis could take place in the same environment ("test and treat"), without requiring transport of samples to a clinical laboratory. These tests require limited skill and equipment to provide a result in 10–30 minutes, thereby influencing prescribing in a physician's office or at the bedside. A diverse range of technologies can be applied, including lateral flow immunochromatography (dipstick), solid phase capture ELISA with optical or colorimetric read-outs (individual small cassette format), and activation of viral neuraminidase (NA) enzyme activity with substrate detection. Some of these technologies are not suitable for the clinical environment, but can be used in nonspecialist laboratories (reviewed in [28]). A specification for the ideal PoCT is to be affordable, sensitive, specific, rapid, robust, and equipment free, with the potential to allow earlier introduction of treatment, infection control, and greater patient convenience.

However, current PoCT formats, originally developed for the detection of human influenza, use antibodies to detect conserved type-specific viral nucleoprotein (NP) or matrix (M) protein present in respiratory secretions. This allows detection of influenza A or B, but may not always distinguish between them and does not indicate which subtype of influenza A is involved. Although influenza PoCT devices are widely used in some countries (e.g., Japan) in conjunction with antiviral drug prescribing for seasonal influenza, and have good levels of specificity, limitations to the global uptake of such tests have related to the cost of the test and their unreliable negative predictive value arising from suboptimal sensitivity of detection. Although PoCT diagnosis for influenza is desired by clinicians and is clearly within reach technically, it is unlikely that the detection technologies (which generally depend on detection of viral protein) used in currently available devices will achieve better sensitivity than the 40–80% recorded in field studies with human influenza. In addition, early data from clinical cases of H5N1 indicate that existing PoCT tests perform poorly in comparison with H5 virus culture investigation, partly because the concentration of H5 virus protein in respiratory secretions from the upper airways is limited and partly because of the inherent sensitivity limitations of the tests.

Improvements in sensitivity for PoCTs will likely come from technologies that concentrate viral antigen from larger sample volumes than can be currently analyzed, coupled with target amplification *in situ* or novel technologies. A promising example is NAAT technology compressed into a dipstick format, with rapid read out [29].

To enhance global influenza diagnostic capability there is an urgent need to develop and deploy subtype-specific PoCT, with much improved performance characteristics and low cost, possibly using handheld devices suitable for nonspecialist clinical laboratories and for use in field settings in countries with low technology infrastructure.

Detection of viral genome: Amplification techniques

The gradual dissemination of NAAT including real time RT-PCR in clinical laboratories has shifted the focus of laboratory diagnosis of influenza from dependency on virus culture, taking several days, to a highly specific and sensitive diagnosis available within several hours. Laboratory automation coupled with machinery for NAAT testing and information systems facilitates and streamlines high throughput molecular diagnostics to provide exquisitely sensitive, specific, quantitative detection of virus nucleic acids, including influenza A, in different body fluids. Molecular assays can be used in conjunction with other diagnostic assays, clinical, and epidemiologic information to:

1. Detect influenza A or B virus in symptomatic patients using viral RNA extracted directly from respiratory specimens, or from culture media inoculated with clinical material. This usually requires an approach that targets a conserved type-specific gene, for example NP, MP, or NS1.

2. Determine the subtype of influenza A virus in clinical material. This requires an approach targeting variable surface protein genes either the HA or NA, or both.

Diagnostic algorithms vary, depending on the laboratory and setting. A clinical laboratory in parts of the developed world outside South-East Asia will focus on detection of seasonal influenza and may employ a multi-step algorithm, combining a screening RT-PCR, which detects whether a sample contains influenza A or B, followed by a subtyping PCR to assess whether it is H1 or H3 using a battery of segment-specific RT-PCR reactions. In contrast, in parts of South-East Asia, it may be important to also consider the possibility of H5 zoonotic infection in the presentation of severe clinical illness, and so the algorithm approach to subtyping may differ.

Updating molecular detection

There is a clear shift towards NAAT for influenza diagnosis, in line with trends in laboratory medicine generally. A number of methods use fluorescent dyes to detect and quantitate in real time the amplification of DNA by PCR. Methods incorporating a labeled oligonucleotide probe dually labeled with a fluorophore and a quencher (such as a TaqMan™ probe) improve the specificity of detection of amplified specific targets on a real-time basis. Methodology is being increasingly commercialized to provide simple "walk away" automated technology solutions for less complex laboratories [28]. However, sensitivity and specificity are primarily dependent on the quality of oligunucleotide primers used.

Ensuring that influenza diagnostic techniques based on NAAT such as RT-PCR are both sensitive and specific requires accurate knowledge of sequence diversity. Portions of gene segments that are highly conserved between subtypes are chosen as detection targets. This is reasonably easy to achieve with targets of NP, MP, and NS1. As genetic sequences differ amongst different types and subtypes of influenza viruses, it is possible to design PCR primers and probes that will differentially recognize only one type or subtype of influenza. Amplification of the gene target regions for influenza A subtype-specific diagnosis requires targeting the highly variable viral HA or NA genes. Optimally configured reagents (primers and probes) are ideally designed from the regions of HA that are most conserved. This may be difficult to achieve with such a highly variable target. All strategies based on detection of HA of any subtype require frequent verification that single base substitutions found in newly emerging drift variants do not affect primer and probe performance, which may need to be done in a coordinated way through national and regional networks of laboratories. Technical expertise and unrelenting attention to quality control are critical to accurate and reliable performance of molecular diagnostics used for influenza diagnosis.

Genetic diversity of circulating strains: Impact on diagnosis

In common with human seasonal influenza strains, circulating H5, H7, and H9 strains comprise several diverse lineages or clades, based on sequence analysis of the HA and other genes. These may represent antigenic differences evolving between different lineages. The westward expansion of the H5 viruses in 2005 and 2006 in the bird reservoir to Europe and Africa has involved H5 viruses from the clade 2 lineage. Human cases of H5 were, until mid-2005, exclusively associated with clade 1 viruses, but recent human cases in Turkey, Egypt, and Azerbaijan have involved clade 2 viruses [23]. Human H7N7 infection in Europe in 2003 were due to Eurasian lineage H7 viruses, whereas H7N3 infection in North America was due to North American H7 lineage [30]. This situation is analogous to detection of human influenza strains, where there are frequently co-circulating lineages of viruses causing infection. It is essential to regularly update critical HA detection reagents for nonhuman viruses to take account of sequence diversity, and different genetic lineages detected in circulating viruses and different animal reservoirs. Thus, efficient and effective subtype HA-specific nucleic acid diagnosis, either for human or zoonotic influenza infection, requires coordination between avian and human surveillance laboratories generating HA or NA sequence data, and clinical laboratories supporting clinicians treating patients. Tracking the emergence of diverse strains and adapting primers and probes frequently is essential, if precise diagnostics are to be applied consistently in clinical laboratories. In turn, this requires a rigorous quality assurance and proficiency testing framework within countries to ensure that laboratories providing a clinical diagnosis of influenza subtype using PCR are constantly updating reagents to take account of genetic drift [31].

Direct PCR sequencing of clinical material containing influenza virus does not require virus cultivation. This approach has been successfully applied to fresh, frozen, and archived human tissue, and has provided important diagnostic information, for example the viroarchaeology of 1918 influenza in exhumed cadavers and preserved sections [32]. Although the influenza virus genome is relatively small, consisting of approximately 15 000 nucleotides, the technologies for whole organism sequencing have not yet been applied to any great extent to determine whole genome variation in influenza virus strains as a surveillance tool. Genomic sequencing of a library of animal viruses indicates the wealth of information that can be obtained from this approach [33]. Similar analysis of human influenza A strains collected from a single locality over several years has also revealed a greater degree of diversity and reassortment than had been expected [34]. Analysis of viral whole genomes direct from clinical material will undoubtedly be part of the future direction of laboratory-based virologic surveillance programs [35].

Recording clinical outcome data and linking it to detailed virologic analysis is essential for tracking transmission of drug resistance viruses and evolution of influenza viruses. One of the risks associated with improving the quality of clinical diagnosis through the use of PoCT devices is that there is a net loss of strain information available for analysis of diversity. It is essential to preserve the capacity for labor intensive, low yield traditional virus isolation in parallel with newer technologies for near patient diagnosis. In addition, creative approaches to recovery of viral nucleic acid from used diagnostic PoCT devices, a technically less demanding task than recovery of material from decomposed humans, could provide additional material for global surveillance and may point the way to highly sophisticated whole viral genome sequencing distant from the clinical arena, as a supplement to existing surveillance activity.

Detection of antiviral resistance

The range of drugs licensed for use in treatment or prophylaxis of influenza is very narrow. Drugs either act to inhibit viral ion channels (M2 channel blockers) of influenza A viruses, or inhibit the NA of influenza A and B viruses (the NI class of drugs). As the majority of seasonal influenza A H3N2 and pandemic H1N1 2009 viruses are now naturally resistant to M2 channel blockers, for practical purposes, the NI drugs (oseltamivir and zanamivir) are the mainstay of treatment and prophylaxis of seasonal influenza A and B, and zoonotic infections globally. Several similar NI drugs (peramivir and laninamivir) are close to licensure or have already been licensed in a few countries.

Monitoring antiviral resistance is relevant for individual patient treatment, but also in minimizing the spread and emergence of transmissible antiviral resistance. Surveillance data on antiviral resistance, arising from cumulated data on clinical testing or enhanced structured surveillance schemes informs public health policy and clinical recommendations on prophylaxis, outbreak management, and clinical therapeutics in complex situations.

Laboratory testing to detect NI drug resistance is usually carried out through a combination of genetic and phenotypic tests [36]. Resistance to NI drugs is both type and subtype specific, and usually conferred by single amino acid point substitutions in the viral NA at key residues in either the catalytic site or the framework. A genetic screen of viral NA in clinical samples using a targeted short read sequence based molecular assay, such as pyrosequencing, is a very good fast method of detecting known mutations such as N275Y in N1 containing influenza A infections [37]. With this mutation, there is an excellent correlation between lack of clinical effectiveness, presence of substitution, and altered IC50 of virus isolate. Genetic screening is therefore sufficient to detect antiviral resistance. However, not all substitutions conferring NI drug resistance are recognized in all subtypes, and the clinical effectiveness of oseltamivir and zanamivir may be retained when there are substitutions which lead to modest or moderate decreases in susceptibility.

Consequently, particularly when dealing with other subtypes besides N1, it is relevant to test cultured isolates as well as analyze gene sequence, as all possible substitutions conferring resistance are probably not yet described and an approach that is limited to genetic analysis may fail to detect novel mutations, although this is preferred in hospital laboratories [36].

Analysis of the original clinical material rather than an isolate derived from cell culture is preferred when considering the clinical implications of detection of a mixed viral population. The proportion of viruses in a mixture in cell culture can vary over time, and there may be preferential selection of host variants. Antiviral susceptibility testing in individual patients is usually performed to address the following questions.

1. Lack of illness resolution in hospitalized patients suggesting emergence of drug resistance.

2. Monitoring persistent shedding in immunocompromised patients to detect the emergence of mixtures of sensitive and resistant viruses.

3. Analysis of pretreatment samples to monitor the frequency with which individuals are infected with a known drug-resistant virus.

The emergence of a drug-resistant virus in an immunocompromised individual reduces the options for continued therapy, but also poses a threat to surrounding individuals. Immunocompromised individuals can shed virus for a very long period, running into months, and frequently have a high viral load so measures need to be taken to prevent transmission from such individuals. Continued monitoring of viruses for resistance and linkage to clinical outcome data are essential to ensure optimum clinical guidance and policy decisions on the use of antivirals.

Serological diagnosis of influenza

Acute viral infection is followed by the development of strain-specific antibodies against the HA protein from about 10 to 14 days post illness onset (Figure 15.3); the detection of such anti HA antibody in convalescent phase sera has been the basis of traditional serologic methods for identifying influenza infections. The use of serology is vital for understanding the transmission dynamics and extent of human infection as well as estimating the true burden of illness caused by seasonal influenza epidemics and infrequent but explosive pandemics [38]. Serology can detect both symptomatic and asymptomatic infections that cannot be determined by either disease surveillance programs or detection of virologically confirmed cases. Both of these methods of ascertainment will vastly underestimate disease burden and overestimate severity [5]. Furthermore, serology may facilitate detection of susceptible persons within the population which can aid in risk assessment for estimating the impact of an emerging virus or, in the case of a pandemic, support vaccine policy decision making in the event of limited vaccine supply. The 2009 H1N1 pandemic exposed limitations in the current global capacity to perform serologic assessment of recent influenza infections and highlighted the need for simpler and more comprehensive approaches for assessing the status of human influenza infection.

Serosurveillance

Despite its merit, the use of serology for influenza surveillance has several limitations. Seasonal influenza infections occur regularly and individuals are reinfected throughout life with related strains. At present two serum samples have to be analyzed in order to evaluate the increase of antibody between the acute and convalescent sample. Usually fourfold increases of functional antibody (i.e., hemagglutination inhibition (HAI) and microneutralization (MN) tests) are used for confirmation of recent infection rather than technically less demanding ELISA analysis to ensure that antibody levels measured can serve as a reasonable surrogate for immunity or exposure.

The prior (lifetime) exposure of individuals to circulating influenza viruses in previous years and a high degree of cross-reactivity between antibodies to related virus strains can lead to results that are difficult to interpret through measurement of antibodies that are not directed to the most recent strain infecting the individual. Furthermore, it is currently impossible to distinguish serologically between recent infection and recent vaccination, which further complicates interpretation of results.

Consequently, seroepidemiologic studies have rarely been used for the investigation of seasonal influenza at a population level. However, when analyzing immunologically naïve individuals, such as young children or the population as a whole at the beginning of a pandemic, serology has the potential to provide valuable information on infection susceptibility in population segments due to lack of prior infection with the emerging virus [39]. Early assessment of the severity of a new influenza strain is essential to ensuring a proportionate response. Severity assessment requires the ability to detect asymptomatic and mild infections to determine the true number of infections, which are the denominator in the calculation of case : fatality and case : hospitalization ratios. The number of infections can be determined if the prevalence of immunity prior to the epidemic and during and after the epidemic are known, so that the number of people infected, and thus no longer susceptible, can be calculated. This assessment can be made in two ways: outbreak investigations in the early stages, and population-based surveys as the epidemic progresses, coupled with modeling analysis.

One of the main obstacles for large-scale population-based serologic investigations is the need for venous blood collections to obtain serum samples. Collection of this specimen type requires trained staff and laboratory equipment such as centrifuges in addition to ensuring a cold chain to preserve and transport the collected material. The majority of samples used for large-scale seroepidemiologic analyses during the 2009 pandemic were opportune sera collected for other investigations, such as discarded diagnostic sera collected in hospitals and diagnostic laboratories, in order to minimize cost [39].

Serologic detection of influenza virus infection is rarely useful in immediate clinical management.

However, retrospective analysis may establish a clinical diagnosis in the absence of virus isolation, antigen detection, or viral nucleic acid detection. In addition, it may be a useful surveillance tool, as described. Combined laboratory reports of serologic detection of influenza provide good corroborative measures of the clinical indices of influenza and influenza activity, which are based on the detection of virus replication during the acute phase of illness or on the upsurge of disease presentation (Figures 15.1a and 15.2). Serologic data provides an excellent, if delayed, marker of influenza epidemic activity, contributing to national surveillance data.

The timing of serum collection depends on knowledge of the kinetics of the class or subclass specific antibody response. The choice of the antibody assay may also depend on the age of the patient. Seroconversion following infection takes 14–28 days to complete (Figure 15.3). One of the difficulties with serologic diagnosis of influenza is the necessity of evaluating paired serum samples to verify a rise in antibody titer in response to infection. This is required because influenza infection is frequently a reinfection. There may already be pre-existing partial immunity to influenza, which is boosted by reinfection, but the predictive value of results of testing single samples for influenza serology are unreliable using the most widely available tests, the complement fixation test (CFT) or HAI. Testing for recent influenza infection by detection of immunoglobulin M (IgM) or other immunoglobulin isotypes has not yet had much impact on serologic diagnosis of influenza [40].

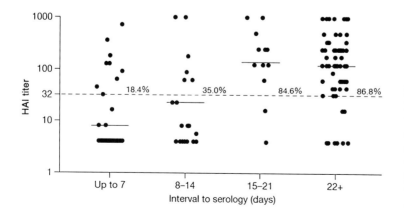

Figure 15.3. Antibody response using hemagglutination inhibition (HAI) tests. A cohort of individuals (N = 148) infected with pandemic influenza H1N1 2009 in 2009, diagnosed using reverse transcription polymerase chain reaction (RT-PCR) were followed up with serology to determine time to seroconversion.

Serologic diagnosis of influenza

The earliest techniques for assessing serologic responses to influenza virus were classic neutralization tests, which are extremely laborious. Nonetheless, it was soon recognized that the results of HAI testing paralleled the results of the far more complex neutralization tests, but were much simpler and cheaper to perform. It was also noted that HAI titers gave a good correlate of protection in human sera [41]. Since then, the assessment of the protective immunity of an individual has been made using serum HAI titers, although CFTs are still widely used in diagnostic laboratories and provide a useful method of testing serum pairs against a number of potential infectious agent antigens to assess serologic profile. CFTs measure antibody responses to the conserved influenza NP rather than HA. These are boosted during infections, and this is manifest as a rise in CFT antibody titer which lasts a few months. They are therefore helpful in differentiating type-specific antibodies to influenza A or B in humans and have an important role when new antigenic variants are circulating, for which there are no subtype-specific reagents available, or when there has been cross-species transmission of influenza A subtypes. Despite this, the rise in CFT titer following infection is slow, the test itself is relatively insensitive, and it measures only the complement fixing classes of antibody. HAI and neutralization assays measure antibodies against subtype-specific and strain-specific antigens and remain the gold standards for the assessment for serologic responses although both tests are susceptible to nonspecific inhibitors, as described below.

Hemagglutination inhibition

The hemagglutination reaction between virus and erythrocyte is susceptible to inhibition. The most useful inhibition, that produced by influenza-specific antibody, is used diagnostically in HAI assays to assess the serologic profile of individuals following infection, and is strain-specific, providing a useful serologic footprint of recent infection (Figure 15.3). The HAI antibody titer present in serum, recognized as a useful correlate of protection for many decades [41], is still probably the most useful measure of susceptibility to influenza and is widely used in assessing responses to vaccines. Excellent review articles,

which remain topical, on the practical considerations of providing diagnostic HAI serology for influenza are to be found in Dowdle et al. [42]. Naturally occurring nonspecific inhibitors of hemagglutination are present in the sera of various animals. The inhibitors act like antibody in HAI tests by interacting with the influenza HA, thus preventing agglutination of erythrocytes by the virus. Inhibitors are heat stable, sialylated glycoproteins that act by competing with cell receptors for binding to the viral hemagglutinin.

Interpretation of hemagglutination and HAI tests requires recognition that nonspecific inhibitors of hemagglutination can produce false positive results in HAI serology. Human sera are usually treated with receptor destroying enzyme (RDE) from *Vibrio cholerae* prior to testing in HAI assay. Partly because of the presence of nonspecific inhibitors in serum and partly because HAI testing uses a biologic "read out," the HAI test, although robust and well used, has many inherently unsatisfactory features, including the lack of reproducibility between different laboratories [43].

The most common source of problems is inadequate removal of nonspecific inhibitors and viability of erythrocyte preparations. The performance of the HAI test is also influenced by the nature of the antigen. Cell culture derived antigens more frequently detect significant titer rises in HAI tests than do egg grown antigens of the same virus strain. Further developments in standardizing and recording HAI tests are occurring with the use of WHO manual for serologic diagnosis [1], preparation of reagent panels, and improved awareness of the variability between laboratories. Although the HAI test is the gold standard for assessment of antibody titers, either following natural infection or vaccination, it does not adequately measure antibody status following human infection with avian viruses [44] or following equine infection with equine strains of influenza [45]. Additional tests needed to be performed or the HAI assay modified [46].

Single radial hemolysis

Single radial hemolysis (SRH) is an alternative test based on the ability of influenza-specific antibodies to lyse antigen-coated red blood cells in the presence of complement. This is recognized to be more reproducible and less error prone than HAI testing of sera [43];

although it is less strain-specific, it may be useful in the assessment of human serologic responses to avian viruses [44]. However, there are significant disadvantages, such as the necessity for high concentrations of purified antigen and uncertainty about the significance of zone sizes seen in the SRH test. The size of the zone of hemolysis is proportionate to the concentration of specific antibody in serum, though this is not an arithmetic relationship. Therefore, results should be standardized and expressed as relative antibody concentrations, which are the proportion or the hemolysis zone diameter induced standard serum. Standardization of SRH for assessment of susceptibility to influenza has not been possible in the way that standardization of SRH as a marker for immunity to rubella has been accomplished, mainly because of the constant necessity to keep updating the test antigens to take account of antigenic drift, although SRH antibody titers may be used as a method for licensing vaccines [44].

Neutralization assays

Classic neutralization methods based on plaque reduction or hemadsorption inhibition are laborious and take several days to complete. They are unsuitable for screening large numbers of serum samples. More recent developments of neutralization-EIA (N-EIA) tests are suitable for accurate titration of neutralizing antibodies in small quantities of serum and neutralizing antibody titers determined in this way correlate very well with titers obtained by HAI. Microneutralization assay formats of this type involve mixing serum and virus strain of interest together for a short period, prior to mixing with cells in suspension of microtiter format or transferring inoculum on to monolyers of MDCK cells [44]. Following single cycle or multiple cycle replication, cells are fixed and stained for the presence of influenza viral antigens by EIA or cytotoxicity index is calculated. Neutralization activity can be calculated either as foci reduction, if an insoluble chromogen is used to stain cells, or, if a soluble substrate is used, spectrophotometric absorbance can be used to calculate an index of neutralizing activity of serum. It is necessary to ensure that detecting antibodies react with new variants of influenza as described above. Use of antibodies directed against the conserved NP gene can obviate this concern. Although limited by strain specificity,

neutralization assays in a modern format provide a sensitive indicator of antibody status following infection with avian hemagglutinin or vaccination with avian strains and have proved an essential tool in estimating person-to-person transmission of H5N1 viruses, occupational exposure to H5N1 or H9N2 viruses [47], and post vaccination responses to H5 vaccines in humans [44].

Measurement of antibody subclasses

Comparison of HAI, CFT, and EIA for the detection of influenza-specific antibody indicates that EIA can detect more antibody rises in serum than either of the other two tests, as would be expected [48] because not all serum antibodies are hemagglutination inhibiting and only a small proportion of antibodies are directed to the influenza NP. Although there is a good correlation between ELISA antibody titer and HAI or neutralizing antibody titer [48], a satisfactory correlation between ELISA IgG detection or IgG subclasses and protection from subsequent challenge with influenza infection has not been derived, despite several studies investigating this using standard ELISA techniques and split virus antigen, whole cell lysate, or recombinant protein as antigen. Although children undergoing primary influenza infections develop high-titered ELISA antibodies to the infecting subtype of virus, they also develop low-titered ELISA, but not HAI antibodies, to other subtypes of influenza HA [49]. Other ELISA assays also detect cross-reactive antibodies. This relative lack of specificity must be borne in mind in interpreting ELISA results.

Although a number of ELISA IgM tests for influenza have been described using egg, tissue culture, and recombinant antigen [50], this kind of test has also not reached widespread use for influenza diagnosis or assessment of vaccine responses, probably because of the difficulty in assessing specificity of responses and the necessity to correlate with HAI titers in order to derive a measure of the protective capacity of individual sera. Similarly, several EIA formats for measuring influenza-specific IgA have been described [50] because of the interest in this molecule as an acute phase response to influenza infection and the possibility that mucosal IgA present in respiratory secretions may be a good correlate of protection from influenza. The optimal collection method for assessing mucosal IgA remains unclear.

Thus, the HAI titer of serum will continue to be a "gold standard" for evaluation of susceptibility or protection from influenza for the foreseeable future, although a reliable test for use on a single serum sample to diagnose recent influenza infection is badly needed. Similar serologic assays are also in use by veterinarians for the diagnosis of influenza in horses, chickens, and pigs.

Conclusions

The entire sequence of influenza viruses has been known since the late 1970s, but the molecular basis of virulence in mammalian hosts is still not understood. It is not known why encephalitis syndromes occur at high frequency following influenza infection in children in Japan [51], why H5N1 viruses are associated with such lethal infection in humans and animals [23], or why unusual clusters of fatalities accompany occasional drift variants of human influenza [4, 35]. Linking viral gene analysis with analysis of host response to infection should be a final step towards understanding influenza pathogenesis in humans and eventually determining predictive markers for clinical outcome and therapeutic intervention. Recent developments in genomic technology, coupled with the study of severe illness which allow investigation of host genome together with infecting viral genome [52], will start to illuminate the relationship between innate human immune response and viral pathogenicity, an elusive goal compared with the clear molecular correlates of virulence seen in avian influenza.

Influenza sequence, combined with knowledge of clinical outcome, will enhance the information available from global surveillance and remove some of the biases inherent in selective sequencing of virus isolates as a consequence of observed antigenic variation. Consideration of zoonotic influenza infection requires a broader diagnostic approach, looking at different body fluids including blood and feces and samples from lower in the respiratory tract. The ability to analyze viruses recovered from different body compartments offers a tantalizing prospect of looking in detail at "within host" variation, and what clues this may yield for better understanding of pathogenesis.

Diagnostic challenges may ultimately become research opportunities, if the technical solution to providing better diagnosis at the point of patient care can be married to the technical achievements of recovery of nucleic acid, sequence reconstruction of viral genomes, and information capture about outcomes of infection.

References

1. World Health Organization website.. WHO Global Influenza Network: Manual for the laboratory diagnosis and virological surveillance of influenza, 2011. Available from http://www.who.int/influenza/gisrs_laboratory/manual_diagnosis_surveillance_influenza/en/index.html (accessed 20 February 2013).

2. World Health Organization. WHO Global Technical Consultation: global standards and tools for influenza surveillance, 2012. Available from http://www.who.int/influenza/resources/documents/technical_consultation/en/index.html (accessed 20 February 2013).

3. Bhat N, Wright JG, Broder KR, Murray EL, Greenberg ME, Glover MJ, et al. Influenza-associated deaths among children in the United States, 2003–2004. N Engl J Med. 2005;353(24):2559–67.

4. Johnson BF, Wilson LE, Ellis J, Elliot AJ, Barclay WS, Pebody RG, et al. Fatal cases of influenza a in childhood. PLoS ONE. 2009;4(10):e7671.

5. Nicoll A, Ciancio BC, Lopez Chavarrias V, Molbak K, Pebody R, Pedzinski B, et al. Influenza-related deaths–available methods for estimating numbers and detecting patterns for seasonal and pandemic influenza in Europe. Euro Surveill. 2012;17(18).

6. Thompson WW, Shay DK, Weintraub E, Brammer L, Cox N, Anderson LJ, et al. Mortality associated with influenza and respiratory syncytial virus in the United States. JAMA. 2003;289(2):179–86.

7. Simonsen L, Clarke MJ, Schonberger LB, Arden NH, Cox NJ, Fukuda K. Pandemic versus epidemic influenza mortality: a pattern of changing age distribution. J Infect Dis. 1998;178(1):53–60.

8. Zambon M. Assessment of the burden of influenza in children. Lancet. 2011;378(9807):1897–8.

9. CDC. Update: influenza A (H3N2)v transmission and guidelines – five states. MMWR Morb Mortal Wkly Rep. 2011;2012(51–52).

10. Capua I, Alexander D. Perspectives on the global threat: the challenge of avian influenza viruses for the world's veterinary community. Avian Dis. 2010;54(1 Suppl.): 176–8.

11. Zambon M, Hays J, Webster A, Newman R, Keene O. Diagnosis of influenza in the community: relationship of clinical diagnosis to confirmed virological, serologic,

or molecular detection of influenza. Arch Intern Med. 2001;161(17):2116–22.

12. Fleming DM, Chakraverty P, Sadler C, Litton P. Combined clinical and virological surveillance of influenza in winters of 1992 and 1993–4. BMJ. 1995;311 (7000):290–1.

13. Bish A, Michie S. Demographic and attitudinal determinants of protective behaviours during a pandemic: a review. Br J Health Psychol. 2010;15(Pt 4):797–824.

14. Evans B, Charlett A, Powers C, McLean E, Zhao H, Bermingham A, et al. Has estimation of numbers of cases of pandemic influenza H1N1 in England in 2009 provided a useful measure of the occurrence of disease? Influenza Other Respir Viruses. 2011;5(6):e504–12.

15. Chan MC, Lee N, Chan PK, To KF, Wong RY, Ho WS, et al. Seasonal influenza A virus in feces of hospitalized adults. Emerg Infect Dis. 2011;17(11):2038–42.

16. Garten RJ, Davis CT, Russell CA, Shu B, Lindstrom S, Balish A, et al. Antigenic and genetic characteristics of swine-origin 2009 A(H1N1) influenza viruses circulating in humans. Science. 2009;325(5937):197–201.

17. de Jong MD, Simmons CP, Thanh TT, Hien VM, Smith GJ, Chau TN, et al. Fatal outcome of human influenza A (H5N1) is associated with high viral load and hypercytokinemia. Nat Med. 2006;12(10):1203–7.

18. Shinya K, Ebina M, Yamada S, Ono M, Kasai N, Kawaoka Y. Avian flu: influenza virus receptors in the human airway. Nature. 2006;440(7083):435–6.

19. Koopmans M, Wilbrink B, Conyn M, Natrop G, van der Nat H, Vennema H, et al. Transmission of H7N7 avian influenza A virus to human beings during a large outbreak in commercial poultry farms in the Netherlands. Lancet. 2004;363(9409):587–93.

20. Gilsdorf A, Boxall N, Gasimov V, Agayev I, Mammadzade F, Ursu P, et al. Two clusters of human infection with influenza A/H5N1 virus in the Republic of Azerbaijan, February-March 2006. Euro Surveill. 2006;11(5): 122–6.

21. Denison AM, Blau DM, Jost HA, Jones T, Rollin D, Gao R, et al. Diagnosis of influenza from respiratory autopsy tissues: detection of virus by real-time reverse transcription-PCR in 222 cases. J Mol Diagn. 2011;13 (2):123–8.

22. Webster RG, Yakhno M, Hinshaw VS, Bean WJ, Murti KG. Intestinal influenza: replication and characterization of influenza viruses in ducks. Virology. 1978;84(2): 268–78.

23. Beigel JH, Farrar J, Han AM, Hayden FG, Hyer R, de Jong MD, et al. Avian influenza A (H5N1) infection in humans. N Engl J Med. 2005;353(13):1374–85.

24. Winters M, Lloyd R Jr, Shahidi A, Brown S, Holodniy M. Use of dried clinical samples for storing and detecting influenza RNA. Influenza Other Respir Viruses. 2011;5(6):413–7.

25. Moore C, Corden S, Sinha J, Jones R. Dry cotton or flocked respiratory swabs as a simple collection technique for the molecular detection of respiratory viruses using real-time NASBA. J Virol Methods. 2008;153(2): 84–9.

26. Ampofo WK, Baylor N, Cobey S, Cox NJ, Daves S, Edwards S, et al. Improving influenza vaccine virus selection: report of a WHO informal consultation held at WHO headquarters, Geneva, Switzerland, 14–16 June 2010. Influenza Other Respir Viruses. 2012;6(2): 142–52, e1–5.

27. Matrosovich M, Matrosovich T, Carr J, Roberts NA, Klenk HD. Overexpression of the alpha-2,6-sialyltransferase in MDCK cells increases influenza virus sensitivity to neuraminidase inhibitors. J Virol. 2003;77(15):8418–25.

28. Tayo A, Ellis J, Linden Phillips L, Simpson S, Ward DJ. Emerging point of care tests for influenza: innovation or status quo. Influenza Other Respir Viruses. 2012;6 (4):291–8.

29. Wu LT, Curran MD, Ellis JS, Parmar S, Ritchie AV, Sharma PI, et al. Nucleic acid dipstick test for molecular diagnosis of pandemic H1N1. J Clin Microbiol. 2010;48 (10):3608–13.

30. Belser JA, Bridges CB, Katz JM, Tumpey TM. Past, present, and possible future human infection with influenza virus A subtype H7. Emerg Infect Dis. 2009;15(6): 859–65.

31. Meijer A, Valette M, Manuguerra JC, Perez-Brena P, Paget J, Brown C, et al. Implementation of the community network of reference laboratories for human influenza in Europe. J Clin Virol. 2005;34(2):87–96.

32. Taubenberger JK, Reid AH, Krafft AE, Bijwaard KE, Fanning TG. Initial genetic characterization of the 1918 "Spanish" influenza virus. Science. 1997;275(5307): 1793–6.

33. Krauss S, Obert CA, Franks J, Walker D, Jones K, Seiler P, et al. Influenza in migratory birds and evidence of limited intercontinental virus exchange. PLoS Pathog. 2007;3(11):e167.

34. Holmes EC, Ghedin E, Miller N, Taylor J, Bao Y, St George K, et al. Whole-genome analysis of human influenza A virus reveals multiple persistent lineages and reassortment among recent H3N2 viruses. PLoS Biol. 2005;3(9):e300.

35. Galiano M, Johnson BF, Myers R, Ellis J, Daniels R, Zambon M. Fatal cases of influenza A(H3N2) in children: insights from whole genome sequence analysis. PLoS ONE. 2012;7(3):e33166.

36. Hurt AC, Chotpitayasunondh T, Cox NJ, Daniels R, Fry AM, Gubareva LV, et al. Antiviral resistance during the 2009 influenza A H1N1 pandemic: public health, laboratory, and clinical perspectives. Lancet Infect Dis. 2012;12(3):240–8.

37. Lackenby A, Thompson CI. Democratis J. The potential impact of neuraminidase inhibitor resistant influenza. Curr Opin Infect Dis. 2008;21(6):626–38.

38. Hardelid P, Andrews NJ, Hoschler K, Stanford E, Baguelin M, Waight PA, et al. Assessment of baseline age-specific antibody prevalence and incidence of infection to novel influenza A/H1N1. Health Technol Assess. 2009;14(55):115–92.

39. Miller E, Hoschler K, Hardelid P, Stanford E, Andrews N, Zambon M. Incidence of 2009 pandemic influenza A H1N1 infection in England: a cross-sectional serological study. Lancet. 2010;375(9720):1100–8.

40. Katz JM, Hancock K, Xu X. Serologic assays for influenza surveillance, diagnosis and vaccine evaluation. Expert Rev Anti Infect Ther. 2011;9(6):669–83.

41. Hobson D, Curry RL, Beare AS, Ward-Gardner A. The role of serum haemagglutination-inhibiting antibody in protection against challenge infection with influenza A2 and B viruses. J Hyg (Lond). 1972;70(4):767–77.

42. Dowdle WR, Schild GC. Influenza: its antigenic variation and ecology. Bull Pan Am Health Organ. 1976;10(3):193–5.

43. Wood JM, Gaines-Das RE, Taylor J, Chakraverty P. Comparison of influenza serological techniques by international collaborative study. Vaccine. 1994;12(2):167–74.

44. Nicholson KG, Colegate AE, Podda A, Stephenson I, Wood J, Ypma E, et al. Safety and antigenicity of non-adjuvanted and MF59-adjuvanted influenza A/Duck/Singapore/97 (H5N3) vaccine: a randomised trial of two potential vaccines against H5N1 influenza. Lancet. 2001;357(9272):1937–43.

45. Sugiura T, Sugita S, Imagawa H, Kanaya T, Ishiyama S, Saeki N, et al. Serological diagnosis of equine influenza using the hemagglutinin protein produced in a baculovirus expression system. J Virol Methods. 2001;98(1):1–8.

46. Stephenson I, Wood JM, Nicholson KG, Zambon MC. Sialic acid receptor specificity on erythrocytes affects detection of antibody to avian influenza haemagglutinin. J Med Virol. 2003;70(3):391–8.

47. Katz JM, Lim W, Bridges CB, Rowe T, Hu-Primmer J, Lu X, et al. Antibody response in individuals infected with avian influenza A (H5N1) viruses and detection of anti-H5 antibody among household and social contacts. J Infect Dis. 1999;180(6):1763–70.

48. Murphy BR, Phelan MA, Nelson DL, Yarchoan R, Tierney EL, Alling DW, et al. Hemagglutinin-specific enzyme-linked immunosorbent assay for antibodies to influenza A and B viruses. J Clin Microbiol. 1981;13(3):554–60.

49. Burlington DB, Wright PF, van Wyke KL, Phelan MA, Mayner RE, Murphy BR. Development of subtype-specific and heterosubtypic antibodies to the influenza A virus hemagglutinin after primary infection in children. J Clin Microbiol. 1985;21(5):847–9.

50. Rimmelzwaan GF, Baars M, van Beek R, van Amerongen G, Lovgren-Bengtsson K, Claas EC, et al. Induction of protective immunity against influenza virus in a macaque model: comparison of conventional and iscom vaccines. J Gen Virol. 1997;78(Pt 4):757–65.

51. Hoshino A, Saitoh M, Oka A, Okumura A, Kubota M, Saito Y, et al. Epidemiology of acute encephalopathy in Japan, with emphasis on the association of viruses and syndromes. Brain Dev. 2012;34(5):337–43.

52. Everitt AR, Clare S, Pertel T, John SP, Wash RS, Smith SE, et al. IFITM3 restricts the morbidity and mortality associated with influenza. Nature. 2012;484(7395):519–23.

16 Epidemiology of influenza

Marc-Alain Widdowson[1] and Arnold S. Monto[2]
[1]International Epidemiology and Research Team, Epidemiology and Prevention Branch, Influenza Division, Centers for Disease Control and Prevention, Atlanta, GA, USA
[2]School of Public Health, University of Michigan, Ann Arbor, MI, USA

Introduction

The epidemiology of influenza is inextricably linked to the virus circulating. "Seasonal" or "interpandemic" influenza occurs every year and is caused by circulating influenza A or B viruses. These seasonal viruses evolve gradually through mutation and consequent antigenic changes in the hemagglutinin and neuraminidase envelope glycoproteins, allowing them to escape host immunity partially; this is termed antigenic drift. Periodically, a whole new gene segment or segments can be introduced through reassortment, resulting in the appearance of a novel type A variant to which there is little population immunity; this is termed antigenic shift, and leads to a pandemic with a high overall attack rate. Pandemic viruses with a novel hemagglutinin may also emerge by mutation of an animal influenza virus and subsequent human transmission, such as occurred in 1918.

Pandemic influenza is further discussed later in this chapter and elsewhere in this textbook. In brief, depending on whether the virus is seasonal or a novel pandemic strain, patterns of infection and disease are different. Characteristics and severity of well-characterized pandemics have varied greatly, but it has been said of seasonal influenza that it is an unchanging disease caused by a changing virus. There is some truth to that, although recognized differences exist in illness patterns produced by the different types and subtypes that circulate from year to year.

By definition, pandemics are only produced by type A viruses which must be novel and have evidence of animal origin. However, because of circulation of similar or related viruses decades before a pandemic, and which have long since have been replaced, there is usually an age above which the population has been exposed to these ancestral viruses and subsequently has some persistence of immunity [1,2]. Therefore, attack rates in such older individuals can be lower than in younger individuals; the specific age involved and degree of protection varies from pandemic to pandemic. While attack rates are always high in pandemics, at least in younger individuals, mortality varies, often dramatically. The devastating 1918 pandemic which killed an estimated 20–50 million people is the benchmark against which the severity of others is measured.

Over the last decade, the greatest perceived threat of a severe pandemic has been influenza A(H5N1) or "avian flu." Sporadic human H5N1 infections have continued to occur over the last 10 years, particularly in Asia and more recently Egypt, but only limited evidence of human-to-human spread has been reported and this transmission has been unsustained. The viral determinants of severity and binding-receptor specificity are well understood for avian influenza A (H5N1) among the sporadic cases occurring in humans [3]. Recent work has shown that as few as five mutations (all of which also occur in nature) can result in current H5N1 strains becoming

Textbook of Influenza, Second Edition. Edited by Robert G. Webster, Arnold S. Monto, Thomas J. Braciale, and Robert A. Lamb.
© 2013 John Wiley & Sons, Ltd. Published 2013 by John Wiley & Sons, Ltd.

transmissible between ferrets and therefore presumed also humans, confirming that H5N1 remains a clear pandemic threat [4].

The vast majority of influenza infection occurs outside of pandemics and is now termed seasonal influenza, in recognition of its occurrence in the colder season of the temperate zones. This term has replaced the expression "inter-pandemic influenza" which might be considered more universal, given that circulation patterns in tropical and subtropical zones often have less clear seasonality. Over the years, the biggest overall public health impact on morbidity and mortality is due to nonpandemic or seasonal influenza, which is the subject for much of this chapter. After a pandemic, the novel influenza A virus will become a new seasonal virus, joining the other seasonal viruses, currently another A subtype virus and type B virus. All will evolve gradually over time by antigenic drift. Because these viruses circulate for years, there is always significant residual immunity in the population from one drifted strain to another and seasonal attack rates will generally be much lower than in a pandemic. However, the extent of spread of a new drifted strain will also be affected by the degree of antigenic change from the previous year's circulating viruses. The relatively severe seasons in 1997 and 2003 occurred because of major drift of influenza A (H3N2) viruses [5]. Unlike the situation during a pandemic when the novel virus typically is predominant, different seasonal influenza types and subtypes can co-circulate. As an example, in 2010–2011, influenza A (H3N2), influenza B, and the 2009 influenza A(H1N1)pdm09 virus, on its way to becoming a seasonal virus, all co-circulated.

In many ways, it is artificial to try to make sharp distinctions between pandemic and seasonal influenza. The pandemic virus typically replaces the previous influenza A strain or subtype and becomes the next seasonal virus. As it does so, the epidemiology of the virus changes as immunity builds in the population.

Seasonal influenza surveillance, epidemiology, and burden

Identifying influenza infection

Influenza viruses cause a wide range of illnesses in persons of all ages which vary from asymptomatic infection to a relatively mild fever and cough, to pneumonia and other complications, and also to death. The fact that there are often common signs and symptoms of seasonal influenza has resulted in development of the concept of "influenza-like illness" (ILI), a syndrome which has often been used as an indirect way to assess the activity of influenza viruses, without the requirement for identification of etiology. As described below, that type of approach is valid in some situations, but not in others where specific identification of etiology is required.

The recent development of real-time polymerase chain reaction (PCR) technology has had a major impact on our ability to recognize the frequency and burden of influenza infection and to conduct experimental or observational epidemiologic studies, such as investigations of vaccine effectiveness where specific identification of etiology is required [6]. Previously, a variety of techniques were used to identify influenza infections, and sensitivity was often a problem. Most techniques could only be performed in a limited number of laboratories and were labor intensive. Isolation was the gold standard, but required the availability of appropriate cell culture systems. Some studies relied on rise in antibody titer in paired sera, an approach that is convenient for looking at attack rates because regular blood collections can be carried out on populations over time. However, we now recognize that serologic conversion cannot distinguish symptomatic from asymptomatic infections. Also, as an outcome it may be biased in situations such as vaccine trials where immune response may vary between vaccines and nonvaccinees [6]. In particular, the change to PCR technology has allowed dramatic improvement in the study of influenza in low-resourced settings [7]. In many of these areas, there is now knowledge about seasonality and initial information on burden which could not have taken place without use of PCR [8]. In developed countries also, the arrival of PCR in major hospital laboratories has greatly improved understanding of influenza burden and risk groups. Rapid antigen tests are also widely used in clinical settings and can provide point-of-care diagnosis that is faster than PCR. However, these generally have lacked sensitivity, though they are reasonably specific. While a positive result can be a strong indication to start antiviral treatment (especially when surveillance suggests influenza is circulating), a negative result in most rapid antigen assays does not discount influenza infection and antivirals or other therapies should still be considered.

Transmission of influenza

Recent studies have found that influenza is not as highly transmissible as previously thought. Using data from past community and household studies, the number of fully susceptible contacts that can be infected by a single case of seasonal influenza (Ro) is under 2, compared with about 15–17 for measles. With seasonal influenza, contacts are usually not fully susceptible because of residual immunity, so the effective reproductive number is lower. Outbreaks may appear intense in crowded settings or institutions, not because of high transmissibility, but because of close contact, the short incubation period, and therefore low case-to-case (serial) interval of 2–4 days.

A more controversial aspect of influenza transmission is the precise mechanism by which the virus spreads from an infected individual to another. Direct contact, small droplet, and aerosol spread all have been thought to be involved; while these distinctions appear theoretical, they are of importance for practical control measures. For instance, if small droplets are significantly involved, then a respirator rather than a surgical mask would be necessary for individual protection. Several lines of evidence, including the effect of interventions, can be used to distinguish among the possibilities. For example, hand hygiene among school children reduces frequency of upper respiratory infections including influenza, suggesting that direct contact is involved to some degree [9], but protection may be enhanced when face masks are added [10]. The most difficult issue relates to distinguishing between large droplet and true aerosol spread. Some evidence suggests that, in certain circumstances, true aerosol transmission might occur [11]. Animal models may also help to examine these mechanisms, especially ferrets because they present with clinical illness similar to humans. However, novel study approaches, such as experiments in which human volunteers are deliberately infected with well-characterized influenza viruses, are also likely necessary. It may be possible to simulate various situations in which spread occurs to help assess the likely size of particles. Whichever the mechanism, influenza transmission is more likely to occur when susceptible persons are brought close together, such as in schools, military installations, and long-term care facilities and, predictably, outbreaks with high attack rates regularly occur in these settings.

Global surveillance of influenza

Countries throughout the world use a variety of different surveillance systems to monitor influenza activity, characterize strains, and document burden. Surveillance of influenza has historically focused on persons seeking care for and presenting with mild influenza disease (fever, cough, and malaise), often termed ILI. This type of surveillance, when performed systematically, can establish seasonality and is a sensitive marker for influenza activity in temperate climes. Moreover, systematic sampling of patients is often added in order to confirm influenza diagnosis, detect viruses that can be antigenically characterized for vaccine selection, or perform antiviral resistance testing. Influenza is also monitored outside of systemized surveillance in countries that routinely use diagnostic tests for influenza in clinical cases, usually in hospital settings. However, additional systems are required to understand the full burden of severe and fatal seasonal influenza infection and associated risk factors. In addition to ILI, many countries now also conduct systematic hospital-based surveillance for influenza disease, screening persons admitted for respiratory illness using a broad case definition of fever and cough or severe acute respiratory illness (SARI). Along with ILI, SARI is now one of the syndromes recommended by the World Health Organization (WHO) for influenza surveillance globally.

Since 2003, global surveillance for influenza has increased dramatically, in part because of the use of PCR. In 2003, just over 70 000 viruses were reported to WHO via the Global Influenza Surveillance and Response System (GISRS) network of accredited National Influenza Centers from 57 countries. In 2011, this had risen to >210 000 viruses from 122 countries including many less developed countries.

Global seasonality

Historically, the seasonality of influenza was recognized in the northern temperate region because of the clear increase of ILI in the colder months. When virologic assays became available, influenza transmission in northern temperate regions was found to occur rarely before November and to wind down in April–May, though substantial year-to-year variation was apparent [12]. In some (but not all) years, influenza A viruses predominated at the beginning of the season, and influenza B viruses took over in later months. This seasonality allowed for recognition of influenza as an important cause of morbidity and mortality, and assessment of the impact of influenza-related hospitalization and death using models without the necessity for laboratory confirmation of individual cases.

In the southern temperate region, the seasons are reversed and influenza seasonal activity is generally underway by June. As is the case in the north, extent of spread is difficult to predict. Seasonality of influenza becomes more complicated, however, at intermediate, subtropical, and tropical latitudes, with variation related to different climate factors and possibly altitude [13]. Generally, in these areas periods of influenza circulation during the year become longer and the timing less predictable, yet some periods of increased spread are maintained. A consistent pattern of two major periods of transmission has been observed in Hong Kong for a number of years, with one peak starting in February and another starting in the Northern Hemisphere summer, but with year-to-year variation in intensity [14]. A somewhat similar pattern has been observed in Singapore. One study has suggested that Brazil, which is largely tropical, has seasonal circulation that peaks first in the north, then the peak seems to move southwards in a "traveling wave" [15].

Environmental factors that may affect transmission and influenza seasonality have been historically difficult to elucidate; they have focused largely on temperature and humidity. For tropical and subtropical regions, a fairly consistent finding has been the association of influenza transmission with the rainy season in areas with little temperature variation. Until recently, animal models and human surveillance data have produced unclear results. However, reanalysis of data from animal models and US surveillance has suggested that a combination of temperature and humidity – absolute humidity or vapor pressure – may be an important environmental driver of infection [16]. Complicating the role of the environment alone are those human activities that drive transmission, such as timing of opening of schools, crowding, and possibly factors such as vitamin D and melatonin levels which may modulate host susceptibility [17].

Overall, with increased surveillance globally, a number of general observations can now be made. Large countries, such as India and China, with diverse climates, can have different regional seasonality. The location of countries to the north or south of the equator should not be confused with seasonal patterns seen in the north or south temperate zones. Influenza circulation in several countries in the Northern Hemisphere (e.g., El Salvador and Senegal) exhibits seasonality June through September [18]. Furthermore, as real-time reverse transcription PCR tests with primers specific for influenza B and A subtypes are increasingly used worldwide, differences in the timing of the circulation of different types and subtypes are becoming apparent. For instance, surveillance in Vietnam suggests that different subtypes of influenza A and influenza B may predominate at different times during the year [19]. Figure 16.1, derived from virologic data reported to WHO, illustrates the unpredictable nature of influenza seasonality globally.

Morbidity

Since 1977, one influenza B virus and two A subtypes have been circulating in human populations. Early studies established that influenza A(H3N2) produced the most severe illnesses, influenza A(H1N1) the least, and influenza B was intermediate. With the replacement in April 2009 of the former seasonal influenza A(H1N1) viruses by influenza A(H1N1)pdm09, the pandemic H1N1, this severity ranking may have been changed, but it is too early to tell. In terms of hospitalizations and deaths, it is clear that influenza A(H3N2) viruses are the subtype most commonly involved. There have been some years in which influenza B has been associated with severe outcomes, but that is less common. The difference might be related to fact that influenza B viruses occur less frequently, and to the more gradual antigenic drift of influenza B viruses, because the greatest impact of influenza A(H3N2) viruses often results from a major drift and subsequent escape from pre-existing protective immunity. Of note, however, a single study from China found an unexpected but clear association between

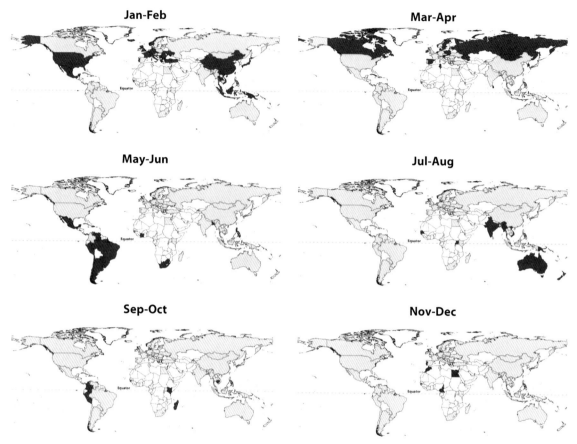

Jan-Feb **Mar-Apr**

May-Jun **Jul-Aug**

Sep-Oct **Nov-Dec**

Figure 16.1. Peak month of transmission of influenza in 81 countries, 1983–2011. Derived from FluNet data [18] and Azziz-Baumgartner et al. [13]. For some countries, the peak months are based on sparse data from few years of observation and which may change over time. Additionally, for large countries there may be regional differences.

increased influenza B circulation and excess mortality, so regional or other differences may exist [20].

A problem in defining total morbidity caused by influenza viruses has been the need for laboratory confirmation, given the overlap of the clinical syndromes produced by respiratory agents, including that of ILI, often used as a surrogate for laboratory-confirmed influenza. Before the advent of PCR, virus culture was difficult to perform in large enough populations to give generalizable results on illness incidence. Other approaches (e.g., rise in antibody titer) were used in order to determine total infection rates. Additional challenges to burden assessment are the long time periods that are necessary to develop stable estimations, due to the major variations in incidence by year in a given country, and the challenge in ascertaining severe outcomes in settings with poor healthcare access. Burden estimates can also vary substantially by site in the same country.

With these considerations in mind, the incidence of infection and illness in the temperate zones has been evaluated over many years, providing robust data on the epidemiology of influenza in these settings. In general, rates are highest in young children and fall with increasing age, with occasional increases sometimes found among young adults when they have greater exposure to their young children. Attack rates of influenza, as measured by serology, can range from 10% to 20% of the general population [12], but are highest in children who can experience annual infection rates of up to 50% in severe influenza A (H3N2) seasons. Though approximately one-third or more of infections may be asymptomatic [21], this high attack rate translates into high rates of outpatient consultation in children. Annually, approximately 6–12% of children under 5 years in the United States will seek clinic or emergency room care for influenza-associated illnesses [22]. Infection rates are usually lower in older adults, in part because of lack of contact with those with the highest frequency of infections, and also because of the presence of broadly reactive antibodies from multiple previous infections. Outbreaks in nursing homes suggest that the frail, institutionalized elderly are also of increased susceptibility to complications because of immune senescence.

Mortality

Understanding the full burden of severe influenza infection is complicated for several reasons. First, influenza disease has a similar presentation to many other respiratory diseases and is seldom tested for in patients, even those that are hospitalized. Moreover, influenza infection can trigger an exacerbation of existing underlying conditions such as cardiovascular illness and chronic obstructive pulmonary disease (COPD) [23]. Secondary bacterial pneumonia can follow an influenza illness; but this initial influenza infection is often not suspected as the trigger of bacterial pneumonia, especially as it can occur 2–3 weeks previous to the bacterial infection. For these reasons, use of influenza-specific diagnoses from hospital discharge and vital statistic data seriously underestimate influenza burden, and so different approaches to assess the burden of influenza have been developed.

Influenza mortality has traditionally been estimated through an excess mortality approach, and estimated largely in developed, northern temperate countries. Several different methods now exist [24], but the core approach is the estimation of the extra (excess) mortality during the influenza season over and above an average expected value or threshold for winter mortality. This baseline threshold is usually derived using vital statistic or multiple-cause-of-death data coded using the International Classification of Disease (ICD) codes. Several categories of mortality codes have been analyzed to estimate excess influenza mortality, including all-cause coded deaths, respiratory and cardiovascular coded deaths, and pneumonia and influenza coded deaths. Several approaches exist for analyzing these data [24], but two types of models are predominant. The first model does not use any viral data, but, using techniques first described by Serfing in the early 1960s, fits a sinusoidal baseline with a 95% confidence interval to a times series of at least 5 years of mortality data. The influenza epidemic period is then defined as when mortality exceeds the upper 95% confidence interval of expected mortality with no influenza epidemic for more than 2 weeks and ends when mortality drops below the epidemic threshold for more than 2 weeks. The observed deaths over this 95% confidence interval during this epidemic period are attributed to influenza. A second, more recent approach uses Poisson regression techniques to incorporate weekly virus surveillance data and the relative activity of influenza into the model. A baseline using a so-called Serfling approach is still created, but with influenza terms set to zero; specific subtype and type terms are then added to the model, including for other pathogens such as respiratory syncytial virus (RSV) that often co-circulate and can confound the apparent association between respiratory mortality and influenza circulation. This approach permits for type and subtype-specific estimates of influenza burden. Other approaches have been used, such as rate difference, where the periods when influenza is not circulating is used as a baseline rate and compared with the rate during periods when the influenza is circulating [24]. Other different approaches include auto-regressive integrated moving average (ARIMA).

An important consideration with regard to these models is the type of mortality data being used. Pneumonia and influenza (P&I) coded deaths are closely correlated to influenza activity, but will only provide an estimate of influenza-associated pneumonia deaths or deaths suspected by a clinician to be influenza. Several earlier studies used these data, but these are likely to underestimate true influenza burden because it is recognized that influenza causes a wide range of severe disease presentations. All-cause mortality conversely may overestimate influenza burden by attributing unrelated deaths (e.g., injuries) to influenza.

One compromise is to use mortality data coded as disease of the respiratory or cardiovascular systems, which should include the majority of influenza-related outcomes with limited misattribution. Of note, however, even these codes would not include potential influenza-associated deaths due to complications of metabolic disorders such as diabetes mellitus. Total respiratory and cardiovascular mortality, and the contribution of influenza infection to this burden, is shown in Figure 16.2a by subtype and type for the years 1981–2009.

Interestingly, different models used on US data have not generated very different mortality estimates, and the following general trends hold true for whichever model is used [25]. First, mortality varies widely each season in part because of different virus attack rates and different strains. Subtype H3N2 in particular is

recognized as associated with increased severity of disease. Second, about 90% of seasonal influenza-associated deaths occur among the elderly 65 years of age and older, and mortality rates rise sharply in those more than 75 years of age. Lastly, the majority of deaths attributed to influenza in these studies are not coded as respiratory deaths, but rather as cardiovascular or other causes, confirming the important role influenza infection has in causing serious complications of a wide range of diseases.

The most recent study by the US Centers for Disease Control and Prevention (CDC) uses Poisson regression techniques to estimate that from 1976 to 2007, 3349–48 614 persons (mean 23 607 persons) died each year from influenza-associated respiratory and circulatory disease in the United States [26]. Of these deaths, 0.5% occurred in persons <19 years of age,

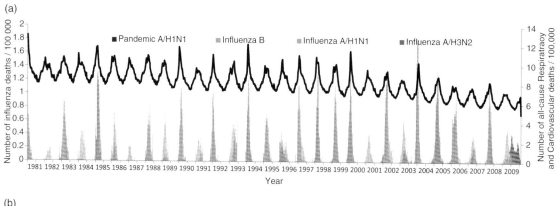

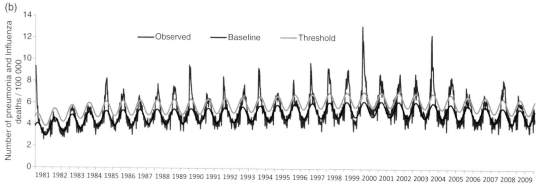

Figure 16.2. (a) Rates of all respiratory and cardiovascular mortality and estimated influenza mortality rate by week and by type and subtype, United States, 1981–2009.

(b) Rates of pneumonia and influenza mortality in 122 cities, United States 1981–2009.

10.1% occurred in persons 19–64 years, and 89.4% occurred in persons ≥65 years. Only 27% of all influenza-associated deaths were coded as P&I; the remaining were coded as either non-P&I respiratory or cardiovascular deaths.

This work, which used viral surveillance data, also found that the average number of deaths in seasons where H3N2 strains were predominant (>20% of all typed and subtyped viruses) was 2.7 times that in seasons when H3N2 was not predominant. Further, over the last 30 years in the United States, the number of deaths has also increased from an average of 17 689 in 1976–1985, to 19 332 in 1986–1995, and finally to 34 584 in 1996–2005. This doubling of the number of influenza-associated deaths well over and above the average population growth rate is due to (i) an expanding aged population (especially the very elderly ≥85 years) at risk of severe influenza disease, (ii) increased circulation of H3N2, and (iii) more persons living with comorbidities.

One major limitation of cause-of-death data is that they are often released several years after collection, and so timely analysis for predictions for any one season is not possible. For this reason (and because P&I data closely correlate with influenza activity), CDC has conducted surveillance since 1970 for P&I deaths in cities throughout the United States, now numbering 122 cities. Weekly, real-time data collected from death certificates helps to assess the severity of any one season as it peaks. P&I surveillance data track patterns of all-cause influenza mortality closely (Figure 16.2b). In addition, after a winter of a particularly virulent H3N2 virus in 2004, laboratory-confirmed influenza deaths among children became notifiable disease events in the United States, allowing for monitoring of severity of illness and risk factors as an influenza season progresses [27].

Hospitalizations

Similar to mortality, the impact of seasonal influenza infection on hospitalizations has been measured largely in temperate regions using robust hospital discharge data, taking advantage of a clear seasonality in influenza transmission. In the United States, the mean estimate of hospitalizations per year from models of hospital discharge data is 55 000–431 000, with considerable variation by year and by predomi-

nant virus [28]. As for mortality, hospitalization rates rise rapidly with age, especially among the elderly, rising from an average of 190 hospitalizations per 100 000 person-years in 65- to 69-year-olds to 1200 per 100 000 person-years in ≥85-year-olds [28]. However, infants and young children, who rarely die of influenza infection in settings with high access to healthcare, also have high rates of influenza-associated hospitalization. Based on hospital discharge data, the highest rates are among children less than 6 months of age; in addition to being at high risk of disease, this group is also not eligible for vaccination. The influenza-attributable hospitalization rates in this group have been reported as high as 1000 per 100 000 child-years, comparable to rates in the very elderly. The rates drop two- to fivefold for ages 6–24 months, and thereafter sharply decrease as age increases [22]. Approximately 10% of hospitalizations among US children will lead to intensive care [29].

Global disease burden

The lack of typical seasonality and diagnosis of influenza illness in tropical and subtropical regions has resulted in a historic under-recognition of the role of influenza globally. However, the expansion of the use of the PCR assay globally is now allowing for a much better appreciation of the potential burden of influenza. Currently, the WHO estimates a total of 250 000–500 000 deaths and 3–5 million cases of severe illness annually due to influenza [30]. These estimates are largely based on simple extrapolation from the US burden estimates and were made when data from nontemperate regions were sparse. Estimation of influenza mortality is complicated in some regions where influenza often circulates throughout the year, or exhibits two or more seasons. Moreover, many tropical and subtropical regions have limited cause-of–death data and sparse virologic data. Nonetheless, several tropical region countries such as Singapore and Hong Kong have estimated influenza-associated mortality using different methods [31,32]. Interestingly, the mortality rates from tropical and temperate regions are generally similar. One exception is South Africa, where the age-adjusted mortality among the elderly over 65 years is 3–4 times higher than estimates from the United States and other higher income countries [33]. The authors state that

40% of the South African population can be considered at or below the poverty line. This raises the concerning issue that the burden of severe influenza may be considerably higher in certain populations, possibly due to comorbidities such as HIV, TB, malnutrition, and poor access to healthcare.

Children in lower resourced settings may experience a higher rate of influenza-associated severe disease than in temperate regions. A recent worldwide meta-analysis of severe influenza-associated disease in children under 5 years found rates of acute lower respiratory tract influenza infections in developing countries to be three times that in developed countries, and also found an increased rate among children 6 months and younger [34]. Influenza-associated hospitalization rates among children in Hong Kong have been reported as several-fold higher than in the United States, though hospitalization rates among the elderly are comparable [35]. Many childhood influenza infections are complicated by secondary infections with *Streptococcus pneumoniae* or *Staphylococcus aureus* and other infections [36]. Lack of appropriate antibiotic treatment, vaccination against bacterial causes of pneumonia, and intensive care in many settings may result in higher rates of severe disease and death.

Groups at special Risk

In addition to extremes of age and institutionalization, certain conditions and comorbidities are associated with a higher risk of influenza-related complications. As defined by the US Advisory Committee on Immunization Practices, these comorbidities include any chronic respiratory condition (including asthma), and hepatic, renal, cardiovascular (except hypertension), hematologic, neurologic/neuromuscular, and metabolic disorders. Among children, the most common underlying risk factor is asthma, whereas among the elderly, chronic obstructive pulmonary disease and other chronic lung conditions are the most common risk factors associated with hospitalization. Rates of hospitalization among adults with one or more of these underlying conditions are four- to 10-fold that of healthy adults. One study reported the rate of hospitalization among adults ≥65 years with comorbidities as 560 per 100 000 person-years compared with 190 per 100 000 person-years in healthy adults [37]. Influenza-related excess deaths have been reported among pregnant

women during pandemics, but pregnant women are also at risk of severe complications from seasonal influenza infection. Also of note, rates of respiratory hospitalization among women during third trimester pregnancy have been found to be several-fold higher during the influenza season than outside the influenza season or among nonpregnant women [38].

During the 2009 H1N1 pandemic, a high body mass index (BMI) of ≥40 was associated with a four- to sevenfold increase in influenza-associated hospitalization, even when controlling for other comorbidities [39]. It remains unclear if morbid obesity is a risk factor for complications only from novel influenza viruses, or also represents a risk group for seasonal influenza. The recent pandemic also highlighted the increased risk of fatal influenza illness among indigenous groups worldwide, which likely applies to seasonal influenza as well. Reported mortality rates were 2–5 times that of nonindigenous populations [40].

One reason for the possibly increased burden of influenza in lower resourced and tropical regions may relate to differences in comorbidities. Low healthcare access results in lack of treatment for the acute episode, but also means that persons are generally living with poorly managed underlying conditions such as asthma, COPD, and cardiovascular disease that will increase the risk of severe influenza disease. In the United States, for instance, lower income populations with comorbidities experience higher influenza-associated hospitalization rates than higher income persons with comorbidities [41]. Some countries may have a high prevalence of HIV infection with low CD4 counts or unrecognized tuberculosis disease and both conditions have been associated with increased risk of severe influenza illness. Sickle cell disease in children has been strongly associated with hospitalization for influenza disease [42], and the sickle cell trait is most common among populations in West and Central Africa. Currently, the lack of data on rates of and risk factors for influenza morbidity and mortality in different settings around the globe and in different subpopulations is a major limitation in our understanding of the full burden, epidemiology, and impact of influenza. This in turn complicates efforts to make informed decisions on vaccination. Table 16.1 outlines some of the differences in influenza epidemiology between temperate and tropical settings.

Table 16.1. Epidemiology and prevention of seasonal influenza in temperate and high and low income tropical countries.

	Temperate	Tropics	
		High to mid income	Low income
Availability of viral surveillance data	Good	Medium–good	Poor–medium Improving rapidly
Availability of surveillance data on mild (ILI) and severe (SARI) disease	ILI: good SARI: good–poor	ILI: good–medium SARI: good–medium	ILI: medium–poor SARI: good–poor
Mortality data for burden estimates	Good	Good–medium	Poor–none
Seasonality	Winter months Good correlation with hemisphere	Some activity throughout much of the year with one or two peaks Poor correlation with hemisphere	Some activity throughout much of the year with one or two peaks Poor correlation with hemisphere
Mortality	Mostly among elderly, approx. 100–150 deaths/100 000 persons. May be higher in low income settings Low among children, although not absent	As temperate in countries that have estimated Low–medium among children	Very little known Unknown among children as impact of low access to healthcare, vaccines and antibiotics unknown
Risk groups for severe disease	Elderly and very young Chronic conditions Immunosuppression Pregnancy Indigenous peoples	As for temperate	As for temperate, with likely addition of malnutrition, HIV/AIDS, tuberculosis, malaria and other risk factors
Antiviral availability	Good	Good–medium	Poor–none
Vaccine used (North or South formulation)	According to hemisphere of country location	According to seasonality of influenza	According to seasonality of influenza
Presence and focus of vaccination recommendations	All countries Risk groups for severe disease and healthcare workers. Increasing focus on young children and pregnant women	Most countries As for temperate, but in flux according to national priorities	Few countries As for temperate, where they exist. Increased focus on maternal immunization as recommended by WHO
Government supported vaccination	Yes	Majority yes	No

ILI, influenza-like illness; SARI, severe acute respiratory illness; WHO, World Health Organization.

Interventions for seasonal influenza

Vaccination timing and target groups

The currently used influenza vaccines need to be given each year, not only because of the requirement to update strains, but also because of the relatively short duration of protection produced by conventional inactivated vaccines. Thus, each year the vaccine needs to be given shortly before the influenza season.

Timing is not an issue in the temperate zones, where influenza is only transmitted during the colder times of the year. However, in the tropics where there may be more unpredictable and year-round transmission, timing of vaccine administration is more problematic, as is the decision regarding which influenza vaccine formulation to use (Northern or Southern Hemisphere formulation). The designation of Northern or Southern formulation does not indicate that different viruses circulate in each hemisphere, but rather represents an update on the most recently prevalent viruses. Timing of vaccination should follow local recommendations, and be based on what is known about seasonality. Generally, vaccination should be given before the likely period of maximal or increased transmission, and as soon as the most recent vaccine formulation is available.

The populations targeted for vaccination have changed over time as epidemiologic evidence of risk groups and burden has increased. In temperate, developed regions, those 65 years and older and those with defined risk conditions were initially identified as priority groups for vaccination. The burden of severe influenza among children has been increasingly recognized, especially after the predominance of a particularly virulent H3N2 strain during the US 2003–2004 influenza season which resulted in a sharp increase in pediatric mortality. The US Advisory Committee on Immunization Practices (ACIP) first recommended vaccination of children 6–23 months of age in 2004; the recommendation was then expanded to children 6–59 months in 2006, and finally to all children in 2008. When these groups and their contacts were added to those previously recommended for vaccination, a majority of the US population was recommended to be vaccinated. To simplify what had become a confusing recommendation, a decision was made in 2010 to make a "universal" recommendation, that all individuals ≥6 months of age should be vaccinated on an annual basis, provided that there are no contraindications. To date, this approach has been essentially limited to the United States. Another important target group is healthcare providers; they are recommended to be vaccinated to protect both themselves and the patients they care for (who are often at high risk of complications from influenza). Also, vaccinating the staff and residents of long-term residential institutions for the elderly can reduce the risk of outbreaks, which can be severe.

Vaccination in less developed settings is often not a priority and coverage is generally very low. However, this situation is changing; in particular, a growing evidence base on the impact of influenza globally has developed, as surveillance and burden data has increasingly become available.

In addition, several less developed countries have been developing local capacity to produce influenza vaccine, in part to be better prepared for a pandemic. Although capacity is still small, it is increasing and will be used to produce seasonal vaccine between pandemics and maintain vaccination programs. One example is the Thai government which is developing capacity for autochthonous production of both trivalent inactivated vaccine and live attenuated vaccine. In the meantime, the government is purchasing externally produced vaccine and recommending vaccination for the elderly, healthcare workers, and those with high risk conditions. From 2003–2011 in Thailand, influenza vaccine coverage has increased 50- to 100-fold.

Different settings may require differing vaccination strategies, especially if opportunities to vaccinate are few. For instance, further study may show that live attenuated influenza vaccines and adjuvanted inactivated vaccines provide a more durable and heterosubtypic protection [43,44]. Even one course of immunizations in early childhood, when the risk of severe illness is highest, may have considerable impact. New strategies such as maternal immunization of pregnant women would not only protect the expectant mothers who are at high risk of influenza complications, but also would protect infants less than 6 months who are too young for direct immunization. Moreover, maternal vaccination may also lower the risk of prematurity and of babies small for gestational age [45]. Such an intervention could be straightforward to incorporate into current antenatal care as an addition to routine measures such as tetanus vaccination.

As a result of these developments in burden estimation, epidemiology, vaccines and vaccine strategies, in 2012 the WHO's Strategic Advisory Group of Experts (SAGE) updated the 2004 influenza vaccination recommendations which were largely based on evidence from developed countries and not very practical or applicable for many countries. The updated SAGE recommendations now include healthcare workers, children under 5 years, the elderly, and those with high-risk conditions, but single out pregnant women as highest priority for vaccination for a variety of reasons, including ease of implementation [46].

Indirect protective effect of vaccination

The concept that vaccinating those with the highest illness frequencies will interrupt transmission and indirectly protect their contacts has been a consideration in establishing policy on vaccine use. Mathematical modeling initially predicted that vaccinating school-age children, who have high infection rates and should be easily accessible for intervention programs, would protect others in the community. When vaccine supply was limited, it was suggested that it might be more efficient to vaccinate this group and rely on indirect effects rather than to vaccinate traditional risk groups such as the elderly.

The first experimental test of this approach was carried out in 1968–1969. At that time, the influenza A (H3N2) virus was spreading, and specific vaccine was only available in limited quantities. The community of Tecumseh, Michigan, was already involved in a study of acute respiratory infection, and a monovalent vaccine was offered to schoolchildren; 86% of them were vaccinated. During the subsequent outbreak, ILI was reduced not only in those who were vaccinated, but also in younger and older age groups, compared with neighboring communities where vaccine was not available. The indirect protective effect seemed to be less in those older than 40 years, suggesting the continued need to directly vaccinate older adults for individual protection [47].

Subsequent household and school-based studies have confirmed the value of "herd immunity" to expand protection beyond those vaccinated. A study in the former Soviet Union using live attenuated vaccine indicated that vaccinating schoolchildren protected both their unvaccinated classmates and teachers. Most recently, children in uniquely closed religious communities in Canada with reduced contact with outside society were given either inactivated influenza vaccine or hepatitis A vaccine and unvaccinated contacts within these communities were strongly protected [48]. Indirect protection likely varies with the setting and is dependent on the contact patterns between different households and communities.

Measuring the impact of vaccination on mortality

The extent of the impact of rising influenza vaccination coverage on elderly mortality has been difficult to ascertain. Placebo-controlled randomized trials of the effect of vaccination on mortality would need to be very large and are generally not ethically possible in settings where vaccine is available. Observational studies have shown strong associations between vaccination and mortality reduction, though some reported reductions of 50% of all-cause winter mortality are most likely confounded because the frail (more likely to die) are often far less likely to be vaccinated. Studies giving more consideration to the issue of confounding have found that vaccination with inadjuvanted trivalent influenza vaccine may be up to 50% effective in reducing influenza-associated deaths; that translates to a 4.6% reduction in risk of mortality of any cause during the influenza season [49]. Adjuvanted and high-dose vaccines with increased immunogenicity and likely efficacy have been developed for the elderly, though are not available in all countries.

Antivirals

Neuraminidase inhibitors (NAIs) are currently the only commonly used antivirals as adamantanes are not effective against influenza B viruses and most influenza A viruses are now resistant to adamantanes. NAIs can be used for treatment, especially in high risk groups, and sometimes for prophylaxis. Antivirals would be the earliest treatment and control measure in the event of a pandemic because a matched vaccine would take several months to develop.

One question raised when antivirals are used for prophylaxis, especially in a pandemic situation, is whether a recipient who is known to be exposed experiences a mild or asymptomatic infection and therefore is subsequently protected or if the recipient will still require vaccination. As many as 50% of prophylaxis recipients may develop asymptomatic infection as shown by increases in antibody titer, but many will also be totally protected from infection, and therefore remain susceptible. Therefore, it is prudent to consider all individuals unprotected and eligible for vaccination after the antiviral medication is discontinued.

Another important question is whether use of the NAIs in treatment reduces transmission to others. NAI treatment reduces virus shedding only modestly, though the reduction may be greater if used early in infection. Influenza is a self-limited infection and the amount of virus shed will decrease over time, with or without treatment, so the added benefit of NAIs for reducing transmission may be marginal. One household study found that oseltamivir, but not zanamivir, reduced transmission among household members [50]. It was hypothesized that this was because zanamivir did not reduce spread of virus from the nose, as it is administered by oral inhalation; however, dissimilarity of the age composition of the households compared may also have influenced the findings. Prophylactic use of NAIs will prevent infection and therefore transmission.

Non-pharmaceutical interventions

Hand hygiene is of general value in preventing infectious respiratory disease including influenza. One school-based study in Egypt found a strong reduction in influenza infections among pupils at intervention schools where children were encouraged to wash their hands [9]. Of particular note is the role of face masks in preventing transmission. Several studies have suggested an effect of surgical masks alone in reducing transmission, but the effect often does not reach statistical significance [51,52] and requires further study. Even a small positive effect could have a large population effect if masks are used extensively. Use of a face mask by an ill person to stop droplet transmission at the source is likely more effective than the use by a healthy person to prevent exposure. However, the major question involves which face mask should be used in healthcare settings: a standard surgical mask, or a N-95 respirator that is designed to fit closely around the face and more effectively filter out particulate matter. This question will be difficult to resolve until transmission mechanics are better understood. Other interventions for seasonal influenza include patient and contact management (e.g., self-isolation of ill persons and exposure avoidance by contacts), as well as community interventions such as closure of schools.

Pandemic influenza

When a novel subtype of influenza A virus emerges, typically of animal origin, low herd immunity will result in a high attack rate in the population. Though pandemics vary, several further features distinguish them from seasonal influenza epidemics. One clear difference is in seasonality; in the temperate zone, seasonal influenza is restricted to the cold season and usually peaks in the winter. Spread of pandemic viruses may be less affected by seasonal factors; in the past, pandemic viruses have emerged outside of established influenza seasons. This may be because herd immunity is low to these novel viruses, allowing out-of-season transmission. Nonetheless, the 2009 H1N1 pandemic showed some seasonality – in the United States there was continued transmission through June and focal transmission over the summer, but the bulk of clinical illness occurred in the wave beginning in August 2009. This was likely related to the reopening of schools, and was months earlier that the typical start of influenza season. This is similar to the situation that was experienced by Japan during the 1957 pandemic, during which there were spring and autumn waves. In contrast, in the Southern Hemisphere the timing of much of the first wave of 2009 pandemic H1N1 was as expected for seasonal influenza because the novel virus arrived there during the colder season.

Although pandemics are characterized by increased relative mortality in the young, especially in those under 2 years, the elderly may still bear the brunt of the mortality as is seen with seasonal influenza; this was the case in the 1957 and 1968 pandemics. The 1918 pandemic was unique among those with well-documented mortality data. The mortality in persons 20–39 years of age appears to be related to virulence factors of that particular virus; deaths also were associated with bacterial superinfection, as was the case in 1957 and 1968.

A study using vital statistics data available during the 1918 pandemic highlights first the heterogeneity of pandemic transmission throughout the world, and also that lower resourced countries may have borne the brunt of the 1918 pandemic. Every 10% decrease of per capita income in a country was associated with a 10% rise in pandemic mortality [53]. As there were no antibiotics or antivirals in 1918, this differential mortality by income level is unlikely to have been caused by access to healthcare and more likely reflects underlying nutritional or health status. Similarly, a study of 2009 H1N1 pandemic mortality using lower respiratory tract mortality risk ratios found that >50% of pandemic deaths occurred in the lowest income countries of Africa and South-East Asia in the first year of the pandemic [54].

Pandemic preparedness and specific planning remain critical even in an era of antibiotic treatment and modern medicine. The high attack rates, rapid global spread, and unpredictable virulence of novel viruses such as influenza A (H5N1) are a real threat. It is helpful to think of influenza impact as being on a continuum, as even seasonal influenza outbreaks sometimes have high impact, particularly after a major drift in antigenic structure of the virus. Certain outbreaks of seasonal influenza in Africa have had alarmingly high fatality proportions, similar to estimates from the 1918 pandemic. Moreover, the number of deaths caused by seasonal influenza exceeds those occurring in a pandemic.

The best ways to detect, monitor, and control the next pandemic are to build strong global surveillance, understand the epidemiology and risk factors for seasonal influenza in different settings, and promote interventions such as vaccination which are underused in many settings. These interventions are the same for seasonal and pandemic influenza and will reduce impact of seasonal influenza, stimulate demand and development of influenza vaccines, and better prepare for a pandemic.

References

1. Kilbourne ED. Influenza pandemics of the 20th century. Emerg Infect Dis. 2006;12:9–14.
2. Nguyen-Van-Tam JS, Hampson AW. The epidemiology and clinical impact of pandemic influenza. Vaccine. 2003;21:1762–8.
3. Hatta M, Gao P, Halfmann P, Kawaoka Y. Molecular basis for high virulence of Hong Kong H5N1 influenza A viruses. Science. 2001;293:1840–2.
4. Herfst S, Schrauwen EJ, Linster M, Chutinimitkul S, de Wit E, Munster VJ, et al. Airborne transmission of influenza A/H5N1 virus between ferrets. Science. 2012; 336:1534–41.
5. Bhat N, Wright JG, Broder KR, Murray EL, Greenberg ME, Likos AM, et al. Influenza-associated deaths among children in the United States, 2003–2004. N Engl J Med. 2005;353:2559–67.
6. Petrie JG, Ohmit SE, Johnson E, Cross RT, Monto AS. Efficacy studies of influenza vaccines: effect of end points used and characteristics of vaccine failures. J Infect Dis. 2011;203:1309–15.
7. World Health Organization. Global Influenza Surveillance and Response System (GISRS).. Available from: http://www.who.int/influenza/gisrs_laboratory/en/index.html (accessed 8 February 2013).
8. Radin JM, Katz MA, Tempia S, Talla Nzussouo N, Davis R, Duque J, et al. Influenza Surveillance in 15 Countries in Africa, 2006–2010. J Infect Dis. 2012;206 (Suppl 1):S14–21).
9. Talaat M, Afifi S, Dueger E, El-Ashry N, Marfin A, Kandeel A, et al. Effects of hand hygiene campaigns on incidence of laboratory-confirmed influenza and absenteeism in schoolchildren, Cairo, Egypt. Emerg Infect Dis. 2011;17:619–25.
10. Cowling BJ, Chan KH, Fang VJ, Cheng CK, Fung RO, Wai W, et al. Facemasks and hand hygiene to prevent influenza transmission in households: a cluster randomized trial. Ann Intern Med. 2009;151:437–46.
11. Moser MR, Bender TR, Margolis HS, Noble GR, Kendal AP, Ritter DG. An outbreak of influenza aboard a commercial airliner. Am J Epidemiol. 1979;110:1–6.
12. Monto AS, Koopman JS, Longini IM Jr. Tecumseh study of illness. XIII. Influenza infection and disease, 1976–1981. Am J Epidemiol. 1985;121:811–22.
13. Azziz-Baumgartner E, Dao CN, Nasreen S, Bhuiyan MU, Mah-E-Muneer S, Al Mamun A, et al. Seasonality, timing and climate drivers of influenza activity globally. J Infect Dis. 2012;206:838–46.
14. Yang L, Wong CM, Lau EH, Chan KP, Ou CQ, Peiris JS. Synchrony of clinical and laboratory surveillance for influenza in Hong Kong. PLoS ONE. 2008;3:e1399.
15. Alonso WJ, Viboud C, Simonsen L, Hirano EW, Daufenbach LZ, Miller MA. Seasonality of influenza in Brazil: a traveling wave from the Amazon to the subtropics. Am J Epidemiol. 2007;165:1434–42.
16. Shaman J, Goldstein E, Lipsitch M. Absolute humidity and pandemic versus epidemic influenza. Am J Epidemiol. 2011;173:127–35.
17. Dowell SF. Seasonal variation in host susceptibility and cycles of certain infectious diseases. Emerg Infect Dis. 2001;7:369–74.
18. World Health Organization. FluNet. . Available from: http://www.who.int/influenza/gisrs_laboratory/flunet/en// (accessed 7 February 2013).
19. Dharan NJ, Beekmann SE, Fiore A, Finelli L, Uyeki TM, Polgreen PM, et al. Influenza antiviral prescribing practices during the 2007–08 and 2008–09 influenza seasons in the setting of increased resistance to oseltamivir among circulating influenza viruses. Antiviral Res. 2010;88:182–6.
20. Feng L, Shay DK, Jiang Y, Zhou H, Chen X, Zheng Y, et al. Influenza-associated mortality in temperate and subtropical Chinese cities, 2003–2008. Bull World Health Organ. 2012;90:279–288B.
21. Carrat F, Vergu E, Ferguson NM, Lemaitre M, Cauchemez S, Leach S, et al. Time lines of infection and

disease in human influenza: a review of volunteer challenge studies. Am J Epidemiol. 2008;167:775–85.

22. Poehling KA, Edwards KM, Weinberg GA, Szilagyi P, Staat MA, Iwane MK, et al. The underrecognized burden of influenza in young children. N Engl J Med. 2006;355:31–40.

23. Warren-Gash C, Smeeth L, Hayward AC. Influenza as a trigger for acute myocardial infarction or death from cardiovascular disease: a systematic review. Lancet Infect Dis. 2009;9:601–10.

24. Thompson WW, Comanor L, Shay DK. Epidemiology of seasonal influenza: use of surveillance data and statistical models to estimate the burden of disease. J Infect Dis. 2006;194(Suppl. 2):S82–91.

25. Thompson WW, Weintraub E, Dhankhar P, Cheng OY, Brammer L, Meltzer MI, et al. Estimates of US influenza-associated deaths made using four different methods. Influenza Other Respi Viruses. 2009;3:37–49.

26. Centers for Disease Control and Prevention. Estimates of deaths associated with seasonal influenza – United States, 1976–2007. MMWR Morb Mortal Wkly Rep. 2010;59:1057–62.

27. Centers for Disease Control and Prevention. Overview of Influenza surveillance in the United States. 2012. Available from: http://www.cdc.gov/flu/weekly/overview.htm (accessed 7 February 2013).

28. Thompson WW, Shay DK, Weintraub E, Brammer L, Bridges CB, Cox NJ, et al. Influenza-associated hospitalizations in the United States. JAMA. 2004;292:1333–40.

29. Schrag SJ, Shay DK, Gershman K, Thomas A, Craig AS, Schaffner W, et al. Multistate surveillance for laboratory-confirmed, influenza-associated hospitalizations in children: 2003–2004. Pediatr Infect Dis J. 2006;25:395–400.

30. World Health Organization. Influenza (Seasonal) Fact sheet 211. Available from http://www.who.int/mediacentre/factsheets/fs211/en/ (accessed 7 February 2013).

31. Wong CM, Chan KP, Hedley AJ, Peiris JS. Influenza-associated mortality in Hong Kong. Clin Infect Dis. 2004;39:1611–7.

32. Lee VJ, Yap J, Ong JB, Chan KP, Lin RT, Chan SP, et al. Influenza excess mortality from 1950–2000 in tropical Singapore. PLoS ONE. 2009;4:e8096.

33. Cohen C, Simonsen L, Sample J, Kang JW, Miller M, Madhi SA, et al. Influenza-related mortality among adults age 25–54 years with AIDS in South Africa and the United States of America. Clin Infect Dis. 2012;55:996–1003.

34. Nair H, Brooks WA, Katz M, Roca A, Berkley JA, Madhi SA, et al. Global burden of respiratory infections due to seasonal influenza in young children: a system-

atic review and meta-analysis. Lancet. 2011;378:1917–30.

35. Chiu SS, Lau YL, Chan KH, Wong WH, Peiris JS. Influenza-related hospitalizations among children in Hong Kong. N Engl J Med. 2002;347:2097–103.

36. Finelli L, Fiore A, Dhara R, Brammer L, Shay DK, Kamimoto L, et al. Influenza-associated pediatric mortality in the United States: increase of Staphylococcus aureus coinfection. Pediatrics. 2008;122:805–11.

37. Mullooly JP, Bridges CB, Thompson WW, Chen J, Weintraub E, Jackson LA, et al. Influenza- and RSV-associated hospitalizations among adults. Vaccine. 2007;25:846–55.

38. Dodds L, McNeil SA, Fell DB, Allen VM, Coombs A, Scott J, et al. Impact of influenza exposure on rates of hospital admissions and physician visits because of respiratory illness among pregnant women. CMAJ. 2007;176:463–8.

39. Morgan OW, Bramley A, Fowlkes A, Freedman DS, Taylor TH, Garguillo P, et al. Morbid obesity as a risk factor for hospitalization and death due to 2009 pandemic influenza A(H1N1) disease. PLoS ONE. 2010;5:e9694.

40. La Ruche G, Tarantola A, Barboza P, Vaillant L, Gueguen J, Gastellu-Etchegorry M; epidemic intelligence team at InVS. The 2009 pandemic H1N1 influenza and indigenous populations of the Americas and the Pacific. Euro Surveill. 2009;14.

41. Glezen WP, Greenberg SB, Atmar RL, Piedra PA, Couch RB. Impact of respiratory virus infections on persons with chronic underlying conditions. JAMA. 2000;283:499–505.

42. Bundy DG, Strouse JJ, Casella JF, Miller MR. Burden of influenza-related hospitalizations among children with sickle cell disease. Pediatrics. 2010;125:234–43.

43. Vesikari T, Knuf M, Wutzler P, Karvonen A, Kieninger-Baum D, Schmitt HJ, et al. Oil-in-water emulsion adjuvant with influenza vaccine in young children. N Engl J Med. 2011;365:1406–16.

44. Ambrose CS, Wu X, Belshe RB. The efficacy of live attenuated and inactivated influenza vaccines in children as a function of time postvaccination. Pediatr Infect Dis J. 2010;29:806–11.

45. Omer SB, Goodman D, Steinhoff MC, Rochat R, Klugman KP, Stoll BJ, et al. Maternal influenza immunization and reduced likelihood of prematurity and small for gestational age births: a retrospective cohort study. PLoS Med. 2011;8:e1000441.

46. World Health Organization. Meeting of the Strategic Advisory Group of Experts on Immunization, November 2011 – conclusions and recommendations. Wkly Epidemiol Rec. 2012;1–16.

47. Monto AS, Davenport FM, Napier JA, Francis T Jr. Modification of an outbreak of influenza in Tecumseh,

Michigan by vaccination of schoolchildren. J Infect Dis. 1970;122:16–25.

48. Loeb M, Russell ML, Moss L, Fonseca K, Fox J, Earn DJ, et al. Effect of influenza vaccination of children on infection rates in Hutterite communities: a randomized trial. JAMA. 2010;303:943–50.

49. Fireman B, Lee J, Lewis N, Bembom O, van der Laan M, Baxter R. Influenza vaccination and mortality: differentiating vaccine effects from bias. Am J Epidemiol. 2009;170:650–6.

50. Halloran ME, Hayden FG, Yang Y, Longini IM Jr, Monto AS. Antiviral effects on influenza viral transmission and pathogenicity: observations from household-based trials. Am J Epidemiol. 2007;165:212–21.

51. Suess T, Remschmidt C, Schink SB, Schweiger B, Nitsche A, Schroeder K, et al. The role of facemasks and hand hygiene in the prevention of influenza transmission in households: results from a cluster randomised trial; Berlin, Germany, 2009–2011. BMC Infect Dis. 2012;12: 26.

52. Aiello AE, Perez V, Coulborn RM, Davis BM, Uddin M, Monto AS. Facemasks, hand hygiene, and influenza among young adults: a randomized intervention trial. PLoS ONE. 2012;7:e29744.

53. Murray CJ, Lopez AD, Chin B, Feehan D, Hill KH. Estimation of potential global pandemic influenza mortality on the basis of vital registry data from the 1918–20 pandemic: a quantitative analysis. Lancet. 2006;368: 2211–8.

54. Dawood FS, Iuliano AD, Reed C, Meltzer MI, Shay DK, Cheng PY, et al. Estimated global mortality associated with the first 12 months of 2009 pandemic influenza A H1N1 virus circulation: a modelling study. Lancet Infect Dis. 2012;12(9):687–95.

PART 5

Immunology of influenza

Section Editor: Thomas J. Braciale

17 Innate immunity

Akiko Iwasaki[1] and Malik Peiris[2]

[1]Department of Immunobiology, Howard Hughes Medical Institute, Yale University School of Medicine, New Haven, CT, USA

[2]Centre of Influenza Research and School of Public Health, The University of Hong Kong, Hong Kong SAR, China

Introduction

The innate immune system is designed to detect microbial infections through recognition of molecular patterns that are specifically present in microorganisms, including viruses. The best characterized microbial sensors are the pattern recognition receptors (PRRs), which detect relatively invariant molecular patterns found in most microorganisms of a given class [1]. These structures are referred to as pathogen-associated molecular patterns (PAMPs) [2], though they are not unique to microbes that can cause disease (pathogens). In humans, influenza viruses replicate in the superficial epithelial cells of the respiratory tract. The cells of the innate immune system, including the viral target (epithelial cells) and sentinel cells (dendritic cells (DCs) and macrophages), recognize influenza virus infection through the use of distinct set of PRRs. The engagement of the PRR initiates a signaling cascade, resulting in secretion of antiviral factors, such as type I interferons (IFNs). The type I IFN molecules bind to the IFNαβ receptor (IFNαβR) on neighboring cells, resulting in the activation of hundreds of antiviral genes. This provides a mechanism for preventing nearby cells from further replicating influenza virus. In addition to type I IFNs, PRR engagement results in the activation of various proinflammatory cytokine genes and co-stimulatory molecules. Co-stimulatory molecules expressed by antigen presenting cells initi-ate activation of adaptive immune responses. The cytokines bind to their respective receptors and induce activation of innate cells, including macrophages, DCs, and natural killer (NK) cells. However, overt production of cytokines often results in inflammation and immune pathologies after influenza virus infection. This is particularly seen after infection with highly virulent influenza strains, causing a "cytokine storm" leading to severe inflammatory damage and pathogenesis [3]. Therefore, the extent and the duration of cytokine responses must be tightly regulated to provide innate defense while avoiding immune-mediated pathology. This chapter describes the nature of influenza virus recognition by PRRs, antiviral functions of type I IFNs, the cell types involved in orchestrating innate defense against influenza virus, and the role of cytokines in immune defense versus pathology upon infection by various strains of influenza viruses.

Innate sensors of influenza virus infection

Various microbial sensor pathways are used by the innate immune system to induce antimicrobial defense mechanisms. Influenza virus is recognized by the innate immune system through at least three distinct classes of PRRs: retinoic acid inducible gene I (RIG-I), Toll-like receptors (TLR3, TLR7, and TLR8), and a

Textbook of Influenza, Second Edition. Edited by Robert G. Webster, Arnold S. Monto, Thomas J. Braciale, and Robert A. Lamb.
© 2013 John Wiley & Sons, Ltd. Published 2013 by John Wiley & Sons, Ltd.

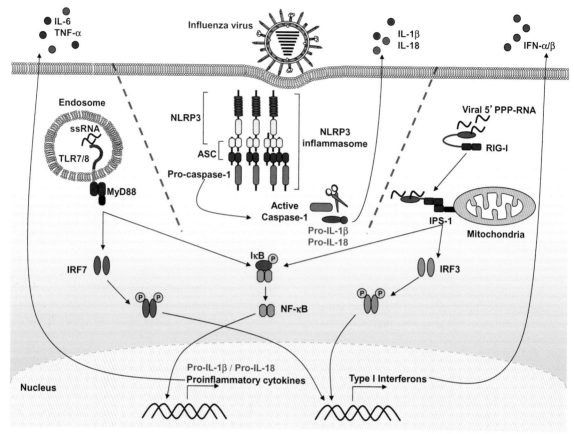

Figure 17.1. Innate sensors of influenza virus infection. Influenza A virus is sensed by at least three different types of pattern recognition receptors. First, viral single-stranded RNA is recognized by TLR-7 and TLR-8 in the endosome. Second, the cytosolic sensor retinoic acid inducible gene I (RIG-I) detects viral ssRNA bearing 5′ triphosphates. TLR-7 and TLR-8 signal through the adaptor protein, MyD88, which leads to the downstream activation of IRF-7 and NF-κB. In contrast, RIG-I signals through the adaptor IPS-I located on the mitochondria for the activation of IRF-3 and NF-κB. Activated IRF-7 and IRF-3 can translocate to the nucleus to activate the production of type I interferons while NF-κB acts as a transcription factor for the induction of a proinflammatory cytokines including IL-6, TNF-α, and the pro-form IL-1β. The TLR-7–TLR-8 pathway is critical for the production of type I IFNs in specialized sentinel cells, while most other virally infected cells utilize the RIG-I pathway. Third, influenza A virus activates the NLRP3 inflammasome in dendritic cells and macrophages leading to the activation of caspase-1, which mediates the processing of pro-IL-1β to mature IL-1β and its subsequent release. Adapted from Pang and Iwasaki [62] with permission from Elsevier.

NOD-like receptor (NLRP3) (Figure 17.1) [4]. Both RIG-I and TLRs induce activation of type I IFN and cytokine genes, while NLRP3 induces the activation of caspase-1 that cleaves and releases cytokines, interleukin 1β (IL-1β), and IL-18. RIG-I and NLRP3 detect virus in the cytosol of infected cells (cell-intrinsic recognition), while TLR3 and TLR7/TLR8 detect virus-infected cells and viral RNA in the endosomes of sentinel cells (cell-extrinsic recognition), respectively.

In virally infected cells, the cytosolic RNA sensor RIG-I detects influenza viral single-stranded RNA (ssRNA) bearing 5′-triphosphates after fusion and replication. Upon binding viral RNA, RIG-I assumes an open conformation, allowing it to interact with its adaptor protein, IPS-1 expressed on the mitochondria. IPS-1 induces activation of NF-κB and IRF3, resulting in transcription of cytokine and IFN genes, respectively.

Cell extrinsic recognition of influenza virus occurs in sentinel cells such as the plasmacytoid dendritic cells (pDCs). There, influenza viral ssRNA is recognized by Toll-like receptor 7 (TLR7) in the endosome. This occurs in the absence of direct infection of pDCs by influenza virus. TLR7 engagement leads to the activation of the adaptor MyD88 and production of proinflammatory cytokines and type I IFNs via NF-kB and IRF7 dependent pathways, respectively. In humans, influenza virus recognition is mediated by another endosomal TLR, TLR8. TLR8 is expressed by myeloid cells including DCs and macrophages. In addition, TLR-3, which recognizes dsRNA in the endosomes, has been shown to mediate proinflammatory cytokine responses, and not type I IFN response, following influenza infection leading to pathology.

Another class of PRR responsible for sensing influenza virus is the cytosolic sensor NLRP3 [4]. NLRP3 forms a multiprotein complex known as the "inflammasome," which acts as a platform for activating caspase-1. NLRP3 recruits the adaptor protein ASC (apoptosis-associated speck-like protein containing a caspase recruitment domain). ASC contains a N-terminal PYD domain and a C-terminal caspase activation and recruitment domain (CARD) which is essential for the binding and recruitment of caspase-1 to the inflammasome (Figure 17.1) [5]. The activation of the NLRP3 inflammasome and the production of IL-1β usually require two signals. The first signal can be triggered by TLR agonists, leading to transcriptional activation of NLRP3 [6]. The second signal is triggered in response to various stress signals associated with damaged-self and non-self molecules. In the case of influenza virus infection of DCs and macrophages, TLR7 engagement by viral genomic RNA triggers the first signal, while the M2 ion channel activity in the trans-Golgi network serves as the second signal in activating NLRP3 [7]. Once activated, caspase-1 can cleave its substrates, which include IL-1β and IL-18, which are released to extracellular environment. Unlike type I IFNs, IL-1β and IL-18 do not induce antiviral resistance. Instead, IL-1β acts on DCs to promote the development of adaptive immune responses [8,9], while IL-18 primes

NK cells and cytotoxic T cells for the production of IFN-γ and enhance their cytolytic activity.

Influenza virus recognition by these PRRs does not represent simply redundant pathways. First, different cell types appear to utilize distinct PRR for influenza detection. In humans, TLR7 is expressed by only a few cell types, namely, pDCs and IFN-stimulated B cells, while RIG-I is expressed ubiquitously. RIG-I is critical for viral detection and IFN-α production in fibroblasts and conventional DCs whereas pDCs use the TLR7 for innate recognition of influenza virus [10]. TLR3 is expressed by a subset of DCs in both humans and mice which are dedicated to stimulating CD8 T-cell responses. NLRP3 is predominantly expressed by DCs, neutrophils, monocytes, and macrophages, but not lymphocytes and other leukocytes [11]. Second, PRRs engage different effector pathways. Mice deficient in RIG-I or TLR7 pathways are able to mount intact adaptive immune responses while those lacking the ASC, caspase-1, IL-1R, and MyD88 are unable to mount strong T-cell and B-cell responses against influenza infection [4]. Thus, inflammasome-mediated IL-1β is critical in inducing adaptive immune responses, while RIG-I and TLR7 induce type I IFNs critical in innate antiviral defense.

Type I interferon-mediated antiviral defense mechanisms

The main host defense strategy against viral pathogens is the elimination of the infected cells and making uninfected cells more refractory to virus infection. This can be achieved by cell-intrinsic mechanisms which are induced by type I IFNs and operate in the infected cells, or with the help of cytotoxic lymphocytes; NK cells and CD8 T cells. Type I IFNs are a family of cytokines that act early in the innate immune response and are key cytokines capable of inducing an antiviral state in infected and uninfected neighboring cells [12]. Type I IFNs trigger expression of hundreds of IFN-stimulated genes (ISGs). Here, a handful of examples of how ISGs provide protection against influenza viruses are provided.

Orthomyxovirus resistance gene (Mx) proteins

Mx proteins belong to a family of GTPases consisting of MxA and MxB in humans and Mx1 and Mx2 in mice [13]. Human MxA is expressed in the cytoplasm, while mouse Mx1 is expressed in the nucleus. The Mx proteins have a large N-terminal GTPase domain, a central interacting domain (CID), and a C-terminal leucine zipper (LZ) domain. Both the CID and the LZ domains are required to recognize target viral structures. Influenza viruses are targeted by Mx proteins. Remarkably, transgenic expression of human MxA in IFNαβR-deficient mice confers full resistance to otherwise fatal infection with influenza virus infection [14,15], indicating that this effector molecule is sufficient for protective innate defense against these viruses. The main viral targets seems to be the viral nucleocapsid-like structures. The MxA protein in the cytosol recognizes viral RNPs, and blocks nucleocapsid transport to the nucleus. In contrast, mouse Mx1 protein is expressed in the nucleus and prevents transcription catalyzed by the virion-associated polymerase (Figure 17.2). It is interesting to note that most inbred strains of mice harbor a defective Mx1 gene [13] and a nonfunctional Mx-2 gene. Therefore, studies using inbred mice must be interpreted with the caveat that they are Mx deficient.

2′-5′ oligoadenylate synthetase and ribonuclease L (RNase L)

2′-5′ Oligoadenylate synthetase (OAS) and ribonuclease L (RNase L) act in concert to degrade viral RNA in the cytosol. While basal levels of OAS and RNase L are found constitutively, stimulation through the IFNαβR dramatically increases their expression levels. Activated by dsRNA, OAS converts ATP into 2′-5′ oligoadenylate, which functions as a second messenger to activate latent ribonuclease RNase L. Activated RNase L degrades viral and cellular ssRNAs, inhibiting protein synthesis and viral growth (Figure 17.2). Mice deficient in RNase L have increased susceptibility to RNA viruses including influenza virus [16].

Protein kinase R

Protein kinase R (PKR) is a serine/threonine kinase that phosphorylates the a-subunit of eukaryotic translation initiation factor 2a (eIF2a). PKR becomes activated through homodimerization upon binding to viral double-stranded RNA (dsRNA) structures via its dsRNA binding domains. This results in inhibition of translation and a decrease in total cellular and viral

protein synthesis, effectively reducing viral production. In addition to its translational regulatory function, PKR has a role in signal transduction and transcriptional control through the IκB–NF-κB pathway [17]. PKR can also mediate apoptosis, cell growth arrest, and autophagy, all of which will serve to curb viral replication and spread in the host [18]. In addition to the virus-restricting function of PKR, recent studies indicate that PKR functions to stabilize IFN-α and IFN-β mRNA, thereby ensuring robust IFN protein production [19]. Mice genetically deficient in PKR are susceptible to infection with a variety of viruses including influenza virus.

ISG15

ISG15 is an ubiquitin-like molecule that can be covalently attached to target proteins using E1, E2, and E3-like enzymes. UBE1L (E1-like ubiquitin-activating enzyme) was shown to be the specific ISG15-activating enzyme [20]. Two E2 ubiquitin-conjugating enzymes, UBCH6 and UBCH8, serve as ISG15 carriers. Subsequently, two E3 ubiquitin ligases, HERC5 (homologous to the E6-associated protein C terminus (HECT) domain and RCC1-like domain containing protein 5) and TRIM25 conjugate ISG15 to protein substrates. All enzymes identified in the ISGylation pathway are coordinately induced by type I IFNs. There are over 150 targets of ISGylation. Interestingly, by physically associating with polyribosomes, HERC5 ensures that ISG15 conjugation is restricted to the newly synthesized pool of proteins, which in infected cells will consist primarily of newly translated viral proteins (Figure 17.2) [21]. Mice deficient in ISG15 are more susceptible to challenge with influenza A and B viruses [22]. The exact cell type and mechanism of the antiviral action of ISG15 against influenza viruses are unclear.

Viperin

Viperin (*v*irus *i*nhibitory *p*rotein, *e*ndoplasmic *r*eticulum-associated, *int*erferon inducible) is another IFN-inducible protein that is known to prevent replication of a variety of viruses including influenza virus [23]. Viperin impairs the release of influenza virus by disrupting lipid rafts via suppression of the activity of farnesyl diphosphate synthase, a key enzyme in iso-

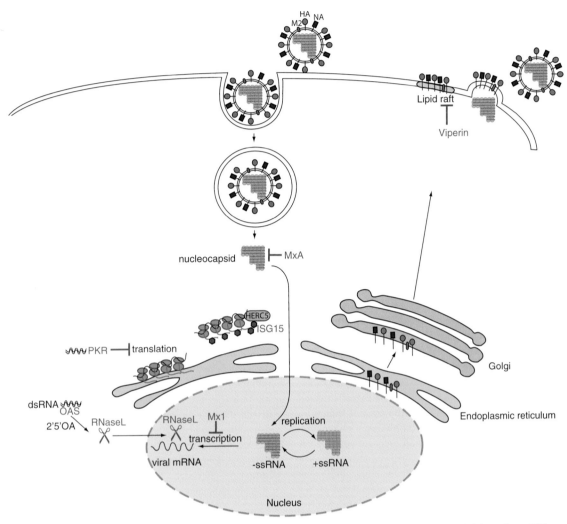

Figure 17.2. Innate antiviral defense mechanisms. Type I interferons (IFNs) induce expression of over 300 IFN-stimulated genes (ISGs). When an IFN-stimulated cell encounters influenza virus, an antiviral program attempts to restrict the virus at multiple steps in viral infection. Human MxA in the cytosol traps viral nucleocapsid and prevents its nuclear import, while mouse Mx1 protein blocks viral transcription in the nucleus. In the cytosol, viral dsRNA activates 2′-5′ oligoadenylate synthetase (OAS) and protein kinase R (PKR). OAS produces 2′5′ oligoadenylate from ATP, which activates a latent ribonuclease, RNaseL. RNaseL can cleave viral mRNA (as well as host mRNA). PKR activated by dsRNA inhibits translation, thereby impairing viral protein synthesis. ISG15 modifies newly synthesized proteins (most of these are viral proteins) by forming complex with HERC5. Viperin impairs viral budding by disrupting lipid rafts.

prenoid biosynthesis [24]. In addition, viperin local-izes to the lipid droplets [23] and through a yet undefined pathway interferes with the replication of other viruses that do not require lipid rafts for synthesis.

Cell types involved in innate defense against influenza virus

The human host employs multiple stages of defense against influenza virus invasion. The first line of defense is provided by the mucus layer that cover the upper and lower respiratory tract. The mucus contains mucins, which are complex high molecular weight glycoproteins with extensive O-glycan attachment. Once within the mucus layer, influenza virus is met with a variety of antimicrobial peptides that can directly bind and kill the virus before it can reach the host epithelial layer. Virions are also phagocytosed and destroyed by the alveolar macrophages that reside within the alveolar space.

Upon successful attachment and entry into the airway epithelial cells, a number of cell types are mobilized to the lung tissue, including neutrophils, monocytes, pDCs, DCs, and NK cells. Recruitment of these cells critically depends on the release of IL-1β by the inflammasome complex [8]. NK cells recognize influenza virus infected cells through natural cytotoxicity receptor 1 (NCR-1) and mediate viral clearance [25]. Monocytes are recruited rapidly to the influenza-infected lung and differentiate into DCs and macrophages. These monocyte-derived DCs are important in restimulating cytotoxic T cells to kill infected cells within the lung [26,27]. A hallmark of inflammation in the influenza-infected lung is the recruitment and accumulation of neutrophils. Neutrophils are a short-lived phagocytic cell population that ingest infected dead cells and clear them from the sites of infection. Together with alveolar macrophages, phagocytic clearance of virus infected dead cells by neutrophils provides an important mechanism of viral clearance [28]. Unlike other innate leukocytes, DCs are capable of initiating adaptive immune responses. After recognizing influenza virus through PRRs, DCs undergo a maturation program and migrate to the draining lymph nodes to prime naïve T and B cells (see below).

Dendritic cells – innate link to adaptive immunity

Dendritic cells have an important role in immune responses at multiple levels. First, they are situated at various sites of pathogen entry, and are among the first cells to recognize the incoming pathogens through a set of PRRs. Engagement of PRRs upon viral recognition induces the expression of genes required to both eliminate the pathogens (innate effectors) and to initiate adaptive immune responses [29]. Second, DCs are the only cell type capable of initiating adaptive

immune responses by activating naïve T lymphocytes. Pathogen recognition through PRRs activates DCs to increase their expression of the chemokine receptor, CCR7, which enables them to migrate from the site of infection to the secondary lymphoid tissues, where naïve lymphocytes recirculate. On transit, DCs undergo a maturation program that results in the upregulation of co-stimulatory molecules and translocation of their major histocompatibility complex (MHC) class II to the cell surface [30]. Once in the lymph node, DCs can present antigens derived from the pathogens to naïve T cells and induce their activation (through co-stimulation) and differentiation (through secretion of appropriate cytokines) [31].

DCs can be broadly divided into two types: those that reside in the peripheral tissues (lung; tissue DCs) and those that reside in the blood and lymphoid tissues (blood DCs) [32]. The blood DCs differentiate from precursors that enter these tissues from peripheral blood. In the mouse lymph nodes and spleen, the blood DCs can be divided into CD8a+ DC (CD8a+ CD11b-), CD4+ DC (CD4+ CD11b+), DN DC (CD4- CD8-), and pDCs. Mouse CD8a+ DCs express TLR3 but lack TLR5 and TLR7 [33]. In contrast, both human and mouse pDCs express TLR7 and TLR9 but not TLR3. In the lung, distinct DC subsets survey the airway and the parenchyma for invading pathogens [34]. The conducting airway epithelia contain DCs that extend dendrites through forming tight junction with the epithelial cells, and are CD103+ CD11b- Langerin+. Beneath the epithelial layer, CD103- CD11b+ DCs survey the lamina propria. The alveolar space also contains MHCII^hi DCs and is easily accessible by bronchoalveolar lavage (BAL). Upon influenza infection, both CD103+ DCs and CD11b+ DCs prime CD8 T-cell responses in the draining lymph nodes [35]. More detailed discussion of DCs involved in generating adaptive immunity to influenza viruses is found in Chapter 19.

Innate immune responses and the pathogenesis of influenza

Innate immune responses in human influenza

Innate immune responses are key components of first line host defense. Here we summarize the available information on innate immune responses in seasonal pandemic H1N1 2009, 1918 influenza, and highly pathogenic avian influenza H5N1 infections in humans, experimental animal models and primary human cells so as to illustrate current understanding and gaps in knowledge on the role of these immune responses in protection and disease.

Influenza in humans ranges from asymptomatic infection, the typical "influenza-like-illness" syndrome, to occasionally severe disease and even death. While viral replication and direct viral pathology associated with most influenza viruses (with the exception of highly pathogenic avian influenza (HPAI) H5N1) is generally restricted to the respiratory tract, the illness manifests with prominent systemic clinical manifestations including fever, myalgia, and fatigue, in addition to the respiratory symptoms of sore throat, cough, and coryza. These systemic manifestations are believed to be mediated largely by innate immune responses elicited by the infection in the respiratory epithelium (see Chapter 24) [36].

In human subjects experimentally infected with influenza, both local and systemic symptoms peak together with viral load and with levels of IL-6 and IFN-α in nasal lavage fluid. Levels of tumor necrosis factor α (TNF-α) and IL-8 also increase in nasal lavage but peaks later than clinical symptoms, while IL-1β and transforming growth factor β (TGF-β) levels did not increase either locally or systemically in these mild influenza infections. Cytokine levels in the plasma or serum were not as great as those observed in the nasal lavage and in some instances (IFN-α, IL-8) no increases in blood levels were detectable although these cytokines were detectable in the nasal lavage [36]. These observations have been regarded as supportive evidence that both direct viral damage and cytokines contribute to symptoms of influenza, particularly to the systemic manifestations of the illness. Similar results have been observed in naturally occurring seasonal and pandemic H1N1 influenza. Elevated plasma levels of IL-6, IL-8, and CXCL-10 peak at day 3–4 of illness and the levels correlate with nasopharyngeal respiratory viral load [37]. Increased levels of IL-6 are independently associated with prolonged hospitalization and more severe disease [37]. In pandemic H1N1, initial viral load, plasma IL-6 levels, and a slower fall in viral load appeared to correlate with disease severity [37]. In comparison with patients with seasonal influenza, those with pandemic influenza have suppressed Th1 and Th17 cytokines

(IL-10, MIG, IL-17A), suggesting weaker adaptive immune responses in pandemic influenza, possibly as a consequence of less effective cross-reactive memory [38,39].

Human H5N1 disease and, to a lesser extent, infection with 1918 influenza were associated with increased progression to acute respiratory distress syndrome (ARDS) and death [40]. Patients with H5N1 disease have had higher levels of CXCL-10, MCP-1, and MIG than those with seasonal influenza and patients who had fatal H5N1 disease had higher levels of these cytokines (as well as IL-8) compared with survivors [41]. Serum cytokine levels were correlated with viral load in the nasopharynx. Thus, the overall picture is one where viral replication, cytokine levels, and adaptive immunity are inextricably linked in the pathogenic process.

Influenza encephalopathy in children and in adults is associated with elevated levels of cytokines such as IL-6, IL-8, MCP-1, and CXCL-10 in the plasma and in cerebrospinal fluid (CSF) in the absence of virus invasion of the central nervous system [42]. Viral load in the nasopharynx was not significantly different from patients with uncomplicated influenza.

Influenza has been identified as a trigger for acute myocardial infarction or death from cardiovascular disease and the role of inflammation and altered vascular endothelial function have been proposed as possible mechanisms [43].

There are few studies comparing cytokine induction patterns between influenza A and B viruses at the clinical, experimental animal, or primary human cell culture levels. Limited data suggest that the ratio of Th2 (IL-4):Th1 (IFN-γ) in children with influenza A is higher than in influenza B infections, suggesting differences in the Th1:Th2 balance between these two virus infections [44]. More studies need to be carried out in this area.

Animal models of influenza to study pathogenesis of influenza virus infections

Ferrets are the most relevant experimental models for understanding the pathogenesis of influenza. However, the paucity of immunologic tools and reagents in ferrets has led to studies on macaques and mice. Avian influenza H5N1 and 1918 influenza viruses both cause markedly more severe respiratory disease in macaques, ferrets, and mice than do seasonal influenza viruses (without prior virus adaptation). The 2009 pandemic H1N1 is associated with intermediate severity in these experimental animal models. The increased virulence of H5N1 and 1918 viruses is associated with higher viral titers in the lungs and more potent proinflammatory innate immune responses (summarized in Table 17.1). As with investigations in humans, it is difficult to dissect the contribution of viral replication competence from that of its effect on innate immune responses.

Experimental studies on mice with specific innate immune gene defects (gene knock-out) are more informative. Experimental H5N1 infection of mice with single gene defects affecting IL-6 and MCP-1 had no obvious phenotype compared with the respective wild-type mice [45]. This is likely because of the redundancy of innate immune signaling pathways. On the other hand, MyD88 [46] and IL-1 receptors [8,9] have a protective effect in PR8 and H5N1 [45] infected mice, respectively, illustrating the important role innate immune responses have as a first host responder to influenza infection. H5N1 virus infection in mice with defects in TNF-receptor 1 signaling had less pronounced weight loss, although this was not associated with overt survival advantage [45]. Triple knock-out mice with defective TNF-1, TNF-2, and IL-1 receptors had delayed mortality and less weight loss than wild-type mice following challenge with HK/483/97 (H5N1) virus but there was no survival advantage following challenge with PR8 (mouse adapted seasonal influenza H1N1) [47]. Improved survival was associated with reduced lung inflammation indicating that these inflammatory responses are associated with pathology that overrides any protective contribution. On the other hand, the triple gene defect was associated with increased dissemination of H5N1 virus to the brain. As HK/483/97 is neurotropic in mice, it would be of interest to see if a greater protective phenotype will be observed with a non-neurotropic H5N1 virus (e.g., HK/486/97). TLR3 [48] and IL-17 [49] signaling is detrimental to survival of influenza virus infected mice.

Interaction between CD200R in alveolar macrophages and CD200 presented on lung epithelial cells contributed to maintaining immune homeostasis in uninfected lungs. Influenza infection in mice deficient in CD200 leads to increased weight loss and mortality [50]. Effector T cells infiltrating the lungs after influenza infection secrete IL-10 along with proinflammatory cytokines. Blocking the IL-10R with monoclonal antibody in influenza infected mice leads to increased and accelerated lethality without affecting viral clearance [51].

Therapeutic strategies that block innate immune signaling pathways have been shown to have some beneficial effects in experimental animal models of influenza disease. A CXCR3 antagonist AMG487 reduced disease severity but failed to reduce mortality in H5N1 virus infected ferrets [52]. Modulation of tipDC trafficking by the peroxisome proliferator-activated receptor γ agonist pioglitazone moderated lung pathology in PR8 (H1N1) infected mice without completely losing the beneficial effects of cytotoxic T-cell recruitment [27]. Combination therapy of the COX2 inhibitor celecoxib and mesalazine together with the antiviral zanamivir significantly enhanced survival in H5N1 infected mice [53].

In summary, while many innate immune responses are protective and beneficial, some can be deleterious, particularly so with viruses such as H5N1 which are potent activators of innate immune responses.

Innate immune responses in primary human cells
in vitro

Studies in primary human cells infected with different influenza viruses provide an experimental model to compare intrinsic differences, if any, in the innate immune host response profile of different influenza viruses. Comparison of the transcriptomic profiles of H5N1 and seasonal H1N1 infected macrophages reveals marked differences in host responses, with H5N1 viruses eliciting more potent proinflammatory responses including TNF-α and IFN signaling and in activating antiapoptotic pathways [54] by activating IRF-3, p38 MAPK, and NF-κB pathways [55]. H5N1 viruses had similar phenotypes in primary human alveolar epithelial cells [56]. As these experiments are carried out with identical virus dose, these results suggest that the markedly proinflammatory responses seen in lungs of H5N1 virus infected mice, ferrets, and macaques as well as the higher levels of these cytokines seen in H5N1 infected patients may be due to intrinsic properties of the H5N1 virus itself rather than overall differences in replication competence. However, there were marked differences among H5N1 viruses in their potency in eliciting these innate immune responses [57].

Table 17.1. Role of innate immunity in the pathogenesis of pandemic H1N1, avian H5N1, and 1918 H1N1 compared with seasonal influenza.

	Pandemic H1N1 2009	H5N1	1918 H1N1
Human clinical and autopsy data			
Viral load in upper respiratory tract	Viral load comparable to seasonal influenza but severe cases have higher viral load and slower clearance of virus than milder disease [37]	Higher and more prolonged viral load than seasonal flu. Fatal disease associated with higher viral load [41]	Not known
Proinflammatory cytokines in serum/plasma	IL-6, IL-8, and CXCL-10 levels higher in patients with severe disease. Correlates with nasopharyngeal viral load. Lower levels of Th1 and Th17 cytokines than seasonal influenza [37,38,63]	Higher in H5N1 than seasonal influenza (IP-10, MIG, MCP-1, IL-8, IL-10, IL-6, IFN-γ) and patients with fatal outcome have higher levels than survivors [41]	Not known
Pathology of fatal disease	Primary viral pneumonia and diffuse alveolar damage (DAD) or secondary bacterial superinfection	Primary viral pneumonia and DAD. Secondary bacterial infection not common [40]	Diffuse alveolar damage due to primary viral pneumonia or secondary to bacterial superinfection [40]
Extra-respiratory dissemination of infectious virus	Rare	Occurs. But lung pathology remains major cause of death [40]	Not known
Experimental animal infections studies			
Macaques	Higher viral titers and more lung pathology than seasonal flu Higher and more prolonged elevation of MCP-1, MIP-1a, IL-6, and IL-18	Severity of pathology H5N1 > 1918 > seasonal flu. Targets type 2 pneumocytes. Stronger and more prolonged innate inflammatory responses (type 1 IFN, IL-1, IL-6, TNF-α, CXCL-10) compared with seasonal flu [64]	Severe respiratory disease with fatal outcome associated with a dysregulated innate immune response. Prolonged activated of IL-6, CCL11 (eotaxin-1), CXCL6 (GCP-2) genes but weaker type 1 IFN response [65]. Seasonal influenza virus with 1918 HA and NA has increased pathogenicity and increased innate immune response compared with seasonal flu [64]
Ferrets	More virus replication in alveoli, more lung pathology but less severe than H5N1 or 1918 Severe seasonal influenza is associated with reduced IFN and increased IL-6 responses [66]	Increased innate immune and IFN signaling (e.g., CXCL-10); T-cell and B-cell signaling pathways downregulated in H5N1 compared with seasonal H3N2 [52]	Severe disease in ferrets [67]

(Continued)

277

Table 17.1. (*Continued*)

	Pandemic H1N1 2009	H5N1	1918 H1N1
Mice	Replicate more efficiently in lung and modestly more lung pathology and weight loss than seasonal flu but not as severe as H5N1 or 1918 H1N1. Lung cytokine induction modest and lower than induced by H5N1, 1918, or a previous triple reassortant H1N1 virus (A/Ohio/2/07) than infected humans	Increased macrophage and polymorph infiltration and increased levels of proinflammatory cytokines (IL-6, IFN-γ, MCP-1, MIP-1α) in mouse lung [68]	Severe disease in mice associated with high replication efficiency and activation of proinflammatory cytokines and apoptotic pathways. Increased macrophage and polymorph infiltration and increased levels of proinflammatory cytokines (IL-6, IFN-γ, MCP-1, MIP-1α) in mouse lung [68]

Infection of primary human cells *in vitro*

	Pandemic H1N1 2009	H5N1	1918 H1N1
Alveolar epithelial cells	Viral replication competence and innate host responses comparable to seasonal influenza	Stronger proinflammatory cytokine responses (IFN-β, CXCL-10, RANTES, IL-6) than seasonal flu [56]. But strain-to-strain variation exists	Enhanced replication competence in human primary broncho-epithelial cells
Peripheral blood monocyte derived macrophages	Viral replication and innate host responses comparable to seasonal influenza	Stronger proinflammatory cytokine responses (TNF-α, IFN-α and IFN-β, CXCL-10, MCP-1, RANTES, MIP-1 α and β) than seasonal flu [68,69]. There is variation between strains of H5N1 [57]	No evidence of increased induction of proinflammatory cytokines [68]
Alveolar macrophages	No data	Productive replication of H5N1 viruses; but abortive replication of seasonal influenza. Cytokine responses less intense than with peripheral blood monocyte derived macrophages [58]	Not known
Bronchial epithelial cells	Marginally increased replication in differentiated cells; enhanced viral replication at 33°C and comparable cytokine induction to seasonal influenza	Less replication of H5N1 in differentiated bronchial epithelium associated with weaker interferon responses [70]	Enhanced replication competence in human primary broncho-epithelial cells
Dendritic cells	Viral replication and innate host responses comparable to seasonal influenza	Stronger IFN-α responses than seasonal flu in pDCs, differences in TNF-α less pronounced, comparable CXCL-10 induction and enhanced replication competence [68]	Comparable viral replication with low pathogenic virus [68]

Modified from Peiris et al. [71] with permission from Elsevier. For those statements without citation of original references, refer to [71] for the citation to relevant original work.

In comparison with peripheral blood derived macrophages, alveolar macrophages are less reactive in production of proinflammatory cytokines following H5N1 virus infection. While alveolar macrophages are equally permissive to infection with both seasonal and H5N1 influenza viruses, only H5N1 virus is able to replicate productively in these cells [58].

In contrast to H5N1 virus infection, pandemic H1N1 infection is not associated with marked differences in transcriptome profile compared with that of seasonal influenza.

Viral reverse genetics has identified that the viral polymerase genes, rather than the surface (hemagglutinin, neuraminidase) genes, as the viral genetic determinants of the high proinflammatory phenotype of H5N1 viruses. Single mutations in the PB2 protein (e.g., PB2 E627K) can dramatically affect the proinflammatory phenotype of an H5N1 virus [59].

Conclusions

Influenza viruses are recognized by multiple innate sensors including the TLRs, RLRs, and NLRs. Type I IFNs provide key defense against influenza virus replication by inducing several ISGs that block various stages of virus infection. In addition, IL-1β released as a result of inflammasome activation has a key role in the initiation of adaptive immune responses against influenza. Various cell types including alveolar macrophages, monocytes, and NK cells provide innate defense, whereas DCs link innate recognition of influenza virus to adaptive immunity. While innate immune responses are crucial components of the protective host responses to influenza infection, under certain conditions innate immune responses can contribute to detrimental pathology. Whether the innate immune system mediate protective versus pathogenic responses to influenza infection depends on multiple factors, including the virulence of the viral strains, the inoculum size, and the immune competence of the host. Viral replication, cytokine levels, and adaptive immunity are inextricably linked to the pathogenic process. Defining the pathways involved in pathogenesis may provide novel therapeutic targets to manage severe influenza diseases, but the challenge is to do so without compromising the key protective roles of the innate and adaptive immune response networks. In this regard, recent findings that influenza virus replication is dependent on NF-κB and the Raf/MEK/ERK and COX-2 pathways is of interest as these would be potential therapeutic targets that block viral replication as well as proinflammatory pathways [60,61]. Future studies are needed to develop preventative and therapeutic agents that can effectively block influenza virus infection and pathology.

References

1. Janeway CA Jr. Approaching the asymptote? Evolution and revolution in immunology. Cold Spring Harb Symp Quant Biol. 1989;54(Pt 1):1–13.
2. Medzhitov R. Toll-like receptors and innate immunity. Nat Rev Immunol. 2001;1(2):135–45.
3. Peiris JS, Cheung CY, Leung CY, Nicholls JM. Innate immune responses to influenza A H5N1: friend or foe? Trends Immunol. 2009;30(12):574–84.
4. Pang IK, Iwasaki A. Control of antiviral immunity by pattern recognition and the microbiome. Immunol Rev. 2012;245(1):209–26.
5. Martinon F, Tschopp J. NLRs join TLRs as innate sensors of pathogens. Trends Immunol. 2005;26(8):447–54.
6. Bauernfeind FG, Horvath G, Stutz A, Alnemri ES, MacDonald K, Speert D, et al. Cutting edge: NF-kappaB activating pattern recognition and cytokine receptors license NLRP3 inflammasome activation by regulating NLRP3 expression. J Immunol. 2009;183(2):787–91.
7. Ichinohe T, Pang IK, Iwasaki A. Influenza virus activates inflammasomes via its intracellular M2 ion channel. Nat Immunol. 2010;11(5):404–10.
8. Ichinohe T, Lee HK, Ogura Y, Flavell R, Iwasaki A. Inflammasome recognition of influenza virus is essential for adaptive immune responses. J Exp Med. 2009;206:79–87.
9. Schmitz N, Kurrer M, Bachmann MF, Kopf M. Interleukin-1 is responsible for acute lung immunopathology but increases survival of respiratory influenza virus infection. J Virol. 2005;79(10):6441–8.
10. Kato H, Sato S, Yoneyama M, Yamamoto M, Uematsu S, Matsui K, et al. Cell Type-Specific Involvement of RIG-I in Antiviral Response. Immunity. 2005;23(1):19–28.
11. Guarda G, Zenger M, Yazdi AS, Schroder K, Ferrero I, Menu P, et al. Differential expression of NLRP3 among hematopoietic cells. J Immunol. 2011;186(4):2529–34.
12. Isaacs A, Lindenmann J. Virus interference. I. The interferon. Proc R Soc Lond B Biol Sci. 1957;147(927):258–67.

13. Haller O, Staeheli P, Kochs G. Interferon-induced Mx proteins in antiviral host defense. Biochimie. 2007;89 (6–7):812–8.

14. Hefti HP, Frese M, Landis H, Di Paolo C, Aguzzi A, Haller O, et al. Human MxA protein protects mice lacking a functional alpha/beta interferon system against La crosse virus and other lethal viral infections. J Virol. 1999;73(8):6984–91.

15. Pavlovic J, Arzet HA, Hefti HP, Frese M, Rost D, Ernst B, et al. Enhanced virus resistance of transgenic mice expressing the human MxA protein. J Virol. 1995;69(7): 4506–10.

16. Silverman RH. Viral encounters with 2′,5′-oligoadenylate synthetase and RNase L during the interferon antiviral response. J Virol. 2007;81(23):12720–9.

17. Kumar A, Haque J, Lacoste J, Hiscott J, Williams BR. Double-stranded RNA-dependent protein kinase activates transcription factor NF-kappa B by phosphorylating I kappa B. Proc Natl Acad Sci U S A. 1994;91(14): 6288–92.

18. Sadler AJ, Williams BR. Structure and function of the protein kinase R. Curr Top Microbiol Immunol. 2007; 316:253–92.

19. Schulz O, Pichlmair A, Rehwinkel J, Rogers NC, Scheuner D, Kato H, et al. Protein kinase R contributes to immunity against specific viruses by regulating interferon mRNA integrity. Cell Host Microbe. 2010;7(5): 354–61.

20. Ritchie KJ, Zhang DE. ISG15: the immunological kin of ubiquitin. Semin Cell Dev Biol. 2004;15(2):237–46.

21. Durfee LA, Lyon N, Seo K, Huibregtse JM. The ISG15 conjugation system broadly targets newly synthesized proteins: implications for the antiviral function of ISG15. Mol Cell. 2010;38(5):722–32.

22. Lenschow DJ, Lai C, Frias-Staheli N, Giannakopoulos NV, Lutz A, Wolff T, et al. IFN-stimulated gene 15 functions as a critical antiviral molecule against influenza, herpes, and Sindbis viruses. Proc Natl Acad Sci U S A. 2007;104(4):1371–6.

23. Fitzgerald KA. The interferon inducible gene: viperin. J Interferon Cytokine Res. 2011;31(1):131–5.

24. Wang X, Hinson ER, Cresswell P. The interferon-inducible protein viperin inhibits influenza virus release by perturbing lipid rafts. Cell Host Microbe. 2007;2(2): 96–105.

25. Gazit R, Gruda R, Elboim M, Arnon TI, Katz G, Achdout H, et al. Lethal influenza infection in the absence of the natural killer cell receptor gene Ncr1. Nat Immunol. 2006;7(5):517–23.

26. McGill J, Van Rooijen N, Legge KL. Protective influenza-specific CD8 T cell responses require interactions with dendritic cells in the lungs. J Exp Med. 2008; 205(7):1635–46.

27. Aldridge JR Jr, Moseley CE, Boltz DA, Negovetich NJ, Reynolds C, Franks J, et al. TNF/iNOS-producing dendritic cells are the necessary evil of lethal influenza virus infection. Proc Natl Acad Sci U S A. 2009;106(13): 5306–11.

28. Hashimoto Y, Moki T, Takizawa T, Shiratsuchi A, Nakanishi Y. Evidence for phagocytosis of influenza virus-infected, apoptotic cells by neutrophils and macrophages in mice. J Immunol. 2007;178(4):2448–57.

29. Medzhitov R, Janeway CA Jr. Innate immune induction of the adaptive immune response. Cold Spring Harb Symp Quant Biol. 1999;64:429–35.

30. Trombetta ES, Mellman I. Cell biology of antigen processing *in vitro* and *in vivo*. Annu Rev Immunol. 2005;23:975–1028.

31. Bancherau J, Steinman RM. Dendritic cells and the control of immunity. Nature. 1998;392(6673):245–52.

32. Itano AA, Jenkins MK. Antigen presentation to naive CD4 T cells in the lymph node. Nat Immunol. 2003;4 (8):733–9.

33. Edwards AD, Diebold SS, Slack EM, Tomizawa H, Hemmi H, Kaisho T, et al. Toll-like receptor expression in murine DC subsets: lack of TLR7 expression by CD8 alpha+ DC correlates with unresponsiveness to imidazoquinolines. Eur J Immunol. 2003;33(4):827–33.

34. Hammad H, Lambrecht BN. Dendritic cells and airway epithelial cells at the interface between innate and adaptive immune responses. Allergy. 2011;66(5):579–87.

35. Braciale TJ, Sun J, Kim TS. Regulating the adaptive immune response to respiratory virus infection. Nat Rev Immunol. 2012;12(4):295–305.

36. Hayden FG, Fritz R, Lobo MC, Alvord W, Strober W, Straus SE. Local and systemic cytokine responses during experimental human influenza A virus infection. Relation to symptom formation and host defense. J Clin Invest. 1998;101(3):643–9.

37. Lee N, Chan PK, Wong CK, Wong KT, Choi KW, Joynt GM, et al. Viral clearance and inflammatory response patterns in adults hospitalized for pandemic 2009 influenza A(H1N1) virus pneumonia. Antivir Ther. 2011;16 (2):237–47.

38. Lee N, Wong CK, Chan PK, Chan MC, Wong RY, Lun SW, et al. Cytokine response patterns in severe pandemic 2009 H1N1 and seasonal influenza among hospitalized adults. PLoS ONE. 2011;6(10):e26050.

39. Jiang TJ, Zhang JY, Li WG, Xie YX, Zhang XW, Wang Y, et al. Preferential loss of Th17 cells is associated with CD4 T cell activation in patients with 2009 pandemic H1N1 swine-origin influenza A infection. Clin Immunol. 2010;137(3):303–10.

40. Taubenberger JK, Morens DM. The pathology of influenza virus infections. Annu Rev Pathol. 2008;3:499–522.

41. de Jong MD, Simmons CP, Thanh TT, Hien VM, Smith GJ, Chau TN, et al. Fatal outcome of human influenza A (H5N1) is associated with high viral load and hyper-cytokinemia. Nat Med. 2006;12(10):1203–7.

42. Kawada J, Kimura H, Ito Y, Hara S, Iriyama M, Yoshikawa T, et al. Systemic cytokine responses in patients with influenza-associated encephalopathy. J Infect Dis. 2003;188(5):690–8.

43. Warren-Gash C, Smeeth L, Hayward AC. Influenza as a trigger for acute myocardial infarction or death from cardiovascular disease: a systematic review. Lancet Infect Dis. 2009;9(10):601–10.

44. Sato M, Hosoya M, Wright PF. Differences in serum cytokine levels between influenza virus A and B infections in children. Cytokine. 2009;47(1):65–8.

45. Szretter KJ, Gangappa S, Lu X, Smith C, Shieh WJ, Zaki SR, et al. Role of host cytokine responses in the pathogenesis of avian H5N1 influenza viruses in mice. J Virol. 2007;81(6):2736–44.

46. Seo SU, Kwon HJ, Song JH, Byun YH, Seong BL, Kawai T, et al. MyD88 signaling is indispensable for primary influenza A virus infection but dispensable for secondary infection. J Virol. 2010;84(24):12713–22.

47. Perrone LA, Szretter KJ, Katz JM, Mizgerd JP, Tumpey TM. Mice lacking both TNF and IL-1 receptors exhibit reduced lung inflammation and delay in onset of death following infection with a highly virulent H5N1 virus. J Infect Dis. 2010;202(8):1161–70.

48. Le Goffic R, Balloy V, Lagranderie M, Alexopoulou L, Escriou N, Flavell R, et al. Detrimental contribution of the Toll-like receptor (TLR)3 to influenza A virus-induced acute pneumonia. PLoS Pathog. 2006;2(6):0526.

49. Crowe CR, Chen K, Pociask DA, Alcorn JF, Krivich C, Enelow RI, et al. Critical role of IL-17RA in immunopathology of influenza infection. J Immunol. 2009;183(8):5301–10.

50. Snelgrove RJ, Goulding J, Didierlaurent AM, Lyonga D, Vekaria S, Edwards L, et al. A critical function for CD200 in lung immune homeostasis and the severity of influenza infection. Nat Immunol. 2008;9(9):1074–83.

51. Sun J, Madan R, Karp CL, Braciale TJ. Effector T cells control lung inflammation during acute influenza virus infection by producing IL-10. Nat Med. 2009;15(3):277–84.

52. Cameron CM, Cameron MJ, Bermejo-Martin JF, Ran L, Xu L, Turner PV, et al. Gene expression analysis of host innate immune responses during Lethal H5N1 infection in ferrets. J Virol. 2008;82(22):11308–17.

53. Zheng BJ, Chan KW, Lin YP, Zhao GY, Chan C, Zhang HJ, et al. Delayed antiviral plus immunomodulator treatment still reduces mortality in mice infected by high inoculum of influenza A/H5N1 virus. Proc Natl Acad Sci U S A. 2008;105(23):8091–6.

54. Lee SM, Gardy JL, Cheung CY, Cheung TK, Hui KP, Ip NY, et al. Systems-level comparison of host-responses elicited by avian H5N1 and seasonal H1N1 influenza viruses in primary human macrophages. PLoS ONE. 2009;4(12):e8072.

55. Hui KP, Lee SM, Cheung CY, Ng IH, Poon LL, Guan Y, et al. Induction of proinflammatory cytokines in primary human macrophages by influenza A virus (H5N1) is selectively regulated by IFN regulatory factor 3 and p38 MAPK. J Immunol. 2009;182(2):1088–98.

56. Chan MC, Cheung CY, Chui WH, Tsao SW, Nicholls JM, Chan YO, et al. Proinflammatory cytokine responses induced by influenza A (H5N1) viruses in primary human alveolar and bronchial epithelial cells. Respir Res. 2005;6:135.

57. Sakabe S, Iwatsuki-Horimoto K, Takano R, Nidom CA, Le MQ, Nagamura-Inoue T, et al. Cytokine production by primary human macrophages infected with highly pathogenic H5N1 or pandemic H1N1 2009 influenza viruses. J Gen Virol. 2011;92(Pt 6):1428–34.

58. Yu WC, Chan RW, Wang J, Travanty EA, Nicholls JM, Peiris JS, et al. Viral replication and innate host responses in primary human alveolar epithelial cells and alveolar macrophages infected with influenza H5N1 and H1N1 viruses. J Virol. 2011;85(14):6844–55.

59. Mok KP, Wong CH, Cheung CY, Chan MC, Lee SM, Nicholls JM, et al. Viral genetic determinants of H5N1 influenza viruses that contribute to cytokine dysregulation. J Infect Dis. 2009;200(7):1104–12.

60. Lee SM, Gai WW, Cheung TK, Peiris JS. Antiviral effect of a selective COX-2 inhibitor on H5N1 infection *in vitro*. Antiviral Res. 2011;91(3):330–4.

61. Ludwig S. Targeting cell signalling pathways to fight the flu: towards a paradigm change in anti-influenza therapy. J Antimicrob Chemother. 2009;64(1):1–4.

62. Pang IK, Iwasaki A. Inflammasomes as mediators of immunity against influenza virus. Trends Immunol. 2011;32(1):34–41.

63. Lee N, Wong CK, Chan PK, Lun SW, Lui G, Wong B, et al. Hypercytokinemia and hyperactivation of phospho-p38 mitogen-activated protein kinase in severe human influenza A virus infection. Clin Infect Dis. 2007;45(6):723–31.

64. Baskin CR, Bielefeldt-Ohmann H, Tumpey TM, Sabourin PJ, Long JP, Garcia-Sastre A, et al. Early and sustained innate immune response defines pathology and death in nonhuman primates infected by highly pathogenic influenza virus. Proc Natl Acad Sci U S A. 2009;106(9):3455–60.

65. Kobasa D, Jones SM, Shinya K, Kash JC, Copps J, Ebihara H, et al. Aberrant innate immune response in lethal infection of macaques with the 1918 influenza virus. Nature. 2007;445(7125):319–23.

66. Svitek N, Rudd PA, Obojes K, Pillet S, von Messling V. Severe seasonal influenza in ferrets correlates with reduced interferon and increased IL-6 induction. Virology. 2008;376(1):53–9.

67. Tumpey TM, Szretter KJ, Van Hoeven N, Katz JM, Kochs G, Haller O, et al. The Mx1 gene protects mice against the pandemic 1918 and highly lethal human H5N1 influenza viruses. J Virol. 2007;81(19):10818–21.

68. Perrone LA, Plowden JK, Garcia-Sastre A, Katz JM, Tumpey TM. H5N1 and 1918 pandemic influenza virus infection results in early and excessive infiltration of macrophages and neutrophils in the lungs of mice. PLoS Pathog. 2008;4(8):e1000115.

69. Cheung CY, Poon LL, Lau AS, Luk W, Lau YL, Shortridge KF, et al. Induction of proinflammatory cytokines in human macrophages by influenza A (H5N1) viruses: a mechanism for the unusual severity of human disease? Lancet. 2002;360(9348):1831–7.

70. Chan MC, Chan RW, Yu WC, Ho CC, Chui WH, Lo CK, et al. Influenza H5N1 virus infection of polarized human alveolar epithelial cells and lung microvascular endothelial cells. Respir Res. 2009;10:102.

71. Peiris JS, Hui KP, Yen HL. Host response to influenza virus: protection versus immunopathology. Curr Opin Immunol. 2010;22(4):475–81.

Antibody-mediated immunity

Nicole Baumgarth,[1] Michael C. Carroll,[2] and Santiago Gonzalez[2]

[1]Center for Comparative Medicine and Department of Pathology, Microbiology, and Immunology, University of California, Davis, CA, USA

[2]Program in Cellular and Molecular Medicine, The Immune Disease Institute, Children's Hospital, Departments of Pediatrics, Harvard Medical School, Boston, MA, USA

Antibody response to influenza virus

The induction of specific antibodies is one of the hallmarks of the adaptive immune response to influenza virus infection. The antibodies are induced quickly, both locally in the respiratory tract as well as systemically. They neutralize the virus, reduce virus replication efficiency and spread, and contribute to complete immune-mediated clearance from influenza infection typically within a week or two of infection. Following acute infection, memory B cells and long-lived plasma cells are also formed, which protect the host from reinfection with the same influenza virus for many years, if not decades. It appears to be a perfect response, yet we remain susceptible to reinfections with influenza viruses on an almost yearly basis. Antibody-mediated immune protection, while highly protective against reinfection with the same virus strain, is vulnerable to the high rate of mutations that occur within the strongly immunodominant spike proteins of influenza virus, particularly the hemagglutinin (HA) gene. Thus, the induction of highly protective antibodies exerts enormous immune pressure on the virus to mutate away from the neutralizing antibodies, causing yearly waves of influenza virus infections with viruses that are distinct from those that caused influenza outbreaks the previous season. However, recent evidence suggests that humans also generate antibodies against very conserved regions of the virus, including virus-neutralizing epitopes on the HA molecule. Such antibodies can provide broadly cross-reactive and cross-protective immunity that may contribute to the eventual disappearance of circulating seasonal influenza virus strains. Harnessing these types of antibody responses through vaccination represents the next major step towards the ultimate goal of designing a universal influenza virus vaccine.

Antibody responses are nonredundant immune components of the response to influenza virus infection

Immune protection following vaccination with the inactivated influenza split-virus vaccine, which contains influenza virus components from usually three currently recirculating influenza A and B strains (see Chapters 20 and 23), is mediated chiefly by the induction of antibodies that neutralize the virus either by blocking entry of the virus into the respiratory tract epithelial cells, or rapidly thereafter. Antibodies to the virus are generated mostly following the interaction of B lymphocytes with "help" from CD4 T lymphocytes; an interaction that ultimately leads to the differentiation of B cells to antibody-secreting plasma cells. Thus, pre-existing antibodies, vaccine or infection induced, can provide complete immune protection against reinfection with the same (homosubtypic) strain of influenza virus.

Clinical observations during the 2009 influenza A H1N1 pandemic provide strong support for earlier

Textbook of Influenza, Second Edition. Edited by Robert G. Webster, Arnold S. Monto, Thomas J. Braciale, and Robert A. Lamb.
© 2013 John Wiley & Sons, Ltd. Published 2013 by John Wiley & Sons, Ltd.

experimental studies that showed that antibodies raised against a heterosubtypic virus (i.e., an influenza virus strain that differs in HA and neuraminidase (NA)) can nonetheless provide partial protection. Despite the emergence of a new H1N1 reassortant ("swine-flu") in 2009, morbidity and mortality rates among the elderly were unexpectedly low that year. This is a group of individuals with a usually high risk for influenza-induced disease and death. The epidemiologic observations indicated that this patient group harbored cross-reactive immunity. Indeed, serologic studies revealed that individuals born before the 1970s were partially protected by the presence of pre-existing cross-reactive antibodies to a previous circulating H1N1 strain (reviewed in [1]). Thus, even the presence of only partially overlapping, cross-reactive antibodies can provide significant levels of protection.

Following acute influenza virus infections complex immune responses are induced in which B cells act synergistically with the cellular arm of the immune system, CD8 cytotoxic T cells, natural killer cells, alveolar macrophages and other effectors, to clear infected cells. They inhibit a further spread of the virus deeper into the respiratory tract and aid the recovery process. Experimental studies going back to the 1970s have demonstrated that B cells are essential components of the recovery process, showing that mice, either depleted or genetically ablated of B cells, have increased levels of mortality and morbidity following live virus challenge [2]. Thus, despite the broad array of immune effectors induced by a live virus infection, B cells are nonredundant in immune protection from disease and death, not just during a recall response after reinfection, but also during a primary infection. While much of the B-cell response to influenza virus is generated following the interaction of antigen-specific B cells with CD4 T cells, CD4 T-cell-independent B-cell responses also seem to contribute significantly to immune protection (reviewed in [2]).

Taken together, antibodies have a nonredundant role both prophylactically and therapeutically. Prophylactically, after induction following vaccination or infection, by blocking infection with homosubtypic strains of influenza virus. Therapeutically, after homosubtypic and heterosubtypic virus infection, by limiting virus burden and pathology associated with infection. This chapter outlines current knowledge on the induction, function, and specificity of the humoral immune response against influenza virus infection and its limitations.

Anatomy and kinetics of the antibody responses to influenza virus infection

Influenza virus in humans and other mammals is typically a respiratory tract infection, transmitted via droplets into the upper respiratory tract. Epithelial cells in the nasal cavity and/or upper pharynx are likely the first targets of seasonal influenza virus strains, although more pathogenic strains might directly infect lower parts of the lung. Lymph nodes draining that site of infection, the cervical lymph nodes, are likely where the specific B-cell responses to influenza are initiated. Antibody-secreting cells are identified in the cervical and mediastinal lymph nodes of mice and ferrets as early as 3 days after initial infection [3,4]. The extremely rapid kinetics of the infection-induced local B-cell responses may explain how antibodies can contribute to clearance of primary influenza infections [2].

In contrast, antibody-secreting cells in the lung are not detected prior to day 7 in wild-type mice and only after they are detected in the spleen [5]. Once induced, however, they are present for life. Their induction pathways are currently unclear. Following infection, B cells may be activated first in the tissue-draining lymph nodes from which they then migrate to the lung. In support, early migration studies showed that precursors of immunoglobulin G (IgG) secreting cells from the mediastinal and bronchial lymph nodes preferentially home to salivary glands and the lung [6]. B cells might also be induced locally in the mucosa of the upper respiratory tract or the lung tissue, however, possibly in the germinal center-like structures that are present within the nose-associate lymphoid tissues (NALT), or adjacent larger airways in the bronchus-associated lymphoid tissue (BALT) [7]. However, BALT structures are not present in the absence of prior inflammation or infection and might not represent permanent structures in humans. Given the likely importance of inducing antibody secretion as close as possible to the site of virus entry, defining precisely the differentiation pathways that induce antibody-secreting cells in the lung or upper respiratory tract is of great importance.

If virus is not contained in the upper respiratory tract, lower parts of the bronchial tree are infected and their draining lymph nodes (mediastinal) participate in B-cell response priming. While influenza virus replication and release of viral progeny is observed only in respiratory tract epithelium, viral antigens are found also in other lung cells, including B cells. Virus replication that is not contained reaches the small airways and alveoli, causing pneumonia.

The highly tissue-restricted nature of the infection results in B (and T) cell responses that are initially also restricted to the lymphoid tissues of the respiratory tract. This can provide an obstacle in accurately assessing early adaptive immunity to the virus in a clinical setting, because local responses are not always adequately represented by blood tests. In fact, antibody levels in the respiratory tract, but not the serum, best correlate with levels of protection from reinfection [8]. A similar challenge exists with establishing correlates of protection induced with the live-attenuated influenza vaccine (LAIV) that causes upper respiratory tract infections. Changes to blood antibody titers might not accurately reflect the levels of protection induced by LAIV. This hurdle might be overcome by measuring antibody-secreting plasmablasts in peripheral blood. Between 6 and 8 days after vaccination or infection, spontaneous antibody-secreting plasma blasts are present transiently in the peripheral blood of humans, apparently representing a wave of memory B cells that are drawn into the acute response [9]. These cells, when identified by flow cytometry and then sort purified and short-term cultured on to ELISPOT plates, will generate highly specific antibodies to the vaccine antigen. Total peripheral blood mononuclear cells (PBMC) might also be cultured directly on ELISPOT plates and then frequencies of antibody-secreting cells can be assessed as percentage of total PBMC. The peak frequencies of antibody-secreting cells, which can amount to nearly 6% of B cells at day 7 after vaccination of humans with the inactivated vaccine [9], tightly correlate with serum antibody titers. Given that serum antibody titers take a few weeks to develop, this sensitive and highly accurate technique allows for a very rapid assessment of the magnitude and specificity of the induced response [10]. The approach has been applied successfully for the detection of influenza-specific IgA plasmablasts among peripheral blood lymphocytes following LAIV, although the transient nature of their appearance requires accurate timing. Thus, once initiated, antigen-specific B-cell responses result in the rapid generation of antibody-producing plasma cells. Apart from the transient appearance in blood, antibody-producing cells are found within the lymph nodes and in the mucosa of the upper respiratory tract during the acute phase of infection.

Following clearance of the virus, antibody secretion continues for months and years. This was particularly apparent during the 2009 pandemic. In the United States, the majority of individuals afflicted were young adults and only 5% were over 51 years old. About 33% of those over 60 years of age had cross-reactive antibodies to 2009 pandemic H1N1 [11]. In Finland, up to 96% of people born between 1909 and 1919 had cross-protective antibodies to the 2009 pandemic strain, likely due to its relationship to the "Spanish flu" H1N1 strain that circulated in the first part of the twentieth century. Two anatomic sites have been associated with this long-term production of influenza-specific antibodies: bone marrow and lung tissue [12]. Whether the lung airway harbors specific niches for these cells and how they are maintained long term are important unresolved questions. Influenza-specific antibodies in the serum are contributed by secreting cells at both locations. In the upper respiratory tract, IgA-secreting plasma cells can also be found in the lamina propria of the mucosa. As smaller bronchi and the alveolar regions of the lung lack a mucosa, antibody secretion in the lower respiratory tract is restricted to the BALT region and much of the locally produced antibody is IgG and IgM, while 95% of antibody-producing cells in the upper respiratory tract are IgA [13].

The other important component of the adaptive response that provides long-term antibody-mediated immunity is the memory B-cell pool. Like plasma cells, memory B cells are maintained for many months locally in the respiratory tract and systemically in most tissues after infection. Memory B cells are typically of high affinity as they arise from B cells that undergo extensive somatic hypermutation and selection. They circulate throughout the body and can rapidly respond to an infection with differentiation to antibody-secreting cells. The transient presence of plasmablasts in the blood following vaccination [9,10] likely represent activated memory B cells, as these cells showed signs of extensive hypermutation [9]. Importantly, memory B cells are not assessed when testing for serum antibody titers. To what extent serum antibody levels correlate with the B-cell response induced in the respiratory tract is currently unknown. Despite the fact that serum hemagglutination inhibition (HAI) see below) titers highly correlate with protection levels [8], this undefined relationship between serum antibody titers and memory B-cell frequencies must be taken into consideration when assessing new vaccine modalities, particularly those that target the respiratory tract, such as the LAIV.

Induction of B-cell responses to influenza antigen

B-cell responses to influenza virus are initiated in the lymph nodes draining the respiratory tract (Figure 18.1). Following their encounter with antigen in the

B-cell follicles likely presented by follicular dendritic cells (FDC; see below), B cells migrate to the border of the T–B cell zone and received "T-cell help" from CD4 T cells. Following this activation step B cells then either form "extrafollicular foci," in which following a brief period of clonal expansion they rapidly differentiate to short-lived plasmablasts, or they return to the B-cell follicle to participate in germinal center responses. While germinal center responses are critically dependent on CD4 T-cell help, extrafollicular foci responses may be induced via T-dependent and T-independent processes. However, at least in mice, the vast majority of the antibody response is produced in a CD4 T cell-dependent manner.

Extrafollicular foci form within about 3–5 days after influenza infection in the draining lymph nodes,

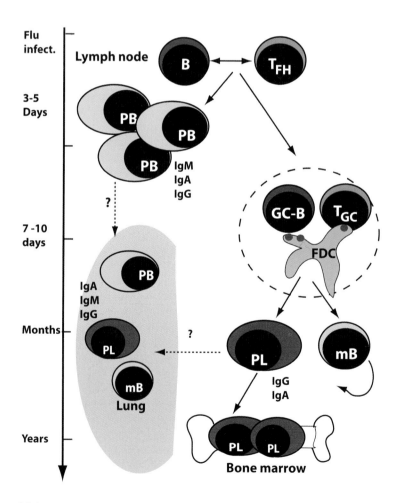

Figure 18.1. Rapid induction of influenza-specific B-cell responses following influenza virus infection. Following influenza virus infection, viral antigen-presentation to CD4 T and B cells and their subsequent interaction leads to the rapid development of IgM, IgG, and IgA antibody-secreting plasmablasts (PB) in extrafollicular foci of the lymph node within 3–5 days. Antibody-secreting cells are found within the lung 7–10 days after infection. Their origins are unknown, but they may arise from B cells in lymph nodes. Germinal centers (GC) develop beginning 1 week after infection and persist for months. In GC, follicular dendritic cells (FDC) present viral antigens to GC B cells. Selection based on antigen binding and CD4 T-cell help results in the selection of high affinity, long-lived plasma cells (PL) and memory B cells (mB). Plasma cells are found in bone marrow and lungs for years – decades after influenza infection. Memory B cells recirculate in the blood and are present also in the lung.

last for about a week, and are the earliest source for virus-specific IgG. These foci may be formed by B cells of relatively high affinity for the antigen, thus not requiring extensive hyperaffinity maturation to bind to the virus [14]. Germinal center responses take at least 1 week to develop(i.e., they develop around the time of influenza virus clearance). They are the birthplaces of memory B cells and long-lived bone marrow plasma cells. In contrast to the extrafollicular B-cell responses, both memory B cells and plasma cells show extensive signs of hyperaffinity maturation and selection. Once initiated, germinal center responses can be found in the draining mediastinal lymph nodes up to 5 months after infection of mice, thus long after virus clearance. The ongoing display of viral antigens on FDC might explain the longevity of this response. Given this time line, the major benefit of germinal center responses is in the development of strong long-lasting immune protection from reinfection. Long-lived plasma cells are responsible for the continuous production of serum antibodies which are measurable for months and years after a primary infection.

Follicular dendritic cells as major sources of antigen for B cells

Despite decades of research into humoral immunity to influenza, until recently little was known of where and how B cells actually acquire viral antigen to initiate B-cell responses in the lymph nodes. As B cells bear antibody receptors, it was assumed that antigen was taken up at diverse sites in the periphery. However, like with T cells, B cells are less likely to take up soluble antigen. Instead, they rely on stromal cells such as the FDC, or on bone marrow-derived dendritic cells (DC) to present antigen to B cells and facilitate antigen uptake and B-cell activation. FDC are not only an efficient source of antigen, they are essential for the organization of the B-cell follicles in secondary lymphoid tissues and within tertiary sites such as the BALT [15].

Growing evidence indicates that FDC in lymphoid tissues are not constitutively active but can respond rapidly to changes in the environment. Inflammatory mediators induce maturation of FDC in primary B-cell follicles to a mature phenotype identified in germinal centers. Manipulation of FDC activation could provide an important approach for regulation or programming of B-cell responses via novel vaccine approaches. This might be particularly important in design of influenza vaccines for the elderly or the very young or individuals with an impaired immune system who often show ineffective vaccine responses. Moreover, efficient FDC activation is known to enhance germinal center responses and because they facilitate somatic hypermutation of B cells, this could lead to an improvement in affinity maturation of influenza-specific antibodies.

Localization of antigen to follicular dendritic cells for B-cell response induction

As FDC as part of the lymph node stroma are sessile, antigen must be delivered to them. It is known that skin draining DC deliver antigen captured in the periphery to both the T-cell areas and B-cell follicles. Antigens administered intranasally, such as following influenza virus infection, are delivered to the cervical and mediastinal lymph nodes via respiratory dendritic cells (RDC). RDC capture viral antigen and migrate from the respiratory tract to the draining lymph nodes via a chemokine-dependent pathway. However, the mechanism by which RDCs acquire influenza virus antigen in the lung is not clearly understood. Early studies suggested that influenza virus infects RDC directly, leading to antigen presentation to CD8+ T lymphocytes and the establishment of cytotoxic T-cell responses (see Chapter 19). Alternatively, immature RDC may acquire antigen from infected epithelial cells within the lung through phagocytosis and then migrate to the lymph nodes for presentation to T and/or B cells. The capacity to capture influenza virus is shared by different RDC subsets, but clear differences exist in their ability to transport virus to the lymph nodes. The RDC subsets facilitating B-cell antigen presentation and activation following influenza virus infection remain to be identified.

To identify possible antigen-presentation pathways, recent studies have used multiphoton-intravital imaging (MP-IVM) to track fluorescent-labeled antigens and immune complexes in peripheral lymph nodes that drain a site of vaccine application. The studies have identified at least three pathways in which antigen is transported or delivered to FDC [16]. In all pathways lymph-borne antigens, including viral particles, are rapidly taken up by macrophages that line the subcapsular and medullary sinuses.

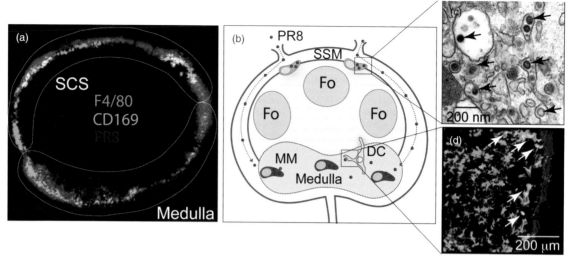

Figure 18.2. Transport of influenza antigen within the lymph nodes after footpad immunization of mice. (a) Multiphoton *in vivo* imaging (MP-IVM) snapshot of draining lymph nodes showing UV-inactivated influenza virus A/Puerto Rico/8/34(A/PR8, red) 7 min after footpad injection. The virus is already present in the subcapsular sinus (SCS) and in the medulla of the lymph node, and it co-localizes with subcapsular sinus macrophages (SSMs) (MOMA-1+, green) and medullary macrophages (MMs) (F4/80+, blue). (b) Schematic drawing showing tracking of A/PR8 in the lymph node. SSMs and MMs and lymph node resident dendritic cells (DC) capture and internalize the virus. (c) Electron micrograph showing influenza virions inside an SSM 30 min after footpad injection. (d) MP-IVM of the capture of A/PR8 by DC in the medulla of popliteal lymph nodes. Arrows indicate virus-bearing eYFP+ DCs. (Panel A adapted from Gonzalez et al. [57] with permission from Nature Immunology).

These sinus-lining phagocytic cells act as guardians to prevent systemic spread of pathogens and help direct movement of the antigen to the B-cell follicles (Figure 18.2). However, their role in transporting antigens to the FDC may be limited. Recent studies using an UV-inactivated strain of influenza (A/Puerto Rico/8/34; H1N1) as a model vaccine identified an essential role for lymph node-resident DC in development of an efficient humoral response [16]. In this model system, ablation of DC resulted in a block in both the T-independent and T-dependent antibody responses, suggesting that DC may act to transport viral antigen into the B-cell and T-cell zones where it is presented directly to the lymphocytes or handed off to other resident DC.

In summary, FDC are essential for maintenance of the B-cell follicles within lymph nodes. Antigen is likely presented to them via DC trafficking from the sites of infection or vaccination, or by hand off from resident antigen-presenting cells. Once antigen is deposited on to FDC, they retain it for relatively long periods of time. FDC are critical for the formation of B-cell responses, including the formation and maintenance of germinal centers and the differentiation of germinal center B cells into long-lived antibody-producing plasma cells and memory B cells.

Shaping of the B-cell response to influenza virus by innate immune signals

Complement system in the adaptive response to influenza

The complement system is best understood for it role in opsonization of microbial pathogens and its participation in mediation of the inflammatory response. Acting as a cascade of serine proteases, the pathway is composed of over 30 distinct proteins found both in the blood and as cell surface receptors [17]. Of the three main pathways for activation of the complement system, only the classic pathway seems to have a major role in enhancement of adaptive immunity. Thus, complement C3 was proposed to act as a natural adjuvant to link innate and adaptive immunity (see Chapters 20–23 for a discussion on use of adjuvants in influenza vaccines) [18].

Indeed, C3 has a critical role in mice infected intranasally with influenza A/Puerto Rico/8/34. In the absence of C3, both CD8 and CD4 T-cell migration into the lung during the early phase of infection were greatly diminished. Characterization of the draining lymph nodes at day 10 post-infection identified a similar impairment in infiltration of influenza-specific T cells and correlated with a significant reduction in specific IgG titers [19]. One explanation for the defect in the adaptive response to influenza in C3–/– mice is that the uptake or transport of viral antigens into the draining lymph nodes is impaired. Induction of long-term immunity to influenza also depends on an intact complement pathway. Mice deficient in either C3 or its receptor CD21 immunized with an inactive form of influenza virus fail to make a protective response when challenged with infectious virus 8 weeks post-vaccination. Notably, survival correlates with IgG anti-influenza titers [20].

FDC are essential for maintenance of the germinal center response as they provide a source of antigen and cytokines such as B-cell activation factor (BAFF). Complement C3 acts both in the retention of antigens via CD21/35 receptors expressed on FDC and for induction of survival signal via the BCR co-receptor (CD21/CD19/CD81) [21]. Therefore, as proposed by Fearon and Carter [22], complement acts as a natural adjuvant to enhance the long-term humoral response to influenza.

Toll-like receptor-mediated regulation of antiviral B-cell responses

Current research has extensively detailed the role of Toll-like receptors (TLRs) in the activation and function of DC (see Chapter 17). However, B cells also express many TLR. TLR signaling might act in synergy with the B-cell receptor to induce B-cell activation. Thus far, TLR signaling has been shown to affect the quality of the B-cell response after influenza virus infection. Specifically, mice lacking TLR-7 or the TLR adaptor molecule MyD88 demonstrated altered IgG subtype profiles [23]. More work is needed to reveal the effects of pattern recognition, receptor-mediated signals on B-cell responses to influenza.

Type I interferon (IFN) is the earliest activator of local B-cell responses following influenza infection. Type I IFN comprises a family of at least 16 cytokines in humans and mice, all of which utilize the same broadly expressed type I IFN receptor (IFNR) [24]. Type I IFN production is induced rapidly during influenza virus infection, corresponding closely with the increase in viral titers in the lung (see Chapter 17). B cells circulating through the sites of infection are stimulated through type I IFNR and accumulate in the regional lymph nodes within 24–48 h after infection, thus prior to cognate T–B interaction and likely even prior to antigen stimulation [25,26].

Type I IFN seems to shape humoral responses against influenza virus via direct and indirect mechanisms. Indirect regulation might entail IFN-mediated stimulation of myeloid DC via induction of interleukin 6 (IL-6) production and thereby alterations in induction of T-cell help. It may also enhance the differentiation of B cells to antibody-secreting plasma cells [27]. Direct type I IFN-mediated B-cell stimulation appears to affect multiple stages of B-cell activation and is required for maximal antibody responses [25,26]. One mechanism appears to be the IFN-mediated induction of CD86 on B cells [28]. Notably, both tissue-specific deletion of the IFNR–/– and CD86 on B cells resulted in altered IgG subtype responses, similar to the findings in influenza infected TLR-7 and MyD88 deficient mice [23]. Together, these findings establish type I IFN as a nonredundant innate signal in the initiation of the early antibody response against influenza virus infection.

Increasingly, data point to direct and indirect effects of infection-induced innate signals on the magnitude and quality of the antiviral B-cell response. Exploiting these signals for vaccine-mediated B-cell activation might enhance vaccine-induced humoral immunity.

Viral targets of the antibody response to influenza virus

Hemagglutinin-specific antibodies

Influenza's two major spike proteins, the glycoproteins HA and NA, protrude from its envelope and make them excellent targets for B-cell responses. The HA protein, with its "lollipop"-like structure consisting of a globular head region and a stalk region (see Chapter 5), is a major target of neutralizing antibodies.

Vaccine efficacy and levels of pre-existing immunity in a population is typically assessed by measuring HA-specific neutralizing and HAI antibodies. Hemagglutination describes the agglutination or clumping of red blood cells. Inhibition of this process, HAI, in the presence of immune serum is used as a measure of serum neutralizing capacity. A more labor-intensive assay that tests the ability of antibodies or serum to inhibit influenza virus infection of either cultured cells or embryonated hens' eggs directly is the virus neutralization assay. HAI titers are excellent correlate measures of protection, as was already noted by Salk and Suriano in 1949 [29]. An HAI titer of 1:40 has been determined as corresponding to a 50% reduction in the risk of contracting influenza in a susceptible adult population [30]. Thus, HA-specific antibodies can prevent virus receptor–host cell interaction and thereby prevent infections (Figure 18.3) (see Chapter 20).

HA-specific neutralizing antibodies bind to distinct regions of the molecule. Four discrete immunodominant antigenic sites have been identified on the H1 (and H3) molecules [31,32]. These four sites, Ca, Cb,

Sa, and Sb, all map to defined antigenic regions that surround the receptor binding pocket in the globular head of the HA molecule, formed by the HA1 polypeptide. As discussed in more detail below, while these antibodies are highly effective at neutralizing the virus, frequent mutations in these parts of the virus reduce their usefulness for protection from subsequent infections.

In addition to antibodies against the receptor-binding pocket, humans and mice also generate HA-specific antibodies directed against the highly sequence-conserved "stalk" region of influenza HA, formed by parts of the HA1 and by the entire HA2 polypeptide (see Chapters 5 and 21). This area includes the cleavage domain, which is required for fusion and productive replication of influenza viruses. It is the most highly conserved region of all influenza HA proteins [33]. The cleavage domain is located in a loop of the HA precursor, and thus is accessible to antibody on the plasma membrane of infected host cells. As expected from the highly conserved nature of the peptide, antibodies binding to the stalk region provide passive protection against a broad range of influenza virus strains [34,35]. Antistalk antibodies prevent fusion of the virus with the host cell (i.e., virus entry) [34].

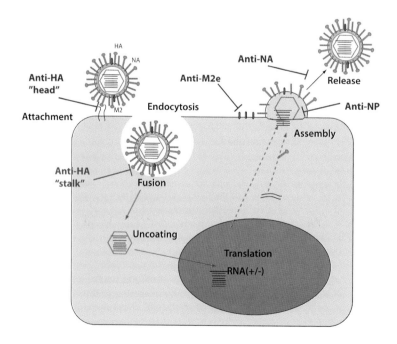

Figure 18.3. Influenza-specific antibodies inhibit influenza virus entry and replication at various points in its replication cycle. The replication cycle of influenza virus reveals distinct peptide targets of influenza-specific antibodies. Neutralizing antibodies to the receptor-binding ("head") region of HA block virus attachment and entry into respiratory tract epithelial cells, whereas anti-HA antibodies binding to its "stalk" may block virus infection by inhibiting fusion of the virus with the host cell membrane. Anti-NP and anti-M2e antibodies reduce the efficiency of influenza virus replications. Finally, antibodies to NA act by inhibiting the release of nascent virus particle from the surface of infected host cells, thereby inhibiting virus spread.

Antibodies against the stalk region are of great potential significance for the design of future broadly neutralizing antibody-inducing vaccines. Given their potential for providing broad levels of heterosubtypic immunity, their induction in infected individuals has recently been suggested to have a role in the dynamics that shape the replacement of a seasonal influenza virus strain with a pandemic strain [36].

Neuraminidase-specific antibodies

Antibodies to NA have received less attention. This is in part because the NA molecule facilitates influenza binding only indirectly and directly only late during infection (see Chapter 5). Indirect effects of antibodies to NA may include the inhibition of NA-mediated cleavage of sialic acids mucus overlying the respiratory tract epithelium, a process that can enhance virus access to host cells. Mostly, however, antibodies to NA, or NA inhibitory drugs, act by blocking the cleavage of newly generated nascent virus particles from the host cell surface. By inhibiting this process, antibodies to NA strongly inhibit replication efficiency of influenza virus and reduce the dissemination of virus particles for infection of neighboring cells and thereby ameliorate disease severity, as shown in recent mouse studies (reviewed in [37]).

Antibodies against nonsurface glycoproteins of influenza

Antibodies against other influenza virus-encoded proteins are induced also following an infection and can provide immune protection. Antibodies to the conserved nucleoprotein (NP) of influenza provided passive protection from death and disease after homosubtypic and heterosubtypic influenza virus challenge [38]. NP might be a promising candidate target for a universal influenza virus vaccine, as it is the frequent target also of cross-protective cytotoxic virus-specific CD8 T cell. However, given that NP is a virus internal antigen, antibodies do not neutralize the virus but act by inhibiting virus replication efficiency.

In contrast to the abovementioned antibodies, which are all induced by natural infections, antibodies to the matrix-2 (M2) protein of influenza virus (see Chapter 6) are not generated in influenza virus infected humans and mice. Immunization experiments with the ectodomain of M2 (M2e), or the passive transfer of monoclonal antibodies to M2e, have provided good evidence, however, that this highly conserved protein may be a good target for vaccine-induced broadly protective antibodies against influenza [39]. While phase I clinical trials have been completed successfully, the efficacy of an M2e vaccine in humans remains to be demonstrated. Recent studies invoked the importance of alveolar macrophages and their expression of Fcγ receptors as crucial for the protective capacity of anti-M2e IgG antibodies [40]. Thus, anti-M2e antibodies seem to be important for opsonization and targeting of infected cells by the cellular arm of the immune system.

In summary, influenza virus infection induces responses against multiple influenza antigens. Protective antibodies include the neutralizing and broadly neutralizing antibodies raised against HA. They also include antibodies to NA, NP, and M2e, which can reduce virus replication efficiency and spread, and, because they are directed often against highly conserved regions of the virus, may provide broad immune protection.

Antibody-mediated immune pressure selects for antigenic "drift" and "shift"

Influenza virus does not appear to have evolved mechanisms to evade and suppress adaptive immune responses; instead, it seems to "outrun" it. Influenza virus loads in the respiratory tract typically peak within 48–72 h, just about the time of first specific antibody generation. Thus, by the time cellular and humoral adaptive immune responses are generated, the virus has already infected other nonimmune hosts. While the infected host typically clears the virus efficiently, immune-mediated clearance does not prevent the virus from continuing its replication and transmission cycle. However, eventually the majority of the exposed nonimmune population will develop HA-specific antibodies that induce "sterilizing" immunity (i.e., prevent the virus from transmitting to other hosts), stopping its progression, and ending the influenza virus epidemic. Vaccination not only protects the individual from infection, it could also effectively stop ongoing epidemics by reducing the number of susceptible hosts to a point at which further virus transmissions become unlikely, inducing "herd immunity." However, the number of individuals who are vaccinated each year is not currently at rates high enough to disrupt the yearly epidemics.

It has to be stressed that the failure to generate long-term protective immunity against influenza infections is not due to a lack of immunity that develops following infection, or even vaccination. These responses are highly effective. The failure is due chiefly to the high rate of mutations of influenza virus's major antibody targets, HA and NA, antigenic drift, and larger exchanges of entire gene segments (antigenic shift), outlined in Chapters 3–5, that render the pre-existing specific antibodies and T cells nonprotective, because they are no longer able to bind to the mutated components of the virus, or do not bind with sufficient avidity. The fact that neutralizing antibodies against the highly conserved HA stalk region are induced as well as against other influenza proteins that can inhibit virus replication demonstrate the importance of defining major and minor B-cell epitopes for exploitation by future vaccines. However, there is some fear that increased immune pressure on the HA stalk region might force mutations to that region. Whether the resulting virus would retain its replication fitness is not known at this point.

Induced mutations that render neutralizing antibodies ineffective can be demonstrated quite easily *in vitro* by culturing viruses in the presence of monoclonal antibodies. The escape mutants emerging from such cultures are resistant to the antibody-mediated blockade in virus replication [31]. A recent study performing repeated transfer into mice with or without pre-existing immunity (i.e., in the presence or absence of polyclonal influenza-specific antibody responses), supports an important role for neutralizing antibodies in inducing antigenic drift. Interestingly, the mutations appeared to affect mainly the binding strengths, or avidity, between HA and the host cells, and thereby infection efficiency [41].

The increased availability and affordability of high-throughput sequencing make it feasible to study the epidemiology and emergence of new influenza viruses escape mutants also in nature, by sequencing large numbers of virus isolates. However, to fully assess the role of antibody-mediated immunity on influenza virus strain emergence and selection requires tools to mark all antibody epitopes on to the three-dimensional structure of viral proteins. This is because epitopes for neutralizing HA-specific antibodies are nearly all discontinuous determinants formed by residues present on different stretches of the HA peptide [42,43]. In general, predictive tools for discontinuous B-cell epitope mapping are in their infancy [44] and progress will likely require the generation of more experimental data, including more crystal structure information. The extensive work that has already been carried out on understanding the relationship between influenza HA and neutralizing antibodies and the availability of many HA-specific monoclonal antibodies [41] could greatly aid such efforts.

Antigenic shift and drift enable the virus to evade neutralization by antibodies. However, these mechanisms do not operate at the level of the individual, as influenza virus is usually cleared within a few days. Instead, these genetic alterations enable the virus to evade antibody-mediated immune protection at the population level, which would be building over time as more and more individuals are infected and develop specific immunity. The outcome are waves of infections with newly emerging variants of previously circulating influenza virus strains that can infect populations that are only partially protected against the newly emerging strain. The partial protection, while ineffective in preventing infection itself, appears a major reason why during seasonal influenza virus outbreaks healthy individuals usually only develop mild disease, while young children without prior immunity, and the elderly, who might have compromised immunity, are vulnerable to developing more severe forms of the disease.

Role of pre-existing antibodies for the outcome after influenza infection

From the above listed experimental and clinical studies it can be concluded that the pre-existence of antibodies in a host will reduce morbidity and mortality following challenge with a variant strain of influenza virus. Such results are in apparent contrast to conclusions drawn from studies pioneered in the 1950s by Francis [45]. These and other studies on antibody responses to influenza virus infection have led to the concept of "original antigen sin" – a concept based on the findings that during a recall response triggered with a variant strain of influenza, antibodies to the second strain used for immunization are lower in magnitude and avidity than the response to the primary virus (see Chapter 20). While often used as an argument for the potential negative impact prior vaccination or infection may have on the outcome from a subsequent infection, in fact, such negative effects have not been documented epidemiologically. This might have to do with the fact that the original studies in principle identified the induction of potent memory B-cell responses to conserved components of the virus. Memory B cells are typically of high affinity for their cognate antigen and will rapidly differentiate to antibody-secreting cells following a challenge, explaining why the "cross-reactive" antigens gave a higher and faster response than antibodies to novel epitopes. Moreover, such high initial responses against cross-reactive epitopes can lower the challenge viral loads, thus reducing the availability of antigen required for mounting a primary response [46], further explaining the reduction in antibody responses to the challenge virus. Indeed, giving increased doses of challenge antigen can largely overcome the response reduction, indicating that the magnitude of the antibody response adjusts according to viral loads [46]. For the outcome of an infection it matters little whether viral loads were reduced due to cross-reactive antibodies or antibodies mounted against the new virus. Thus, while interesting as an immunologic concept, whether and to what extent "original antigen sin" really is a "sin" and not a "virtue" might not be as easy to answer.

A recent study suggests that the avidity of pre-existing antibodies is crucial for infection outcome [1]. During the 2009 H1N1 pandemic, as in previous pandemics, middle-aged subjects without pre-existing conditions and who had neutralizing antibodies to seasonal influenza strains could become severely ill. The study indicated that these individuals may have generated only low avidity nonprotective antibodies to the pandemic strain, which formed pathogenic lung immune complexes with C4 deposition that strongly correlated with disease. Whether pre-existing B-cell immunity to seasonal influenza strains contributed to, or even caused the lack of high avidity antibody generation, remains an open question. The answer might ultimately determine the clinical relevance and/or context for the phenomenon of "original antigen sin."

Function of antibodies in infection with and clearance from influenza virus

Role and function of IgA antibodies against influenza

There is strong evidence that the local presence of virus-specific IgA on mucosal surfaces of the respiratory tract can completely prevent influenza virus infection [47,48]. IgA producing plasma cells are present in the lamina propria of the respiratory tract mucosa, which overlays the upper respiratory tract, reaching down to the larger bronchi. Small bronchi no longer express a mucosa. Mucosa-resident plasma cells produce dimeric IgA, which aids their transport on to the lumen of the airways via a sophisticated transport mechanism. This first involves its binding to the polymeric Ig receptor, expressed on the basolateral surface of the epithelial cells. Receptor IgA internalization and transcytoses is followed by an enzymatic cleavage process that releases the IgA from the epithelial surface into the lumen. A 60-kd component of the receptor, the "secretory component," however, remains attached to the antibody to generate "secretory IgA." The secretory component can protect the IgA against proteolytic cleavage. It may also anchor the antibody in the mucus overlaying the epithelial cells by selectively binding to mucins (reviewed in [49]). Secretory IgA is thought to provide a highly specific and effective barrier preventing influenza virus from reaching the epithelial cells.

While this directed transport mechanism from the lamina propria into the lumen has long been known to benefit the dissemination of IgA on to the mucosal surface, more recent studies have suggested that it may have additional functions [49]. First, *in vitro* studies showed that during transcytosis IgA can bind to and neutralize virus inside epithelial cells. Intracellular neutralization occurs where endosomes carrying the IgA from the basolateral surface fuse with endosomes from the apical surface containing endocytosed virus. Finally, the transport on to the lumen might also facilitate the removal of virus material from the tissue into the lumen for uptake and degradation by alveolar macrophages, or removal by the mucociliary escalator. That latter process might be of particular importance during the later phase of the infection, when the continued presence of viral antigens could propagate potentially harmful proin-flammatory responses. Thus, locally produced IgA might not only prevent influenza infection, but might also facilitate the "clean-up" process.

From the above, it appears clear that the induction of IgA responses is likely to contribute significantly to protection from influenza virus infection and to prevent or inhibit infection-induced tissue damage. It is thought that one of the main advantages of the LAIV over inactivated influenza virus (IAV) vaccination is that local application of a vaccine could induce protective IgA responses, which the IAV does not. Indeed, the live-attenuated vaccine has been shown to elicit strong IgA responses in the lung. Somewhat surprisingly, however, experimental evidence for the importance for IgA as a *necessary* component of the antiviral humoral response has been difficult to obtain. Studies involving IgA-deficient mice have shown only some rather modest increases in mortality after influenza virus infection compared with wild-type mice [50]. However, IgA-deficient mice show compensatory increases in other immunoglobulin iso-types, particularly the pentameric IgM, which can use the above outlined transport mechanism for secretion on to the lumen of the respiratory tract. Thus, the exact contribution of IgA to immune protection is unclear from those studies.

Likewise, in a relatively small prospective study with IgA-deficient humans, a relatively prevalent primary immunodeficiency particularly in Scandina-via, IgA-deficient individuals exhibited no increase in influenza-induced mortality or morbidity compared with immunocompetent controls [51]. In a related study, the same group did find slight increases in IgG levels against influenza and other local infections in the serum of IgA-deficient individuals, potentially indicating that those individuals had a higher rate of infections than immunocompetent control subjects [52]. Nonetheless, there is little evidence that IgA-deficient individuals develop increased morbidity or mortality after influenza virus infection.

Role and function of IgG antibodies to influenza

Thus, there seems to be a discrepancy in the literature with regard to the potency of IgA to prevent influenza virus infections on the one hand, and the lack of a clear effect by its absence on the other. The impor-tance of IgG antibodies in providing immune protec-tion against influenza and other infectious insults in the respiratory tract may provide an explanation for this apparent discrepancy. Because the lower parts of the respiratory tract lack a lamina propria and associ-ated local plasma cell population, humoral protection comes from the inflammatory transudate that carries mainly IgG antibodies on to the epithelial surfaces, thus providing humoral immune protection in the parts of the respiratory tract that lack a mucosa. Given the large surface areas of the alveoli is 800 times larger than the epithelial cell surfaces overlying a mucosa, it can be seen how the presence of IgG may compensate for much of any loss in IgA [53]. This also explains why IAV represents a highly effective vaccine approach, despite its inability to induce mucosal IgA production.

Thus, influenza virus specific antibodies of the IgG isotype are highly important in the protection of the nonmucosal compartments of the respiratory tract. IgG-producing cells can be found during acute infec-tion in the draining lymph nodes, short term in the spleen and somewhat later also in the lung and even-tually in the bone marrow, where they remain for years [5]. Most influenza-specific memory B cells both in the lung and in the periphery have class switched to IgG and their rapid recall responses have been demonstrated [9]. They are the predominant immune mechanism induced by IAV and their titers strongly correlate with immune protection [8]. While IgG has no active transport mechanisms for its secre-tion on to mucosal surfaces or into tissues, it rapidly reaches inflamed tissues via the transudate from the blood. Indeed, it is by far the most prevalent immu-noglobulin in the secretion in the lower airways after influenza virus infection [53]. Relevant for clearance from influenza virus infection, IgG antibodies can facilitate natural killer (NK) cell-mediated clearance of infected cells and opsonize virus for uptake by alveolar macrophages. There are few if any studies selectively depleting only IgG antibodies without also affecting IgM or IgA responses, but given the above it can be generally concluded that antibodies of the IgG isotype are of great importance in provid-ing immune protection from challenge infection. Indeed, it is likely that at least some of the effects attributed to the local production of IgA might come from the rapid influx of IgG into the respiratory tract [53].

Role and function of virus-binding IgM

When considering antibodies of the IgM isotype, one has to distinguish between those induced in response to infection by antigen-specific B cells and the "natural" IgM (i.e., antibodies that are generated in the absence of prior antigenic stimulation but nonetheless can bind to and neutralize influenza virus). Natural IgM is of interest, as these antibodies are often polyreactive and have been shown to bind broadly to numerous influenza A and B strains [54].

In mice, B cells responsible for producing natural antibodies, mainly IgM and also IgA, have been identified as "B-1 cells", a small B-cell subset that is generated from B-cell precursors that are distinct from those generating the majority of the conventional B cells and that are generated predominantly early in ontogeny (reviewed in [55]). While it is undisputed that humans harbor natural antibodies similar to mice, the cell population responsible has not been as clearly defined yet. Natural IgM was shown to be a nonredundant component of the humoral response to influenza virus infection, as mice that only lacked B-1 cell-derived IgM succumbed to infection at higher rates than controls. Natural IgM might control influenza virus infection by complement-mediated lysis. However, it is likely that IgM might have other important regulatory functions, as IgM-deficient mice showed reduced virus binding IgG responses.

Influenza virus-induced IgM has received little attention. It is widely seen as a "first" line of immune defense, as adaptive B-cell responses usually show a rapid induction of IgM followed by a somewhat slower induction of IgG. However, at least in mouse and ferret models of infection, IgG and IgM responses in the regional lymph nodes seem to appear at similar times, about 3 days after infection. A recent study in humans naturally infected with pandemic influenza H1N1 found a correlation between early virus-specific IgM in the serum and the later development of robust neutralizing IgG responses [56], consistent with the abovementioned studies in mice. That same study also found that the early IgM did not have HAI activity, in contrast to the later IgG response.

Antibodies of the IgM isotype do not harbor the frequent somatic mutations in the immunoglobulin locus seen among the IgG responses. This is because B cells secreting IgM may not, or at least not often, participate in germinal center responses. Because IgM is typically a pentamer and thus harbors 10 antigen binding sites, IgM antibodies might bind antigen with relatively high avidity, despite their overall lower affinity. This multimeric structure also allows IgM to be transported via the polymeric Ig receptor on to the airway lumen of the respiratory tract. Although its affinity for binding to the receptor is lower than that of the dimeric IgA [49].

Conclusions

Influenza virus infection induces a powerful humoral immune response both locally and eventually also systemically, supported by specialized cells that provide antigen to B cells. Local responses are induced and/or maintained by the presence of tertiary lymphoid structures in the respiratory tract. While the local production of IgA and to a lesser degree IgM in the upper respiratory tract may block influenza virus entry, the presence of serum IgG provides a strong and effective mechanism for preventing influenza virus dissemination into the lower respiratory tract. Even non-neutralizing antibodies have important roles in reducing virus dissemination and disease induction, and potentially regulating B-cell responses. By reducing virus burden and eliminating virus antigen from the respiratory tract, antibodies likely reduce inflammatory responses and thereby the extent of tissue damage and disease. For the development of universal influenza vaccines, emphasis has been on the induction of the cellular arm of the immune system. However, given the recent evidence that the stalk of HA can induce broadly neutralizing antibody responses, continued exploration of the function and induction pathways of neutralizing antibodies remains an important area of research into protective immunity to influenza virus.

References

1. Monsalvo AC, Batalle JP, Lopez MF, Krause JC, Klemenc J, Hernandez JZ, et al. Severe pandemic 2009 H1N1 influenza disease due to pathogenic immune complexes. Nat Med. 2011;17:195–9.
2. Gerhard W, Mozdzanowska K, Furchner M, Washko G, Maiese K. Role of the B-cell response in recovery of mice from primary influenza virus infection. Immunol Rev. 1997;159:95–103.

3. Sangster MY, Riberdy JM, Gonzalez M, Topham DJ, Baumgarth N, Doherty PC. An early CD4+ T cell-dependent immunoglobulin A response to influenza infection in the absence of key cognate T–B interactions. J Exp Med. 2003;198:1011–21.

4. Sealy R, Surman S, Hurwitz JL, Coleclough C. Antibody response to influenza infection of mice: different patterns for glycoprotein and nucleocapsid antigens. Immunology. 2003;108:431–9.

5. Jones PD, Ada GL. Persistence of influenza virus-specific antibody-secreting cells and B-cell memory after primary murine influenza virus infection. Cell Immunol. 1987;109:53–64.

6. McDermott MR, Bienenstock J. Evidence for a common mucosal immunologic system. I. Migration of B immunoblasts into intestinal, respiratory, and genital tissues. J Immunol. 1979;122:1892–8.

7. Randall TD. Bronchus-associated lymphoid tissue (BALT) structure and function. Adv Immunol. 2010;107:187–241.

8. Couch RB, Kasel JA. Immunity to influenza in man. Annu Rev Microbiol. 1983;37:529–49.

9. Wrammert J, Smith K, Miller J, Langley WA, Kokko K, Larsen C, et al. Rapid cloning of high-affinity human monoclonal antibodies against influenza virus. Nature. 2008;453:667–71.

10. Lee FE, Halliley JL, Walsh EE, Moscatiello AP, Kmush BL, Falsey AR, et al. Circulating human antibody-secreting cells during vaccinations and respiratory viral infections are characterized by high specificity and lack of bystander effect. J Immunol. 2011;186:5514–21.

11. Dawood FS, Jain S, Finelli L, Shaw MW, Lindstrom S, garten RJ, et al. Emergence of a novel swine-origin influenza A (H1N1) virus in humans. N Engl J Med. 2009;360:2605–15.

12. Jones PD, Ada GL. Influenza-specific antibody-secreting cells and B cell memory in the murine lung after immunization with wild-type, cold-adapted variant and inactivated influenza viruses. Vaccine. 1987;5:244–8.

13. Tamura S, Kurata T. Defense mechanisms against influenza virus infection in the respiratory tract mucosa. Jpn J Infect Dis. 2004;57:236–47.

14. Paus D, Phan TG, Chan TD, Gardam S, Basten A, Brink R. Antigen recognition strength regulates the choice between extrafollicular plasma cell and germinal center B cell differentiation. J Exp Med. 2006;203:1081–91.

15. Cyster JG, Ansel KM, Reif K, Ekland EH, Hyman PL, Tang HL, et al. Follicular stromal cells and lymphocyte homing to follicles. Immunol Rev. 2000;176:181–93.

16. Gonzalez SF, Degn SE, Pitcher LA, Woodruff M, Heesters BA, Carroll MC. Trafficking of B cell antigen in lymph nodes. Annu Rev Immunol. 2011;29:215–33.

17. Reid KB, Porter RR. The proteolytic activation systems of complement. Annu Rev Biochem. 1981;50:433–64.

18. Fearon DT, Locksley RM. The instructive role of innate immunity in the acquired immune response. Science. 1996;272:50–3.

19. Kopf M, Abel B, Gallimore A, Carroll M, Bachmann MF. Complement component C3 promotes T-cell priming and lung migration to control acute influenza virus infection. Nat Med. 2002;8:373–8.

20. Fernandez Gonzalez S, Jayasekera JP, Carroll MC. Complement and natural antibody are required in the long-term memory response to influenza virus. Vaccine. 2008;26(Suppl. 8):I86–93.

21. Fischer MB, Goerg S, Shen L, Prodeus AP, Goodnow CC, Kelsoe G, et al. Dependence of germinal center B cells on expression of CD21/CD35 for survival. Science. 1998;280:582–5.

22. Fearon DT, Carter RH. The CD19/CR2/TAPA-1 complex of B lymphocytes: linking natural to acquired immunity. Annu Rev Immunol. 1995;13:127–49.

23. Heer AK, Shamshiev A, Donda A, Uematsu S, Akira S, Kopf M, et al. TLR signaling fine-tunes anti-influenza B cell responses without regulating effector T cell responses. J Immunol. 2007;178:2182–91.

24. Theofilopoulos AN, Baccala R, Beutler B, Kono DH. Type I interferons (alpha/beta) in immunity and autoimmunity. Annu Rev Immunol. 2005;23:307–36.

25. Coro ES, Chang WL, Baumgarth N. Type I IFN receptor signals directly stimulate local B cells early following influenza virus infection. J Immunol. 2006;176:4343–51.

26. Le Bon A, Thompson C, Kamphuis E, Durand V, Rossmann C, Kalinke U, et al. Cutting edge: enhancement of antibody responses through direct stimulation of B and T cells by type I IFN. J Immunol. 2006;176:2074–8.

27. Le Bon A, Schiavoni G, D'Agostino G, Gresser I, Belardelli F, Tough DF. Type i interferons potently enhance humoral immunity and can promote isotype switching by stimulating dendritic cells in vivo. Immunity. 2001;14:461–70.

28. Rau FC, Dieter J, Luo Z, Priest SO, Baumgarth N. B7-1/2 (CD80/CD86) direct signaling to B cells enhances IgG secretion. J Immunol. 2009;183:7661–71.

29. Salk JE, Suriano PC. Importance of antigenic composition of influenza virus vaccine in protecting against the natural disease; observations during the winter of 1947–1948. Am J Public Health Nations Health. 1949;39:345–55.

30. Hobson D, Curry RL, Beare AS, Ward-Gardner A. The role of serum haemagglutination-inhibiting antibody in protection against challenge infection with influenza A2 and B viruses. J Hyg (Lond). 1972;70:767–77.

31. Gerhard W, Yewdell J, Frankel ME, Webster R. Antigenic structure of influenza virus haemagglutinin defined by hybridoma antibodies. Nature. 1981;290:713–7.

32. Caton AJ, Brownlee GG, Yewdell JW, Gerhard W. The antigenic structure of the influenza virus A/PR/8/34 hemagglutinin (H1 subtype). Cell. 1982;31:417–27.

33. Chun S, Li C, Van Domselaar G, Wang J, Farnsworth A, Cui X, et al. Universal antibodies and their applications to the quantitative determination of virtually all subtypes of the influenza A viral hemagglutinins. Vaccine. 2008;26:6068–76.

34. Ekiert DC, Bhabha G, Elsliger MA, Friesen RH, Jongeneelen M, Throsby M, et al. Antibody recognition of a highly conserved influenza virus epitope. Science. 2009;324:246–51.

35. Wrammert J, Koutsonanos D, Li GM, Edupuganti S, Sui J, Morrissey M, et al. Broadly cross-reactive antibodies dominate the human B cell response against 2009 pandemic H1N1 influenza virus infection. J Exp Med. 2011;208:181–93.

36. Pica N, Hai R, Krammer F, Wang TT, Maamary J, Eggink D, et al. Hemagglutinin stalk antibodies elicited by the 2009 pandemic influenza virus as a mechanism for the extinction of seasonal H1N1 viruses. Proc Natl Acad Sci U S A. 2012;109:2573–8.

37. Marcelin G, Sandbulte MR, Webby RJ. Contribution of antibody production against neuraminidase to the protection afforded by influenza vaccines. Rev Med Virol. 2012.

38. Carragher DM, Kaminski DA, Moquin A, Hartson L, Randall TD. A novel role for non-neutralizing antibodies against nucleoprotein in facilitating resistance to influenza virus. J Immunol. 2008;181:4168–76.

39. Treanor JJ, Tierney EL, Zebedee SL, Lamb RA, Murphy BR. Passively transferred monoclonal antibody to the M2 protein inhibits influenza A virus replication in mice. J Virol. 1990;64:1375–7.

40. El Bakkouri K, Descamps F, De Filette M, Smet A, Festjens E, Birkett A, et al. Universal vaccine based on ectodomain of matrix protein 2 of influenza A: Fc receptors and alveolar macrophages mediate protection. J Immunol. 2011;186:1022–31.

41. Hensley SE, Das SR, Bailey AL, Schmidt LM, Hickman HD, Jayaraman A, et al. Hemagglutinin receptor binding avidity drives influenza A virus antigenic drift. Science. 2009;326:734–6.

42. Caton AJ, Brownlee GG, Yewdell JW, Gerhard W. The antigenic structure of the influenza virus A/PR/8/34 hemagglutinin (H1 subtypes). Cell. 1982;31:417–27.

43. Knossow M, Skehel JJ. Variation and infectivity neutralization in influenza. Immunology. 2006;119:1–7.

44. Ponomarenko JV, Bourne PE. Antibody-protein interactions: benchmark datasets and prediction tools evaluation. BMC Struct Biol. 2007;7:64.

45. Francis T Jr. Influenza: the new acquayantance. Ann Intern Med. 1953;39:203–21.

46. Kim JH, Skountzou I, Compans R, Jacob J. Original antigenic sin responses to influenza viruses. J Immunol. 2009;183:3294–301.

47. Renegar KB, Small PA Jr. Passive transfer of local immunity to influenza virus infection by IgA antibody. J Immunol. 1991;146:1972–8.

48. Renegar KB Jr, Immunoglobulin PAS. A mediation of murine nasal anti-influenza virus immunity. J Virol. 1991;65:2146–8.

49. Strugnell RA, Wijburg OL. The role of secretory antibodies in infection immunity. Nat Rev Microbiol. 2010;8:656–67.

50. Arulanandam BP, Raeder RH, Nedrud JG, Bucher DJ, Le J, Metzger DW. IgA immunodeficiency leads to inadequate Th cell priming and increased susceptibility to influenza virus infection. J Immunol. 2001;166:226–31.

51. Aho K, Pyhala R, Koistinen J. IgA deficiency and influenza infection. Scand J Immunol. 1976;5:1089–92.

52. Pyhala R, Aho K, Kantanen ML, Koistinen J. Virus antibody levels in IgA deficiency. Scand J Immunol. 1976;5:1093–6.

53. Ito R, Ozaki YA, Yoshikawa T, Hasegawa H, Sato Y, Suzuki Y, et al. Roles of anti-hemagglutinin IgA and IgG antibodies in different sites of the respiratory tract of vaccinated mice in preventing lethal influenza pneumonia. Vaccine. 2003;21:2362–71.

54. Baumgarth N, Herman OC, Jager GC, Brown L, Herzenberg LA, Herzenberg LA. Innate and acquired humoral immunities to influenza virus are mediated by distinct arms of the immune system. Proc Natl Acad Sci U S A. 1999;96:2250–5.

55. Baumgarth N. The double life of a B-1 cell: self-reactivity selects for protective effector functions. Nat Rev Immunol. 2011;11:34–46.

56. Qiu C, Tian D, Wan Y, Zhang W, Qiu C, Zhu Z, et al. Early adaptive humoral immune responses and virus clearance in humans recently infected with pandemic 2009 H1N1 influenza virus. PLoS ONE. 2011;6:e22603.

57. Gonzalez SF, Lukacs-Kornek V, Kuligowski MP, Pitcher LA, Degn SE, Kim YA, et al. Capture of influenza by medullary dendritic cells via SIGN-R1 is essential for humoral immunity in draining lymph nodes. Nat Immunol. 2010;11(5):427–34.

19

Cell-mediated immunity

Stephen J. Turner,[1] Peter C. Doherty,[1] and Anne Kelso[1,2]

[1]Department of Microbiology and Immunology, The University of Melbourne, Victoria, Australia

[2]WHO Collaborating Centre for Reference and Research on Influenza, Victoria, Australia

Introduction

The immune response to the influenza A viruses starts with activation of the innate immune system at the time of initial exposure. The infected cells produce type 1 interferons and other defence molecules, and natural killer (NK) cells, NK T cells, monocyte–macrophages and neutrophils traffic to the site of invasion to deliver cytokines and other effector proteins at close range (see Chapter 17). In a naïve individual, the adaptive response is slower, with the first immunoglobulin M (IgM) antibodies being detected after about 4 or 5 days. Produced by B lymphocytes and plasma cells, antibodies have a critical role in protection by binding to the major surface glycoproteins of the virus (see Chapters 18 and 20).

In this chapter, we discuss the other arm of the adaptive response, cell-mediated immunity (CMI), delivered by thymus-derived CD4[+] and CD8[+] T lymphocytes and directed against virus-infected and antigen-presenting cells (APCs). Activated CD4[+] and CD8[+] T cells have distinct roles in the control of influenza virus infections. The CD4[+] T cells secrete cytokines and other mediators that help antibody-producing B lymphocytes and optimize CD8[+] T-cell responses in the lymphoid tissue. The CD8[+] T cells produce cytotoxic molecules as well as cytokines, enabling them to destroy virus infected cells. This limits virus spread, contributes to clearance, and reduces disease severity.

T-cell recognition of viral antigens

Antigen presentation

Whereas antibodies generally bind to conformational structures on proteins and other antigens, CD8[+] and CD4[+] T cells recognize peptide fragments (p) bound to self major histocompatibility complex class I (MHCI) and class II (MHCII) glycoproteins, respectively [1]. Non-self pMHCI complexes can be displayed on the surface of any cell type while presentation of pMHCII complexes is generally limited to professional APCs, such as dendritic cells (DCs) and macrophages (Figure 19.1a) [2].

The MHC molecules are, after the antibodies, the most diverse (polymorphic) proteins produced by mammals. As humans and mice have three MHCI loci (HLA-A, B, C in humans; H-2 K, D, L in mice), each with two alleles, any cell can potentially present peptides complexed with six different MHCI molecules. With this degree of polymorphism and polyallelism, the likelihood that a pathogen does not contain an immunogenic peptide is low (within the individual) to infinitesimal (across the species).

The peptides that bind to MHCI molecules are normally derived from proteins synthesized within the cytoplasm of infected cells. Following degradation in the proteasome, peptide fragments move via a selective channel (the TAP transporter) to the endoplasmic reticulum where best-fit peptides (usually

Textbook of Influenza, Second Edition. Edited by Robert G. Webster, Arnold S. Monto, Thomas J. Braciale, and Robert A. Lamb.
© 2013 John Wiley & Sons, Ltd. Published 2013 by John Wiley & Sons, Ltd.

7–12 amino acids) are loaded into the groove of the MHCI glycoprotein. By contrast, peptides derived from phagocytosed or endocytosed proteins processed via the endosomal/lysomal compartment bind to MHCII molecules. These pMHCI and pMHCII complexes are then translocated to the cell surface.

T-cell receptor

Antigen-specific T cells recognize pMHC complexes [1] via clonally expressed T-cell receptor (TCR) αβ heterodimers (Figure 19.1b). Functional TCR generation occurs during lymphocyte development in the thymus through the random rearrangement of vari-

able (V), diversity (D), and junctional (J), or V and J, gene segments from the TCRβ and TCRα gene loci, respectively. As for immunoglobulin molecules, the hypervariable complementarity determining regions (CDR) encoded within the Vα and Vβ gene segments form the sites that bind different pMHC complexes. The CDR3 regions are formed at the junction of different V(D)J germline segments after somatic recombination, whereas the TCR Vα and Vβ CDR1 and 2 regions are germline constructs.

Unlike the immunoglobulin molecules, the TCRs do not undergo somatic hypermutation. Thus, building a comprehensive TCR repertoire relies on the use of different gene segments and both combinatorial

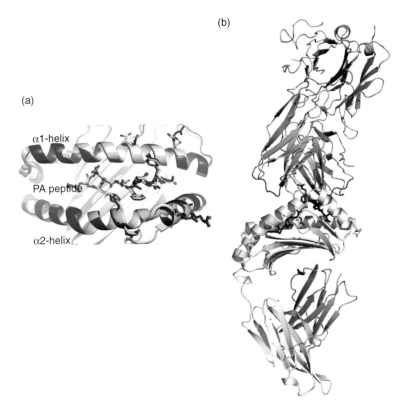

(b)

(a)

α1-helix

PA peptide

α2-helix

Figure 19.1. Structure of peptide–MHC class I complex. (a) Structural representation of the MHC class I H-2D^b molecule complexed to the acid polymerase peptide, residues 224–233, amino acid sequence SSLENFRAYV (D^{b}PA$_{224}$). Shown is top-down view with the α1 helix at the top, the PA$_{224-233}$ peptide in the middle, and the α2 helix at the bottom. (b) A ribbon representation of the PA TCR/D^{b}PA$_{224-233}$ complex [59], showing the TCRα chain in pale pink, the TCRβ chain in pale blue, H-2D^b in white and the PA$_{224-233}$ peptide in dark purple. The CDR regions of the PA TCR are colored purple (CDR1α), green (CDR2α), yellow (CDR3α), red (CDR1β), blue (CDR2β), and orange (CDR3β). The TCR sit atop the H–2D^{b}PA$_{224}$ complex.

and junctional diversity in the association of TCRαβ heterodimers [1]. The TCR repertoire is further expanded by the lack of precision during V(D)J gene rearrangement and by the addition of nontemplate encoded nucleotides at V(D)J junctions. Mathematical estimates suggest that there are 10^{12}–10^{15} different TCRs. However, thymic selection ensures that the number of distinct TCRαβ pairs within an individual is reduced to approximately 2×10^7 (human) or 2×10^6 (mouse) [3,4]. Interestingly, the naïve TCR repertoires of different individuals do not overlap to any great extent, so the potential TCR diversity is much greater at the population level. The essential constraint is that the immunoglobulin and TCR repertoires together must be able to recognize any novel, or familiar, pathogen, while minimizing autoimmunity, the "horror autotoxicus" first recognized at the turn of the twentieth century by Paul Ehrlich.

Primary T-cell response to influenza viruses

The T-cell response to influenza viruses begins with the recruitment of naïve precursors to the regional lymph nodes draining the site of infection in the respiratory tract. The structure and microenvironment of the lymph nodes brings naïve CD8+ and CD4+ T cells into contact with pMHCI and pMHCII presenting DCs in a cytokine-rich milieu provided, at least in part, by the responding CD4+ population. Once activated, T cells undergo differentiation and clonal expansion (cell division), with the progeny cells eventually exiting in the efferent lymph and blood to transit to the site of antigen deposition, in this case the infected lung. Most of what we know about T-cell immunity to the influenza viruses is derived from experiments in mice.

Role of DCs in priming CD8+ and CD4+ T cells

The DCs are generally considered to be the main antigen processing and/or presenting cells in the murine influenza model [5]. Both lung and lymph node resident DCs have parts to play in the induction of influenza virus-specific T-cell immunity. A primary role for tissue-resident DCs is the continual sampling of their environment for invading pathogens. Following influenza A virus infection, lung resident DCs are

activated via their pathogen pattern receptors, such as Toll-like receptor (TLR)-9, TLR-7 and intracellular sensors such as RIG-I or MDA-5, then exit the lung and traffic via afferent lymph to the regional lymph nodes. Further activation via the TLR/RIG-I/MDA-5 DCs carry antigen from the infected tissue to the draining node and provide secondary signals that promote the activation of naïve and memory antigen-specific CD4+ and CD8+ T cells [6].

Specificity of T cell responses to the influenza A viruses

Whereas antibodies are mainly directed towards the highly variable surface glycoproteins of the influenza virus, the hemagglutinin (HA) and the neuraminidase (NA), both mouse and human T cells preferentially recognize peptides derived from the internal viral proteins. The selection pressure exerted by human CD8+ T cells seems to be less than that associated with the immunoglobulin response (see Chapter 18), with the consequence that many T-cell epitopes are highly conserved within and between influenza A subtypes.

For the most thoroughly analyzed C57BL/6J (B6, H-2^b) mouse model, influenza-specific CD8+ T cells recognize peptides [7–11] derived from the nucleoprotein (NP$_{366-374}$), acid polymerase (PA$_{224-233}$), basic polymerase subunit 1 (PB1$_{703-711}$), basic polymerase subunit 1 frameshift 2 protein (PB1-F2$_{62-70}$), non-structural protein 2 (NS2$_{114-121}$), and matrix protein 1 (M1$_{128-135}$). The CD4+ T-cell response is particularly broad, with H-2 I-A^b-restricted peptides being derived from both conserved internal proteins and the more variable HA and NA surface molecules [7]. A prime and challenge protocol with serologically different (for HA and NA) influenza A viruses allows analysis of the recall of T-cell-mediated immunity, particularly for CD8+ cells [8], mimicking the situation for a new pandemic virus.

Tracking and analyzing T-cell respones

Once they receive appropriate activation signals from DCs and other cells in the lymph node, virus-specific CD4+ and, especially, CD8+ T cells undergo marked clonal expansion. Antigen-specific T cells that recognize a given pMHC can be readily identified by the binding of isolated pMHC complexes [9]. These complexes are produced in the laboratory and used as fluorochrome-labeled dimers or tetramers, allowing antigen-specific T cells to be quantified, characterized, and purified using a flow cytometer or sorter. Immune T-cell numbers can also be measured by *in vitro* stimulation with the relevant peptide in an inhibitor of cytokine secretion, followed by fixation and staining with a fluorochrome-labeled monoclonal antibody to a given cytokine. Intracellular cytokine-staining (ICS) for interferon-γ (IFN-γ) gives T-cell numbers similar to those found using pMHC tetramers. In a variant of the ICS approach, CD4+ T cells are stimulated in the wells of plastic plates to produce IFN-γ which is then captured by a plate-bound antibody. This ELISpot technique has also been used to count CD8+ T cells where the numbers are too low to detect with tetramers.

Numbers, kinetics, and immunodominance hierarchies

In B6 mice, virus replication is generally maximal by day 3–5 after infection and starts to decrease within another 2–3 days (Figure 19.2). This drop in virus titers coincides with the emergence of an expanded pool of antigen-specific CD8+ T cells, first in the draining lymph node and then in the lung. These cells reach peak numbers in the respiratory tract around day 10 then decrease following virus elimination (between day 8 and 10), leaving an identifiable, long-lived population of memory T cells that can be recalled rapidly to effector function on virus challenge (Figure 19.2). A characteristic of the B6 mouse model is that the influenza-specific CD8+ T-cell response follows a reproducible hierarchy, with the D^{b}NP and D^{b}PA epitope-specific sets being the most prevalent (immunodominant), while numbers specific for the D^{b}PB1-F2 and K^{b}NS2 epitopes remain at lower levels (sub-dominant).

Recent technical advances have enabled the isolation of naïve epitope-specific (pMHC tetramer binding) T cells for the first time. In young adult B6 mice (8–12 weeks), the numbers of naïve CD8+ T cells specific for the different influenza pMHCI complexes ranged from about 20 to 500 per mouse [10]. Unexpectedly, naïve CD8+ T-cell numbers do not necessarily mirror the antigen driven immunodominance hierarchy. Immunodominance can, in fact, reflect greater antigen driven proliferation from a smaller set

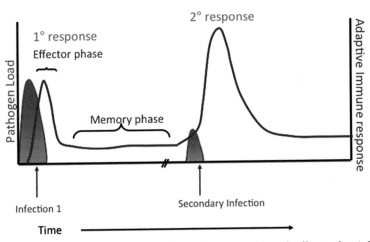

Figure 19.2. Kinetics of T-cell responses after primary and secondary influenza A virus infection. Intranasal influenza A virus infection in mice results in peak viral titers at around day 3 (red shade); at around day 4–5 influenza-specific T-cell numbers start to increase (blue line) and this coincides with a decrease in viral titer. Virus-specific T-cell numbers peak at day 10 after infection, at about the same time virus is cleared (effector phase). Upon clearance of infection, virus-specific T-cell numbers contract to establish a pool of long-lived, readily identifiable memory T cells (memory phase). Upon secondary infection, virus-specific T-cell numbers rapidly increase mediating more rapid effector function ensuring viral growth is limited.

of naïve precursors, while subdominant populations may be incompletely recruited from the naive pool [10]. Although many factors shape CD8+ T-cell immunodominance hierarchies, there is now strong evidence that the magnitude of the primary CTL response to virus is related more to the duration and timing of antigen availability than to naïve T-cell precursor frequency [10]. However, while immune T cell counts are readily quantified by tetramer binding, it is much harder to measure antigen levels *in vivo*, a problem that is currently a focus of intense analysis using mass spectrometry-based approaches [11].

Mechanisms of T-cell-mediated viral control

Immune CD8+ cytotoxic T lymphocytes (CTLs) are generally considered to be the main effectors of influenza A virus clearance, although it is likely that CD4+ T cells play a part beyond the provision of help to B cells and for the promotion of CTL memory. Early evidence that CD8+ T cells are important for recovery from influenza virus infection came from studies demonstrating delayed virus clearance after primary infection of MHCI-deficient (and thus CD8+ T-cell-deficient) mice [12]. Furthermore, Ig$^{-/-}$ "knockout" mice cleared influenza A viruses via a CD8+ T-cell-dependent mechanism [13] and adoptive transfer of activated influenza-specific TCR transgenic CD8+ T cells into naïve hosts resulted in faster virus clearance and improved survival [14].

Antigen-specific CD4+ and CD8+ T cells undergo a program of proliferation and differentiation leading to the acquisition of specific effector functions [15,16]. Cytotoxic function is characteristic of the CD8+ subset, while both CD4+ and CD8+ T cells produce various cytokines, particularly IL-2, IFN-γ, and TNFα [17]. While there are still many questions about the relative significance of these different mechanisms *in vivo*, it is likely that the various effector pathways function together to mediate virus clearance and recovery.

Cytotoxic T-cell activity

Effector CD8+ CTLs contain large cytoplasmic granules [18] loaded with serine proteases known as granzymes (grz) and the pore-forming protein per-

forin (pfp) (Figure 19.3). The best characterized grz and most abundant proteins in CTL granules are grzB and grzA [19]. Following TCR ligation of pMHCI complexes on the surface of infected cells, granules are exocytosed, releasing pfp and grz at the synaptic interface in a unidirectional transit that spares the CTL while inducing programmed cell death in the infected target [20].

The development of CD8+ CTL effector function begins soon after TCR/pMHCI ligation on the antigen-presenting DC in the draining lymph node [21]. This process is both progressive with cell division and stochastic, with single-cell analysis for grz A, B, C, K, and pfp mRNA demonstrating initial heterogeneity of effector gene expression that becomes more homogeneous as the differentiating CTL precursor expresses more of these genes and develops into a fully functional effector [22]. Broadly speaking, the acquisition of pfp and grz mRNA correlates with cytotoxic potential and effector differentiation [22,23]. Delayed pfp expression may serve to limit the killing of antigen-presenting DCs early in the immune response, ensuring that the CTL response is not terminated prematurely. Moreover, mechanisms regulating the expression of the various grz and pfp expression are different and specific to the particular gene.

While the optimal, rapid control of influenza A virus infection by CTLs is pfp dependent [24], the role of the individual grzs is less clear and Fas–Fas ligand-mediated interactions may also play a part under some circumstances. Mice lacking grzA and grzB showed no defect in influenza virus clearance and in fact, grzA/B-deficient CD8+ T cells can still mediate lysis of influenza virus-infected cells [25]. Thus, there maybe a role for other less studied grz such as grzK or grzC; for example, grzK mRNA is expressed at high frequency by influenza-specific CD8+ effectors [25]. Activated CD4+ T cells can also express grzB and pfp [26], and while mouse experiments have indicated this does not normally happen during an influenza A virus infection, recent analysis suggests that this is not necessarily the case for human CD4+ T cells [27].

Cytokines

The localization to the infected lung of influenza A virus specific CD8+ CTLs expressing proinflammatory

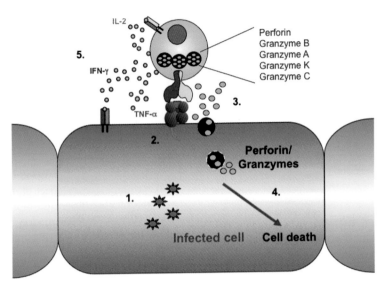

Figure 19.3. Influenza A virus-specific CD8+ CTLs exhibit functional heterogeneity. 1. Upon infection, cytosolic viral proteins are processed and presented at the cell surface bound to MHC class I molecules. 2. The pMHCI complexes are recognized by specific T-cell receptors expressed on activated effector CTLs. 3. TCR-dependent activation of effector CTLs results in release and deposition of cytolytic proteins, such as granzymes and perforin, from effector CTLs on to the infected cell. 4. Perforin-dependent uptake of granzymes by the target cell initiates a proteolytic cascade that results in apoptosis of the target cell. 5. Upon TCR-mediated recognition of pMHC, effector CTLs can secrete a number of effector cytokines, such as IFN-γ, TNF-α, and IL-2. Both IFN-γ and TNF-α have direct antiviral and inflammatory effects, whereas IL-2 is considered a proliferative and/or survival factor for effector CTLs.

cytokines is thought to be important for both protection and recovery [14]. Activated influenza virus-specific CD8+ and CD4+ T cells synthesize a number of cytokines, particularly IFN-γ, TNF-α, and IL-2 (Figure 19.3) [17]. In contrast to pfp/grz expression, cytokine production at both the mRNA and protein level is a transient response to TCR/pMHCI ligation limiting their action to sites of antigen presentation.

In addition to having a direct effector role [26], the CD4+ helpers promotes effective antibody responses and durable CD8+ CTL memory (see below). As CD8+ T cells do not express the pMHCII complexes recognized by the CD4+ set, this latter effect is presumably indirect. Inflammatory cytokines produced by activated CD4+ T cells set DCs up to be optimal stimulators, help shape the environment within the lymph node, trigger B-cell isotype switching (via IFN-γ and IL-4), produce the IL-21 that drives germinal center formation, and ensure both B-cell affinity maturation and the generation of B-cell memory [28].

Risks of immunopathology

The potent effector mechanisms used by activated T cells have the potential to cause severe damage to virus-infected hosts (reviewed in [29]). The severe, acute complications observed in human H5N1 virus infection, for example, are associated with an innate immune response that leads to fulminant inflammation, neutrophilia, and an acute lung pathology characteristic of cytokine shock [30] (see Chapter 17). However, in other instances, excessive cytokine production, in particular IFN-γ, may be associated with protection and diminished immunopathology [31]. Prime and boost experiments with different influenza A viruses in the B6 mouse model can induce massive secondary CTL responses that cause little clinical impairment. In fact, there is recent evidence that the balance between efficacy and pathology is self-regulated within the CD8+ T-cell compartment. Braciale et al. showed that lung-resident influenza A virus-specific CD8+ T cells are major producers of IL-10 (a potent anti-inflammatory mediator) which, if inhibited within the infected lung, led to greater respiratory compromise due to increased inflammation and enhanced lethality [32]. This CD8+ T-cell-mediated regulatory function required the participation of both innate immune cells producing IL-27 and virus-specific CD4+ T cells [33]. A vaccine strategy that selectively promotes CD8+ T-cell memory might need to prime for the rapid induction of this self-regulatory mechanism.

T-cell memory to influenza viruses

Generation of T-cell memory

Memory CTLs are long-lived, antigen-experienced cells capable of responding rapidly on subsequent infection with heterotypic viruses [34]. Acute influenza A virus infections are associated with the establishment of long-lived memory CTL precursors that endure for the life of a laboratory mouse [35]. However, the origin of these memory cells remains a matter of debate.

After primary activation, the differentiation and clonal expansion of CD8+ CTLs and virus clearance, there is a marked contraction of the effector population. It has been thought that the survivors form the memory CD8+ T-cell pool [36]. Recently, however, there are suggestions that CD8+ CTL memory can be established very early after T-cell activation [37,38], indicating that there may be distinct pathways of effector and memory T-cell differentiation. These indications that optimal T-cell memory can be established early after vaccination without effector differentiation obviously have important implications for the design of broad-spectrum vaccines [37]. In addition, CD4+ T-cell memory needs to be factored into the equation, as immune CD4+ T cells are essential for the generation and maintenance of effective CD8+ CTL memory through the actions of cytokines such as IL-2 [39] and other stimulatory signals that promote optimal DC function.

In the mouse model, following secondary respiratory challenge in the absence of neutralizing antibody, memory T cells that are present in physiologic numbers (<0.1% or less) can be recalled to the virus-infected lung approximately 2 days earlier and in 5-

to 10-fold greater numbers than in the primary response (Figure 19.2) [8]. This is true for the immunodominant pMHCI-specific sets (such as D^{b}NP$_{366-374}$-specific CD8+ T cells) but others (such as the K^{b}PB1$_{703-711}$-specific population which are prominent in primary responses) expand little, if at all [40]. For the design of T-cell-activating vaccines, it will be important to understand the mechanisms underlying this profound difference in recall responses and to define what constitutes an optimal protective T-cell epitope.

While there is little impact on the first few days of virus growth, the faster and more robust secondary CTL response accelerates virus clearance, perhaps due to the presence of significant numbers of CD8+ memory CTLs in the respiratory tract before challenge [41]. Influenza-specific CD4+ T cells can also be found in the resting lung and are thought to provide some measure of protection [42]. These and other experiments indicate that priming influenza-specific T-cell memory can limit virus growth and significantly diminish morbidity and death, but they also highlight the need for a more sophisticated understanding of how to optimize such protection.

Lung-resident memory T cells

Some memory T cells persist long term within the lung after the resolution of infection [43] where they are thought to constitute a frontline defence against secondary challenge. There is evidence that retention in the respiratory tract is dependent on VLA1-1 [44] and that, rather than being a static population, these lung-resident memory cells are constantly refreshed from the recirculating memory pool [45]. Following secondary challenge, any lung-resident memory T cells are supplemented by two waves of CTL recruitment to the infected respiratory tract. The first occurs rapidly (1–3 days) after infection, with CD62L^{lo} effector memory cells being drawn from the blood into the damaged lung via a CCR5-dependent mechanism [45]. Evidently these CTLs do not undergo further proliferation, although they rapidly acquire cytotoxic activity and likely contribute to early virus elimination [46]. The second wave relies on the expansion and further differentiation of CD62L^{hi} central memory T cells in the lymph node and their subsequent migration in large numbers to the site of pathology. Strategies that promote and sustain high effector memory

T-cell numbers in the lung after infection are likely to limit the impact of influenza A virus infection, though there must be a fine balance so as not to compromise the physiologic integrity of this delicate tissue.

Human immunity to influenza viruses

Role of human T cells in protection against influenza viruses

While influenza A virus-specific T cells are readily identifiable in humans [47,48], evidence for their role in the control of infection has been largely circumstantial. A retrospective analysis demonstrated that prior symptomatic influenza A (H1N1) infection was associated with increased protection from the 1957 influenza A (H2N2) pandemic virus in adults but not children, suggesting the accumulation of heterosubtypic immunity with age [49]. Whether this was T-cell-mediated is not known. The most direct evidence for a role for CTL in recovery in human influenza comes from an early study in which inducible virus-specific cytotoxic T-cell activity was correlated with diminished viral shedding in seronegative individuals [50]. It has been widely assumed that these cytotoxic effectors were CD8+ CTLs, but a recent study has suggested that CD4+ T cells may have been involved [27]. Most work on CD4+ T cells in human influenza virus infection has focused on their role in promoting robust antibody responses to homologous viruses or vaccines. However, Wilkinson et al. [27] recently reported that the numbers of pre-existing memory CD4+ rather than CD8+ T cells in the blood correlated with reduced severity of disease following challenge with a heterologous influenza A virus. Further work is needed to establish the relative significance of CD4+ and CD8+ T cells and to define their effector mechanisms in immunity to human influenza viruses.

Specificities of human T cells

The studies cited above support the idea that the recall of established, influenza-specific CD8+ and CD4+ T-cell memory can limit the damage caused by primary infection with a novel influenza A virus subtype (or antigenic drift variant) expressing antigenically different HA and NA glycoproteins. Such cross-protective T cells may play their most important part in reducing morbidity and mortality during a pandemic. For this reason, there has been considerable interest in defining the cross-reactivities of human T cells for different influenza A viruses.

A recent study examined influenza-specific memory T-cell reactivity against all viral proteins of a former seasonal influenza A (H1N1) virus and a highly pathogenic influenza A (H5N1) virus. There were three major observations: (i) reactivity was largely directed towards the more conserved viral proteins, particularly NP and M1; (ii) memory T cells in people who could never have been exposed to H5N1 recognized conserved peptides from H5N1-derived proteins, confirming the potential for heterosubtypic immunity in humans; and (iii) both CD4+ and CD8+ T-cell responses were specific for these conserved viral components [48]. The findings for CD4+ T cells raised particular interest as most of the discussion about heterosubtypic immunity against novel pandemic influenza A viruses had hitherto focused on priming the CD8+ CTL compartment.

Implications of T-cell immunity for the design of influenza vaccines

Specific antibodies provide the most effective immune defence against the influenza viruses. This is the basis of conventional influenza vaccines in which formalin- or β-propiolactone-inactivated viral antigens induce neutralizing antibodies against the HA and NA of the homologous virus strain. Such vaccines do not induce detectable CTL memory although they may achieve modest boosting of an existing memory CTL pool. As CD8+ and CD4+ T cells commonly recognize peptides that are highly conserved between different influenza A subtypes and strains and may thus offer some heterosubtypic protection in humans, there is now considerable interest in developing vaccine technologies that induce cross-protective T cells as adjuncts to antibody-based vaccines [51]. Primed T cells cannot prevent infection but they may lessen the impact of future pandemic influenza A viruses by promoting early virus clearance and reducing disease severity.

Challenges in designing T-cell vaccines

There are a number of barriers to the design of an effective cross-protective T-cell vaccine for influenza

A viruses. One is the delivery of virus proteins to the cytosol of APCs in a way that ensures appropriate peptide processing and access to the MHCI pathway [2]. Another is the activation of DCs to provide appropriate co-stimulation for optimal CD8$^+$ T-cell priming [6]. Inappropriate DC activation may yield smaller CD8$^+$ CTL responses, poor memory CD8$^+$ CTL precursor generation and diminished functional capacity, exemplified by the decreased production of proinflammatory mediators and inefficient trafficking to the site of infection.

Another major issue is epitope selection. Because of MHC allele specificity, an optimal immunogenic peptide for one individual may be irrelevant for another. There is little doubt that there are many more immunogenic peptides to be discovered. As several of the known prominent responses are specific for sequences that lack the typical features identified by predictive algorithms, systematic screening will be needed to identify the spectrum of immunodominant peptides associated with a range of MHC alleles. A successful vaccine would deliver a broad spectrum of protective specificities, at least providing coverage for a particular ethnic group. There might be some justification for developing targeted vaccines to protect people, including indigenous populations, who are at particular risk. One way to achieve a broad spectrum of specificities is to include full-length proteins from the conserved, internal components of the influenza A virus, perhaps delivered via a third-party virus vector. Another possibility is to pursue a more targeted strategy by incorporating determinants that can bind to related groups of MHC alleles (termed supertypes) [52]. Such an approach could limit the number of determinants required to protect a given population. It may also be useful to develop vaccine strategies that amplify subdominant CD8$^+$ T-cell responses and memory in light of evidence that such T cells can play a significant part in the control of other virus infections [53].

Vaccine technologies for the induction of cross-protective T-cell immunity

At present, while virus-vectored systems and live attenuated viruses (like the cold adapted Flumist®) offer the most physiologic way to activate CD4$^+$ and CD8$^+$ T-cell immunity to influenza, the prospects for

the development of a noninfectious cross-protective vaccine continue to improve (see Chapter 21). In addition to promoting antibody responses, some adjuvants already in human use (such as MF59 and AS03) enhance the ability of (for example) inactivated H5N1 influenza vaccines to activate cytokine-producing human CD4$^+$ T-cell responses, though they are generally ineffective when it comes to priming CD8$^+$ T-cell memory [54].

Other strategies with potential for human use include virus-like particles [49], immunostimulatory complexes (ISCOMs) [55] and virosomes [56]. Another novel approach is the use of minimal CD4$^+$ and CD8$^+$ T-cell epitopes conjugated to a lipid moieties, termed lipopeptides, to induce to induce robust cellular immunity [57,58]. For example, Pam2Cys, derived from *Mycoplasma fermentans* and a potent TLR2 ligand and DC activator [57], is capable of inducing robust influenza-specific CD4$^+$ and CD8$^-$ T-cell responses [57]. Of course, the use of peptide vaccines has the potential to be limited for reasons stated earlier, so it will be of particular interest to see whether such approaches can be used with whole protein vaccine preparations to ensure broad coverage for different HLA backgrounds.

Conclusions

Immune CD4$^+$ and CD8$^+$ T-cell responses have long been known to be essential for the control of influenza A virus infections. Technological developments over the past 15 years or so have greatly improved our capacity to quantitate and to monitor these immune lymphocyte sets, while at the same time allowing us to probe naïve, effector, and memory T cells for differential patterns of gene expression and epigenetic control. While such analyses are greatly enhancing our understanding of both molecular regulation and immune mechanisms, the practical challenge of how best to manipulate both CD4$^+$ and CD8$^+$ T-cell memory to achieve a measure of long-term, if partial, heterosubtypic protection remains. The challenge from the aspect of humoral and cellular immunity is to evolve immunization strategies that would, in the face of challenge with a novel, virulent and rapidly spreading pandemic strain, greatly diminish the incidence of severe disease and mortality. That would represent a real advance.

Acknowledgments

We would like to thank Dr. Stephanie Gras and Professor Jamie Rossjohn for the structural figures. Some of the findings discussed here were supported by National Health and Medical Research Program Grant No. 567122 (awarded to P.C.D., A.K., and S.J.T.); National Institute Health Grant AI70251 (P.C.D.), an Australian Research Council Future Fellowship (S.J.T.) and the American Lebanese Syrian Associated Charities (ALSAC). The Melbourne WHO Collaborating Centre for Reference and Research on Influenza is supported by the Australian Government Department of Health and Ageing.

References

1. Davis MM, Chien YH. T cell antigen receptors. In: Paul WE, editor. Fundamental Immunology. Philadeliphia: Lippincott-Raven; 1999. p. 341–66.

2. Yewdell JW, Haeryfar SM. Understanding presentation of viral antigens to CD8$^+$ T cells in vivo: the key to rational vaccine design. Annu Rev Immunol. 2005;23:651–82.

3. Casrouge A, Beaudoing E, Dalle S, Pannetier C, Kanellopoulos J, Kourilsky P. Size estimate of the alpha beta TCR repertoire of naive mouse splenocytes. J Immunol. 2000;164:5782–7.

4. Arstila TP, Casrouge A, Baron V, Even J, Kanellopoulos J, Kourilsky P. A direct estimate of the human alphabeta T cell receptor diversity. Science. 1999;286:958–61.

5. Crowe SR, Turner SJ, Miller SC, Roberts AD, Rappolo RA, Doherty PC, et al. Differential antigen presentation regulates the changing patterns of CD8$^+$ T cell immunodominance in primary and secondary influenza virus infections. J Exp Med. 2003;198:399–410.

6. Belz GT, Smith CM, Kleinert L, Reading P, Brooks A, Shortman K, et al. Distinct migrating and nonmigrating dendritic cell populations are involved in MHC class I-restricted antigen presentation after lung infection with virus. Proc Natl Acad Sci U S A. 2004;101:8670–5.

7. Crowe SR, Miller SC, Brown DM, Adams PS, Dutton RW, Harmsen AG, et al. Uneven distribution of MHC class II epitopes within the influenza virus. Vaccine. 2006;24:457–67.

8. Flynn KJ, Belz GT, Altman JD, Ahmed R, Woodland DL, Doherty PC. Virus-specific CD8$^+$ T cells in primary and secondary influenza pneumonia. Immunity. 1998;8:683–91.

9. Altman JD, Moss PA, Goulder PJ, Barouch DH, McHeyzer-Williams MG, Bell JI, et al. Phenotypic analysis of antigen-specific T lymphocytes. Science. 1996;274:94–6.

10. La Gruta NL, Rothwell WT, Cukalac T, Swan NG, Valkenburg SA, Kedzierska K, et al. Primary CTL response magnitude in mice is determined by the extent of naive T cell recruitment and subsequent clonal expansion. J Clin Invest. 2010;120:1885–94.

11. Tan CT, Croft NP, Dudek NL, Williamson NA, Purcell AW. Direct quantitation of MHC-bound peptide epitopes by selected reaction monitoring. Proteomics. 2011;11:2336–40.

12. Eichelberger M, Allan W, Zijlstra M, Jaenisch R, Doherty PC. Clearance of influenza virus respiratory infection in mice lacking class I major histocompatibility complex-restricted CD8$^+$ T cells. J Exp Med. 1991;174:875–80.

13. Doherty PC, Topham DJ, Tripp RA, Cardin RD, Brooks JW, Stevenson PG. Effector CD4$^+$ and CD8$^+$ T-cell mechanisms in the control of respiratory virus infections. Immunol Rev. 1997;159:105–17.

14. Cerwenka A, Morgan TM, Dutton RW. Naive, effector, and memory CD8 T cells in protection against pulmonary influenza virus infection: homing properties rather than initial frequencies are crucial. J Immunol. 1999;163:5535–43.

15. Kaech SM, Ahmed R. Memory CD8$^+$ T cell differentiation: initial antigen encounter triggers a developmental program in naive cells. Nat Immunol. 2001;2:415–22.

16. Gett AV, Hodgkin PD. Cell division regulates the T cell cytokine repertoire, revealing a mechanism underlying immune class regulation. Proc Natl Acad Sci U S A. 1998;95:9488–93.

17. La Gruta NL, Turner SJ, Doherty PC. Hierarchies in cytokine expression profiles for acute and resolving influenza virus-specific CD8$^+$ T cell responses: correlation of cytokine profile and TCR avidity. J Immunol. 2004;172:5553–60.

18. Peters PJ, Borst J, Oorschot V, Fukuda M, Krahenbuhl O, Tschopp J, et al. Cytotoxic T lymphocyte granules are secretory lysosomes, containing both perforin and granzymes. J Exp Med. 1991;173:1099–109.

19. Smyth MJ, Kelly JM, Sutton VR, Davis JE, Browne KA, Sayers TJ, et al. Unlocking the secrets of cytotoxic granule proteins. J Leukoc Biol. 2001;70:18–29.

20. Stinchcombe JC, Griffiths GM. Secretory mechanisms in cell-mediated cytotoxicity. Annu Rev Cell Dev Biol. 2007;23:495–517.

21. Jones CM, Cose SC, Coles RM, Winterhalter AC, Brooks AG, Heath WR, et al. Herpes simplex virus type 1-specific cytotoxic T-lymphocyte arming occurs within lymph nodes draining the site of cutaneous infection. J Virol. 2000;74:2414–9.

22. Jenkins MR, Kedzierska K, Doherty PC, Turner SJ. Heterogeneity of effector phenotype for acute phase and

memory influenza A virus-specific CTL. J Immunol. 2007;179:64–70.

23. Johnson BJ, Costelloe EO, Fitzpatrick DR, Haanen JB, Schumacher TN, Brown LE, et al. Single-cell perforin and granzyme expression reveals the anatomical localization of effector CD8+ T cells in influenza virus-infected mice. Proc Natl Acad Sci U S A. 2003;100:2657–62.

24. Topham DJ, Tripp RA, Doherty PC. CD8+ T cells clear influenza virus by perforin or Fas-dependent processes. J Immunol. 1997;159:5197–200.

25. Jenkins MR, Trapani JA, Doherty PC, Turner SJ. Granzyme K expressing cytotoxic T lymphocytes protects against influenza virus in granzyme AB–/– mice. Viral Immunol. 2008;21:341–6.

26. Brown DM, Lee S, Garcia-Hernandez Mde L, Swain SL. Multifunctional CD4 cells expressing gamma interferon and perforin mediate protection against lethal influenza virus infection. J Virol. 2012;86:6792–803.

27. Wilkinson TM, Li CK, Chui CS, Huang AK, Perkins M, Liebner JC, et al. Preexisting influenza-specific CD4+ T cells correlate with disease protection against influenza challenge in humans. Nat Med. 2012;18:274–80.

28. Linterman MA, Beaton L, Yu D, Ramiscal RR, Srivastava M, Hogan JJ, et al. IL-21 acts directly on B cells to regulate Bcl-6 expression and germinal center responses. J Exp Med. 2010;207:353–63.

29. La Gruta NL, Kedzierska K, Stambas J, Doherty PC. A question of self-preservation: immunopathology in influenza virus infection. Immunol Cell Biol. 2007;85:85–92.

30. Cheung CY, Poon LL, Lau AS, Luk W, Lau YL, Shortridge KF, et al. Induction of proinflammatory cytokines in human macrophages by influenza A (H5N1) viruses: a mechanism for the unusual severity of human disease? Lancet. 2002;360:1831–7.

31. Wiley JA, Hogan RJ, Woodland DL, Harmsen AG. Antigen-specific CD8(+) T cells persist in the upper respiratory tract following influenza virus infection. J Immunol. 2001;167:3293–9.

32. Sun J, Madan R, Karp CL, Braciale TJ. Effector T cells control lung inflammation during acute influenza virus infection by producing IL-10. Nat Med. 2009;15:277–84.

33. Sun J, Dodd H, Moser EK, Sharma R, Braciale TJ. CD4+ T cell help and innate-derived IL-27 induce Blimp-1-dependent IL-10 production by antiviral CTLs. Nat Immunol. 2011;12:327–34.

34. Harrington LE, Galvan M, Baum LG, Altman JD, Ahmed R. Differentiating between memory and effector CD8 T cells by altered expression of cell surface O-glycans. J Exp Med. 2000;191:1241–6.

35. Marshall DR, Turner SJ, Belz GT, Wingo S, Andreansky S, Sangster MY, et al. Measuring the diaspora for virus-specific CD8+ T cells. Proc Natl Acad Sci U S A. 2001;98:6313–8.

36. Kaech SM, Hemby S, Kersh E, Ahmed R. Molecular and functional profiling of memory CD8 T cell differentiation. Cell. 2002;111:837–51.

37. Badovinac VP, Messingham KA, Jabbari A, Haring JS, Harty JT. Accelerated CD8+ T-cell memory and prime-boost response after dendritic-cell vaccination. Nat Med. 2005;11:748–56.

38. Kedzierska K, Stambas J, Jenkins MR, Keating R, Turner SJ, Doherty PC. Location rather than CD62L phenotype is critical in the early establishment of influenza-specific CD8+ T cell memory. Proc Natl Acad Sci U S A. 2007;104:9782–7.

39. Williams MA, Tyznik AJ, Bevan MJ. Interleukin-2 signals during priming are required for secondary expansion of CD8+ memory T cells. Nature. 2006;441:890–3.

40. Bennett SR, Carbone FR, Karamalis F, Flavell RA, Miller JF, Heath WR. Help for cytotoxic-T-cell responses is mediated by CD40 signalling. Nature. 1998;393:478–80.

41. Christensen JP, Doherty PC, Branum KC, Riberdy JM. Profound protection against respiratory challenge with a lethal H7N7 influenza A virus by increasing the magnitude of CD8(+) T-cell memory. J Virol. 2000;74:11690–6.

42. Teijaro JR, Turner D, Pham Q, Wherry EJ, Lefrancois L, Farber DL. Cutting edge: tissue-retentive lung memory CD4 T cells mediate optimal protection to respiratory virus infection. J Immunol. 2011;187:5510–4.

43. Kohlmeier JE, Woodland DL. Immunity to respiratory viruses. Annu Rev Immunol. 2008.

44. Ray SJ, Franki SN, Pierce RH, Dimitrova S, Koteliansky V, Sprague AG, et al. The collagen binding alpha1beta1 integrin VLA-1 regulates CD8 T cell-mediated immune protection against heterologous influenza infection. Immunity. 2004;20:167–79.

45. Kohlmeier JE, Miller SC, Smith J, Lu B, Gerard C, Cookenham T, et al. The chemokine receptor CCR5 plays a key role in the early memory CD8+ T cell response to respiratory virus infections. Immunity. 2008;29:101–13.

46. Kohlmeier JE, Cookenham T, Roberts AD, Miller SC, Woodland DL. Type I interferons regulate cytolytic activity of memory CD8(+) T cells in the lung airways during respiratory virus challenge. Immunity. 2010;33:96–105.

47. Forrest BD, Pride MW, Dunning AJ, Capeding MR, Chotpitayasunondh T, Tam JS, et al. Correlation of cellular immune responses with protection against culture-confirmed influenza virus in young children. Clin Vaccine Immunol. 2008;15:1042–53.

48. Lee LY, Ha do LA, Simmons C, de Jong MD, Chau NV, Schumacher R, et al. Memory T cells established by seasonal human influenza A infection cross-react with avian influenza A (H5N1) in healthy individuals. J Clin Invest. 2008;118:3478–90.

49. Kang SM, Yoo DG, Lipatov AS, Song JM, Davis CT, Quan FS, et al. Induction of long-term protective immune responses by influenza H5N1 virus-like particles. PLoS ONE. 2009;4:e4667.

50. McMichael AJ, Gotch FM, Noble GR, Beare PA. Cytotoxic T-cell immunity to influenza. N Engl J Med. 1983;309:13–7.

51. Doherty PC, Kelso A. Toward a broadly protective influenza vaccine. J Clin Invest. 2008;118:3273–5.

52. Sidney J, Peters B, Frahm N, Brander C, Sette A. HLA class I supertypes: a revised and updated classification. BMC Immunol. 2008;9:1.

53. Frahm N, Kiepiela P, Adams S, Linde CH, Hewitt HS, Sango K, et al. Control of human immunodeficiency virus replication by cytotoxic T lymphocytes targeting subdominant epitopes. Nat Immunol. 2006;7:173–8.

54. Galli G, Medini D, Borgogni E, Zedda L, Bardelli M, Malzone C, et al. Adjuvanted H5N1 vaccine induces early CD4+ T cell response that predicts long-term persistence of protective antibody levels. Proc Natl Acad Sci U S A. 2009;106:3877–82.

55. Rimmelzwaan GF, Baars M, van Beek R, van Amerongen G, Lovgren-Bengtsson K, Claas EC, et al. Induction of protective immunity against influenza virus in a macaque model: comparison of conventional and iscom vaccines. J Gen Virol. 1997;78(Pt 4):757–65.

56. Gluck R, Burri KG, Metcalfe I. Adjuvant and antigen delivery properties of virosomes. Curr Drug Deliv. 2005;2:395–400.

57. Jackson DC, Lau YF, Le T, Suhrbier A, Deliyannis G, Cheers C, et al. A totally synthetic vaccine of generic structure that targets Toll-like receptor 2 on dendritic cells and promotes antibody or cytotoxic T cell responses. Proc Natl Acad Sci U S A. 2004;101: 15440–5.

58. Nguyen DT, de Witte L, Ludlow M, Yuksel S, Wiesmuller KH, Geijtenbeek TB, et al. The synthetic bacterial lipopeptide Pam3CSK4 modulates respiratory syncytial virus infection independent of TLR activation. PLoS Pathog. 2010;6:e1001049.

59. Day EB, Guillonneau C, Gras S, La Gruta NL, Vignali DA, Doherty PC, et al. Structural basis for enabling T-cell receptor diversity within biased virus-specific CD8+ T-cell responses. Proc Natl Acad Sci U S A. 2011;108:9536–41.

20 Immunogenicity, efficacy of inactivated/live virus seasonal and pandemic vaccines

Wendy A. Keitel,[1] Kathleen M. Neuzil,[2] and John Treanor[3]

[1]Departments of Molecular Virology and Microbiology and Medicine, Baylor College of Medicine, Houston, TX, USA

[2]Vaccine Access and Delivery Global Program, PATH and University of Washington, Seattle, WA, USA

[3]Department of Medicine, Microbiology and Immunology, University of Rochester Medical Center, Rochester, NY, USA

Introduction

Immunization against influenza serves as the primary approach for control of influenza in persons and populations. Since the recognition of influenza as a disease caused by a virus, both parenterally administered killed or inactivated vaccines as well as intransally administered live attenuated vaccines have been developed and licensed for human use worldwide (Table 20.1). These approaches share the general goal of inducing immunity to the hemagglutinin (HA) and possibly to the neuraminidase (NA) of the virus, and are therefore reformulated frequently so that the components of the vaccine match as closely as possible the anticipated circulating influenza virus(es). The potential roles of other immune responses induced by vaccination in disease protection remain largely unknown.

The specific details of individual vaccines and the rationale for current vaccine recommendations in the United States have been extensively reviewed elsewhere [1]. This chapter briefly reviews the safety and immunogenicity of seasonal influenza vaccines, available data on vaccine protection, and discusses candidate pandemic influenza vaccines.

Inactivated influenza vaccine

Inactivated influenza vaccines (IIVs) were first licensed for use in civilian populations in 1945 based on dem-

onstration of efficacy in healthy military recruits. The development of the zonal gradient centrifuge provided the methodology to produce more highly purified vaccines in which reactogenic contaminants had been removed. Current vaccines are chemically inactivated and administered as either "whole virus" (WV) preparations or detergent disrupted and partially purified "split-product," "split-virion," or "subunit" (SV) vaccines. In the late 1970s the single radial immunodiffusion (SRID) test was developed to quantify the antigenic content of the vaccine, leading to more consistent standardization and the consensus to use a dose of 15 µg HA antigen per strain. Young children have traditionally received half of the adult dose; recent studies have suggested that increased dose vaccines may be of benefit in seniors. Intradermal immunization with standard or lower doses of antigen has also been approved.

The composition of the vaccine has changed to reflect the ongoing evolution of influenza viruses. Since 1977, influenza vaccines have contained a representative A/H3N2, A/H1N1, and B virus: trivalent influenza vaccine (TIV). Since 2004, two antigenically distinct lineages of influenza B viruses have co-circulated: the Victoria and the Yamagata lineages. Therefore, quadrivalent formulations of vaccine containing both lineages are being licensed for use in the 2013–2014 influenza season and beyond.

Growth of virus in embryonated hens' eggs has been the preferred method for production of both inactivated and live vaccines for decades. However,

Textbook of Influenza, Second Edition. Edited by Robert G. Webster, Arnold S. Monto, Thomas J. Braciale, and Robert A. Lamb.
© 2013 John Wiley & Sons, Ltd. Published 2013 by John Wiley & Sons, Ltd.

Table 20.1. Vaccines licensed for prevention of seasonal influenza worldwide.

Type of vaccine	Adjuvant (no/yes)	Types of preparations	Substrate for production	Route(s) of administration
Inactivated	No	Whole virus	Eggs	IM
			Cell culture	IM
		Subvirion	Eggs	IM, ID
			Cell culture	IM
	Yes	Whole virus (alum)	Eggs	IM
		Subvirion (MF-59)	Eggs	IM
		Virosomal	Eggs	IM
Live, attenuated	N/A	Influenza A or B; Ann Arbor-based	Eggs	IN
		Influenza A or B; Leningrad-based	Eggs	IN

ID, intradermal; IM, intramuscular; IN, intranasal.

eggs have many potential drawbacks for vaccine production, including limited availability and potential for scale-up, vulnerability of the chicken population to potential pandemic strains of influenza, and selection of egg-adapted viruses that may differ antigenically from wild-type (wt) strains. Therefore, alternative substrates for vaccine production have been explored, including various mammalian cell culture systems, insect cells, and plant cells (see Chapter 23).

Safety considerations and reactions following immunization

Influenza vaccines are among the safest medical interventions known. Hundreds of millions of doses of TIV are administered to people of all ages each year, and the vast safety database confirms the safety of contemporary IIV. For example, no increase in clinically important medically attended events has been noted among over 251 000 children <18 years of age who were enrolled in one of five health maintenance organizations within the Vaccine Safety Datalink, the largest published post-licensure population-based study of vaccine safety [2].

Injection site reactions

The most common adverse events reported following immunization with TIV are tenderness and/or pain at the injection site. Redness and/or swelling at the injection site occasionally occur. Injection site reactions typically develop within the first day after injection and resolve within a day or two. Most injection site reactions are mild and rarely interfere with daily activities. In placebo-controlled clinical trials among healthy adults, injection site discomfort has been more frequent in subjects given IIV than among subjects given placebo, and more frequent in younger than in older subjects. Generally, the frequencies of injection site reactions are higher in females than males. Among young children, 3–7% experience an injection site reaction. Minor injection site reactions may occur more frequently with higher doses of vaccine or when vaccine is administered intradermally (ID) rather than intramuscularly (IM).

Systemic reactions

Systemic reactions following immunization of adults with contemporary IIV preparations are uncommon. Mild to moderate transient temperature elevations occur in less than 1% of adults, typically within the day or two after immunization, and may be more common with higher dose vaccine. Headache, generalized myalgia, and malaise may occasionally occur; however, in placebo-controlled clinical trials in younger and elderly adults, rates of systemic reactions were similar among groups given IIV or placebo [3,4].

While WV and SV vaccines are similarly reactogenic in adults, WV vaccines are associated with fever in children. Among children younger than 6 years of age enrolled in randomized clinical trials of SV vaccines, systemic symptoms occur in 4–16%, with fever being the most common reaction [5]. This is likely an upper estimate as there is no placebo control to estimate the baseline occurrence of these events. An increased frequency of fever and febrile seizures was observed among young children given one specific TIV during the 2010 influenza season in Australia. The risk for febrile seizure was estimated to be as high as 9 per 1000 children vaccinated. The pathogenesis of these reactions is not known, and surveillance has not identified increases in febrile seizures in subsequent years. However, this vaccine is not currently recommended for use among children <9 years of age in the United States [6]. Concomitant immunization of young children with TIV and pneumococcal conjugate vaccine (PCV) was shown to be associated with an increased risk of developing febrile seizures. Because the magnitude of this risk was low and the risk of acquiring influenza among young children is high, no changes in current recommendations have been made.

Immediate hypersensitivity reactions

Immediate hypersensitivity reactions (hives, wheezing, angioedema, or anaphylactic shock) following IIV occur rarely. The pathogenesis of these reactions is attributed to immunoglobulin E (IgE) mediated hypersensitivity to egg protein or other vaccine components. IIV is contraindicated for persons who experienced an anaphylactic reaction following prior receipt of an IIV. Generally, if persons can eat eggs or egg-containing products, vaccination is safe. Recent studies support the safety of IIV among persons who experience mild allergic reactions to eggs such as hives. Clinical protocols have been proposed to administer TIV to persons who are at high risk for severe or complicated influenza who also have a history of immediate hypersensitivity to eggs, if the benefit of immunization is judged to outweigh the risk [1].

Adverse events of special interest

Guillain–Barré Syndrome (GBS), an acute inflammatory demyelinating polyneuropathy, has been associated with a variety of infectious agents. During the 1976 swine influenza vaccination campaign, an elevated risk of GBS was noted; the risk of developing GBS was estimated to be 1 per 100 000 vaccinees. In most years since 1976 no significant increase in the number of cases of GBS has been observed in association with IIVs; however, in a study conducted during the 1992–1993 and 1993–1994 seasons, the relative risk for GBS was higher during the 6 weeks after vaccination (relative risk = 1.7), representing about 1 additional case per 1 million persons vaccinated [7]. The most recent studies have suggested a statistically significant but very slight increased relative risk of GBS within 7 weeks of influenza vaccination.

The oculorespiratory syndrome (ORS) is a syndrome of red eyes, facial edema, and/or respiratory symptoms such as coughing, wheezing, sore throat, hoarseness, difficulty breathing, or chest tightness that develop within 2–24 hours after vaccination. The onset is acute and the course is self-limited. ORS was first described in the 2000–2001 season in Canada and subsequent investigations have identified ORS in association with a variety of influenza vaccines. The pathogenesis is not known, but is not believed to be IgE-mediated. Persons with a history of ORS after prior immunization with IIV can be revaccinated safely if IgE-mediated hypersensitivity can be excluded.

Adverse pregnancy outcomes have not been associated with influenza immunization and immunization during all trimesters of pregnancy is considered safe [8]. Immunization during pregnancy also results in transplacental transfer of antibody to the infants that may confer protection to infant as well as the mother (see below).

Immunogenicity

The primary mediator of protection against influenza following immunization with IIV is probably antibody to the HA. Antibodies to the NA, mucosal antibodies, cell-mediated immune (CMI) responses and antibody responses to other influenza antigens are also observed. The roles of these responses in protection have not been clearly defined.

Serum HA-specific responses

The serum antibody responses to the HA are well characterized and serve as benchmarks for licensure of IIVs. Vaccine and host factors are associated with HA-specific responses. Important vaccine factors include vaccine type, number of doses, HA content, inclusion of adjuvant, and route of immunization; important host factors include age, prior priming, and underlying health status.

Responses in healthy adults The immunogenicity of seasonal IIVs among healthy adults <65 years of age has been studied extensively: one dose of TIV containing 15 µg HA/strain given IM stimulates hemagglutination inhibition (HAI) antibody responses in most subjects whose pre-existing antibody levels are low. Immune response frequencies are lower among persons with high pre-existing levels of HAI antibody. Serum HAI antibody levels peak 2–4 weeks after immunization, and titers decline by ~50% over 6–12 months.

Responses in seniors HA-specific serum antibody responses decline with advancing age, possibly attributable to loss or alteration of T-cell function. When compared with younger adults, the proportions of elderly subjects who achieve a putative protective HAI antibody titer are lower. Both age and underlying conditions may contribute to these lowered responses. A higher dose vaccine, containing 60 µg HA/stain elicits post-vaccination antibody titers approximately 1.5- to twofold greater than those seen with standard dose [9], although the effect of these higher responses on protection have not yet been demonstrated.

Responses in children Because adults and older children have usually experienced many prior influenza infections and/or vaccinations with related influenza viruses, they require only a single dose of vaccine for annual immunization. Such primed individuals also generally respond with antibody that recognizes a broader range of antigenic variants than do unprimed individuals. In contrast, unimmunized young children generally require two doses of IIV given at least 4 weeks apart to generate substantial serum antibody responses.

Once a child has been primed with two doses of vaccine, a single dose of vaccine is recommended in subsequent seasons regardless of age. However, predicting immune responses of young children who have received single doses in two consecutive seasons is more complex. In studies performed in immunologically naïve children, responses among children who received the first dose of vaccine in the spring and the second dose in the fall were similar when compared with those who received both doses in the fall when vaccine antigens did not change. However, when the vaccine components change between seasons, the response to a single dose in the spring and a single dose of the new antigen in the fall is clearly inferior to the response to two doses of the new antigen in the fall [10].

Most children ≥6 months old develop putative protective levels of HAI antibody after receiving the recommended number of doses. However, antibody responses in young infants are reduced compared with older children. Reduced responses among very young children may be related to a combination of immaturity of the immune system and a lower degree of priming.

Responses in other populations

HIV infected persons: While immunization of HIV infected persons with IIVs is safe and well tolerated, the immunogenicity among HIV-positive children and adults is generally lower than among immunocompetent persons. The lowest response rates are observed among patients with advanced immunosuppression (CD4 count <200 and/or AIDS). A second dose has not been demonstrated to improve response rates; however, increasing the dose of antigen may be helpful [11].

Other immunocompromised populations: Many studies have assessed the immunogenicity of IIVs among diverse immunocompromised populations, including persons with chronic rheumatologic disease, solid organ transplant recipients, renal failure patients, and persons with chronic hematologic disorders. While there is some variability in results, serum HAI antibody response rates and geometric mean titers of antibody after immunization are generally lower when compared with healthy age-matched controls, and responses are lowest among the most highly immunocompromised patients. To be maximally effective, immunizations should be given before immunosuppression or transplantation, avoiding the nadir of white counts, and should include vaccination of close contacts. Most patients with chronic obstructive pulmonary disease (COPD) respond reasonably well to vaccination, and steroids at doses commonly used to treat reactive airways disease do not appear to preclude vaccine responses.

Serum NA-specific responses

Despite evidence that NA-specific antibody responses contribute to protection, neither the NA content nor the enzymatic activity of the vaccine is standardized, and NA-specific antibody responses are not routinely assessed. One reason for this has been the difficulty in standardization of assays. Antibody responses to the NA develop, albeit at a lower rate than those to the HA. High dose vaccine has also been reported to induce significantly higher frequencies of response and higher levels of antibody to the NA in the elderly when compared with a standard dose of TIV [12].

Mucosal antibody responses

Mucosal anti-influenza antibodies can also be detected in 30–60% of adults following immunization with IIVs. Antibody to the HA in nasal secretions peaks 2–4 weeks after immunization in primed, healthy adults and falls over the next 3–6 months. Dose-related increases in mucosal HA-specific antibody responses have been observed following IM immunization with increasing doses of a monovalent influenza A/H1N1 vaccine [13].

Cellular immune responses

Antibody-secreting cells (ASC) appear in blood and tonsils as early as 2 days after vaccination, and are detected in the blood of adults and older children more frequently than in young children after immunization [14]. An increase in cytotoxic T lymphocytes, directed primarily at the conserved internal proteins, has been shown in healthy adults with a peak at 14 and 21 days after vaccination and return to baseline at 6 months. An increase in HA-specific $CD8^+$ T cells on day 7 after vaccination has also been detected by tetramer staining in adults receiving inactivated influenza vaccine (see Chapter 19) [15]. Baseline frequencies of influenza-specific, interferon γ-producing memory $CD4^+$ T cells are higher in children who received more previous vaccinations [16].

Biomarkers of immune responsiveness

In studies using intensive systems biology approaches to characterize the early response to vaccination, several early markers of immune activation have been shown to correlate quite closely with the ultimately development of HAI antibody responses in healthy adults receiving influenza vaccine. These "biomarkers" of the immune response have included genes consistent with upregulation of the interferon response and antigen processing, and other genes involved in the innate immune response [17,18]. These approaches may ultimately prove useful in the rapid evaluation of new influenza vaccines, as well as in understanding the individual factors that are responsible for the diversity of immune responses seen in clinical trials.

Revaccination

Recent clinical trials have demonstrated that there are no consistent differences in post-vaccination titers or proportion of subjects with putative protective titers when compared with subjects immunized for the first time, and that there is no consistent decrease or increase in the level of protection against influenza when multiple vaccination groups are compared with single vaccination groups [19].

Efficacy and effectiveness

The ability of influenza vaccines to prevent influenza has been assessed in numerous clinical studies which vary greatly in design, populations, and endpoints. These studies have included prospective randomized controlled studies, in which case they are referred to as efficacy studies, as well as a wide variety of nonrandomized cohort and retrospective study designs which assess vaccine effectiveness. Studies have assessed both laboratory-confirmed influenza, and nonlaboratory-confirmed endpoints. It has been recognized that studies that utilize a serologic definition of influenza infection may overestimate the efficacy of influenza vaccine, because it is harder to demonstrate post-vaccination to post-season antibody increases in the vaccinated group [20].

Randomized studies of efficacy against laboratory-confirmed influenza

Healthy adults A number of prospective randomized studies of IIV using culture-confirmed influenza

317

endpoints have recently been conducted in healthy adults aged 18–64 as vaccine manufacturers have carried out post-licensure responsibilities for regulatory agencies (reviewed in [21]). These studies have shown a wide range of efficacy of approximately 40–80%, with lower levels of efficacy typically seen in years with apparent antigenic mismatch. A recent meta-analysis of eight randomized controlled trials in healthy adults during 2004–2008 estimated the pooled efficacy of TIV against culture-confirmed influenza to be 59% (95% CI, 51–67%) among those aged 18–64 years. The role of antigenic mismatch in the efficacy observed in these trials is unclear, and some studies in young adults have demonstrated high levels of efficacy (76%) despite a degree of antigenic mismatch. Recent studies using virus culture and/or polymerase chain reaction (PCR) endpoints have demonstrated similar levels of efficacy for both egg-grown and cell culture-grown TIVs [22].

Randomized trials of vaccine in adults have also assessed nonlaboratory-confirmed endpoints. For example, vaccination of healthy adults is associated with decreased absenteeism from work or school, decreased numbers of physician visits and overall antibiotic use [23]. These benefits may not extend to years when there is not a good match between vaccine and circulating viruses. Immunization of healthcare workers has also been shown to be effective in reducing days of absence from work and febrile respiratory illness rates in such trials.

Children Relatively few recent prospective trials have assessed inactivated vaccine efficacy in children. In a randomized controlled trial in healthy children aged 6–23 months, vaccine efficacy was 66% (95% CI, 34–82%) in the first year, but efficacy could not be assessed in the second year due to a very low influenza attack rate (efficacy –7%; 95% CI, –247 to 67). Immunization of asthmatic children has also been shown to reduce the incidence of influenza. More recently, the efficacy of TIV against PCR-confirmed influenza was assessed in a randomized placebo-controlled trial in healthy children aged 6–72 months [24]. Efficacy of TIV against all influenza strains was 43% compared with the placebo group.

Elderly and high-risk groups Although annual vaccination of the elderly and other high-risk persons has been recommended for many years, there are very few randomized trials demonstrating efficacy in these groups, in part because the existing vaccine recommendations make it difficult to perform studies using a placebo group. In the most commonly referenced study, TIV was 58% (95% CI, 26–77%) efficacious in preventing serologically documented influenza illness in a population of adults 60 years of age and older [3]. When the groups were further stratified by age, efficacy estimates against serologically documented influenza illness were 59% (95% CI, 20–79%) in those 60–69 years and 23% (95% CI, –36 to 87%) in those ≥70 years old.

Other high-risk groups IVV has also been shown to be protective in limited studies in other high-risk groups, including those with HIV infection. In one recent randomized double-blind placebo-controlled trial conducted in South Africa, immunization of HIV-infected adults with TIV conferred 76% (95% CI, 9–96%) protection against virologically confirmed illness [25]. Influenza vaccination has also been shown to be of benefit in randomized trials in patients with COPD, heart disease, and other risk conditions.

Effectiveness against laboratory-confirmed influenza Monitoring influenza vaccine efficacy (VE) on an annual basis by conducting randomized placebo-controlled studies would clearly be a very difficult undertaking, and is probably not possible in children, the elderly, and other high-risk groups. Therefore, a number of observational study designs have been used for this purpose. Many recent studies have utilized a test-negative, case–control design, in which individuals meeting a particular case definition are tested for influenza using a highly sensitive and specific diagnostic test, and the vaccination exposure of test-positive cases and test-negative controls is determined. Large surveillance networks for this purpose have been established in Canada, the United States, Europe, and Australia for purposes of making interim and end-of-season estimates of VE.

Studies using this design have shown variable results with estimates generally ranging from as low as 20% or, in some cases, no effectiveness, to as high as 70%. While the various networks vary in their study design and the specific selection criteria for subject inclusion, a few overall generalizations can be stated. Failure to detect VE has typically occurred in studies with very low prevalence of influenza in the study population, or in years with substantial antigenic mismatch between the vaccine and circulating strains, most often involving influenza B lineage mismatch. The relationship of antigenic mismatch with VE for influenza A/H1N1 and A/H3N2 viruses is not as consistent, but even in situations of antigenically matched viruses VE remains in the 60–70% range in these studies. In some cases, these viruses have been shown to have substantial changes on a HA sequence level despite appearing well matched by traditional HAI tests [26].

Most studies have not enrolled enough subjects in a single season to make age-specific estimates of VE. However, there is a trend towards decreased VE in elderly, not surprising given their diminished immune response to vaccination. After accumulating cases over several seasons, it is possible to use the same test-negative case–control design to demonstrate VE of approximately 60% against influenza-related hospitalization in a population of community dwelling older adults [27].

While the use of a study design in which testing is performed without knowledge of vaccination status may eliminate some biases related to healthcare access and health seeking behavior, the results are influenced by the accuracy of the diagnostic testing, because errors in assignment to the case or control group will bias VE towards nil. Recently, in a study carried out in children, it was demonstrated that using the test-negative case–control approach, estimates of VE were substantially higher when children with documented infections with viruses other than influenza were used as a control group, rather than using all children who were test-negative for influenza [28].

Other observational studies
A larger body of data exists from nonrandomized or observational studies of VE. These studies have suggested that influenza vaccination can reduce pneumonia and influenza (P&I) hospitalizations and death among the elderly regardless of whether they have other conditions that place them at high risk for complications following influenza. While post-licensure observational studies are important tools for monitoring VE, such studies relating to IIV in the elderly are particularly challenging to perform and interpret. Frailty selection bias (a higher baseline risk of hospitalization and death among unvaccinated versus vac-

cinated subjects) and nonspecific endpoints may overestimate VE in cohort studies.

Studies in the pediatric population may be less susceptible to some of the potential biases identified for older adults. Immunization of infants and children is associated with decreased rates of medically attended acute respiratory illness, pneumonia, acute otitis media, school absenteeism, work days lost by parents, and/or antibiotic use during influenza epidemics. Vaccination of asthmatic children may shorten somewhat the duration of influenza-related asthma exacerbations. A retrospective study conducted in Japan demonstrated that universal vaccination of schoolchildren reduced the number of class cancellation days and absenteeism when compared with years during which the immunization program was abandoned [29].

Protection of infants
Infants less than 6 months of age are at substantial risk for influenza-related morbidity, but are too young to receive influenza vaccine. One strategy to protect vulnerable infants is maternal immunization, with protection mediated both by transfer of maternal antibody as well as reduced potential for contact with an influenza-infected mother. In a randomized study of maternal immunization, infants born to mothers immunized with influenza vaccine had substantially lower rates of laboratory documented influenza in the first 6 months of life than did infants born to mothers immunized with pneumococcal vaccine [30]. Similarly, in a retrospective case–control study, the frequency of influenza immunization was substantially lower in the mothers of infants hospitalized with PCR-confirmed influenza than in mothers infants hospitalized who were PCR negative, with an estimated protective effect of 92% [31].

Pandemic formulations

Vaccines created in response to the pandemics of 1957 (Asian flu, A/Japan/57, H2N2), 1968 (Hong Kong flu, A/Hong Kong/68, H3N2) and 1977 (Russian flu, A/Russia/77, H1N1) were essentially updated versions of the then licensed forms of IIVs containing the new pandemic antigens. In the 1980s there was growing recognition of the potential role of avian influenza viruses in providing novel HAs for pandemic viruses, and since the initial detection of severe human disease due to avian H5N1 influenza viruses in 1997 (see Chapters 11 and 17) there have been significant efforts to generate vaccine candidates representing the viruses felt to have the greatest pandemic potential.

Initial approaches for H5N1 and other avian pandemic candidates (H7, H9) tried to mimic as closely as possible licensed seasonal vaccines. However, because highly pathogenic avian viruses are rapidly lethal for eggs and require high levels of containment, these first attempts used antigenically related low pathogenicity strains or recombinant proteins. It quickly became apparent that IIVs based on avian HAs were poorly immunogenic [32].

Several general findings have subsequently emerged from studies carried out with candidate inactivated H5N1 vaccines. As expected, two doses were required to generate immune responses in naïve subjects. Higher doses are more immunogenic than lower doses, with a more dramatic dose–response relationship than seen with seasonal vaccine. In contrast to seasonal vaccine, WV preparations may be more immunogenic than SV vaccines, although differences in immunogenicity are marginal. Administration of vaccine by the ID route does not provide better immune responses nor allow substantial dose-sparing. Finally, aluminum-based adjuvants generally are not effective for avian influenza vaccines, as seen with seasonal influenza vaccines. Aluminum-containing adjuvants have been shown to modestly enhance responses to some pandemic formulations. In contrast, oil-in-water based emulsions have repeatedly been shown to enhance the magnitude and the breadth of immune responses to avian influenza vaccines (see below).

A second strategy for enhancing the immunogenicity of IIVs for avian pandemic influenza viruses has been the use of prime–boost regimens. Although these unadjuvanted pandemic vaccines have not generated substantial immune responses when administered as a primary series, surprisingly vigorous responses have been seen to booster doses. A key characteristic appears to be the duration of time between priming and boosting, as the studies demonstrating significant boosting have generally administered the third dose ≥1 year after the primary series [33], while administration of a booster dose at 6 months did not have as great an effect. The interesting observation has been that boosting can be observed in subjects who did not respond to the primary series. Most studies demonstrating the prime–boost phenomenon have used different antigenic variants for priming and boosting, and demonstrated increased antibody against both strains [34].

Adjuvants

For many years, licensed inactivated influenza vaccines have been administered without adjuvants. However, it is clear that the immune response to vaccination and the protective effects of vaccine are suboptimal, particularly in some groups at high risk for influenza-related complications including young children and the elderly. Thus, there has been significant interest in the potential use of adjuvants to enhance the protective effects of vaccination (see Chapters 18 and 19). Although influenza vaccines adsorb well to aluminum salts, these compounds have not been effective adjuvants for influenza, for unknown reasons. Early studies suggested that water-in-oil emulsions using mineral oil could very substantially improve antibody responses in military recruits. However, use of these adjuvants was restricted by substantial local side effects including the development of sterile abscesses at the site of administration, and a suggested association of vaccination with the development of plasmacytomas.

Subsequently, oil-in-water emulsions based on the metabolizable oil squalene have been shown to substantially improve immune responses with an excellent safety profile. While there is relatively little effect on the immune response to seasonal vaccines in healthy adults, the oil-in-water emulsion MF59 results in an approximately 50% increase in antibody titers in older adults [35], and MF59 adjuvanted seasonal inactivated vaccines have been licensed for use in the elderly in Italy for several years. Recently, a large randomized trial in young children compared MF59-adjuvanted inactivated vaccine with unadjuvanted subvirion vaccine over two seasons (different unadjuvanted vaccines were used in each season). Absolute efficacy against all influenza strains was 86% in the group given TIV-MF59 and 43% in the group given unadjuvanted TIVs when compared with the placebo group [24].

Oil-in-water emulsions have demonstrated especially striking improvements in the antibody responses to candidate H5 pandemic vaccines. These studies have shown higher titers of antibody against the vaccine virus, as well as against antigenic variants, the development of B cells that recognize a larger variety of HA epitopes, and broadened and more vigorous CD4 T-cell responses [36,37].

Live influenza vaccines

The use of live attenuated virus as a vaccine for influenza was suggested very shortly after influenza virus was first recognized as the cause of the human disease, and a number of live vaccine candidates have been evaluated in clinical trials. The most common strategy has been to utilize a single attenuated vaccine virus, or master donor virus (MDV) in which the mutations responsible for attenuation reside in one or more of the six internal, non-HA or NA gene segments. New attenuated viruses representing the most recent influenza strains can then be generated rapidly through reassortment, and as long as the MDV attenuating mutations do not interact with the HA or NA genes, the new reassortants should maintain the same level of attenuation.

A number of MDV have been evaluated, but both currently licensed live attenuated influenza vaccines (LAIV) utilize a MDV generated by serial passage in cell culture at low temperature, resulting in a cold-adapted (ca) virus. In the United States and European Union, LAIV have been licensed utilizing the ca influenza A/Ann Arbor/6/60 (H2N2) and B/Ann Arbor 1/66 MDVs. Other MDVs developed in Russia utilizes the ca A/Leningrad/134/17/57 and B/USSR/60/69 viruses. These ca viruses and their reassortants display three characteristic phenotypes: (i) the *ca* phenotype, defined as the ability to replicate efficiently at 25°C, a restrictive temperature for *wt* influenza viruses; (ii) the temperature-sensitive (*ts*) phenotype, defined as significant ($>2 \log_{10}$) restriction of virus replication at 38–39°C; and (iii) the attenuation (*att*) phenotype, defined as restricted replication in the lower respiratory tract of experimental animals. Multiple mutations appear to be involved in the attenuation of these donor viruses.

Safety

Common side effects

LAIV-T or closely related formulations of LAIV have been well tolerated in adults, even among those with low levels of prevaccination antibody. Nasal symptoms (runny nose, nasal congestion, or coryza) and sore throat were the most frequently identified adverse symptoms attributable to vaccination in these studies.

LAIV-T have also been shown to be safe and well tolerated in children. Children under 8 years have had slightly increased rates of low grade fever, runny nose, and abdominal symptoms in the 7 days following vaccination than placebo recipients. However, when considering all the pediatric studies in aggregate, no consistent symptom was significantly more common in LAIV than placebo recipients. In older children, 11 to <16 years of age, sore throat was observed slightly more frequently in LAIV recipients than in IIVs. Prelicensure formulations of bivalent and trivalent LAIV have also been observed to be safe and well tolerated in children with the most common symptoms following vaccine noted as runny nose or coryza, cough, headache, chills, vomiting, and abdominal pain.

Adverse events of special interest

In larger studies, wheezing has been consistently identified as a vaccine-associated side effect in young children, although occurring at low rates. In the largest trial, medically significant wheezing within 42 days of vaccination was reported in 3.8% of children <2 years old after receipt of LAIV compared with 2.1% in those who received TIV [38]. Wheezing generally occurs in the youngest, previously unvaccinated children following the first dose of vaccine. Because of this observation, LAIV is currently approved for use in the United States for children ≥2 years old who do not have a history of asthma.

No significant vaccine-related adverse events have been seen in studies of children with cystic fibrosis or asthma, and vaccinated children with asthma have not experienced significant changes in FEV1, use of beta-adrenergic rescue medications or asthma symptom scores compared with placebo recipients. LAIV has also been well tolerated in adults with asthma or COPD.

Potential for transmission

Because LAIV is a live vaccine, there is the potential for transmission of vaccine virus to contacts. LAIV can be recovered from nasal secretions of about half of adult recipients, although generally shedding of LAIV by adults is of low titer and short duration. Although young children shed much higher levels of vaccine virus, no transmission of LAIV from vaccine recipients to susceptible contacts was detected in studies of young children involved in daycare-like settings where LAIV and placebo recipients played together for up to 8 hours a day for 7–10 days after vaccination. In the largest study, 197 children aged 8–36 months were randomized to receive trivalent LAIV or placebo intranasally (IN), and vaccine virus shedding was assessed for 21 days after vaccination. Although 80% of LAIV recipients shed at least one vaccine strain, for a mean of 7.6 days, clear evidence of transmission was detected in only one placebo recipient.

Immunogenicity

Serum and mucosal antibody responses

Studies of the immunogenicity of LAIVs have been carried out in children, adults, and in the elderly. The results of these studies are consistent with the hypothesis that the replication of these vaccines in the upper respiratory tract, and hence their immunogenicity, is influenced by the susceptibility of the host at the time of vaccination. The frequency and magnitude of detectable immune responses to vaccination is therefore highest in young children, intermediate in adults, and lowest in elderly subjects who have been repeatedly infected with influenza viruses throughout their lifetimes. In addition, the LAIV given IN is generally more effective than parenterally administered IIV at inducing nasal HA-specific IgA, while IIV usually induces higher titers of serum HAI and HA-specific IgG antibody.

Most susceptible children will demonstrate measurable serum and mucosal HA-specific antibody responses. Mucosal responses have been demonstrated in up to 85% of young children following LAIV-T. In contrast, adults generally have a low rate of serum antibody response following LAIV, and relatively lower rates of mucosal responses. Even in those with low pre-vaccination vaccine-specific influenza antibody, the rates of serum antibody responses to LAIV in adults and the elderly are low. However, the significance of these findings is unclear, as protection can be demonstrated in some circumstances in the absence of detectable mucosal responses, and the specific levels of mucosal antibody required for protection are unknown [39].

Cellular immune responses

B-cell responses to both TIV and LAIV in infants, children, and adults have recently been reported [14]. Influenza-specific IgA and IgG ASC peak on days 7–12 after either LAIV or TIV in both adults and older children, consistent with other studies in adults showing peak of ASC after TIV around days 7–8. In contrast to children, IgG ASC were significantly higher in adults after TIV than LAIV. Antibody responses were also significantly lower after LAIV than TIV in both adults and children, and generally development of ASC seemed to be a more sensitive indicator of vaccine "take" after LAIV than was antibody response. The levels of pre-vaccination memory B cells were low in all age groups, but numbers of pre-vaccination memory B cells were higher in adults than children. TIV, but not LAIV, increased the numbers of circulating memory B cells at 1 month.

Influenza-specific interferon-γ (IFN-γ) producing CD4$^+$ and CD8$^+$ lymphocytes have also been detected following both LAIV or TIV [40,41]. In children 5–9 years of age, TIV resulted in increases in the numbers of CD4$^+$ but not in the numbers of CD8$^+$ cells on day 10 following vaccination. There were no significant changes in natural killer (NK) cells following TIV. In contrast, administration of LAIV resulted in increases in both IFN-γ producing CD4$^+$ and CD8$^+$ cells as well as in NK cells. In children 6–35 months old, only children who received LAIV developed influenza-specific CD4$^+$, CD8$^+$ and $\gamma\delta$ T cells, whereas serum HAI responses were similar in the two groups [42]. An analysis of data collected during a large field trial evaluation of LAIV concluded that the post-vaccination level of influenza virus-specific IFN-γ producing T cells by Elispot analysis was the best correlate of vaccine-induced protection [43].

Efficacy and effectiveness

Randomized studies of efficacy against laboratory-confirmed influenza

Children LAIV-T was demonstrated to be efficacious in the prevention of influenza in a pivotal 2-year randomized, placebo controlled trial conducted in 1314 children aged 15 to <72 months [44]. Efficacy against culture-confirmed influenza illness in the first year of this trial was 95% (95% CI, 88–97%) against influenza A/H3N2 and 91% (95% CI, 79–96%) for influenza B. In the second year of the trial, the H3 component of the vaccine (A/Wuhan/93) was not a close match with the predominant H3 virus that season, A/Sydney/95. However, the efficacy of LAIV against this variant was 86% (95% CI, 75–92%) [45]. Overall, the efficacy of LAIV to prevent any influenza illness during the 2-year period of surveillance in this field study was 92% (95% CI, 88–94%). The overall efficacy of LAIV against culture-confirmed influenza among children 6 to <36 months who were attending daycare was recently shown to be 85% and 89% in the first and second year of the study, respectively [46]. Significant protection against influenza-associated acute otitis media also was demonstrated (>90% in both years). Studies in Asia have reached similar conclusions, with an efficacy of LAIV compared with placebo of 64–84% over multiple seasons, depending on the antigenic match with the vaccine [47].

Adults Relatively few placebo-controlled trials of the efficacy of LAIV-T have been conducted in adults. In the human challenge model, cold-adapted and inactivated influenza vaccines were of approximately equal efficacy in prevention of experimentally induced influenza A (H1N1), A (H3N2), and B. The combined efficacy in preventing laboratory-documented influenza illness due to the three wild-type influenza strains was 85% for LAIV. In a randomized controlled study in healthy persons aged 1–64 years, of whom most of the participants were adults, the efficacy of a pre-licensure bivalent preparation of LAIV for preventing culture-confirmed influenza A illness in adults was 85% (95% CI, 70–92%) for H1N1 and 58% (95% CI, 29–75%) for H3N2.

Elderly and high-risk In a recently reported randomized, double-blind, placebo-controlled clinical trial of LAIV among community-dwelling ambulatory adults ≥65 years old, the overall efficacy of LAIV against viruses that were antigenically similar to the vaccine was 42% [48]. While at the time of the study, that was felt to indicate inferior efficacy of LAIV, in light of subsequent studies showing similar levels of effectiveness for TIV in this population, perhaps this concept should be re-evaluated.

Administration of LAIV (IN) and TIV (IM) simultaneously was shown to result in an approximately 60% decrease in cases of laboratory-confirmed influenza in an elderly nursing home population compared with TIV alone [49]. However, this protective effect of combined vaccination could not be demonstrated in a population of adults with COPD [50].

Efficacy studies against clinical endpoints
The LAIV-T was also evaluated in a large study against clinical endpoints performed in 4561 healthy working adults [51]. In this study, the effectiveness of LAIV-T in preventing severe febrile respiratory illness of any cause during the influenza season was 29%.

Pandemic formulations of live influenza vaccines

Limited clinical trials of candidate cold-adapted pandemic vaccines have been performed under isolation conditions in order to prevent transmission of vaccine virus to others. Based on the available information, it appears that viruses with the avian HA and NA genes on the the A/Ann Arbor/6/60 cold-adapted background exhibit extremely restricted replication in humans [52]. Despite nasal drop administration of 10^7 $TCID_{50}$ to susceptible young adults, virus can be detected by PCR only, and only on the first day after administration. Relatively few serum antibody responses have been detected. Data from preliminary results of candidate cold-adapted H7 and H9 viruses has been slightly more promising [53]. Although virus replication still appears to severely compromised, higher frequencies of antibody responses were seen with neutralizing antibody responses seen in the majority of subjects receiving the H7N3 vaccine. IgG and nasal IgA antibody responses have also been detected.

Comparisons of inactivated and live influenza vaccines

While relatively few randomized direct comparisons of the efficacy of live and inactivated vaccines have been performed, the available studies are consistent with the observed effects of age and prior influenza experience on immunogenicity. When these vaccines have been compared in young children 12–59 months of age, LAIV-T has shown consistently superior protection, with an approximately 50% greater protective efficacy than inactivated vaccine [38,54]. Studies conducted in healthy young children have generally concluded that LAIV-T may be more efficacious than TIV, including both against viruses which are well matched antigenically to the vaccine virus and those which are antigenically drifted [38].

In contrast to young children, studies that have directly compared the vaccines in adults have suggested that the vaccines have similar efficacy, or that TIV vaccine is slightly more efficacious than live vaccine. In one three-armed study, the efficacy of LAIV compared with placebo for prevention of laboratory-confirmed influenza in healthy adults was 57%, while the efficacy of the IIV was 77%, but the difference between the two vaccines was not statistically significant [55]. In a subsequent season in the same population, the absolute efficacies of TIV and LAIV were 68% and 36%, respectively [56]. Similar results have been reported from a retrospective study evaluating the effectiveness of IIV and LAIV against medical visits for pneumonia and influenza-related diagnoses in the US military [57]. Generally, rates of such visits were lower in recipients of IIV, except for personnel who had not been vaccinated in previous years, in which there was no apparent difference in the effectiveness of the two types of vaccines. In recent effectiveness studies that have included both LAIV and TIV recipients, there were no clear-cut differences in effectiveness between the two vaccines [58].

References

1. CDC. Prevention and control of influenza with vaccines: recommendations of the Advisory Committee on Immunization Practices (ACIP), 2010. MMWR Morb Mortal Wkly Rep. 2010;59(RR–8):1–62.
2. France EK, Glanz JM, Xu S, Davis RL, Black SB, Shinefield HR, et al. Safety of the trivalent inactivated influenza vaccine among children – a population-based study. Arch Pediatr Adolesc Med. 2004;158(11): 1031–6.
3. Govaert TM, Thijs CT, Masurel N, Sprenger MJ, Dinant GJ, Knottnerus JA. The efficacy of influenza vaccination in elderly individuals. A randomized double-blind placebo-controlled trial. JAMA. 1994;272 (16):1956–61.
4. Nichol KL, Margolis KL, Lind A, Murdoch M, McFadden R, Hauge M, et al. Side effects associated with influenza vaccination in healthy working adults. A randomized, placebo-controlled trial. Arch Intern Med. 1996;156(14):1546–50.
5. Neuzil KM. Influenza vaccine for children. Clin Infect Dis. 2004;38:689–91.
6. CDC. Update: recommendations of the Advisory Committee on Immunization Practices regarding use of CSL seasonal influenza vaccine (Afluria) in the United States during 2010–11. MMWR Morb Mortal Wkly Rep. 2010;59:989–92.
7. Lasky T, Tarracciano GJ, Magder L, Koski CL, Ballesteros M, Nash D, et al. The Guillan–Barre syndrome and the 1992–1993 and 1993–1994 influenza vaccines. N Engl J Med. 1998;339(25):1797–802.
8. Tamma PD, Sult KS, delRio D, Steinhoff MC, Halsey NA, Omer SB. Safety of influenza vaccination during pregnancy. Am J Obstet Gynecol. 2009;201:547–53.
9. Falsey AR, Treanor JJ, Tornieporth N, Capellan J, Gorse GJ. Superior immunogenicity of high dose influenza vaccine compared with standard influenza vaccine in adults >65 years of age: a randomized double-blined controlled phase 3 trial. J Infect Dis. 2008;200: 172–80.
10. Englund JA, Walter EB, Fairchok MP, Monto AS, Neuzil KM. A comparison of 2 influenza vaccine schedules in 6- to 23-month-old children. Pediatrics. 2005 April 1;115(4):1039–47.
11. El Sahly HM, Davis C, Kotloff K, Meier J, Winokur PL, Wald A, et al. Higher antigen content improves the immune response to 209 H1N1 influenza vaccine in HIV-infected adults: a randomized clinical trial. J Infect Dis. 2012;205:703–12.
12. Cate TR, Rayford Y, Nino D, Winokur PL, Brady RC, Belshe R, et al. A high dosage influenza vaccine induced significantly more neuraminidase antibody than standard vaccine amont elderly subjects. Vaccine. 2010;28: 2076–8.
13. Keitel WA, Couch RB, Cate TR, Hess KR, Baxter B, Quarles JM, et al. High doses of purified influenza A virus hemagglutinin significantly augment serum and nasal secretion antibody responses in healthy young adults. J Clin Microbiol. 1994;32(10):2468–73.
14. Sasaki S, Jaimes MC, Holmes TH, Dekker CL, Mahmood K, Kemble GW, et al. Comparison of the influenza-specific effector and memory B cell responses to immunization of children and adults with live attenuated or inactivated influenza vaccines. J Virol. 2007;81: 215–28.
15. Kosor Krnic E, Gagro A, Drazenovic V, Kuzman I, Jeren T, Cecuk-Jelicic E, et al. Enumeration of haemagglutinin-specific CD8+ T cells after influenza vaccination using MHC class I peptide tetramers. Scand J Immunol. 2008; 67(1):86–94.

16. Zeman AM, Holmes TH, Stamatis S, Tu WW, He XS, Bouvier N, et al. Humoral and cellular immune responses in children given annual immunization with trivalent inactivated influenza vaccine. Pediatr Infect Dis J. 2007;26(2):107–15.

17. Bucasas KL, Franco LM, Shaw CA, Bray MS, Wells JM, Nino D, et al. Early patterns of gene expression correlate with the humoral immune response to influenza vaccination in humans. J Infect Dis. 2011;203: 921–9.

18. Nakaya HI, Wrammert J, Lee EK, Racioppi L, Marie-Kunze S, Haining WN, et al. Systems biology of vaccination for seasonal influenza in humans. Nat Immunol. 2011;12:786–95.

19. Keitel WA. Repeated immunization of children with inactivated and live attenuated influenza virus vaccines: safety, immunogenicity, and protective efficacy. Semin Pediatr Infect Dis. 2002;13(2):112–9.

20. Petrie JG, Ohmit SE, Johnson E, Cross RT, Monto AS. Efficacy studies of influenza vaccines: effect of end points used and characteristics of vaccine failures. J Infect Dis. 2011;203(9):1309–15.

21. Osterholm MT, Kelley NS, Sommer A, Belongia E. Influenza vaccine efficacy and effectiveness: a new look at the evidence. Lancet Infect Dis. 2012;12:36–44.

22. Frey S, Vesikari T, Szymczakiewicz-Multanowska A, Lattanzi M, Izu A, Groth N, et al. Clinical efficacy of cell culture-derived and egg-derived inactivated subunit influenza vaccines in healthy adults. Clin Infect Dis. 2010;51:997–1004.

23. Bridges CB, Thompson WW, Meltzer MI, Reeve GR, Talamonti WJ, Cox NJ, et al. Effectiveness and cost-benefit of influenza vaccination of healthy working adults: a randomized controlled trial. [see comments]. JAMA. 2000 Oct 4;284(13):1655–63.

24. Vesikari T, Knuf M, Wutzler P, Karvonen A, Kieninger-Baum D, Schmitt H-J, et al. Oil-in-water emulsion adjuvant with influenza vaccine in young children. N Engl J Med. 2011;365:1406–16.

25. Mahdi SA, Maskew M, Koen A, Kuwanda L, Besselaar TG, Naidoo D, et al. Trivalent inactivated influenza vaccine in African adults infected with human immunodeficiency virus: double blind, randomized clinical trial of efficacy, immunogenicity, and safety. Clin Infect Dis. 2011;52:128–37.

26. Skowronski DM, Janjua NZ, de Serres G, Winter A-L, Dickinson JA, Gardy JL, et al. A sentinel platform to evaluate influenza vaccine effectiveness and new variant circulation, Canada 2010–2011 season. Clin Infect Dis. 2012;55:332–42.

27. Talbot HK, Griffin MR, Chen Q, Zhu Y, Williams JV, Edwards KM. Effectiveness of seasonal vaccine in preventing confirmed influenza-associated hospitalizations in community dwelling older adults. J Infect Dis. 2011;203:500–8.

28. Kelly H, Jacoby P, Dixon G, Carcione D, Williams S, Moore HC, et al. Vaccine effectiveness against laboratory-confirmed influenza in healthy young children. Pediatr Infect Dis J. 2011;30:107–11.

29. Kawai S, Nanri S, Ban E, Inokuchi M, Tanaka T, Tokumura M, et al. Influenza vaccination of schoolchildren and influenza outbreaks in a school. Clin Infect Dis. 2011;53:130–6.

30. Zaman K, Roy E, Arifeen SE, Rahman M, Raquib R, Wilson E, et al. Effectiveness of maternal influenza immunization in mothers and infants. N Engl J Med. 2008;359:1555–64.

31. Benowitz I, Esposito DB, Gracey KD, Shapiro ED, Vazquez M. Influenza vaccine given to pregnant women reduces hospitalization due to influenza in their infants. Clin Infect Dis. 2010;51:1355–61.

32. Treanor JJ, Campbell JD, Zangwill KM, Rowe T, Wolff M. Safety and immunogenicity of an inactivated subvirion influenza A (H5N1) vaccine. N Engl J Med. 2006;354:1343–51.

33. Goji NA, Nolan C, Hill H, Wolff M, Rowe T, Treanor JJ. Immune respones of healthy subjects to a single dose of intramuscular inactivated influenza A/Vietman/1203/04 (H5N1 vaccine after priming with an antigenic variant. J Infect Dis. 2008;198:635–41.

34. Belshe RB, Frey SE, Graham I, Mulligan MJ, Eduparanti S, Jackson LA, et al. Safety and immunogenicity of influenza A H5 subunit vaccines: effect of vaccine schedule and antigenic variant. J Infect Dis. 2011;203: 666–73.

35. Podda A. The adjuvanted influenza vaccines with novel adjuvants: experience with the MF59-adjuvanted vaccine. Vaccine. 2001;19:2673–80.

36. Galli G, Hancock K, Hoschler K, DeVos J, Praus M, Bardelli M, et al. Fast rise of broadly cross-reactive antibodies after boosting long-lived human memory B cells primed by an MF59 adjuvanted prepandemic vaccine. Proc Natl Acad Sci U S A. 2009;106:7962–7.

37. Khurana S, Verma N, Yewdell JW, Hilbert AK, Castellino F, Lattanzi M, et al. MF59 adjuvant enhances diversity and affinity of antibody-mediated immune response to pandemic influenza vaccines. Sci Transl Med. 2011;3: 85ra48.

38. Belshe RB, Edwards KM, Vesikari T, Black SV, Walker RE, Hultquist M, et al. Live attenuated versus inactivated influenza vaccine in infants and young children. N Engl J Med. 2007;356(7):685–96.

39. Belshe RB, Gruber WC, Mendelman PM, Mehta HB, Mahmood K, Reisinger K, et al. Correlates of immune protection induced by live attenuated, cold-adapted,

trivial, intranasal influenza virus vaccine. J Infect Dis. 2000;181:1133–7.

40. He X-S, Holmes TH, Zhang C, Mahmood K, Kemble GW, Lewis DB, et al. Cellular immune responses in children and adults receiving inactivated or live attenuated influenza vaccines. J Virol. 2006;80(23):11756–66.

41. He X-S, Holmes TH, Mahmood K, Kemble GW, Dekker CL, Arvin AM, et al. Phenotypic changes in influenza-specific CD8+ T cells after immunization of children and adults with influenza vaccines. J Infect Dis. 2008;197(6):803–11.

42. Hoft DF, Babusis E, Worku S, Spencer CT, Lottenbach K, Truscott SM, et al. Live and inactivated influenza vaccines induce similar humoral responses, but only live vaccines induce diverse T cell responses in young children. J Infect Dis. 2011;204:845–53.

43. Forrest BD, Pride MW, Dunning AJ, Rosario M, Capeding Z, Chotpitayasunondh T, et al. Correlation of cellular immune responses with protection against culture-confirmed influenza virus in young children. Clin Vaccine Immunol. 2008;15:1042–53.

44. Belshe RB, Mendelman PM, Treanor J, King J, Gruber WC, Piedra P, et al. The efficacy of live attenuated cold-adapted trivalent, intranasal influenzavirus vaccine in children. N Engl J Med. 1998;358:1405–12.

45. Belshe RB, Gruber WC, Mendelman PM, Cho I, Reisinger K, Block SL, et al. Efficacy of vaccination with live attenuated, cold-adapted, trivalent, intranasal influenza virus vaccine against a variant (A/Sydney) not contained in the vaccine. J Pediatr. 2000;136(2):168–75.

46. Vesikari T, Fleming DM, Aristegui JF, Vertruyen A, Ashkenazi S, Rappaport R, et al. Safety, efficacy, and effectiveness of cold-adapted influenza vaccine-trivalent against community-acquired, culture-confirmed influenza in young children attending day care 10.1542/peds.2006-0725. Pediatrics. 2006;118(6):2298–312.

47. Tam JS, Capeding MR, Lum LC, Chotpitayasunondh T, Jiang Z, Huang LM, et al. Efficacy and safety of a live attenuated, cold-adapted influenza vaccine, trivalent against culture-confirmed influenza in young children in Asia. Pediatr Infect Dis J. 2007;26(7):619–28.

48. DeVilliers PJT, Steele AD, Hiemstra LA, Rappaport R, Dunning AJ, Gruber WC, et al. Efficacy and safety of a live attenuated influenza vaccine in adults 60 years of age and olcer. Vaccine. 2010;28:228–34.

49. Treanor JJ, Mattison HR, Dumyati G, Yinnon A, Erb S, O'Brien D, et al. Protective efficacy of combined live intranasal and inactivated influenza A virus vaccines in the elderly. Ann Intern Med. 1992;117(8):625–33.

50. Gorse GJ, O'Connor TZ, Young SL, Mendelman PM, Bradley SF, KNichol KL, et al. Efficacy trial of live, cold-adapted and inactivated influenza virus vaccines in older adults with chronic obstructive pulmonary disease: a VA cooperative study. Vaccine. 2003;21:2133–44.

51. Nichol KL, Mendelman PM, Mallon KP, Jackson LA, Gorse GJ, Belshe RB, et al. Effectiveness of live, attenuated intranasal influenza virus vaccine in healthy, working adults: a randomized controlled trial. JAMA. 1999;282(2):137–44.

52. Karron RA, Talaat KR, Luke CJ, Callahan KA, Thumar B, diLorenzo SC, et al. Evaluation of two live attenuated cold-adapted H5N1 influenza virus vaccines in healthy adults. Vaccine. 2009;27:4953–60.

53. Talaat KR, Karron RA, Callahan KA, Luke CJ, diLorenzo SC, Chen GL, et al. A live attenuated H7N3 influenza virus vaccine is well tolerated and immungenic in a phase I trial in healthy adults. Vaccine. 2009;27:3744–53.

54. Ashkenazi S, Vertruyen A, Aristegui J, Esposito S, McKeith DD, Klemola T, et al. Superior relative efficacy of live attenuated influenza vaccine compared with inactivated influenza vaccine in young children with recurrent respiratory tract infections. Pediatr Infect Dis J. 2006;25(10):870–9.

55. Ohmit SE, Victor JC, Rotthoff JR, Teich ER, Truscon RK, Baum LL, et al. Prevention of antigenically drifted influenza by inactivated and live attenuated vaccines. N Engl J Med. 2006;355(24):2513–22.

56. Monto AS, Ohmit SE, Petrie JG, Johnson E, Truscon R, Teich E, et al. Comparative efficacy of inactivated and live attenuated influenza vaccines. N Engl J Med. 2009;361:1260–7.

57. Wang Z, Tobler S, Roayaei J, Eick A. Live attenuated or inactivated influenza vaccines and medical encounters for respiratory illnesses among US military personnel. JAMA. 2009;301:945–53.

58. Treanor JJ, Talbot HK, Ohmit SE, Coleman L, Thompson MG, Cheng P-Y, et al. Effectiveness of seasonal influenza vaccine in the United States during a season with circulation of all three vaccine strains. Clin Infect Dis. 2012;55:951–9.

21 New approaches to vaccination

Chih-Jen Wei,[1]* Damian C. Ekiert,[2]* Gary J. Nabel,[1,4] and Ian A. Wilson[2,3]

[1]Vaccine Research Center, NIAID, National Institutes of Health, Bethesda, MD, USA

[2]Department of Integrative Structural and Computational Biology, The Scripps Research Institute, La Jolla, CA, USA

[3]IAVI Neutralizing Antibody Center and Scripps Center for HIV/AIDS Vaccine Immunology and Immunogen Discovery, The Scripps Research Institute, La Jolla, CA, USA

[4]Sanofi, Cambridge, MA, USA

Introduction

Effective vaccination remains the most effective tool to support the public health efforts to reduce influenza-associated morbidity and mortality. However, as influenza virus evolves through genetic mutations, new vaccines are needed almost every year. The current annual vaccination approach with trivalent inactivated or live-attenuated vaccines, although effective, is costly, estimated at 2–4 billion dollars annually. Furthermore, its protective efficacy varies, depending on whether there is a good antigenic match between the circulating viruses and the vaccine strains [1]. Moreover, the emergence of completely new strains, such as the pandemic 2009 H1N1, the threat of highly pathogenic avian H5N1, and the potential re-emergence of H2N2 subtype virus [2], underscore the need for a broadly protective influenza vaccine [3]. The recent identification of broadly neutralizing antibodies to influenza virus in humans provides a path towards antibody-mediated cross protection that might be elicited by vaccination (see Chapters 5 and 19) [4–11]. In this chapter, we focus on the structural basis of influenza recognition by these broad and potent neutralizing antibodies and discuss novel vaccine approaches that might elicit such protective antibodies in humans in an effort to develop a universal influenza vaccine.

*These authors contributed equally to this work.

Structural basis for development of universal influenza vaccines

Broadly neutralizing antibodies have been studied extensively for several viruses and, in particular, in the search for an effective vaccine for the human immunodeficiency virus (HIV). Given the well-established role of antibodies in protection against many viral pathogens [12] and the diversity of viruses, such as influenza and HIV-1, an effective prophylactic vaccine will likely need to induce a robust neutralizing antibody response that confers protection against numerous subtypes, clades, and strains. The discovery in the early 1990s of broadly neutralizing antibodies against HIV-1, such as b12 [13], which recognize the CD4 binding site on the viral envelope protein gp120, confirmed that rare broadly protective antibodies can be generated in some infected individuals. By understanding the molecular basis of their recognition in the context of B-cell development, it is hoped that a vaccine can be designed that will re-elicit similar antibodies. Since then, hundreds of antibodies targeting several additional sites of vulnerability on gp120 and gp41 have been identified. Many of these antibodies have been structurally characterized, including 2F5 [14], 4E10 [15, 16], and z13 [16, 17], against the membrane-proximal external region (MPER); 2G12 against a high mannose cluster on the glycan shield [18]; VRC01 against the CD4 binding site [19]; PG9 and PG16 against glycans and V1/V2 loop [20–23];

and PGT127 and PGT128 against glycans and V3 loop [24]. Applying structural information on bnAbs to vaccine development has been challenging, particularly in the absence of a crystal structure of the complete HIV envelope spike (gp160). However, our understanding of the humoral response against the virus, particularly among long-term nonprogressors and elite controllers, has helped to define some possible immune correlates of protection that likely must be achieved in a successful vaccine candidate and has laid the foundation for diverse vaccine efforts.

Although the first broadly neutralizing antibodies against influenza were identified around the same time as the report of the isolation of b12, progress to identify and understand bnAbs against influenza has been curiously slow until very recently. In 1993, Okuno et al. [25] described an unusual antibody called C179, which was reported to neutralize multiple H1 and H2 viruses, and later H5, H6, and H9 viruses [26]. The activity of C179 was remarkably broad compared with other antibodies that were known at the time, and it was the first neutralizing antibody whose recognition mapped to the more conserved HA2 subunit of HA. In subsequent studies that took advantage of the existing crystal structures of influenza A hemagglutinin (HA) surface glycoprotein [27], some of the same researchers engineered HA constructs with most of the immunodominant regions of the HA1 head deleted, but retaining most of HA2, including the C179 epitope [28]. Immunization of mice with this "headless" HA immunogen derived from the H2 subtype induced heterosubtypic immunity against challenge with an H1N1 virus. In effect, the pioneering work from Okuno et al. and Sagawa et al. had already proved the potential power of using broadly neutralizing antibodies as a guide for the development of improved vaccines. However, despite the exciting potential of the body of work on C179, more than a decade passed with little apparent interest in bnAbs against influenza.

Despite this slow start, interest in bnAbs against influenza has exploded since 2008, following the discovery of human antibodies that are capable of neutralizing multiple virus subtypes, and these bnAbs included CR6261 [29, 30], F10 [8], and A06 [31]. These antibodies, along with hundreds of similar antibodies identified subsequently, are very similar in

sequence and use the same V_H1-69 germline. Members of this family of V_H1-69 antibodies generally cross-react widely across most group 1 subtypes, including two of the three human virus subtypes (H1 and H2), two zoonotic subtypes (H5 and H9), and several avian subtypes. This pattern of reactivity is reminiscent of that of C179, suggesting that C179 and the V_H1-69 mAbs may recognize a similar epitope on HA. Crystal structures of CR6261 [29], F10 [8] and C179 [32] in complex with HA revealed that both antibodies bind to a similar epitope on the HA stem, in close proximity to the viral membrane (Figure 21.1).

The hallmark of the V_H1-69 family is a hydrophobic CDR H2, which inserts into a hydrophobic pocket in the HA stem region. The epitope on HA is highly conserved across all 16 virus subtypes. Recently, a non-V_H1-69 clone called FI6 was reported to bind or neutralize multiple group 2 subtypes (including the third of the human subtypes, H3, that have caused pandemics, and an additional zoonotic subtype, H7, that has sporadically infected humans), in addition to having broad activity against group 1 influenza viruses [10]. Consequently, the high degree of sequence conservation in this region on HA makes this surface an ideal target for therapeutic interventions. Importantly, many V_H1-69 mAbs have a relatively small number of somatic mutations from the germline sequence, and individuals with detectable serum titers of stem antibodies occur at a modest frequency. This situation contrasts with many of the extremely rare and heavily mutated bnAbs against HIV, which may be more challenging to re-elicit by vaccination. Thus, most individuals are expected to carry V_H1-69 anti-HA stem antibodies in their immune repertoire, and the challenge is to develop vaccination strategies to promote the expansion and maturation of these B-cell clones.

In addition to the epitope recognized by the V_H1-69 family of antibodies, two other conserved regions in the HA have been identified that can be targeted by neutralizing antibodies: (i) a second epitope in the stem recognized by another human mAb, CR8020; and (ii) a region in HA1 recognized by S139/1 that may include the receptor binding site (Figure 21.1).

First, human antibody CR8020 was found to cross-react with all six group 2 influenza virus subtypes and protect mice from lethal challenge with H3 and H7

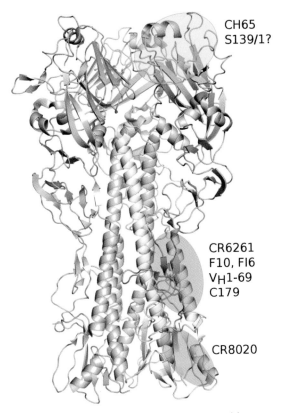

CH65
S139/1?

CR6261
F10, FI6
V_H1-69
C179

CR8020

Figure 21.1. Epitopes on HA that are recognized by bnAbs. Crystal structures of a number of HA antibody complexes have defined three distinct epitopes that are targeted by broadly neutralizing antibodies. These epitopes are mapped on to the crystal structure of the trimeric HA ectodomain from A/Puerto Rico/8/1934 (H1N1) (PDB code 1RUZ) [33], which is depicted as ribbons with a single HA1 subunit highlighted in pink and an HA2 subunit in cyan (the remaining protomers are colored gray for clarity). The first major class to be characterized structurally recognizes an epitope on the HA stem (red oval), and includes CR6261/F10/C179, other V_H1-69 mAbs, and the more recently discovered FI6 and CR9114. The second unique epitope identified is also located on the stem (blue oval), and is recognized by CR8020. Finally, a third epitope near the receptor binding site (yellow) is recognized by CH65, C05, S139/1, and most likely by other mAbs.

viruses [11]. Thus, the activity of CR8020 (group 2 specific) is complementary to CR6261/F10 and other V_H1-69 mAbs (group 1 specific), and a cocktail of CR6261/F10 and CR8020 (or a two component vaccine) would provide protection against most influ-

enza A viruses. Biochemical and structural studies of CR8020 bound to H3 HA have produced a clear picture of the molecular details of this epitope. CR8020 also recognizes an epitope on the HA stem that is well conserved among group 2 viruses. It is noteworthy that the CR8020 is largely distinct from the V_H1-69 stem epitope, thereby defining an alternative site that can be targeted on group 2 viruses. Further, the CR8020 epitope, apart from the surrounding glycans, is also relatively well conserved among group 1 HAs and is moderately well conserved between groups 1 and 2, raising the possibility that other antibodies may be found that could target this site and possibly achieve group 1-specific (or even pan influenza A) cross-reactivity. Such antibodies would be analogous to the case of FI6, which recognizes essentially the same surface on HA as group 1-specific VH1-69 antibodies but with extended breadth that also includes group 2 HAs [10].

Second, murine monoclonal S139/1 was identified and found to neutralize viruses from several subtypes from both groups 1 and 2, including H1, H2, H3, H5, H9, and H13 [34]. In contrast to stem antibodies, which block membrane fusion but not receptor binding, S139/1 inhibits hemagglutination and attachment, suggesting that it binds an epitope in the HA1 "head," close to the receptor binding site. Indeed, virus escape variants that are no longer sensitive to S139/1 neutralization have mutations close to the sialic acid binding pocket. Although it is more variable than epitopes on the HA stem, the receptor binding site is moderately well conserved compared with the surrounding hypervariable loops recognized by most other strain-specific antibodies against the head. A recent crystal structure of S139/1 bound to an H3 HA has now provided an understanding of the molecular basis of this cross-reactivity. S139/1 inserts its CDR H2 into the conserved receptor binding site where sialic acid binds and the overall footprint of the Fab of the antibody avoids some of the hypervariable residues surrounding the site, which enables it to be more broadly neutralizing [35]. Furthermore, previous structural work on CH65, a moderately cross-reactive, subtype-specific antibody confirmed that antibodies targeting the receptor binding site do exist and can take advantage of the relatively high conservation of the receptor binding site to increase their breadth of activity [36]. The extension of CH65's footprint outside this conserved region likely limits its

329

activity to a subset of the H1 subtype, and the challenge in the future will be to explore strategies that allow the targeting of the most conserved residues in the receptor binding site while avoiding surrounding variable regions. An example of this strategy is exemplified by cross-neutralizing antibody C05 that inserts a single CDR loop, CDR H3, into the receptor binding site with minimal contact from only one other CDR H1; this H1 contact is not required for neutralization of various influenza viruses [37]. The footprint of this antibody then more closely matches that of the relatively small receptor binding site. Thus, the identification of other cross-reactive mAbs against the head will be of great interest, as well as acquiring further structural information on how such antibodies can selectively target the relatively small and shallow HA receptor binding site. Thus, a total of three sites on HA have been identified – middle stem (V_H1-69), lower stem (CR8020), and receptor binding site – as targets of broadly neutralizing antibodies, and efforts to improve the breadth of protection after vaccination can take advantage of the knowledge of these three classes of antibodies and their epitopes (Figure 21.1).

New approaches to elicit cross-protective immunity against influenza virus

Gene-based prime-boost vaccination to elicit antibodies to the conserved HA stem region

DNA vaccination has been developed as a potential immunization platform in animals and humans for various infectious diseases, including HIV, Ebola, severe acute respiratory syndrome, West Nile, and pandemic influenza [38–46]. Unlike the traditional inactivated or live-attenuated virus vaccines, which require production of infectious virus in chicken eggs or cell cultures, DNA vaccines against influenza virus can be easily and quickly manufactured as soon as the genetic sequences of the strains of interest become available. DNA vaccines encoding conserved epitopes of influenza HA, NP, or M proteins elicit both antibody and T-cell responses and conferred protective immunity in various animal models [47–58].

Although safe and well tolerated in humans, the efficacy of DNA vaccines by themselves against influenza virus from several clinical trials has not been very promising [59–61]. However, prime–boost immunization utilizing DNA vaccines as priming agents has induced improved HA antibody responses in several animal studies. For example, priming with DNA vaccines encoding H1 or H3 HAs significantly increases the HAI and microneutralization titers against the homologous virus when a trivalent inactivated vaccine was used as a boost [62]. Similarly, an H5 DNA vaccine prime followed by live-attenuated vaccine boost induces protective immunity against an antigenically distinct H5N1 virus in ferrets [63]. A broadly neutralizing antibody (12D1) against H3 subtype viruses that span 40 years was identified in mice immunized sequentially with DNA vaccines encoding three different H3 HAs followed by a boost with a fourth H3 virus [64]. Of most relevance to the development of a universal influenza vaccine, priming with a DNA vaccine encoding H1 HA from a relatively contemporary seasonal strain, followed by boosting with seasonal inactivated vaccine or HA-adenoviral vector, stimulated production of antibodies that cross-neutralize not only H1N1 strains dating from 1934 to 2007, but also HAs from other subtype viruses, such as H2N2 and H5N1 [65]. This prime–boost combination conferred protection against divergent H1N1 virus challenge in mice and ferrets (Figure 21.2). Importantly, it was shown to elicit antibodies to the conserved stem region of HA and can be induced in nonhuman primates [65], suggesting a potential application in humans.

This gene-based, prime–boost approach was further assessed in two recent phase I clinical trials [7], providing proof of concept that such antibodies can be elicited by vaccination in humans. Priming with an H5 DNA vaccine enhanced H5 specific antibody titers following an inactivated H5N1 vaccine boost. The strongest antibody response was observed with a longer prime–boost interval, and broadly neutralizing antibodies directed to the conserved stem epitope were induced in some individuals. However, the mechanism of DNA priming remains poorly understood. Notwithstanding, it has been suggested that gene-based vaccination increases T-cells' responses by expanding the number and diversity of CD4 clones, which in turn stimulate B cells to secret antibody of greater magnitude and breadth [7, 65, 66]. In addition, the delivery of the viral HA by a gene-based vector, such as a DNA vaccine, allows expression of HA in the absence of

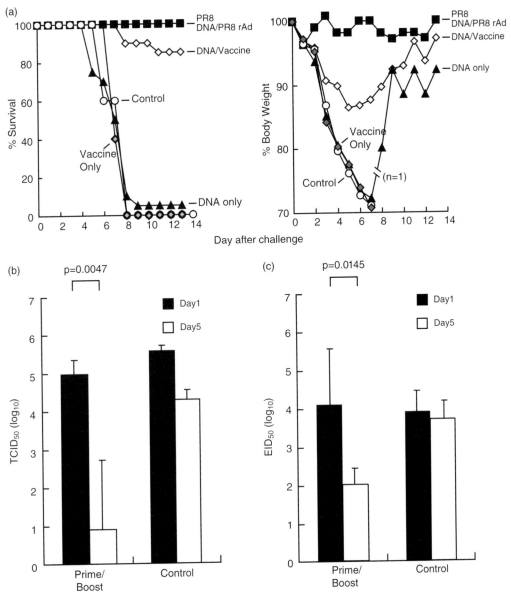

Figure 21.2. Gene-based prime–boost immunization protects mice and ferrets from H1N1 viral challenge. (a) Protection of prime–boost immune mice after heterologous virus challenge. Mice were immunized with control vector (n = 5), H1 (A/PR/8/1934, 1934 PR8) HA DNA/rAd5 (n = 5), H1 (A/New Caledonia/20/1999, 1999 NC) HA DNA (n = 20), seasonal vaccine (n = 5), or H1 1999 NC HA DNA/seasonal vaccine (n = 20). After challenging the animals with 50 LD$_{50}$ H1N1 1934 PR8 virus, survival (left) and weight loss (right) were recorded and evaluated. $P = 0.3713$ between the PR8 DNA/PR8 rAd and DNA/Vaccine groups; $P < 0.0001$, DNA/Vaccine compared with DNA only or Vaccine only groups by Kaplan–Meyer analysis. (b) Protection of ferrets from H1N1 A/Brisbane/59/2007 (2007 Bris) viral challenge. Two groups of four ferrets were immunized with 1999 NC HA DNA/seasonal flu vaccine or control vector and challenged with heterologous 2007 Bris virus (10$^{6.5}$ EID$_{50}$). Virus titers in the nasal swabs from days 1 and 5 post challenge were determined by means of end-point titration in MDCK cells. $P = 0.0104$ between day 5 control and day 5 prime–boost. (c) Protection of ferrets from H1N1 1934 PR8 viral challenge. Two groups of six ferrets were immunized with 1999 NC HA DNA/rAd5 vaccine or control vector and challenged with heterologous 1934 PR8 virus (10$^{6.5}$ EID$_{50}$). Virus titers in the nasal swabs from days 1 and 5 post challenge were determined in eggs from an initial dilution of 1 : 10 in phosphate buffered saline and expressed as EID$_{50}$/mL. The limit of virus detection was 10$^{1.5}$ EID$_{50}$/mL. $P = 0.0004$ between day 5 control and day 5 prime–boost. Adapted with permission from Wei et al. [65] with permission from the American Association for the Advancement of Science.

other viral proteins that may mask its presentation to the immune system or increase the accessibility of the HA molecules compared with that on the viral surface, thus providing a stimulus that otherwise cannot engage this region of the molecule. Taken together, these studies suggest that broadly neutralizing antibodies to influenza virus can be elicited through an alternative vaccination approach using vaccines currently available in humans. A gene-based prime–boost immunization may then serve as a platform for the first generation of universal influenza vaccine.

Structure-based immunogen design to elicit broadly neutralizing HA antibodies

Although broadly neutralizing antibodies against the conserved epitopes of HA have been identified in humans [5, 6, 9–11, 36], the level of these antibodies circulating in the human sera remains relative low even after repeated influenza infection and immunization [4]. One possible explanation for this phenomenon is that the viral HA spikes are not presented optimally to the host immune system. Traditional influenza vaccines, as with circulating influenza viruses, expose the highly immunodominant head region of the HA trimeric proteins on the surface. Due to the density of HA spikes on the viral surface, the conserved broadly neutralizing stem epitopes that are more proximal to the membrane are significantly less accessible than the HA heads and are also surrounded in part by the other main surface glycoprotein, neuraminidase. This restricted access likely limits the recognition of these conserved neutralization sites by the host immune system. However, antibodies that target the conserved stem epitopes protect animals from viral infection [5, 6, 8–11, 29, 64, 67], suggesting that this region is not inaccessible to these bnAbs when given a passive therapy. Recently, the genetic and structural basis for development of bnAbs to this epitope have been elucidated. In humans, the uniquely hydrophobic CDRH2 region of germline heavy chain VH1-69 specifically contacts the conserved stem site and is activated to direct Ab affinity maturation towards this epitope [68]. Thus, the question that arises is whether alternative presentation of these conserved epitopes in a nonphysiologic state would generate bnAbs with a sufficiently high titer to confer protection.

Recent studies of the molecular nature of these epitopes provide some insights that may lead to new structure-based design of novel immunogens [8, 10, 11, 29]. For example, a prefusion form of HA2 expressed in *Escherichia coli* has been shown to be immunogenic in mice and protects animals against a homologous viral challenge and also provides heterologous protection within the same subtype [70]. Vaccination with a "headless" HA, an immunogen lacking the globular head and comprising only the conserved stem region of HA, also confers protection against lethal H1 or H3 viral challenge in mice, although it so far has failed to demonstrate elicitation of broadly neutralizing activity *in vitro* [71]. This latter result is of particular interest, as it suggests that non-neutralizing antibodies may have some utility *in vivo*, perhaps due to Fc-mediated effector functions. Studies on FI6 [10] and on anti-HIV antibody b12 [72] have demonstrated that mutations in the Fc region that interfere with complement deposition and Fc-receptor engagement may reduce the efficacy of antibody therapy in passive immunization experiments, suggesting that direct inactivation of virus particles does not completely account for the protective efficacy of at least some antibodies *in vivo*. Consistent with the potential role of Fc, non-neutralizing antibodies against neuraminidase have also been demonstrated to be protective *in vivo* [73], suggesting that NA may also be a useful target for future vaccine design efforts. Antisera from mice immunized with a synthetic peptide vaccine based on the binding site of the aforementioned 12D1 mAb react with a broad range of HAs including H2, H3, H5, H7, and the pandemic 2009 H1N1, and this vaccine induces protective neutralizing antibodies against both H1 and H3 subtype viruses [74]. Together, these findings with the recent identification of another stem-directed bnAb that binds and neutralizes group 1 and 2 HAs [10], as well as antibody CR9114 that cross-reacts with influenza A and B viruses [75] suggest the possibility of inducing such cross-protective immunity in humans with immunogens designed to elicit the desired immune response. The information gained from atomic-level structures will no doubt facilitate an understanding of the vaccine-induced immune response to influenza and provide structural parameters to guide further vaccine design.

Conclusions

Due to the rapid accumulation of mutations in influenza virus and the unpredictability of new influenza pandemics, current immunization strategies that rely on the strain-matched vaccines constantly struggle to keep abreast of the unrelenting antigenic changes that occur in influenza viruses. The present influenza vaccine approach also provides marginal immune responses for those who need them the most, the elderly and the very young. Furthermore, in pandemics, such as 1918 and 2009 H1N1, young adults are often more adversely affected than the elderly. The difficulty of rapidly manufacturing virus-based vaccines using dated technology also hinders influenza preparedness, as witnessed in the 2009 H1N1 outbreak. Despite valiant efforts, the 2009 H1N1 vaccine was not available early in the epidemic and, when it was supplied, it was accessed by only a very small percentage of the world's population [76]. Thus, there is clearly room for improvement.

Recent advances in understanding heterosubtypic immunity, identification of various conserved epitopes on HA, and the generation of bnAbs by different vaccination platforms or immunogens, suggest a pathway to a broader, stronger, and longer-lasting protective vaccine that can be produced quickly and more efficiently. The pursuit of a vaccine that targets the common sites of vulnerability among the enormous diversity of influenza strains and subtypes will substantially benefit from the development of new vaccine technologies. It is not inconceivable given the exciting advances in identification of novel epitopes in the past few years that a universal vaccine that protects against diverse influenza viruses can be developed in the foreseeable future.

References

1. Osterholm MT, Kelley NS, Sommer A, Belongia EA. Efficacy and effectiveness of influenza vaccines: a systematic review and meta-analysis. Lancet Infect Dis. 2011;12(1):36–44.
2. Nabel GJ, Wei CJ, Ledgerwood JE. Vaccinate for the next H2N2 pandemic now. Nature. 2011;471(7337):157–8.
3. Nabel GJ, Fauci AS. Induction of unnatural immunity: prospects for a broadly protective universal influenza vaccine. Nat Med. 2010;16(12):1389–91.
4. Sui J, Sheehan J, Hwang WC, Bankston LA, Burchett SK, Huang CY, et al. Wide prevalence of heterosubtypic broadly neutralizing human anti-influenza A antibodies. Clin Infect Dis. 2011;52(8):1003–9.
5. Corti D, Suguitan AL Jr, Pinna D, Silacci C, Fernandez-Rodriguez BM, Vanzetta F, et al. Heterosubtypic neutralizing antibodies are produced by individuals immunized with a seasonal influenza vaccine. J Clin Invest. 2010;120(5):1663–73.
6. Wrammert J, Koutsonanos D, Li GM, Edupuganti S, Sui J, Morrissey M, et al. Broadly cross-reactive antibodies dominate the human B cell response against 2009 pandemic H1N1 influenza virus infection. J Exp Med. 2011;208(1):181–93.
7. Ledgerwood JE, Wei CJ, Hu Z, Gordon IJ, Enama ME, Hendel CS, et al. DNA priming and influenza vaccine immunogenicity: two phase 1 open label randomised clinical trials. Lancet Infect Dis. 2011;11(12):916–24.
8. Sui J, Hwang WC, Perez S, Wei G, Aird D, Chen LM, et al. Structural and functional bases for broad-spectrum neutralization of avian and human influenza A viruses. Nat Struct Mol Biol. 2009;16(3):265–73.
9. Friesen RH, Koudstaal W, Koldijk MH, Weverling GJ, Brakenhoff JP, Lenting PJ, et al. New class of monoclonal antibodies against severe influenza: prophylactic and therapeutic efficacy in ferrets. PLoS ONE. 2010;5(2):e9106.
10. Corti D, Voss J, Gamblin SJ, Codoni G, Macagno A, Jarrossay D, et al. A neutralizing antibody selected from plasma cells that binds to group 1 and group 2 influenza A hemagglutinins. Science. 2011;333(6044):850–6.
11. Ekiert DC, Friesen RH, Bhabha G, Kwaks T, Jongeneelen M, Yu W, et al. A highly conserved neutralizing epitope on group 2 influenza A viruses. Science. 2011;333(6044):843–50.
12. Plotkin SA. Correlates of protection induced by vaccination. Clin Vaccine Immunol. 2010;17(7):1055–65.
13. Burton DR, Pyati J, Koduri R, Sharp SJ, Thornton GB, Parren PW, et al. Efficient neutralization of primary isolates of HIV-1 by a recombinant human monoclonal antibody. Science. 1994;266(5187):1024–7.
14. Bryson S, Julien JP, Hynes RC, Pai EF. Crystallographic definition of the epitope promiscuity of the broadly neutralizing anti-human immunodeficiency virus type 1 antibody 2F5: vaccine design implications. J Virol. 2009;83(22):11862–75.
15. Cardoso RM, Zwick MB, Stanfield RL, Kunert R, Binley JM, Katinger H, et al. Broadly neutralizing anti-HIV antibody 4E10 recognizes a helical conformation

of a highly conserved fusion-associated motif in gp41. Immunity. 2005;22(2):163–73.

16. Zwick MB, Labrijn AF, Wang M, Spenlehauer C, Saphire EO, Binley JM, et al. Broadly neutralizing antibodies targeted to the membrane-proximal external region of human immunodeficiency virus type 1 glycoprotein gp41. J Virol. 2001;75(22):10892–905.

17. Nelson JD, Brunel FM, Jensen R, Crooks ET, Cardoso RM, Wang M, et al. An affinity-enhanced neutralizing antibody against the membrane-proximal external region of human immunodeficiency virus type 1 gp41 recognizes an epitope between those of 2F5 and 4E10. J Virol. 2007;81(8):4033–43.

18. Calarese DA, Scanlan CN, Zwick MB, Deechongkit S, Mimura Y, Kunert R, et al. Antibody domain exchange is an immunological solution to carbohydrate cluster recognition. Science. 2003;300(5628):2065–71.

19. Zhou T, Georgiev I, Wu X, Yang ZY, Dai K, Finzi A, et al. Structural basis for broad and potent neutralization of HIV-1 by antibody VRC01. Science. 2010;329 (5993):811–7.

20. McLellan JS, Pancera M, Carrico C, Gorman J, Julien JP, Khayat R, et al. Structure of HIV-1 gp120 V1/V2 domain with broadly neutralizing antibody PG9. Nature. 2011;480(7377):336–43.

21. Pancera M, McLellan JS, Wu X, Zhu J, Changela A, Schmidt SD, et al. Crystal structure of PG16 and chimeric dissection with somatically related PG9: structure-function analysis of two quaternary-specific antibodies that effectively neutralize HIV-1. J Virol. 2010;84(16): 8098–110.

22. Pejchal R, Walker LM, Stanfield RL, Phogat SK, Koff WC, Poignard P, et al. Structure and function of broadly reactive antibody PG16 reveal an H3 subdomain that mediates potent neutralization of HIV-1. Proc Natl Acad Sci U S A. 2010;107(25):11483–8.

23. Julien JP, Lee JH, Cupo A, Murin CD, Derking R, Hoffenberg S, et al. Asymmetric recognition of the HIV-1 trimer by broadly neutralizing antibody PG9. Proc Natl Acad Sci U S A. 2013;110:4351–6.

24. Pejchal R, Doores KJ, Walker LM, Khayat R, Huang PS, Wang SK, et al. A potent and broad neutralizing antibody recognizes and penetrates the HIV glycan shield. Science. 2011;334(6059):1097–103.

25. Okuno Y, Isegawa Y, Sasao F, Ueda S. A common neutralizing epitope conserved between the hemagglutinins of influenza A virus H1 and H2 strains. J Virol. 1993;67 (5):2552–8.

26. Smirnov YA, Lipatov AS, Gitelman AK, Okuno Y, Van Beek R, Osterhaus AD, et al. An epitope shared by the hemagglutinins of H1, H2, H5, and H6 subtypes of influenza A virus. Acta Virol. 1999;43(4): 237–44.

27. Wilson IA, Skehel JJ, Wiley DC. Structure of the haemagglutinin membrane glycoprotein of influenza virus at 3 Å resolution. Nature. 1981;289(5796):366–73.

28. Sagawa H, Ohshima A, Kato I, Okuno Y, Isegawa Y. The immunological activity of a deletion mutant of influenza virus haemagglutinin lacking the globular region. J Gen Virol. 1996;77(Pt 7):1483–7.

29. Ekiert DC, Bhabha G, Elsliger MA, Friesen RH, Jongeneelen M, Throsby M, et al. Antibody recognition of a highly conserved influenza virus epitope. Science. 2009;324(5924):246–51.

30. Throsby M, van den Brink E, Jongeneelen M, Poon LL, Alard P, Cornelissen L, et al. Heterosubtypic neutralizing monoclonal antibodies cross-protective against H5N1 and H1N1 recovered from human IgM+ memory B cells. PLoS ONE. 2008;3(12):e3942.

31. Kashyap AK, Steel J, Rubrum A, Estelles A, Briante R, Ilyushina NA, et al. Protection from the 2009 H1N1 pandemic influenza by an antibody from combinatorial survivor-based libraries. PLoS Pathog. 2010;6(7):e1000990.

32. Dreyfus C, Ekiert DC, Wilson IA. Structure of a classical broadly neutralizing stem antibody in complex with a pandemic H2 hemagglutinin. J Virol. 2013 Apr 3. [Epub ahead of print]

33. Gamblin SJ, Haire LF, Russell RJ, Stevens DJ, Xiao B, Ha Y, et al. The structure and receptor binding properties of the 1918 influenza hemagglutinin. Science. 2004; 303(5665):1838–42.

34. Yoshida R, Igarashi M, Ozaki H, Kishida N, Tomabechi D, Kida H, et al. Cross-protective potential of a novel monoclonal antibody directed against antigenic site B of the hemagglutinin of influenza A viruses. PLoS Pathog. 2009;5(3):e1000350.

35. Lee PS, Yoshida R, Ekiert DC, Sakai N, Suzuki Y, Takada A, et al. Heterosubtypic antibody recognition of the influenza virus hemagglutinin receptor binding site enhanced by avidity. Proc Natl Acad Sci U S A. 2012;109(42):17040–5.

36. Whittle JR, Zhang R, Khurana S, King LR, Manischewitz J, Golding H, et al. Broadly neutralizing human antibody that recognizes the receptor-binding pocket of influenza virus hemagglutinin. Proc Natl Acad Sci U S A. 2011;108(34):14216–21.

37. Ekiert DC, Kashyap AK, Steel J, Rubrum A, Bhabha G, Khayat R, et al. Cross-neutralization of influenza A viruses mediated by a single antibody loop. Nature. 2012;489(7417):526–32.

38. Martin JE, Sullivan NJ, Enama ME, Gordon IJ, Roederer M, Koup RA, et al. A DNA vaccine for Ebola virus is safe and immunogenic in a phase I clinical trial. Clin Vaccine Immunol. 2006;13(11):1267–77.

39. Tavel JA, Martin JE, Kelly GG, Enama ME, Shen JM, Gomez PL, et al. Safety and immunogenicity of a

Gag-Pol candidate HIV-1 DNA vaccine administered by a needle-free device in HIV-1-seronegative subjects. J Acquir Immune Defic Syndr. 2007;44(5):601–5.

40. Graham BS, Koup RA, Roederer M, Bailer RT, Enama ME, Moodie Z, et al. Phase 1 safety and immunogenicity evaluation of a multiclade HIV-1 DNA candidate vaccine. J Infect Dis. 2006;194(12):1650–60.

41. Kibuuka H, Kimutai R, Maboko L, Sawe F, Schunk MS, Kroidl A, et al. A phase 1/2 study of a multiclade HIV-1 DNA plasmid prime and recombinant adenovirus serotype 5 boost vaccine in HIV-Uninfected East Africans (RV 172). J Infect Dis. 2010;201(4):600–7.

42. Ledgerwood JE, Pierson TC, Hubka SA, Desai N, Rucker S, Gordon IJ, et al. A West Nile virus DNA vaccine utilizing a modified promoter induces neutralizing antibody in younger and older healthy adults in a phase I clinical trial. J Infect Dis. 2011;203(10): 1396–404.

43. Martin JE, Pierson TC, Hubka S, Rucker S, Gordon IJ, Enama ME, et al. A West Nile virus DNA vaccine induces neutralizing antibody in healthy adults during a phase 1 clinical trial. J Infect Dis. 2007;196(12): 1732–40.

44. Jaoko W, Karita E, Kayitenkore K, Omosa-Manyonyi G, Allen S, Than S, et al. Safety and immunogenicity study of Multiclade HIV-1 adenoviral vector vaccine alone or as boost following a multiclade HIV-1 DNA vaccine in Africa. PLoS ONE. 2010;5(9):e12873.

45. Catanzaro AT, Roederer M, Koup RA, Bailer RT, Enama ME, Nason MC, et al. Phase 1 clinical evaluation of a six-plasmid multiclade HIV-1 DNA candidate vaccine. Vaccine. 2007;25(20):4085–92.

46. Martin JE, Louder MK, Holman LA, Gordon IJ, Enama ME, Larkin BD, et al. A SARS DNA vaccine induces neutralizing antibody and cellular immune responses in healthy adults in a Phase I clinical trial. Vaccine. 2008; 26(50):6338–43.

47. Kim JH, Jacob J. DNA vaccines against influenza viruses. Curr Top Microbiol Immunol. 2009;333:197–210.

48. Epstein SL, Tumpey TM, Misplon JA, Lo CY, Cooper LA, Subbarao K, et al. DNA vaccine expressing conserved influenza virus proteins protective against H5N1 challenge infection in mice. Emerg Infect Dis. 2002;8(8): 796–801.

49. Tompkins SM, Zhao ZS, Lo CY, Misplon JA, Liu T, Ye Z, et al. Matrix protein 2 vaccination and protection against influenza viruses, including subtype H5N1. Emerg Infect Dis. 2007;13(3):426–35.

50. Jimenez GS, Planchon R, Wei Q, Rusalov D, Geall A, Enas J, et al. Vaxfectin-formulated influenza DNA vaccines encoding NP and M2 viral proteins protect mice against lethal viral challenge. Hum Vaccin. 2007;3(5): 157–64.

51. Robinson HL, Boyle CA, Feltquate DM, Morin MJ, Santoro JC, Webster RG. DNA immunization for influenza virus: studies using hemagglutinin- and nucleoprotein-expressing DNAs. J Infect Dis. 1997;176 (Suppl. 1):S50–5.

52. Laddy DJ, Yan J, Kutzler M, Kobasa D, Kobinger GP, Khan AS, et al. Heterosubtypic protection against pathogenic human and avian influenza viruses via in vivo electroporation of synthetic consensus DNA antigens. PLoS ONE. 2008;3(6):e2517.

53. Rao SS, Kong WP, Wei CJ, Van Hoeven N, Gorres JP, Nason M, et al. Comparative efficacy of hemagglutinin, nucleoprotein, and matrix 2 protein gene-based vaccination against H5N1 influenza in mouse and ferret. PLoS ONE. 2010;5(3):e9812.

54. Cox RJ, Mykkeltvedt E, Robertson J, Haaheim LR. Non-lethal viral challenge of influenza haemagglutinin and nucleoprotein DNA vaccinated mice results in reduced viral replication. Scand J Immunol. 2002;55(1): 14–23.

55. Ulmer JB, Donnelly JJ, Parker SE, Rhodes GH, Felgner PL, Dwarki VJ, et al. Heterologous protection against influenza by injection of DNA encoding a viral protein. Science. 1993;259(5102):1745–9.

56. Epstein SL, Kong WP, Misplon JA, Lo CY, Tumpey TM, Xu L, et al. Protection against multiple influenza A subtypes by vaccination with highly conserved nucleoprotein. Vaccine. 2005;23(46–47):5404–10.

57. Okuda K, Ihata A, Watabe S, Okada E, Yamakawa T, Hamajima K, et al. Protective immunity against influenza A virus induced by immunization with DNA plasmid containing influenza M gene. Vaccine. 2001;19 (27):3681–91.

58. Saha S, Yoshida S, Ohba K, Matsui K, Matsuda T, Takeshita F, et al. A fused gene of nucleoprotein (NP) and herpes simplex virus genes (VP22) induces highly protective immunity against different subtypes of influenza virus. Virology. 2006;354(1):48–57.

59. Drape RJ, Macklin MD, Barr LJ, Jones S, Haynes JR, Dean HJ. Epidermal DNA vaccine for influenza is immunogenic in humans. Vaccine. 2006;24(21):4475–81.

60. Jones S, Evans K, McElwaine-Johnn H, Sharpe M, Oxford J, Lambkin-Williams R, et al. DNA vaccination protects against an influenza challenge in a double-blind randomised placebo-controlled phase 1b clinical trial. Vaccine. 2009;27(18):2506–12.

61. Smith LR, Wloch MK, Ye M, Reyes LR, Boutsaboualoy S, Dunne CE, et al. Phase 1 clinical trials of the safety and immunogenicity of adjuvanted plasmid DNA vaccines encoding influenza A virus H5 hemagglutinin. Vaccine. 2010;28(13):2565–72.

62. Wang S, Parker C, Taaffe J, Solorzano A, Garcia-Sastre A, Lu S. Heterologous HA DNA vaccine

prime–inactivated influenza vaccine boost is more effective than using DNA or inactivated vaccine alone in eliciting antibody responses against H1 or H3 serotype influenza viruses. Vaccine. 2008;26(29–30):3626–33.

63. Suguitan AL Jr, Cheng X, Wang W, Wang S, Jin H, Lu S. Influenza H5 hemagglutinin DNA primes the antibody response elicited by the live attenuated influenza A/Vietnam/1203/2004 vaccine in ferrets. PLoS ONE. 2011;6(7):e21942.

64. Wang TT, Tan GS, Hai R, Pica N, Petersen E, Moran TM, et al. Broadly protective monoclonal antibodies against H3 influenza viruses following sequential immunization with different hemagglutinins. PLoS Pathog. 2010;6(2):e1000796.

65. Wei CJ, Boyington JC, McTamney PM, Kong WP, Pearce MB, Xu L, et al. Induction of broadly neutralizing H1N1 influenza antibodies by vaccination. Science. 2010;329(5995):1060–4.

66. Wu L, Kong WP, Nabel GJ. Enhanced breadth of CD4 T-cell immunity by DNA prime and adenovirus boost immunization to human immunodeficiency virus Env and Gag immunogens. J Virol. 2005;79(13):8024–31.

67. Prabhu N, Prabakaran M, Ho HT, Velumani S, Qiang J, Goutama M, et al. Monoclonal antibodies against the fusion peptide of hemagglutinin protect mice from lethal influenza A virus H5N1 infection. J Virol. 2009;83(6):2553–62.

68. Lingwood D, McTamney PM, Yassine HM, Whittle JR, Guo X, Boyington JC, et al., Structural and genetic basis for development of broadly neutralizing influenza antibodies. Nature 2012; 489(7417):566–70.

69. Kanekiyo M, Wei CJ, Yassine HM, McTamney PM, Boyington JC, Whittle JRR et al. Nature. 2013; In press.

70. Bommakanti G, Citron MP, Hepler RW, Callahan C, Heidecker GJ, Najar TA, et al. Design of an HA2-based Escherichia coli expressed influenza immunogen that protects mice from pathogenic challenge. Proc Natl Acad Sci U S A. 2010;107(31):13701–6.

71. Steel J, Lowen AC, Wang TT, Yondola M, Gao Q, Haye K, et al. Influenza virus vaccine based on the conserved hemagglutinin stalk domain. MBio. 2010;1(1).

72. Hessell AJ, Hangartner L, Hunter M, Havenith CE, Beurskens FJ, Bakker JM, et al. Fc receptor but not complement binding is important in antibody protection against HIV. Nature. 2007;449(7158):101–4.

73. Sandbulte MR, Jimenez GS, Boon AC, Smith LR, Treanor JJ, Webby RJ. Cross-reactive neuraminidase antibodies afford partial protection against H5N1 in mice and are present in unexposed humans. PLoS Med. 2007;4(2):e59.

74. Wang TT, Tan GS, Hai R, Pica N, Ngai L, Ekiert DC, et al. Vaccination with a synthetic peptide from the influenza virus hemagglutinin provides protection against distinct viral subtypes. Proc Natl Acad Sci U S A. 2010;107(44):18979–84.

75. Dreyfus C, Laursen NS, Kwaks T, Zuijdgeest D, Khayat R, Ekiert DC, et al. Highly conserved protective epitopes on influenza B viruses. Science. 2012;337(6100):1343–8.

76. Stohr K. Vaccinate before the next pandemic? Nature. 2010;465(7295):161.

22 Control of influenza in animals

Ilaria Capua[1] and Dennis J. Alexander[2]

[1]OIE/FAO Reference Laboratory for Avian Influenza and Newcastle Disease, Istituto Zooprofilattico Sperimentale delle Venezie, Viale dell'Università 10, Padua, Italy

[2]Virology Department, Animal Health and Veterinary Laboratories, Weybridge, Addlestone, Surrey, UK

Introduction

National and international regulations subdivide animal diseases into two groups: notifiable diseases, outbreaks of which must be reported to the national or international authority, and non-notifiable diseases, those for which there is no such requirement. By and large an animal disease is classified as notifiable to veterinary authorities if it endangers animal or public health, and will particularly include the emergence of previously "unknown" variants of the pathogen. The reason notification is necessary is to allow the rapid implementation of measures at national and international levels to avoid spread of infection through practices linked to husbandry and management of animals and through international trade of animals or their commodities (e.g., meat, sperm, eggs, and feathers).

The national or international regulations for the control of animal diseases include the methods, tools, and procedures used in diagnosis and control of the disease.

Influenza A viruses (IAVs) are known to infect birds and mammals, in which they may cause a mild or severe clinical condition depending on the host and on the characteristics of the virus. Some animal species undergo only sporadic or self-limiting infections, while in other species, such as certain birds, dogs, pigs, and horses, infection results in adaptation of the virus to the host and endemic disease.

Birds

In birds, IAV infections cause one of two clinical conditions: mild, termed low pathogenicity avian influenza (LPAI), or severe, known as highly pathogenic avian influenza (HPAI). LPAI is a usually nonlethal disease which may be caused by any subtype of avian influenza virus (H1–H16). In contrast, HPAI is one of the most devastating diseases of animals, as in certain avian species (e.g., chickens and turkeys) it can cause flock mortality close to 100% in 48–72 hours. For this reason most national animal health regulations include strict control measures for HPAI outbreaks. To date, only viruses of H5 and H7 subtype have been shown to cause HPAI in susceptible species, but not all H5 and H7 viruses are virulent. In recent times it has become evident that the nonvirulent viruses are the precursors of the HPAI strains, and have been included in national and international control legislation [1].

From a legislative point of view, the only IAVs that are notifiable to the official veterinary services of a given country or to the World Organisation for Animal Health (OIE) are viruses belonging to H5 or H7 subtypes. These subtypes are the subject of regulation, both by the OIE and by most national authorities, which ensure the disease must be managed according to specified provisions which include direct control measures (biosecurity, movement restriction, and stamping out) and indirect measures (vaccination) [1].

Mammals

Mammalian species in which influenza infections are transmissible and established include pigs, horses, and dogs. In other species infection is a rare and self-limiting event, which is usually considered to have occurred as a spill-over from species in which infections are established.

Swine influenza (SI) is widespread globally and is not a notifiable disease, unless it is caused by a new variant (such as H1N1pdm 2009). In any case, national and international regulations do not stipulate any specific control measure for the endemic strains of SI, and vaccination is widely applied [2].

Equine influenza (EI) as a clinical disease has been recorded for many years, but in the virologic era has been shown to be caused by viruses of H7N7, first isolated in 1956, and H3N8 subtypes, first isolated in 1963, although the former now appears to be extinct, not having been isolated for over 20 years. It is a highly contagious, respiratory, self-limiting disease, which may result in significant loss in performance of racing, show, and event horses for a number of weeks. It is a notifiable disease in some countries but not in others, and is included among OIE's listed diseases [3]. EI has been reported worldwide and is endemic in the United States and European Union. Only a handful of island countries such as New Zealand and Iceland have never reported infection, and others, such as Australia, Japan, Hong Kong, and South Africa, experience only occasional outbreaks and EI cannot be considered endemic [4]. Vaccination is recommended and practiced widely. Other control measures include movement restriction and quarantine and are established on a country-by-country basis, also taking into account the status (free or infected) of the country. In some countries, the United Kingdom for example, horse racing authorities have made EI vaccination mandatory [5] and similar regulations have been applied by show and event authorities.

Canine influenza emerged in 2004 in the United States [6] and is caused by an H3N8 subtype IAV, closely related to the equine H3N8 strain. It is now endemic across the United States. Sporadic spill-overs of equine H3N8 have occurred in dogs in the United Kingdom and in Australia [7], but infection does not appear to have become established in dogs in these countries. Vaccines are available in the United States.

An avian origin H3N2 virus has also been reported in dogs in South Korea [7]. More recently, infections of dogs with H1N1 pdm2009 virus have been reported [8].

Canine influenza is not an OIE listed disease, therefore there are no international guidelines for canine influenza for the regulation of trade in animals.

The multifaceted characteristics of IAV infections in animals inevitably result in different approaches in managing and controlling the disease, which are based both on the virus involved and the species affected. For some species, such as dogs and pigs, influenza is not notifiable and therefore disease control measures are usually applied on a voluntary basis by the farmer, breeder, or owner. Vaccination may be used without any major restrictions. For equids, influenza infections are notifiable at an international level and in some cases at a country level, and the use of vaccine is recommended. Trade of infected animals or commodities may result in spread into free areas, thus laboratory testing and quarantine may be imposed by the importing country.

Infections of birds with any influenza subtype other than H5 or H7 are non-notifiable, while provisions and regulations must be implemented in case of infections caused by viruses of H5 or H7 subtypes. Vaccination for these subtypes therefore cannot be used in an unregulated manner, particularly by countries that want to export live poultry and poultry commodities [3].

Control strategies for influenza in mammals

Swine

Since SI is endemic in all intensive pig farming areas, industrialized countries implement vaccination programs to limit the severity of the clinical condition. Commercially available vaccines are oil-adjuvanted whole virus preparations. The virus seeds contained in the vaccine are of the same subtype and lineage as the viruses that are circulating in the population to be vaccinated. For this reason, strains contained in US vaccines are different from those contained in European vaccines [2, 9]. In the European Union, vaccines for SI that are licensed in most countries were developed in the late 1980s to early 1990s with the H1N1 and H3N2 viruses that were circulating in pigs at that time. To date, their antigenic content has not been updated, and the original 20-year-old seed strains are still used for vaccine manufacture. Following the emergence and spread of the human-like H1N2 viruses in the late 1990s, a trivalent vaccine including this "novel" strain was developed and licensed in 2010. At the time of writing, EU experts have recommended against the inclusion of H1N1pdm2009 in commercial vaccines against influenza of pigs.

In the United States, licensing of SI vaccines is less cumbersome than in the European Union, and for this reason there is a greater availability of products on the market and these are also updated on a regular basis [2]. The first SI vaccine was licensed in 1994 in the United States, and contained the classic swine H1N1 virus. A monovalent H3N2 vaccine was made available soon after the emergence and spread of this strain in the US pig population in 1998. The co-circulation of different strains, and the necessity of reducing the number of administrations, resulted in the development and marketing of combined H1–H3 vaccines. As a result of the emergence of the H1N1pdm2009 virus and of its spill-over into pigs, the US Department of Agriculture (USDA) approved and licensed a monovalent vaccine in 2009 [10]. Some commercially available vaccines in the United States contain representatives of different intrasubtypic clusters (e.g., H1α cluster, H1β cluster) [2].

There has been significant debate on the necessity to update the seed viruses contained in SI vaccines regularly because of the occurrence of antigenic drift. The general consensus is that unless a completely new variant emerges, vaccines currently available appear to be efficacious. This has to be correlated with a variety of factors such as the adjuvant – which enhances the breadth of immune response, and to other factors that go beyond the properties of the vaccine itself, including the presence of herd immunity, derived from previous exposures or maternally derived antibodies.

Vaccination schemes for fattening pigs are based on a double intramuscular administration (2–4 weeks apart). Sow herds are vaccinated twice as gilts, with a booster shot 3–6 weeks before farrowing.

There are a variety of products currently under development that exploit novel technology systems. These are not licensed yet and cannot compete for efficacy, safety, and cost with conventional vaccines.

They have been reviewed by Ma and Richt [9] and Van Reeth and Ma [2].

Equids

Although causative virus of EI was first described in 1956, outbreaks of what is now recognized as EI have been recorded throughout history, including a significant outbreak in the United States in 1872. Because of the considerable impact EI has on the horse industry, following the recognition of EI virus, specific vaccines were developed and have been available since the 1960s. Conventional, whole virus, adjuvant vaccines have been used throughout the years and are still commercially available. Subunit "split" vaccines were developed at a later stage and are widely used. In the past decade novel vaccines, most notably canary-pox vectored and live-attenuated vaccines, have been developed and marketed and are now commercially available in some countries. None of the EI vaccines are proven to afford sterile immunity, and thus clinically healthy, infected animals may carry the virus and spread infection to naïve or unprotected animals.

As with other influenza infections of mammals, especially humans, EI viruses undergo antigenic variation by antigenic drift, and thus an international effort is necessary to make recommendations on the updating of vaccines for horses worldwide, bearing in mind the international mobility of horses. This is achieved by the Expert Surveillance Panel (ESP), which includes experts on EI and representatives of the OIE and World Health Organization [11]. This group reviews existing data on surveillance and on viral antigenicity and phylogeny on a regular basis and makes recommendations which are published in the *OIE Bulletin*.

The majority of vaccines against EI contain both EI subtypes (i.e., H7N7 and H3N8). Given that there has been no evidence of circulation of viruses of H7N7 subtype in the last 20 years and its presence in the horse population has been questioned for some time [12], the ESP recommended that H7N7 should no longer be included in EI vaccines some years ago and continue that recommendation to date [13].

In contrast, viruses of H3N8 subtype are still widespread and have undergone substantial antigenic and genetic evolution since their initial isolation. By the mid-1990s it appeared that the original 1963 A/

Equine/Miami/63 strain had diverged into two lineages – the American and Eurasian – based on the original geographic distribution. The American lineage has evolved subsequently into three sublineages: Argentina, Kentucky, and Florida. The Florida sublineage has evolved further into two clades: clade 1 viruses, which were responsible for important disease outbreaks in South Africa in 2003 and Australia and Japan in 2007, and clade 2 viruses, which have been circulating in Europe since 2003 and have caused recent outbreaks in Mongolia, China, and India [4]. Viruses of the two clades do not show strict geographic limitations and isolates of both clades have been reported from countries across the world. This complex epidemiologic situation has led the ESP to recommend in 2010 that both clade 1 and 2 viruses of the Florida sublineage are included in vaccines for the international market [4].

Vaccination for EI is practiced widely and is used for different purposes. In endemic countries, vaccination is seen as a tool for reducing the clinical impact of EI, especially in performance horses such as race, eventing, and show horses. Some equestrian bodies have made vaccination against EI mandatory for the participation in shows and competitions. In countries that are infection-free, vaccination is usually only allowed under well-defined circumstances to protect genetic stock or horses of value from incursions of the virus. The risk of incursions is minimized in these countries by requiring vaccination and quarantine of imported horses. Notwithstanding strict import regulations in free countries, incursions of EI viruses do occur, and may result in an emergency for the veterinary services and a disaster for the equine industry. It is estimated that the EI outbreak in Australia in 2007 cost over 1 billion Australian dollars.

Dogs

The US canine influenza epidemic is the result of a rare event of adaptive evolution of an influenza virus to a new host. The H3N8 virus, which has spread rapidly and become established in the US dog population, is of equine origin and in marked contrast to the H3N2 avian origin North Korean virus incursion into dogs [7].

Initially, the H3N8 virus infected racing greyhounds in which it became widespread. In 2 months, infection spread from Florida to tracks in six states,

and within the next couple of years spread across the entire United States.

Direct control measures such as avoiding contact with infected dogs and kennel hygiene are useful and recommended; however, they have often appeared to be insufficient to prevent infection [14].

In May 2009, USDA approved the first licensure of a canine influenza vaccine, based on an inactivated whole virus preparation. The vaccine is able to reduce the severity of clinical signs and to diminish shedding levels during infection, but, as with influenza vaccines developed for other species, sterile immunity is not achieved and infected vaccinated dogs may infect naïve dogs.

This vaccine is recommended by the American Veterinary Medical Association (AVMA) as a "lifestyle" vaccine which is useful for a subpopulation of dogs that is at risk of infection. This includes racing greyhounds and also dogs that participate in shows and exhibitions or dogs that are housed in communal facilities [14]. Currently, there is no vaccine licensed for canine influenza outside the United States.

Control strategies for influenza in birds

The existence of two clinical forms of influenza in birds, one of which is a deadly disease, complicates the regulatory aspects both for control and for trade purposes. The intrinsic variability in the behaviour of IAV in animal models adds outliers to the categorization adopted. In order to understand the scientific rationale behind regulation the biology of influenza viruses must be understood.

For all IAV the hemagglutinin glycoprotein is produced as a precursor, HA0, which requires post-translational cleavage by host proteases before it is functional and virus particles are infectious [15]. The HA0 precursor proteins of IAV of low virulence for poultry (LPAI viruses) have a single arginine at the cleavage site and another basic amino acid at position −3 or −4 from the cleavage site. These viruses are limited to cleavage by extracellular host proteases such as trypsin-like enzymes and thus restricted to replication at sites in the host where such enzymes are found (i.e., the respiratory and intestinal tracts). HPAI viruses possess multiple basic amino acids (arginine and lysine) at their HA0 cleavage sites either as a result of apparent insertion or apparent substitution [16–18] and appear to be cleavable by an intracellular ubiquitous protease(s), probably one or more proprotein-processing subtilisin-related endoproteases of which furin is the leading candidate [19]. HPAI viruses are able to replicate throughout the bird, damaging vital organs and tissues, which results in disease and death. Viruses of all H (H1–H16) subtypes cause LPAI; only some H5 and H7 viruses cause HPAI.

It appears that HPAI viruses arise by mutation after a LPAI precursor has been introduced into poultry. It follows that all HPAI viruses should have a LPAI progenitor, although the latter have only been isolated in a limited number of cases. Several mechanisms appear to be responsible for this mutation. Most HPAI viruses appear to have arisen as result of spontaneous duplication of purine triplets which results in the insertion of basic amino acids at the HA0 cleavage site and that this occurs due to a transcription fault by the polymerase complex [20]. However, as pointed out by Perdue et al. [20], this is clearly not the only mechanism by which HPAI viruses arise as some appear to result from nucleotide substitution rather than insertion while others have insertions without repeating nucleotides. The Chile 2002 [21] and the Canada 2004 [22] H7N3 HPAI viruses have unusual cleavage site amino acid sequences, which appear to have arisen as a result of recombination with other genes (nucleoprotein gene and matrix gene, respectively) resulting in an insertion at the cleavage site of 11 amino acids for the Chile virus and 7 amino acids for the Canadian virus.

The factors that bring about mutation from LPAI to HPAI are not known. In some instances mutation seems to have taken place rapidly (at the primary site) after the assumed introduction from wild birds; in others the LPAI virus has circulated in poultry for months before mutating. Therefore it is impossible to predict if and when this mutation will occur. However, it can be reasonably assumed that the wider the circulation of LPAI of H5 or H7 subtypes in poultry, the higher the chance that mutation to HPAI will occur.

The marked variation in disease caused by LPAI and HPAI viruses of the same subtype and the fact that, to date, two subtypes H5 and H7 have been shown to be responsible for HPAI means that careful, specific definition is required for statutory control and trade purposes.

Until 2005, European Union and OIE regulations for statutory control purposes and trade only included HPAI viruses. However, the increasing evidence that HPAI viruses emerged in domestic poultry from LPAI progenitors of H5 and H7 subtype viruses and the unpredictability of when the mutation to virulence would occur led to the conclusion that not only HPAI viruses, but also their LPAI progenitors should be controlled in domestic poultry [23, 24]. As a result, the European Union Scientific Committee on Animal Health and Animal Welfare put forward a proposal for a new definition [25]: "an infection of poultry caused by either any influenza A virus that has an intravenous pathogenicity index in 6-week-old chickens greater than 1.2 or any influenza A virus of H5 or H7 subtype." A very similar definition was adopted by the OIE during its 73rd General Session [26].

For the purposes of this Terrestrial Code, avian influenza in its notifiable form (NAI) is defined as an infection of poultry caused by any influenza A virus of the H5 or H7 subtypes or by any AI virus with an intravenous pathogenicity index (IVPI) greater than 1.2 (or as an alternative at least 75% mortality) as described below. NAI viruses can be divided into highly pathogenic notifiable avian influenza (HPNAI) and low pathogenicity notifiable avian influenza (LPNAI):

a) HPNAI viruses have an IVPI in 6-week-old chickens greater than 1.2 or, as an alternative, cause at least 75% mortality in 4- to 8-week-old chickens infected intravenously. H5 and H7 viruses which do not have an IVPI of greater than 1.2 or cause less than 75% mortality in an intravenous lethality test should be sequenced to determine whether multiple basic amino acids are present at the cleavage site of the haemagglutinin molecule (HA0); if the amino acid motif is similar to that observed for other HPNAI isolates, the isolate being tested should be considered as HPNAI.

b) LPNAI are all influenza A viruses of H5 and H7 subtype that are not HPNAI viruses. The term low pathogenicity avian influenza [LPAI] is then used to define all infections caused by AI viruses that are not NAI viruses.

The most significant change in trading regulations with reference to AI, is that in order to export, countries/zones/compartments must demonstrate that they are free from infection. In the past, when only HPNAI was notifiable, freedom from infection relied primarily on the absence of clinical cases. With LPNAI being included in the definition, it follows that it is not possible to rely on clinical evidence alone and that freedom must be demonstrated through appropriate surveillance programs.

The revision of the definition of avian influenza has resulted in modified trade requirements, as these now also apply for LPAI of H5 and H7 subtypes [27]. However, these differ between LPAI and HPAI and are recommended proportionate to the risks posed by the various commodities. Linked to the application of these new requirements guidelines for AI surveillance and for the implementation of the concept of "compartmentalization" have now been included in the Terrestrial Code for 2005.

Direct control measures for poultry

Biosecurity

The term biosecurity refers to any physical barrier or work practice that is put in place to prevent the introduction of virus to susceptible birds or the spread from infected birds. The extent to which total exclusion can be achieved clearly varies with the way birds are reared. There is also a need to balance the cost of biosecurity against the value of the birds. For example, high value elite and grandparent poultry flocks may be reared in high security bird- and rodent-proofed buildings with filtered air, treated food, and regimens of disinfection, clothes changing, and showering for staff and fomites entering the building. In marked contrast, birds such as ducks in much of Asia and ostriches in South Africa tend to be reared extensively with little or no biosecurity measures in place. The reservoir for all LPAI viruses, including H5 and H7 subtypes that potentially may mutate to HPAI viruses, is wild birds, and there is some evidence of spread of Asian H5N1 HPAI virus from wild birds to poultry. Measures aimed at prevention of primary introduction will therefore involve the exclusion from the flock of wild birds or items, including drinking water and food that could be contaminated with infective wild bird excreta. Once an outbreak has occurred measures need to be put in place on infected premises to contain the outbreak to a minimum. Although

there is some evidence that secondary spread of Asian HPAI H5N1 virus may have been the result of wild bird movements in nearly all other avian influenza outbreaks that have been investigated and documented the primary cause of secondary spread has been the movement of personnel between infected and susceptible birds. It is important that personnel access to flocks should be minimized and controlled at all times, not just during disease outbreaks, and regimens of clothing change, equipment disinfection, and other basic hygiene controls enforced before access to the birds is allowed. It is especially important to ensure thorough disinfection of trucks, such as those delivering food, and other vehicles before entering a farm.

Quarantine

When moving live birds, especially between countries, a measure for controlling the possible spread of specified diseases is to move the birds to secure holdings for a prescribed length of time during which they can be monitored and tested for the absence of the causative organism (i.e., quarantine). For most movements of commercial poultry quarantine is not a practicable option primarily because of the length of time involved. However, because of their link to the spread of Newcastle disease virus in the 1970s quarantine of captive caged birds has been practiced since that time in many countries. In the European Union countries quarantine of captive caged birds was required from 2000 by a Commission Decision [28]. This involved moving imported birds to designated, officially approved, quarantine premises where they are held for 30 days and subjected to at least two veterinary inspections at the beginning and the end of this period before release. During the 30-day period either the imported birds or sentinel birds must undergo laboratory testing for Newcastle disease and avian influenza. In addition, birds becoming sick or those that have died have to be tested for virus isolation and detection. Similar quarantine is required in the United States [29].

Since the 1970s, avian influenza viruses have been isolated regularly from captive caged birds held in quarantine, usually these have been LPAI viruses of H3 or H4 subtype, although occasionally virus of H5 or H7 have been isolated [30]. The effectiveness of quarantine of caged birds was both tested and demonstrated in England 2005 when birds held in quarantine showing high mortality were shown to be infected with Asian HPAI H5N1 virus. As a result of this outbreak and other evidence of HPAI virus in wild and wild captured birds, imports of such birds were suspended in the European Union and many other countries.

Control in live bird markets

Live bird markets (LBMs), which usually involve multiple bird species, rapid turnover of birds and usually nonexistent biosecurity have long been recognized as a source and reservoir of avian influenza viruses. During the recent spread of viruses of H5N1 and H9N2 subtypes surveys of LBMs in countries experiencing epizootics have often revealed the presence of one or both of these viruses [31–34]. Samaan et al [35]. identified five critical control points for limiting H5N1 infections in LBMs, which essentially involved imposing biosecurity and hygiene measures.

In Hong Kong in 2001 and 2003 the strategy of having one and then two monthly rest days in which the LBMs were depopulated and subjected to thorough cleansing and disinfected was implemented [36, 37]. Lau et al [37]. reported a 58% reduction in the isolation rate of H9N2 viruses in minor poultry species, but only a 27% reduction in chickens; the second rest day appeared to have little affect on isolation rates.

In the United States LBMs in north-eastern states have been known to be sources of LPAI influenza viruses, including those of H5 and H7 subtypes for some time, and surveillance since 1986 has regularly resulted in virus isolations. LBMs have also been the origins of notifiable LPAI infections occurring in commercial poultry [38, 39]. Initial attempts at controlling avian influenza in LBMs included enforced depopulation and temporary closure [40], which proved to be effective for a limited period. More recently, the US Veterinary Services have drawn up measures to be implemented in a cooperative program incorporating LBMs, the commercial poultry industry, and state and US veterinary services for the control of avian influenza in LBMs. These measures include testing for avian influenza at any time, but at least quarterly; regular quarterly closing for a minimum of 24 hours with depopulation and disinfection and cleaning; and a series of biosecurity measures including training of staff and regular inspections [41].

Vaccination

Background and rationale for using vaccines

In poultry and other birds the main protective immune response against influenza viruses is the result of antibodies produced primarily against the functional surface glycoprotein hemagglutinin. There is some evidence that antibodies to the other important surface glycoprotein, neuraminidase, of which there are nine subtypes (N1–N9) may also confer some protection, but this is to a much lesser extent.

Historical reservations concerning the use of vaccination against avian influenza viruses of H5 and H7 subtypes because it was considered that it would interfere with the rapid diagnosis of HPAI have been modified in recent times in a number of countries where avian influenza in poultry has become endemic as a result of the spread of Asian lineage H5N1 virus across Asia and into Europe and Africa, and the spread of H9N2 infections across Asia. To date, only the use of vaccines against avian influenza viruses of H5 and H7 subtypes is regulated. Vaccines against any other subtype must be licensed and approved, but their use does not impact international trade.

Vaccination of poultry has proved to be a means by which the clinical signs may be reduced or nullified, and a means by which the duration and extent of shedding are reduced. The vaccination of susceptible animals will result in survival in the face of a HPAI challenge and the preservation of a healthy status in case of LPAI. Vaccination has also been shown to increase the resistance of poultry to field challenge; that is, infection may be achieved in vaccinated birds but only with a higher dose of challenge virus than needed to infect fully susceptible birds [42]. However, currently available vaccines do not afford sterile immunity, and subsequent field challenge may result in shedding of viable virus. For this reason, trade regulations for notifiable avian influenza (NAI), allow the export of vaccinated birds or their commodities but only if it is proven that they originate from nonexposed flocks. This requires the application of a DIVA (differentiating infected from vaccinated animals) vaccination strategy, which demonstrates by serologic or virologic diagnosis that field challenge has not occurred. From a disease control and eradication perspective, a DIVA approach also allows the identification of active circulation of virus in the vaccinated population and thus the ability to intervene with appropriate complementary measures (e.g., movement restriction, quarantine, controlled marketing, and stamping out) if a clinically healthy flock is proven to be exposed to field challenge. Targeted elimination of vaccinated or exposed flocks is a means by which infection may be eradicated from a given area. It is important therefore that, if eradication is the ultimate goal, vaccination is seen as a tool to maximize the impact of other control measures, especially good biosecurity, and never the sole method of disease control.

Before a decision is made to vaccinate, consideration must be given to a number of variable factors that will impact on the efficacy of the vaccine and for which there may not be good evidence on which to reach a valid conclusion. Assumptions may have to be made on:

• Whether the level of desirable immunity will be achieved and how long it is likely to last after vaccination.
• How frequently vaccination should take place.
• How close antigenically are the vaccine and the field virus.
• Whether the vaccine will be effective in the host in which it is to be used.

The latter point is particularly pertinent as usually vaccine efficacy studies have been performed in chickens and turkeys but of necessity it has been assumed that similar immune responses will give similar protection in other species, including zoo birds [43]. The danger of such extrapolation was shown in experimental work using HPAI H7N7 as a challenge virus in which van der Goot et al [44, 45]. showed for chickens and ringed teal ducks (*Callonetta leucophrys*) that optimal vaccination reduced excretion and increased the infective dose so that transmission between birds was dramatically reduced. However, in golden pheasants (*Chrysolophus pictus*), while clinical protection was achieved, vaccination had no effect on excretion of challenge virus and no influence on transmission [45]. The problem this creates is that, similar to suboptimal or inappropriate use of vaccine, vaccination of some species may remove or reduce clinical disease without reducing transmission, leading to uncontrolled viral circulation in a given population [46].

When vaccination has been used it has usually been within the context of one of three strategies [47]:
1. *Routine* The routine, or prophylactic, use of vaccination has been usually applied, sometimes com-

pulsorily, in countries where the disease is already considered endemic. If routine vaccination is employed without the application of monitoring systems, strict biosecurity, and depopulation in the face of infection, it seems probable that, if not already endemic, the virus would become so in vaccinated poultry populations. Long-term circulation of virus in a vaccinated population may result in both genetic and antigenic changes in the virus. This has proved to be the case in Mexico where LPAI virus of H5N2 subtype has circulated for over 10 years in the face of widespread prophylactic use of vaccines [48]. Recently, Cattoli et al [49]. have shown the HA gene of HPAI H5N1 viruses are evolving much more rapidly in countries using mass vaccination than viruses in countries that are not.

2. *Preventive* Preventive vaccination is usually applied when there is a perceived serious threat of introduction of avian influenza virus and risk assessments or past experience suggests that other control measures are unlikely to be successful. Alternatively, it could be used when the virus has been introduced in to one avian sector and as a consequence represents a significant threat to another sector. If this strategy is employed, eradication of any subsequent introduction will only be achieved if vaccinated birds are subjected to careful monitoring, preferably based on a strategy for detecting infected vaccinated birds (DIVA).

3. *Emergency* This would normally be employed once an outbreak has occurred as an addition to normal biosecurity and stamping out measures, probably by vaccinating within a restriction zone and outside that in a buffer zone, the aim being to reduce spread within those areas. In these circumstances and in the absence of a DIVA program it would be usual for vaccinated birds to be slaughtered. As an alternative the vaccinated population could be closely monitored and field exposure excluded, this would result in a "vaccination to live" policy as commodities could still be marketed.

Types of avian influenza vaccines

Most avian influenza vaccines currently being produced and marketed have been prepared conventionally by emulsifying infective allantoic fluid inactivated by beta-propiolactone or formalin with mineral oil.

In the past, vaccines have been either prepared from the virus isolate(s) causing the epizootic [50, 51] – autogenous vaccines – or from LPAI viruses possessing the same hemagglutinin subtype as the field virus that yield high concentrations of antigen when grown [52]. Conventional inactivated vaccines aimed at H5, H7, and H9 subtypes are commercially available and have been licensed for use in a number of countries. The H5 and H7 vaccines have been prepared from LPAI viruses so that high biosecurity facilities are not required during their manufacture, but there is some debate on the importance of the degree of antigenic match to field virus of the same subtype.

The application of reverse genetics technology has enabled the generation of entirely avian or avian–human reassortant viruses (see Chapter 9) [53–57]. These viruses have all been further modified to have a LPAI HA0 cleavage site and have been used experimentally or in the field as inactivated vaccines. One of these products based on PR8 virus genes, to allow optimum growth in eggs, with H5 and N1 genes from A/goose/Guandong [56], is being used extensively in the People's Republic of China.

An alternative strategy has been to create avian influenza vaccines by inserting genes from avian influenza viruses, usually the HA gene, in to a live vector virus, resulting in production of the hemagglutinin and a host immune response to it when the "recombinant vaccine" vector virus is used to infect a host. One of the main advantages of recombinant vaccines is that usually both humoral and cellular immune responses are stimulated. The earliest of these types of vaccine were produced by inserting an H5 gene in to fowl poxvirus [58–61] and, following field trials, several of these have been licensed for use in a number of countries. Other viruses that have been used as vectors for expressing avian influenza HA genes are infectious laryngotracheitis virus, vaccinia [62], human adenovirus 5, Venezuelan encephalitis virus, retrovirus, and Newcastle disease (ND) virus [63]. Most of these have only been used experimentally, but the idea of using ND virus to express avian influenza HA genes [64] has been developed further, not least because the recombinant virus has been shown to protect against both HPAI and virulent ND viruses [65]. A recombinant virus based on ND virus vaccine strain La Sota and expressing the Asian lineage H5 HA gene was produced in China [66] and reported to be efficacious in protection studies with either

virus. This virus has been licensed as a vaccine and billions of doses have been used in China in recent years [67].

Despite the advantages of recombinant vaccines there are also problems, chief amongst these are if birds to be vaccinated already have immunity to the vector or if the vector virus has a limited host range.

Due to antigenic variation, seed viruses to be used in avian influenza vaccines need to be carefully selected. Antigenic and genetic evolution occurring for example within the H5N1 viral population requires ongoing update of seed strains for use in given areas [68]. The OIE/FAO network of expertise on animal influenza (OFFLU) has established technical working groups that make recommendations to national authorities and vaccine manufacturers on this issue [69].

Use of avian influenza vaccines

It is not the intention in this section to produce a list of the use of vaccines against avian influenza in different countries and especially not the use and circumstances in which vaccination against HPAI H5N1 and LPAI H9N2 viruses are currently used in many countries; an excellent detailed review was produced by Swayne et al [67]. to which the reader is referred.

Until recent years use of inactivated vaccines against avian influenza was fairly limited. Vaccination had been used in the United States on an emergency basis against LPAI H7 viruses [70, 71] or prophylactically against contemporaneous LPAI viruses of wild birds [50, 72]. More recently, the inactivated vaccine has been used in breeder turkeys in the United States to protect against H1 and H3 swine influenza viruses [73], although this has not been without problems caused by antigenic variation between vaccine and field strains [73].

An inactivated vaccine against H5N2 subtype virus was first used in Mexico in response to HPAI outbreaks in 1994–1995. The HPAI virus appears to have been eradicated; but LPAI virus of H5N2 subtype has continued to circulate, despite the use of billions of doses of inactivated H5N2 vaccine and an almost equal number of doses of a recombinant fowlpox-AI-H5 vaccine [74, 75]. Vaccination strategies employed in Pakistan also appear to have had only limited success. Initially, vaccination was used as part of the control of HPAI H7N3 virus in 1995 [76], but H7N3 HPAI outbreaks re-occurred in 2003–2004 [77]. Although these HPAI H7N3 outbreaks appear to have been brought under control, Naeem et al. [77]. reported that control measures, including use of inactivated vaccine, were unsuccessful in controlling LPAI H9N2 outbreaks first seen in Pakistan in 2005.

In Italy, vaccination was used successfully a part of the emergency control measures to combat several introductions of H5 and H7 LPAI viruses, although other measures including a DIVA strategy and stamping out of infected vaccinated birds were also put in place [78].

The spread of LPAI H9N2 virus across Asia has resulted in the employment of vaccination using inactivated virus in many countries including Pakistan [77], Iran [79], and the People's Republic of China [80], and several countries in the Middle East.

The emergence and spread of HPAI H5N1 resulted in the adoption of vaccination strategies in a number of countries, including the implementation of prophylactic vaccination policies in several. The amount of vaccine used to combat HPAI viruses is enormous. Swayne et al [67]. estimated that between 2002–2010 more than 113 billion doses, mainly against H5 viruses but including a small proportion of H7 vaccines, were used in 15 countries with a combined poultry population of more than 131 billion birds. Most of the vaccine (>90%) has been used in China, but significant amounts have been used in Egypt, Indonesia, and Vietnam [67] in each of these four countries HPAI H5N1 is considered to be enzootic or there are recurring outbreaks [81]. Mass vaccination in countries where there are large poultry populations requires an enormous commitment in terms of finance and resources. In China, the poultry population is in excess of 15 billion birds, requiring the use of nearly 24 billion doses of vaccine in 2010 [67].

In the European Union, "preventive" vaccination against H5 viruses has been allowed in outdoor poultry and in zoo birds in several countries in recent years. For zoo birds this is something of a lottery, and while vaccination results in an immune response in most bird species [43] the efficacy of vaccination in these hosts is unknown. This practice has been discontinued following epidemiologic evidence of a low risk of H5N1 incursion.

Detection of infection in vaccinated flocks and vaccinated birds

Many national and international authorities advocate that any use of vaccination should involve a DIVA strategy with a goal of eradication rather than containment, which is unlikely to be achieved by vaccination alone. The attractiveness of such a strategy is that vaccination would allow the slowing down of the spread of virus so that it can be contained more easily, but the detection of infected vaccinated birds would allow them to be removed from the poultry population. Eradication could be achieved without massive losses from widespread outbreaks or resorting to large-scale pre-emptive culling, thus minimizing the economic impact that has often resulted from HPAI epizootics [82]. A DIVA strategy is necessary because, while field virus is able to infect vaccinated birds and be excreted, there is usually a marked lack of clinical signs seen in infected vaccinated birds, which would mean that HPAI or LPAI viruses of H5 or H7 subtypes could infect a flock and circulate for some time in that flock unnoticed.

A method for detecting whether field virus has infected a vaccinated flock would be to leave a portion of the flock unvaccinated and monitor these sentinel birds regularly for clinical signs and the presence of virus or antibodies. In practice, identifying and sampling sentinel birds raises some management problems and this has led to the development of several different systems that would allow the detection of field challenge of vaccinated birds.

• In Italy in 2000 vaccination was used to supplement direct control measures to combat outbreaks of LPAI caused by a H7N1 virus. The vaccine used contained H7N3 virus and vaccinated and field exposed birds were differentiated using a serologic test to detect specific anti-N1 antibodies [23, 78, 83]. The same strategy was used to control LPAI caused by H7N3 in Italy in 2002–2003 [83], in this case with an H7N1 vaccine. In both cases vaccination with stamping out using this DIVA strategy resulted in eradication of the field virus. Although successful on these two occasions, the use of antibodies to the neuraminidase of the field virus would be jeopardized if a new field virus with a different N-antigen arises or if other viruses with different N subtypes are already circulating.

- The use of vaccines containing only HA (e.g., recombinant vaccines) allows classic immunodiffusion tests or ELISA tests based on nucleoprotein or matrix protein to be used to detect infection in vaccinated birds.
- If inactivated whole virus vaccines are used it has been suggested that detection of antibodies to the nonstructural virus proteins that are only produced during natural infection could be used in a DIVA strategy. However, field validation of this system is lacking [84].

Conclusions

If an animal disease is not considered a sufficient threat to trade or human health that outbreaks do not require notification to national or international authorities, then it is inevitable that treatment and control be developed on a voluntary basis and the goal will be to reduce the clinical impact of the disease, mainly for reasons that are linked to the economic repercussions of infection and will not aim at eradication. In endemic countries, vaccination for swine, equine, and canine influenza aim at preventing viral respiratory damage, with a view to safeguarding animal performances. For pigs, a viral respiratory infection such as influenza will result in reduced food consumption, and therefore diminished food conversion ratios, and possibly the occurrence of a bacterial superinfection with a resulting pneumonia, which would require antibiotic treatment and would worsen production indicators. For horses and dogs, an influenza infection would prevent the animal from racing or participating at any show or exhibition with associated economic damage, and may also be linked to veterinary interventions in severe outbreaks or if there are bacterial complications. By and large, the same situation exists for all non-notifiable subtypes of avian influenza (i.e., H1–H4, H6, H8–H16). This approach to control will not result in eradication and is most likely to sustain the status of endemicity.

For notifiable influenza viruses (i.e., equine influenza in free areas and avian influenza H5 and H7 subtype viruses) control policies in most countries have been be designed with the ultimate goal of eradication. Vaccination can have an important role in such control provided it is linked to careful monitoring and surveillance strategies that ensure vaccination is used correctly and optimally and allow the detection animals that subsequently become infected with the field virus. If reliance is placed on vaccination alone for the control of clinical disease it seems inevitable that not only will the virus spread to free areas (as in the Australian equine influenza outbreak in 2007), but it will become or remain endemic, as HPAI H5N1 virus has in a number of countries.

The perpetuation of a zoonotic influenza infection in vast animal populations, such as poultry, is not only a significant cost in terms of animal health and loss of production, but also a potential serious risk in terms of human health, as one of these viruses could become transmissible in humans and ignite a pandemic. It would seem imperative that to reduce the animal health burden and public health threat, national and international efforts to control animal influenza virus infections should be aimed at eradication rather than limiting the economic impact of disease.

Acknowledgment

The authors wish to acknowledge Francesca Ellero for editorial assistance.

References

1. Capua I, Alexander DJ. The challenge of avian influenza to the veterinary community. Avian Pathol. 2006;35: 189–205.
2. Van Reeth K, Ma W. Swine influenza virus vaccines: to change, or not to change – that's the question. Curr Top Microbiol Immunol. 2012:Sept 13 [Epub ahead of print].
3. Terrestrial Animal Health Code. Criteria for listing diseases. Chapter 1.2. OIE Manual 2010. http://web. oie.int/eng/normes/mcode/en_chapitre_1.1.2.pdf (accessed 12 March 2013).
4. Cullinane A, Elton D, Mumford J. Equine influenza – surveillance and control. Influenza Other Respi Viruses. 2010;4:339–44.
5. British Horseracing Authority. The control of equine influenza in British horseracing. 2011. Available from: http://www.britishhorseracing.com/resources/equine -science-and-welfare/equine-influenza-control.asp (accessed 18 February 2013).
6. Crawford PC, Dubovi EJ, Castleman WL, Stephenson I, Gibbs EP, Chen L, et al. Transmission of equine influenza virus to dogs. Science. 2005;310:482–5.

7. Gibbs EPJ, Anderson TC. Equine and canine influenza: a review of current events. Anim Health Res Rev. 2010; 11(1):43–51.

8. Song D, Lee C, Bokyu K, Jung K, Oh T, Kim H, et al. Experimental infection of dogs with avian-origin canine influenza A virus (H3N2). Emerg Infect Dis. 2009;15: 56–8.

9. Ma W, Richt JA. Swine influenza vaccines: current status and future perspectives. Anim Health Res Rev. 2010;11(1):81–96.

10. United States Department of Agriculture. USDA issues conditional license for pandemic H1N1 vaccine for swine. 2009. Available from: http://www.aphis.usda.gov/newsroom/content/2009/12/h1n1_vaccine.shtml (accessed 18 February 2013).

11. Mumford JA. Biology, epidemiology and vaccinology of equine influenza. Quality control of equine influenza vaccines. Proceedings of the International Symposium organised by the European Directorate for the Quality of Medicines (EDQM), Budapest, 2001:7–12.

12. Webster RG. Are equine 1 influenza viruses still present in horses? Equine Vet J. 1993;25:537–8.

13. OIE Expert Surveillance panel on Equine Influenza Vaccing Composition. 2011. Available from: http://www.oie.int/doc/ged/D10847.PDF (accessed 18 February 2013).

14. American Veterinary Medical Association. Canine influenza virus backgrounder. 2009. Availaible from: https://www.avma.org/KB/Resources/Backgrounders/Pages/Canine-Influenza-Backgrounder.aspx (accessed 11 February 2013).

15. Rott R. The pathogenic determinant of influenza virus. Vet Microbiol. 1992;33:303–10.

16. Senne DA, Panigrapy B, Kawaoka Y. Survey of the haemagglutinin (HA) cleavage site sequence of H5 and H7 avian influenza viruses: amino acid sequence at the HA cleavage site as a marker of pathogenicity potential. Avian Dis. 1996;40:425–37.

17. Vey M, Olrich M, Adler S, Klenk HD, Rott R, Garten W. Haemagglutinin activation of pathogenic avian influenza viruses of serotype H7 requires the recognition motif R-X-R/K-R. Virology. 1992;188:408–13.

18. Wood GW, McCauley JW, Bashiruddin JB, Alexander DJ. Deduced amino acid sequences at the haemagglutinin cleavage site of avian influenza A viruses of H5 and H7 subtypes. Arch Virol. 1993;130:209–17.

19. Stieneke-Grober A, Vey M, Angliker H, Shaw E, Thomas G, Roberts C, et al. Influenza virus hemagglutinin with multibasic cleavage site is activated by furin, a subtilisin endoprotease. EMBO J. 1992;11:2407–14.

20. Perdue ML, Crawford JM, Garcia M, et al. Occurrence and possible mechanisms of cleavage site insertions in the avian influenza hemagglutinin gene. Proceedings of the 4th International Symposium on Avian Influenza, Athens, Georgia. US Animal Health Association 1997; 182–93.

21. Suarez DL, Senne DA, Banks J, Brown IH, Essen SC, Lee CW, et al. Recombination resulting in virulence shift in avian influenza outbreak, Chile. Emerg Infect Dis. 2004;10(4):693–9.

22. Pasick J, Handel K, Robinson J. Intersegmental recombination between the haemagglutinin and matrix genes was responsible for the emergence of a highly pathogenic H7N3 avian influenza virus in British Columbia. J Gen Virol. 2005;86:727–31.

23. Capua I, Marangon S. The avian influenza epidemics in Italy, 1999–2000: a review. Avian Pathol. 2000;29: 289–94.

24. Alexander DJ. Should we change the definition of avian influenza for eradication purposes? Proceedings of the 5th International Symposium on Avian Influenza, Athens, Georgia. 2003;47:976–81.

25. Scientific Committee on Animal Health and Animal Welfare (SCAHAW). The definition of avian influenza: the use of vaccination against avian influenza. Report 17 of the European Scientific Committee on animal health and animal welfare adopted 27.06.2000, Sanco/B3/AH/R17/2000, p. 38. 2000.

26. OIE World Health Organization for Animal Health, Terrestrial Animal Health Code, 14th ed Chapter 2.7.12, 2005. OIE, Paris. p. 294–300.

27. OIE Terrestrial Animal Health Code. 2011. Available from: http://www.oie.int/international-standard-setting/terrestrial-code/access-online/ (accessed 11 February 2013).

28. Commission Decision. 2000/666/EC laying down animal health requirements and the veterinary certification for the import of birds, other than poultry, and the conditions for quarantine. Off J Eur Comm. 2000; L278:26–34.

29. United States Department of Agriculture. Animal and Animal Product Import. 2013. Available from: http://www.aphis.usda.gov/import_export/animals/nonus_pet_bird.shtml (accessed 18 February 2013).

30. ESFA Scientific Panel on Animal Health and Animal Welfare. Animal health and welfare aspects of avian influenza. Annex to The EFSA J 2005;266:1–21.

31. Amonsin A, Choatrakol C, Lapkuntod J, Tantilertcharoen R, Thanawongnuwech R, Suradhat S, et al. Influenza virus (H5N1) in live bird markets and food markets, Thailand. Emerg Infect Dis. 2008;14:1739–42.

32. Negovetich NJ, Feeroz MM, Jones-Engel L, Walker D, Alam SM, Hasan K, et al. Live Bird Markets of Bangladesh: H9N2 Viruses and the Near Absence of Highly Pathogenic H5N1 Influenza. PLoS ONE. 2011;6(4): e19311.

33. Mona AM, Samaha HA, Galal SA, Ahmed Z, Schwabenbauer K. Study on the presence of highly pathogenic avian influenza (HPAI) virus and Newcastle disease virus in live bird markets in Tanta District, Gharbia Governorate, Egypt. AHBL 2009.Promoting strategies for prevention and control of HPAI. 2008. Available from: http://www.fao.org/docrep/013/al685e/al685e00.pdf (accessed 11 February 2013).

34. Abdelwhab EM, Selim AA, Arafa A, Galal S, Kilany WH, Hassan MK, et al. Circulation of avian influenza H5N1 in live bird markets in Egypt. Avian Dis. 2010;54(2):911–4.

35. Samaan G, Gultom A, Indriani R, Lokuge K, Kelly PM. Critical control points for avian influenza A H5N1 in live bird markets in low resource settings. Prev Vet Med. 2011;100(1):71–8.

36. Kung NY, Guan Y, Perkins NR, Bissett L, Ellis T, Sims L, et al. The impact of a monthly rest day on avian influenza virus isolation rates in retail live poultry markets in Hong Kong. Avian Dis. 2003;47:1037–41.

37. Lau EH, Leung YH, Zhang LJ, Cowling BJ, Mak SP, Guan Y, et al. Effect of interventions on influenza A (H9N2) isolation in Hong Kong's live poultry markets, 1999–2005. Emerg Infect Dis. 2007;13:1340–7.

38. Senne DA, Pearson JE, Panigrahy B. 1993 live bird markets: a missing link in the epidemiology of avian influenza. In Proceedings of the 3rd International Symposium on Avian Influenza 1992;50–80.

39. Senne DA, Pedersen JC, Panigrahy B. Live-bird markets in the Northeastern United States: a source of avian influenza in commercial poultry. In: Schrijver RS, Koch G, editors. Avian Influenza, Prevention and Control, Springer: Dordrecht, the Netherlands. 2005. p. 19–24.

40. Mullaney R. Live bird market closure activities in the Northeastern United States. Avian Dis. 2003;47:1096–8.

41. APHIS Veterinary Services Fact Sheet. Protecting America's Live Bird Markets. 2007. Available from: http://www.aphis.usda.gov/publications/animal_health/content/printable_version/fs_livebirdmarket.pdf (accessed 18 February 2013).

42. Capua I, Terregino C, Cattoli G, Toffan A. Increased resistance of vaccinated turkeys to experimental infection with an H7N3 low-pathogenicity avian influenza virus. Avian Pathol. 2004;33:158–63.

43. Philippa J, Baas C, Beyer W, Fouchier R, Smith D, Schaftenaar W, et al. Vaccination against highly pathogenic avian influenza H5N1 virus in zoos using an adjuvant inactivated H5N2 vaccine. Vaccine. 2007;25:3800–8.

44. van der Goot JA, Koch G, de Jong MCM, van Boven M. Quantification of the effect of transmission of avian influenza (H7N7) in chickens. Proc Natl Acad Sci. 2005;102:18141–6.

45. van der Goot JA, Koch G, van Boven M, de Jong MC. Variable effect of vaccination against highly pathogenic avian influenza (H7N7) virus on disease and transmission in pheasants and teals. Vaccine. 2007;25:8318–25.

46. Webster RG, Peiris M, Chen H, Guan Y. H5N1 outbreaks and enzootic influenza. Emerg Infect Dis. 2006; 12:3–8.

47. Bruschke C, Bruckner G, Vallat B. International standards and guidelines for vaccination of poultry against highly pathogenic avian influenza. Dev Biol. 2007;130: 23–30.

48. Lee CW, Senne DA, Suarez DL. Effect of vaccine use in the evolution of Mexican lineage H5N2 avian influenza virus. J Virol. 2004;78(15):8372–81.

49. Cattoli G, Fusaro A, Monne I, Coven F, Joannis T, El-Hamid HS, et al. Evidence for differing evolutionary dynamics of A/H5N1 viruses among countries applying or not applying avian influenza vaccination in poultry. Vaccine. 2011;29:9368–75.

50. Halvorson DA. Strengths and weaknesses of vaccines as a control tool. Proceedings of the Fourth International Symposium on Avian Influenza, Athens, Georgia, USA. In: Swayne DE, Slemons RD (editors). US Animal Health Association. 1998; 223–7.

51. Zanella A, Poli G, Bignami M. Avian influenza: Approaches in the control of disease with inactivated vaccines in oil emulsion. Proceedings of the First International Symposium on Avian influenza, 1981. Carter Composition Corporation, Richmond, USA. 1981; p. 180–3.

52. Bankowski RA. Report of the Committee on Transmissible Diseases of Poultry and Other Avian Species. Proceedings of the 88th Annual Meeting of the US Animal Health Association. 1985; p. 474–83.

53. Shi H, Liu XF, Zhang X, Chen S, Sun L, Lu J. Generation of an attenuate H5N1 avian influenza virus vaccine with all eight genes from avian viruses. Vaccine. 2007; 25:7379–84.

54. Song JM, Lee YJ, Jeong OM, Kang HM, Kim HR, Kwon JH, et al. Generation and evaluation of reassortant influenza vaccines made by reverse genetics for H9N2 avian influenza in Korea. Vet Microbiol. 2008; 130(3–4):268–76.

55. Subbarao K, Chen H, Swayne D, Mingay L, Fodor E, Brownlee G, et al. Evaluation of a genetically modified reassortant H5N1 influenza A virus vaccine candidate generated by plasmid-based reverse genetics. Virology. 2003;305:192–200.

56. Tian G, Zhang S, Li Y, Bu Z, Liu P, Zhou J, et al. Protective efficacy in chickens, geese and ducks of an H5N1-inactivated vaccine developed by reverse genetics. Virology. 2005;341:153–62.

57. Webster RG, Webby RJ, Hoffmann E, Rodenberg J, Kumar M, Chu HJ, et al. The immunogenicity and efficacy against H5N1 challenge of reverse genetics-derived H5N3 influenza vaccine in ducks and chickens. Virology. 2006;351:303–11.

58. Beard CW, Schnitzlein WM, Tripathy DN. Protection of chickens against highly pathogenic avian influenza virus (H5N2) by recombinant fowlpox viruses. Avian Dis. 1991;35:356–9.

59. Garcia-Garcia J, Rodriguez VH, Hernandez MA. Experimental studies in field trials with recombinant fowlpox vaccine in broilers in Mexico. Proceedings of the Fourth International Symposium on Avian Influenza, Athens, Georgia, USA. In: Swayne DE, Slemons RD (editors). US Animal Health Association. 1998; 245–52.

60. Qiao CL, Yu KZ, Jiang YP, Jia YQ, Tian GB, Liu M, et al. Protection of chickens against highly lethal H5N1 and H7N1 avian influenza viruses with a recombinant fowlpox virus co-expressing H5 haemagglutinin and N1 neuraminidase genes. Avian Pathol. 2003;32:25–31.

61. Swayne DE, Mickle TR. Protection of chickens against highly pathogenic Mexican-origin H5N2 avian influenza virus by a recombinant fowlpox vaccine. Proceedings the 100th Annual Meeting of the US Animal Health Association, Little Rock, USA. 1997;557–63.

62. Lüschow D, Werner O, Mettenleiter TC, Fuchs W. Protection of chickens from lethal avian influenza A virus infection by live-virus vaccination with infectious laryngotracheitis virus recombinants expressing the hemagglutinin (H5) gene. Vaccine. 2001;19:4249–59.

63. Kapczynski DR, Swayne DE. Influenza vaccines for avian species. Curr Top Microbiol Immunol. 2009;333: 133–52.

64. Nakaya T, Cross J, Park MS, Nakaya Y, Zheng H, Sagrera A, et al. Recombinant Newcastle disease virus as a vaccine vector. J Virol. 2001;74:11868–73.

65. Veits J, Wiesner D, Fuchs W, Hoffmann B, Granzow H, Starick E, et al. A. Newcastle disease virus expressing H5 hemagglutinin gene protects chickens against Newcastle disease and avian influenza. Proc Natl Acad Sci U S A. 2006;103:8197–202.

66. Ge J, Deng G, Wen Z, Tian G, Wang Y, Shi J, et al. Newcastle disease virus-based live attenuated vaccine completely protects chickens and mice from lethal challenge of homologous and heterologous H5N1 avian influenza viruses. J Virol. 2007;81:150–8.

67. Swayne DE, Pavade G, Hamilton K, Vallat B, Miyagishima K. Assessment of national strategies for control 3 of high pathogenicity avian influenza and low 4 pathogenicity notifiable avian influenza in 5 poultry, with emphasis on vaccines and 6 vaccination. Rev Sci Tech. 2011:30:839–70.

68. Beato MS, Monne I, Mancin M, Bertoli E, Capua I. A proof-of-principle study to identify suitable vaccine seed candidates to combat introductions of Eurasian lineage H5 andH7 subtype avian influenza viruses. Avian Pathol. 2010;39:375–82.

69. World Organisation for Animal Health. Avian Influenza Portal. 2013. Available from: http://www.oie.int/ animal-health-in-the-world/web-portal-on-avian -influenza/offlu/ (accessed 18 February 2013).

70. Halvorson DA, Frame DD, Friendshuh AJ, et al. Outbreaks of low pathogenicity avian influenza in USA. Proceedings of the 4th International Symposium on Avian Influenza, Athens, Georgia. US Animal Health Association 1998;36–46.

71. Swayne DE, Akey B. Avian influenza control strategies in the United States of America. In: Schrijver RS, Koch G, editors. Proceedings of the Frontis Workshop on Avian Influenza Prevention and Control. Wageningen, The Netherlands: Springer; 2004. p. 113–32.

72. McCapes RH, Bankowski RA. Use of avian influenza vaccines in California turkey breeders: medical rationale. Proceedings of the Second International Symposium on Avian Influenza, Athens, Georgia, USA. US Animal Health Association, 1985;271–8.

73. Yassine HM, Lee CW, Suarez DL, Saif YM. Genetic and antigenic relatedness of H3 subtype influenza A viruses isolated from avian and mammalian species. Vaccine. 2007;26:966–77.

74. Villarreal-Chavez C. Experience of the control of avian influenza in the Americas. Dev Biol. 2007;130: 53–60.

75. Villareal-Chavez C, Rivera Cruz E. An update on avian influenza in Mexico. Avian Dis. 2003;47:1002–5.

76. Naeem K. The avian influenza H7N3 outbreak in South Central Asia. Proceedings of the Fourth International Symposium on Avian Influenza, Athens, Georgia, USA. In: Swayne DE, Slemons RD, editors. US Animal Health Association, Kennet Square, 1998;31–5.

77. Naeem K, Siddique N, Ayaz M, Jalalee MA. Avian influenza in Pakistan: outbreaks of low- and high-pathogenicity avian influenza in Pakistan during 2003–2006. Avian Dis. 2007;50:189–93.

78. Capua I, Marangon S. The use of vaccination to combat multiple introductions of notifiable avian influenza viruses of the H5 and H7 subtypes between 2000 and 2006 in Italy. Vaccine. 2007;25:4987–95.

79. Vasfi Marandi M, Bozorgmehri Fard MH, Hashemzadeh M. Efficacy of inactivated HPN2 avian influenza vaccine against non-highly pathogenic A/chicken/Iran/ZMT-173/1999. Arch Razi Inst. 2002;53:23–32.

80. Liu HQ, Peng DX, Cheng J, et al. Genetic mutations of the haemagglutinin genes of H9N2 subtype avian influenza viruses. J Yangzhou Univ In: Agric Life Sci (ed). 2002;23:6–9.

81. FAO. Approaches to controlling, preventing and eliminating H5N1 highly pathogenic avian influenza in endemic countries. 2011. Available from: http://www.fao.org/docrep/014/i2150e/i2150e.pdf (accessed 18 February 2013).

82. Food and Agriculture Organization of the United Nations. FAO Recommendations on the Prevention, Control and Eradication of Highly Pathogenic Avian Influenza (HPAI) in Asia September 2004. FAO Position paper. 2004. Available from: http://web.oie.int/eng/AVIAN_INFLUENZA/FAO%20recommendations%20on%20HPAI.pdf (accessed 12 March 2013).

83. Capua I, Alexander DJ. Avian influenza: recent developments. Avian Pathol. 2004;33:393–404.

84. Tumpey TM, Alvarez R, Swayne DE, Suarez DL. A diagnostic aid for differentiating infected from vaccinated poultry based on antibodies to the nonstructural (NS1) protein of influenza A virus. J Clin Microbiol. 2005;43:676–83.

23 Influenza vaccine production

Klaus Stöhr

Novartis Vaccines and Diagnostics, Inc., Cambridge, MA, USA

Influenza vaccines derived from embryonated hens' eggs have been produced for more than 60 years. However, never in history has the production capacity increased so rapidly as in the last decade. At the same time new manufacturing platforms have emerged that could allow for faster and more efficient production of influenza vaccines containing inactivated or live-attenuated virus or recombinant protein containing influenza vaccines. Annual influenza vaccine supply increased to more than 450 million doses and it is estimated that more than 21 companies produced influenza vaccines in 2010; some of this recent production also took place in developing countries. Although the first cell culture derived influenza vaccines have become more widely commercially available since 2010, the majority of influenza vaccines are still inactivated and egg derived. They are produced and used mainly in Europe and North America and in Japan and Australia.

Enormous progress in influenza vaccine manufacturing

The first influenza vaccine was successfully tested in clinical trials in the United States in 1943 and eventually licensed in 1945. The vaccine contained formalin inactivated influenza virus derived from the allantoic fluid from embryonated hens' eggs. This relatively crude preparation caused frequent local and systemic reactions but was 70% protective against H1N1 influenza virus [1]. Today, a large diversity of influenza vaccines has been licensed and successfully marked; the situation is not paralleled by any other human vaccine. Since the middle of the last century progress in influenza vaccine development has been significant. It has been driven by a multitude of factors beyond advancing production technologies:

- Improved productivity: introduction of mechanized egg handling (e.g. inoculation; allantoic fluid harvesting).
- Reduced reactogenicity of the initial relatively crude vaccines:
  - introduction of virus purification methods to reduce egg protein in late 1960s–1970s (continuous flow sharples centrifuges were replaced by continuous high-speed ultracentrifugation; introduction of sucrose density gradient virus purification)
  - additional downstream processing to move away from whole-virion to split and subunit vaccines during the 1970s–1980s.
- Accelerated and optimized production: introduction of cell culture derived surface protein based and cell, bacteria, and plant derived recombinant candidate vaccines from the 1990s to today.
- Enhanced clinical efficacy and breadth of protection particularly in the elderly and children: live-attenuated vaccines, adjuvantation, increased hemagglutinin (HA) antigen content, intradermal application.

Textbook of Influenza, Second Edition. Edited by Robert G. Webster, Arnold S. Monto, Thomas J. Braciale, and Robert A. Lamb.

- Rapidly ramped up production during a pandemic with potential for reducing idle capacities in the inter-pandemic period: cell, plant, and bacteria derived candidate vaccines.

In addition, egg quality control and supply have significantly improved over the years. Virus seed preparation has also evolved not only to address regulatory requirements, but also to improve virus yield per egg and thus productivity. These production process improvements and the introduction over the years of good manufacturing practice (GMP), quality assurance and control systems, and regulatory control have resulted in the high quality inactivated and live-attenuated influenza vaccines currently available [2,3].

For 35 years, all available influenza vaccines contained three antigens: against the currently circulating influenza A viruses H3 and H1 and against B influenza virus. The H3 virus evolved from the H3N2 virus that caused the 1968 pandemic. The H1 variant virus was added to then bivalent vaccine after the emergence and continuous spread of an H1N1 virus after 1977 which was closely related to the influenza A H1 virus that circulated between 1947 and 1957. The virus spread quickly globally and caused a relatively mild epidemic mainly in the young as older persons had acquired some immunity by earlier infection. By the end of the 1990s, two antigenically distinct influenza B lineages (Victoria and Yamagata) were frequently found to co-circulate regionally or globally. Consequently, an increasing number of companies are developing quadrivalent seasonal influenza vaccines containing antigens or viruses for the two B lineage viruses in addition to two influenza A H3 and H1 variant strains. This has required significant developmental investment as regulators in the United States and Europe consider these vaccines as new, and clinical safety and efficacy comparisons to existing vaccines are required demanding extensive clinical trials. The first of these quadrivalent vaccines (live-attenuated) was licensed by AstraZeneca in the United States in 2012. Other companies also have quadrivalent formulations in development for launch in the United States, likely between 2013 and 2015. When quadrivalent vaccines will be introduced in Europe is uncertain.

The combined effect of vaccine producers to capture emerging technologic advancements in production, increase in demand, improvements in vaccine presentation, and some advances in immunogenicity/efficacy, for example by adjuvantation or live-attenuated vaccines, has resulted in the large numbers of licensed influenza vaccines offered in various presentations (e.g., intramuscular, intradermal, intranasal; single dose, multidose; 0.5 mL, 0.25 mL) for different age groups. In the United States alone, nine different inactivated influenza vaccines from six different producers are available in the 2012–2013 influenza season [4]. Globally, at least 21 companies manufacture influenza vaccine [5]. Table 23.1 provides an overview of the major types of influenza vaccines and examples of manufacturers.

Vaccine development differs from that of pharmaceutical products

The successful development of human vaccines, including those against influenza, differs in many ways from that of chemical compounds or other pharmaceutical products. Clinical trials with vaccines often require tens of thousands of participants. In addition, as vaccines are intended to prevent disease rather than to treat an ill individual, clinical trial subjects are healthy which poses additional ethical challenges. Vaccine development risks and costs are also high as national regulatory and other requirements (e.g., plant certification, process validation, GMP auditing) often stipulate that a production plant is in place perhaps 5 years or more in advance of the (uncertain) approval of the vaccine. The long production cycle of vaccines poses two additional challenges: production must start at the manufacturer's risk often 1–2 years ahead of registration to ensure vaccine availability after approval. Second, customer demand needs to be anticipated 1–2 years in advance and rapid responses to emergencies are very difficult without stockpiling vaccines which often have a short shelf-life.

A sophisticated development "machinery" is required because of the duration and costs of vaccine development and very complex production. Well-coordinated processes and business structures are essential to manage global research, clinical development, regulatory, and manufacturing units in a company producing vaccine. Although part of the vaccine development process can be outsourced (e.g., to clinical research organizations), most large vaccine

Table 23.1. The major types of licensed/late stage influenza vaccines and examples of manufacturers.

Vaccine type/application		Egg-derived							Cell-derived			
		Petering out	CSL	GSK	Sanofi*	Novartis	Solvay	Medimmune	Baxter (VERO)	Novartis (MDCK)	Protein Sciences	Novavax
Inactivated	whole virus											
	split											
	subunit											
	adjuvanted											
	liposomal											
	intradermal			*								
	high HA dose			*								
life-attenuated	whole virus											
Recombinant	recombinant											
	VLP											
	VLP											

VLP, virus-like particle.

Legend:

TEXT: cell line used for production.

Licensed vaccine;
Additional vaccine version licensed.
Additional vaccine version in development.
Vaccine in clinical development phase III.

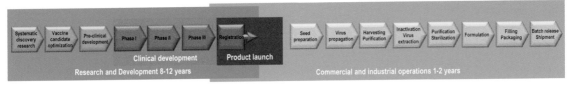

Figure 23.1. Stages and timelines for vaccine development.

companies have to employ several thousands of highly specialized associates to ensure that safe and effective vaccines are developed to meet the most pressing public health needs and fulfill individual national regulations. Scope of preparation and cost of receiving marketing approval in all important markets also increases as the major national regulatory agencies such as the European Medicines Agency, US Food and Drug Administration, Australia's Therapeutic Goods Administration, China's State Food and Drug Administration, Korean Food and Drug Administration, and the Pharmaceutical and Medical Safety Bureau of the Ministry of Health and Welfare Japan each have individual requirements and often request clinical trials in their respective local populations.

Vaccine development including research, clinical development, and registration may take 8–12 years (Figure 23.1). After a medical need has been identified, systematic research is the first phase in the lengthy process to launch a vaccine successfully. During this first exploratory phase, pathogens, genomes, or immunogens are systematically screened to identify suitable antigens for subsequent initial prioritization and proof of concept in animal models or *in vitro* assays.

During the vaccine candidate optimization phase, a few selected antigens are engineered and expressed in hosts that are suitable for later industrial scale up. For each new antigen or substrate, specific release assays have to be developed and standardized, a very time, skill, and resource consuming step for newly introduced vaccines. At that time (6–9 years before launch of the vaccine) the composition of the vaccine is already decided and subsequent production adapted to industrial scale up in an appropriate replication or expression system (cells, eggs, yeasts, bacteria, plants) compliant with GMP requirements. Systematic research, vaccine candidate optimization, and

preclinical technical development up to this stage take on average 3–6 years.

Subsequently, the first vaccine lots are produced and tested for stability and teratogenicity and other toxicologic parameters. After submission of requested documentation and approval by national regulatory agencies and an institutional review board, the first vaccine doses are tested for safety and proof of concept in healthy adults (10–100 subjects) or directly in the target population when ethically necessary. Decisions taken up to this development point on formulation, components, and presentation are often only reversible with enormous costs. For instance, if special requirements for use in developing countries (temperature stability; multi-dose vials; different posology) were reconsidered at a later development stage, any ensuing changes in formulation, composition, delivery, and presentation would likely require setting the development clock back to the preclinical stage.

Further clinical development of influenza vaccines through phases II and III is described elsewhere in this book.

Vaccine production is complex: Barriers to entry are exceptionally high

The setting up and running of an influenza vaccine production facility (and for that matter any vaccine production plant) is generally very complex and extremely resource and time consuming. However, there are differences in terms of capital investment, operational costs, need for know-how, and technology transfer depending upon the methods of production and types of vaccine produced.

Challenges for vaccine production that create hurdles for new players to enter the field are as follow:
• Very long product development cycles lasting up to 8–12 years at costs between $300 million to $1

355

billion. Most vaccine companies invest 10–25% of their revenues into research and development.

• High regulatory hurdles. Vaccines are used for prevention and not for treatment. Therefore safety requirements are naturally extremely rigorous. demanding large clinical trials and the highest production quality resulting in exceptionally high and further increasing regulatory needs. In addition, some regulatory agencies (e.g., US FDA) may require that vaccines already licensed, for example in Europe or Australia, must still go through clinical trials to achieve approval in the United States.

• Complex, experience dependent vaccines environment. Success in the global vaccine market requires not only exceptional technologic and vaccine development capacity, but also a network of relationships with governments, national tender agencies, and global policy and funding organizations such as GAVI, UNICEF, World Health Organization (WHO), Bill and Melinda Gates Foundation [6].

Establishing an influenza vaccine production facility for inactivated egg or cell-derived influenza vaccines takes at least 4–5 years but might be slightly shorter for live-attenuated egg-derived vaccines. In addition, because of national regulatory and other requirements (e.g., plant certification, process validation, GMP auditing), manufacturing facilities have to be in place often 5 years before the vaccine product even launches. The capital investment required establishing a plant for large-scale production of inactivated influenza vaccine in eggs on an existing vaccine manufacturing campus is estimated at approximately $1 per dose of capacity, that is $20 million investment for a plant capable of producing 20 million doses of trivalent vaccine per year. A completely new facility would cost significantly more, and the cost and required time further increases for setting up a new production process. Resources for a cell-culture facility are estimated to be five- to 10-fold more than an equivalent facility for inactivated egg-based production. Because of the simplicity of the scale up process, a nonautomated or semi-automated plant for a live-attenuated egg-derived vaccine can be established for a much smaller investment [7].

Much lower funding seem to be required for the establishment of manufacturing sites for the recently emerging plant-derived influenza candidate vaccines. A facility recently established in North Carolina, United States, in less than 18 months with costs of approximately $36 million produced significantly more than 10 million doses of plant-derived monovalent influenza vaccine bulk in less than 1 month. Considering the lower workforce requirement (less than 100 people for full-scale operation), the high level of automatization of the facility, and lower raw material costs, eventual production costs (cost of goods) for this plant-derived vaccine may be significantly reduced (Medicago; personal information).

Regardless of the production technology, ensuring current good manufacturing practices (cGMP) and implementing appropriate quality control and quality assurance functions is estimated to be around one-third of the operational cost of a modern vaccine plant.

Vaccine production capacities unevenly distributed globally

Although human vaccines are produced in 44 countries by 146 producers (1990: 63 countries), the majority of vaccine production and sales is concentrated in a small number of players and countries. Between 1997 and 2011, 95% of the number of vaccine doses was produced in only 15 countries (Belgium; Brazil; Canada; China; Cuba; Denmark; France; India; Indonesia; Italy; Japan; Korea; Russia; Senegal; United States) [8]. Five companies (GSK; Sanofi; Merck; Pfizer; Novartis) own more than 80% of the global vaccine market; sales reached $25.7 billion in 2011. The rest of the vaccine companies belong to a group of smaller vaccine divisions that are part of larger pharma companies (e.g., Abbott; AstraZeneca; Baxter; CSL; Johnson & Johnson; Takeda) or belong to a host of smaller players. Although vaccine sales above $25 billion might seem enormous, vaccines make up only around 3% of the global pharma market, and are also small in comparison with other economic sectors [6].

Influenza vaccine production has more than doubled in the first decade of the twenty-first century to more than 450 million doses in 2009, with a total potential capacity in the range of 850 million doses [5]. Despite this increase, more than 75% of the annually supplied vaccine doses are still used by approximately 12 countries in North America and Europe. About one-quarter is delivered to the Western Pacific region with Japan and Australia receiving the lion's share. Influenza vaccine use in developing countries is very limited [9]. With the help of GAVI, the 50 least developed countries are still focusing on the introduction of basic pediatric vaccines (diphtheria, tetanus, pertussis, *Haemophilus influenzae* type B, hepatitis B) or on a stable expansion to include MMR (measles, mumps, and rubella), rotavirus, pneumococcal and human papillomavirus vaccine [10].

An estimated 21 companies produced seasonal influenza vaccines in 2009 [5]. In the past, significant strides have been made by these companies in increasing global influenza vaccine production capacity to match projected higher vaccine demands. However, it was clear even during the early stages of the 2009 H1N1 pandemic that there were still significant gaps in the availability and supply of vaccines, with many developing countries receiving pandemic vaccine much later than developed countries, if at all. The WHO outlined a global action plan to increase pandemic vaccine production capacity. Certainly, the most important factor to consider is the need to ensure the sustainability of such enhanced production capacity during inter-pandemic periods [11].

Recently, a study by McKinsey [12] commissioned by the WHO estimated that the seasonal production capacity might further increase up to 1.76 billion doses in 2015. This growth in capacity is said to be due to the upgrade of existing manufacturing facilities or the building of new plants. However, authors also note that the completion of these plans would result in 560–900 million doses of excess seasonal capacity compared with seasonal demand. Manufacturers indicated that such an excess could result in expansion plans not materializing or existing capacity being shut down.

Influenza vaccine production: Driven by disease seasonality and virus evolution

Since their introduction after World War II, the annual production of influenza vaccines has always been a race against time: seasonal influenza outbreaks and rapid evolution of new variant viruses leave only a small window of 4–6 months every year between the recommendation of vaccine prototype viruses by WHO in February and September and delivery of first doses before the beginning of the influenza seasons. Table 23.2 outlines the public health imperatives that derive from influenza virus biology and disease epidemiology. The impact of these public health imperatives on the production of influenza vaccines are manifold but in essence put enormous time pressure on manufacturing:

- Supply must be available ahead of the Northern and Southern Hemisphere influenza outbreaks. To this end, vaccine production must usually commence by January and September, respectively, that is before the WHO strain recommendations. On the other hand, WHO can only make its vaccine candidate strain recommendations in mid-February and September to allow time for robust virus surveillance in countries and WHO Collaborating Centers (CC) and subsequent data analysis.

- As the three (or, in some regions in the future, four) vaccine strains contained in the vaccine are produced consecutively, companies will naturally choose to begin production with the strain that in their assessment is the least likely to be updated by WHO later on. However, when this assessment is inaccurate up to 6–8 weeks of vaccine production may be wasted.

- High growth reassortants derived from the dominating wild viruses are to be available at least 1 month before production begins (to allow for seed virus preparation).

- Standardizing reagents (serum) must always be updated when strains change. Reagents are needed to measure strain yield and to calibrate antigen before bulk blending and for final vaccine formulation. If reagents are not available in time, companies will have to switch production to the next vaccine strain without knowing how much of the first one has already been produced.

- Standardizing reagents are prepared in sheep which takes 1–2 months and requires antigen from virus production or small pilot plants for initiation. Therefore, these reagents are often only available late in the production process and become rate limiting, particularly if small-scale clinical trials are required before licensing (see below).

- Formulated and filled vaccine doses need to be available in June in order to perform clinical trials in certain territories where they are still required after a strain change (e.g., European Union and Canada). This further constrains timelines and adds complexity, forcing companies to formulate small batches immediately from first bulks [2].

Table 23.2. Public health imperatives derived from influenza disease and virus biology.

Influenza disease/virus epidemiology and biology	Public health imperatives
• Virus neutralizing HA antibodies offer best protection but they vane quickly (within months) below the level considered protective • Seasonal, recurrent (winter) influenza outbreaks in the Northern and Southern Hemisphere; influenza viruses circulate at low levels year around in Equatorial region	• Annual revaccination needed shortly before influenza season. Vaccine required in NH before Nov/December and in SH: before April/May
• Dominant drift variant influenza viruses emerge frequently in humans • Three influenza viruses are concurrently circulating in humans: H1; H3 and B viruses. In the past years, two antigenetically distinct B virures circulated concommitantly.	• WHO global influenza virus surveillance needed to detect newly emerging dominating variant viruses • Vaccine must be produced with currently circulating or emerging dominant virus to maintain high vaccine efficacy. • All medically important strains should be integrated into the seasonal influenza: likely global increase from three (H1; H3; B) to 4 strains (adding a second, antigenically distinct B virus lineage)
• Influenza viruses grow in eggs but require adaptation for high yield which is condition for efficient production • Some regulatory agencies require small clinical trials before approval to market after a strain has changed in the influenza vaccine.	• Wild viruses must be reassorted in laboratory to increase yield which is time consuming (different technologies available) • Clinical trials are to be executed during the narrow window between availability of first vaccine doses and annual immunization campaigns.

Prerequisites for vaccine production

Virus surveillance and variant prototype vaccine virus selection

To address influenza virus drift, a global institutional network was created in the late 1940s to ensure that the manufacturers always use the most prevalent influenza variant viruses for production. It has evolved into a universal network of WHO global and national influenza laboratories and several specialized national centers. They have working relationships with several vaccine manufacturers and national and regional licensing agencies. There is no formal contract that governs the seamless cooperation of these institutions but they work in a concerted fashion and support the timely delivery of effective influenza vaccines every year by:

• Sampling patients with respiratory tract infection and typing and isolating influenza viruses. Isolates or original swabs of antigenically significantly different viruses are sent to WHO (national influenza centers).
• Conducting further antigenic and genetic analyses and characterization (WHO CCs, affiliated national and regional specialized institutions).
• Making recommendations on which variant viruses should be used for vaccine production (WHO since 1973; WHO CCs; affiliated national and regional specialized institutions).
• Preparation of candidate high growth reassortants (HGR), assessing antigenic and genetic characteristics of vaccine candidate virus, and developing vaccine calibrating reagents (WHO CCs; affiliated national and regional specialized institutions).

- Vaccine production, registration and licensing (vaccine manufacturers; specialized laboratories of national/regional regulatory agencies) [2].

Preparation of high growth reassortants

The efficacy of influenza vaccine manufacturing is driven by many factors; one of the most important is the yield of the vaccine strain used. It determines the number of doses produced per egg and thus influences the overall capacity of a manufacturing site that is capped by the number of eggs that can be processed per day. As a consequence, strain yield is also an important determinant of the production costs per vaccine dose. To improve the often poor growth characteristics of human isolates of wild-type influenza A viruses, high growth reassortants (HGRs) have been developed since the early 1970s [13,14]. B virus HGRs have not been frequently used in the past but were reintroduced in 2012 [15]. These reassortants possess the genes coding for the surface proteins (HA and neuraminidase (NA)) of the wild-type variant virus selected for vaccine production and one to six of the internal genes of a high growth donor virus (e.g., A/PR/8/34 or for B viruses B/Lee/40 or B/Panama/45/90). The recombination of these genes is achieved by co-infection of eggs with the wild-type virus and the PR8 or B/Lee viruses in the presence of antisera against PR8 or B/Lee surface proteins. At the same time, selection for growth occurs with reassortant viruses with the property of high growth in eggs out-competing slower growing viruses [16].

Preparation of standardizing reagents:

Influenza vaccine seed viruses often grow at very different rates; including HGR strains. Therefore, antigen content in the final monobulk material may vary greatly depending upon individual strain growth characteristics and other factors, particularly in the downstream process. To ensure that each vaccine dose contains the minimum content of 15 µg HA per dose and strain, a reproducible test is needed for vaccine potency standardization of the HA content in the vaccine.

To this end, the single radial immunodiffusion (SRD) assay was developed for influenza vaccine potency assessment in the late 1970s. It became established in 1979 after vaccine clinical trials in the United States and the United Kingdom first demonstrated that HA antigen content of inactivated influenza vaccines as measured by SRD correlates well with vaccine immunogenicity. The assay depends on the availability of an antiserum reagent (usually sheep) and a calibrated antigen standard for each vaccine component. These reagents are supplied worldwide by four essential regulatory laboratories [17].

The influenza HA reacts with antibody to HA in an agarose gel to produce a precipitin ring and the size of the ring depends on the amount of HA. The HA content of an influenza vaccine is calculated by comparison of the precipitin ring formed by the vaccine with that formed by the antigen standard [18,19].

Manufacturing of influenza vaccines

Many more different influenza vaccines are licensed than is the case with other human vaccines. Similarly, the spectrum and number of influenza vaccine in development is unprecedented [20,21] (see also Chapters 21 and 22). Reasons for this progress are manifold (see earlier) and have been driven mainly by the need for vaccine improvements in efficacy and safety as well as differentiation, increasing vaccine demand particularly during the first decade of the twenty-first century, but also by efforts to improve productivity.

Despite these developments, the overwhelming majority of influenza vaccine used nowadays is still produced in embryonated hens' eggs and is inactivated (2009 estimated +90%) [5,12]. As long as quality eggs are in good supply, egg-based influenza vaccines will likely continue to be a very competitive commercial product for several years.

Irrespective of the production process, all inactivated egg-derived (but also cell culture, plant, yeast and bacterial expressed protein, and virus-like particle candidate vaccines) are standardized and will be released by the national regulatory agencies by the content of the influenza surface protein HA for each of the vaccine strains (15 µg HA of each vaccine strain and dose). NA is required to be present in the vaccine but its absolute content is not specified. Live-attenuated influenza vaccines (LAIV) are standardized and released by national regulatory agencies according to the quantity of the vaccine viruses contained.

359

Manufacturing of egg-derived, inactivated influenza vaccines

Despite the large number of licensed inactivated influenza vaccines, the major processing steps of egg-derived inactivated vaccines are relatively similar. Although the vaccines have fundamentally not changed for the past 60 years, many improved and additional process steps have been introduced, such as whole virus antigen disruption, zonal centrifugation, and additional purification of the surface antigens (HA; NA) as well as the use of high growth reassortants. The manufacturers may perform these stages in different sequences in the downstream process (after allantoic fluid harvesting and clarification) and may also use different chemicals and kinetics for virus inactivation, additional concentration steps such as diafiltrations, or specific virus splitting substances and processes. The typical automated

vaccine manufacturing process shown in Figure 23.2 takes approximately 6–7 days to complete.

Seed virus preparation

The quality of the final vaccine and also the efficacy of production is substantially determined by the seed virus material each company prepares and uses for virus propagation. As a first step, specialized WHO affiliated laboratories provide wild-type or high growth reassortants of verified antigenic and genetic characteristics (producers of live-attenuated vaccines generate HGR themselves; see below). The production of vaccine in most countries is based on a seed lot system. Each company prepares a master and several working seed lots by serial virus passaging at high dilution in specific pathogen-free (SPF) eggs or suitable primary cell lines obtained from SPF eggs. This will select for virus that grows at higher yield

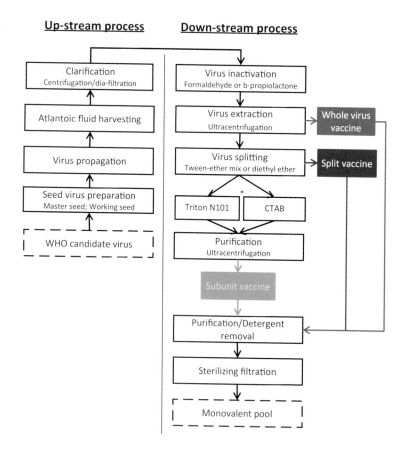

Figure 23.2. Upstream and downstream process of egg-derived inactivated influenza vaccine production. HA, hemagglutinin; NA, neuraminidase; WHO, World Health Organization. *options for HA and NA through virus lipid layer solubilization.

but also aims at diluting out any contaminating agent. Most regulatory agencies require that working seed virus lots should not be passaged more than 15 times from the HGR virus to reduce the probability that the antigenic characteristics of the virus drift significantly from the original reference strain. The final vaccine virus should only be one passage removed from the working seed lot. Each seed lot must be tested for the presence of the recommended HA and NA as well as for freedom from bacteria and fungi (sterility test), viruses and mycoplasma and be released by the local quality assurance function [22].

Egg supply

While live-attenuated vaccines require SPF eggs to be used for production (e.g., in the United States), this is not a requirement for inactivated influenza vaccines. Most companies use incubated embryonated hens' eggs from regular healthy flocks. However, as large numbers are needed (some manufacturers can process more than 150 000 eggs per site per day), a continuous supply throughout the vaccine production campaign is required. Recently, some companies have restructured their egg supply to ensure year round availability in order to provide cover in the event of an influenza pandemic [23].

Most manufacturers disinfect the surface of the incubated embryonated egg before inoculation to reduce contamination, although the influenza virus production process in its entirety must be set up and validated to inactivate any extraneous agent (e.g., viruses, bacteria) present in the harvested allantoic fluid.

Inoculation, virus propagation, and allantoic fluid harvesting

Suitably diluted working seed virus is inoculated into the air space of commercial pre-incubated 10- to 11-day-old embryonated eggs. All major influenza vaccine producers have introduced automatic egg inoculators and allantoic fluid harvesters to speed up the production process and increase capacity per site.

After inoculation, eggs are incubated for up to a further 72 hours, normally at 35°C for influenza A viruses and at 33°C for influenza B virus to enable the virus to replicate. The eggs may then be candled to make sure there are no cracks or contamination, and subsequently chilled to +4°C which kills the embryo and constricts blood vessels to aid the harvest process as influenza virus can hemadsorb to red blood cells. The allantoic fluid is collected in a harvesting vessel, usually by a machine that removes the top of the egg and aspirates the fluid via a harvesting probe that enters the egg. Once harvested, the fluid passes through a low speed clarification centrifuge and is sometimes concentrated by ultrafiltration.

Virus inactivation and sucrose density gradient virus purification

To limit the possibility of contamination, inactivation is typically initiated as soon as possible after harvesting the bulk fluid. The virus is inactivated by the addition of formaldehyde or beta-propiolactone for a time and temperature validated to kill the influenza virus. Validation studies are also required to evaluate the inactivation process on avian leucosis virus and mycoplasmas.

After inactivation, the influenza virus is removed from the allantoic fluid by purification in an ultracentrifuge containing a sucrose density gradient.

The purified virus collect at this stage has purity from egg protein of 85–95%. It could be used to prepare a whole virus influenza vaccine if the subsequent virus splitting were omitted with only a final dia-filtration and sterilizing filtration required before the concentrated monovalent pool stage.

Virus splitting process

Split vaccines Most of the splitting agents (e.g., diethyl ether; Tween-ether combinations; tri (*N*-butyl) phosphate; TritonX100; ammonium deoxycholate; sodium dodecyl sulfate (SDS) or sodium cholate) were tested and introduced in the 1960s and 1970s and are still in use today. They are either solvents or detergents that dissolve or disrupt the lipid coat of the virus. Most of the producers have developed a specific virus splitting process for their licensed vaccines and actual methods used vary widely. Optimal conditions have to be established by each company and sometimes even for each strain.

Some producers add an additional clarification after splitting to remove large particles followed by an additional inactivation step by for example formaldehyde.

An additional purification step by sucrose–density gradient may follow and the HA-rich fraction is harvested. Alternatively, the detergent or solvent may be removed by diafiltration.

Subunit vaccines After it had been shown in the 1970s that HA and NA alone would be sufficient to stimulate a robust immune response against influenza infection, several groups assessed the feasibility of further purifying and concentrating HA and NA in split monovalent pooled harvest. Currently available subunit vaccines that contain mainly HA and NA are produced by adding trimethyl-cetyl-ammonium bromide (CTAB; a quarternary ammonium detergent) or Triton N101 (polyoxyethylene branched nonylcy-clohexyl ether) to the inactivated whole virus produce. These substances strip the HA and NA from the virus core through solubilization of the virus lipid layer. The detergent CTAB is subsequently removed by binding to an absorbent resin and the Triton N101 by salting out in the presence of phosphate.

Final purification and sterilization

Depending upon the manufacturer, a dia-filtration stage to remove sucrose and enable a change to the final buffer may take place either before or after the splitting stage. The sterilizing filtration stage of the monovalent bulk is completed as close as technically possible to the trivalent blending stage for sterility assurance, as these concentrates have to be held until potency values are known, which is dependent on availability of SRD potency reagents.

Testing of the monovalent bulk and formulation of trivalent vaccine

Once SRD reagents are available the potency of individual monovalent bulks can be determined and formulated by addition of diluent to achieve the required antigenic content per strain (H1, H3, and B-Yamagata and/or B-Victoria lineage virus) in the final vaccine. Monovalent bulk must contain at least 90 µg HA per mL (for adjuvanted vaccines: 180 µg) so as not to exceed the 0.5 mL volume of the trivalent vaccine dose.

Extensive testing is required before monovalent bulks may be used in the preparation of the final bulk material. In addition to determining HA antigen content and confirmation of presence and type of NA, this also typically includes sterility testing, testing for the absence of residual infectious virus by serial passaging in embryonated eggs, purity (proportion of HA and NA relative to the total protein content), and approved limits of presence of chemicals used during the product manufacture, for example for inactivation, virus disruption, and purification.

The final bulk vaccine will be tested again for sterility and, where applicable, for the amount of antimicrobial preservative. It is then distributed into sterile closed containers. Quality control testing of the final container comprises several labor-intensive testing regimens to ensure that all release requirements have been met. Typically, this includes confirmation of HA content (15 µg per strain), absence of residual infectious virus, antimicrobial preservative content; residual inactivating agent, ovalbumin, total protein, sterility, and bacterial endotoxins.

Fill–finish and packaging activities

Product can either be filled in multi-dose vials or prefilled syringes depending on market requirements. Sterile filling of vials or syringes and subsequent inspection of the filled vials or syringes are usually completely automated. Prefilled single-use syringes are preservative free. However, multi-dose vials must contain a preservative, which is usually thiomersal. The labeling and packaging process is also automated; individually labeled vials are placed into cartons along with relevant product inserts, leaflets, and syringes [2,7,22–25].

Manufacturing of cell-derived, inactivated influenza vaccines

Egg-derived vaccines have had an extraordinarily long and successful track record of safety and efficacy in Europe, the United States, and elsewhere. Despite the longstanding and remarkable success of egg-derived vaccines, introduction of alternative virus replication platforms have been pursued for several decades. Of particularly interest has been the use of tissue culture cell lines. Their potential practical and theoretical advantages and disadvantages [7,26–28] can be summarized as follows.

• Independence from supply of eggs. Seed cells can be stockpiled and production is initiated at any time and extended for a prolonged period if needed.

• Use of a controlled cell seed lot system, with uniform production of cells. Reduced risk of introduction of exogenous or endogenous adventitious agents.

• Vaccine production process more consistent and reproducible. More easily scalable to larger production capacity.

- Vaccines (whole virus; split or subunit; live-attenuated) which can be released with the same assays as for egg-derived inactivated influenza vaccines.
- Elimination of egg components in the vaccine and the resultant risk of potential allergic reactions.
- The capability of producing influenza vaccines with highly pathogenic avian strains because of higher bio-containment conditions.
- Avoidance of selection of egg-adapted variant virus that may be antigenically distinct from the original source strain thereby potentially improving the specificity and potential avidity of antibody formation and cell-mediated immunity in humans.

However, cell culture influenza vaccine production may also have several challenges compared with egg-derived production.

- Initial capital investment for a cell-based production facility may be several times higher [7,29,30] but also operational costs, particularly for quantities below approximately 25 million doses per year.
- Licensing pathways that are significantly more challenging. Extensive testing of cell banks to demonstrate freedom from adventitious agents and meet oncogenicity and tumorigenicity requirements as laid out in various guidelines and regulations. Extensive measurement and identification of cell-derived proteins [31–34].

The difficulties in finding cells that replicate viruses to sufficient titer and the massive investment for the very time-consuming and resource-intensive seed cell characterization are certainly the main reasons for the small number of human and animal derived permanent cell lines used in human vaccine production. However, they serve as source for a significant number of human viral vaccines. For instance, several hepatitis A, rabies, and herpes zoster vaccines are derived from MRC-5. Another human diploid cell line, WI-8 (also from lung fibroblast), is used for rubella and adenovirus type 4+7 (production ceased) vaccine manufacturing. Influenza, Japanese encephalitis, polio, rabies, rota, and vaccinia vaccines are produced in Vero cell lines (animal origin; African green monkey). Vero cells are certainly the most widely accepted continuous cell lines by regulatory authorities for the manufacture of viral vaccines.

The first licensed and commercialized cell-derived influenza vaccine has been produced from a Madin–Darby canine kidney (MDCK) cell line [27,35–37].

Various continuous cell lines have been tested for replication of influenza viruses such as BHK-21 and HKCC (hamster), PER.C6 (immortalized human retinoblasts), SJPL (porcine lung epithelia cell), EB14, EB66 (both immortalized avian embryonic-derived stem cell lines), PBS-1 (immortalized chicken embryo), MRC-5, WI-38, MDCK, Vero, and NIH-3T3. Of those, only MDCK, Vero, and PER.C6 have consistently yielded influenza virus titers for a large spectrum of different influenza variant viruses sufficiently high enough to be considered commercially viable. In addition, cell lines should grow ideally in synthetic media-free from animal-derived components. They have several advantages including reduced lot-to-lot variability, lower risk of contamination including from prions, easier and less expensive purification of the desired protein, and robust supply [38].

One influenza vaccine has been successfully licensed and commercialized based on a MDCK cell produced in suspension [35] and on one Vero cell line cultivated on microcarrier that uses wild-type influenza A viruses as seeds rather than high growth reassortant strains [36]. Several other companies have developed proprietary master and working cell banks of MDCK cell lines that grow under serum-free conditions (growing freely in suspension or on microcarrier). They all derived from the original MDCK from 1958 [26,27,39,40].

Unlike egg-derived vaccines where individual eggs serve as "mini-bioreactor," the biomass for virus replication – the cell culture – has to be cultivated to sufficient volume before virus inoculation. To this end, industry has developed two primary approaches: mass cell cultivation in suspension or on microcarriers. Each of these approaches has its advantages and disadvantages [35,39].

In suspension, cell lines grow freely while suspended in the nutrient medium in bioreactors. This process can be easily scaled up by simply adding fresh medium and transferring to larger fermenters. Examples are the PER.C6 and an MDCK-33016-PF cell line, the latter developed by Novartis for its licensed seasonal and several pandemic influenza vaccines [35].

"Adherent" or "anchorage dependent" cell lines are mass cultivated in roller bottles, multilayer stacked plate systems, or stirred tank bioreactors using microcarriers. They offer the support that is needed in bioreactors for cells that only grow when adhered to a matrix. These carriers vary in size (typically 100–400 μm) and density (typically 1.02–1.1 g/mL) and can be based of various materials (e.g., dextran matrix also coated with collagen, plastic, glass, or cellulose). For cell passaging, trypsin has to be added for cell dislodging from the microcarriers. Recent overviews on microcarriers can be found in [41,42].

In general, suspension cells seem to be preferred, with easier and faster processing, fewer supplements needed (trypsin, proteins in medium to accommodate adherence), and less stress for cells during passaging. However, both systems have advantages and disadvantages and might be superior to the other depending upon the cell line used. In general, cell density is smaller with microcarrier systems and thus larger or more fermenters are needed. This might have only a small impact on capital investment. Both systems can be run in completely closed systems. Baxter Vaccines' recently licensed seasonal influenza vaccine is produced on adherent Vero cells [36]. In 2001, Influvac® TC, a split-virus influenza vaccine produced in MDCK cells (Solvay Pharmaceuticals), was approved in the Netherlands, but never commercially distributed.

Seed virus preparation

Fundamentally, requirements for seed virus preparation for cell-derived vaccines are comparable as described for egg-derived vaccines. However, there are a few distinct differences:

• Supported by the International Federation of Pharmaceutical Manufacturers (IFPMA), some WHO affiliated laboratories are also generating HGR seed viruses that are passaged in cell culture only (MDCK-33016-PF) to avoid selection of egg-adapted variants with potentially different antigenicity [28].

• In addition to SPF eggs or derived primary cell cultures, diploid and continuous cell lines can also be used for seed virus propagation. The final passage for establishment of the working seeds has to be prepared in the cell line used for routine production.

• Baxter Vaccines uses for its Vero cell-derived influenza vaccine wild-type influenza A viruses as seeds rather than HGR strains. They are subject to the same rigorous testing for seed viruses as HRG.

• Most importantly, several regulators (e.g., European Pharmacopoeia) require companies to provide a comprehensive risk assessment and validation package to demonstrate absence of extraneous agents or stipu-

late approaches with comparable objectives [32,43]. This includes more general considerations on potential contaminants of the virus isolates, the susceptibility of the cell substrate to such viruses, and the capacity of the production process for viral removal or inactivation. Validation includes also comparative data on testing of the seeds with established or rapid assays that may be applied for the demonstration of freedom from extraneous agents because of the long duration of *in vivo* tests.

Cell culture expansion and virus propagation

Working seed cells are thawed and initially cultivated in laboratory sized flasks or roller cultures (for microcarrier system) in a cell culture laboratory. The cells are subsequently expanded stepwise in stainless steel or in disposable bioreactors (see below) of increasing size (e.g., 20–200–1500–5000 L) until the optimal cell density has been reached. In microcarrier based systems, medium is removed at the end of each step and trypsin added for cell detachment from microcarriers. High cell densities and reproducible cell growth are important to increase HA yield per batch and thus production efficiency and process stability. Cell culture at this scale requires a large amount of consumables and media.

Virus from an established seed lot is used for cell infection in the last (largest) bioreactor at reach of the optimal cell density. Various influenza vaccines in development and already licensed have been grown in fermenters of sizes between less than 1 L up to 6000 L [36,39]. As an example for microcarrier systems [36], reports that amplification takes 8 weeks from a single 1-mL ampoule of cells to achieve a fully confluent microcarrier culture at a 6000-L scale. MDCK suspension cells may be scaled up to some 1000 L volumes within 3–4 weeks.

The subsequent downstream steps after virus propagation in commercial production differ between companies but are in general very similar to that of egg-derived vaccines. Fluid is harvested, cells are removed, the virus inactivated (some companies use two separate steps: formalin and ultraviolet treatment), and the whole virus is further purified and split often by continuous sucrose gradient centrifugation and ultrafiltration and/or diafiltration steps. For subunit vaccines, the extracted surface proteins are further purified. Often a final purification and sterilization step is added [35,36].

As viable Vero and also MDCK cells (and, in principle, all continuous cell lines) have the potential to be tumorigenic, demonstration of removal of intact cells from the final product and DNA removal or inactivation to reduce the risk for oncogenicity are fundamental requirements. Therefore, multiple redundant processes have to be part of the downstream process to ensure complete removal of any intact cells (such as by centrifugation, filtration, chemical inactivation and/or disruption) [34,35]. The amount of DNA in the final product must be below 10 ng/dose. The remaining DNA should be degraded to less than 200 base pairs which can be achieved by virus inactivation with β-propriolactone or nuclease treatment [44]. In addition, removal and/or inactivation must be proven of adventitious agents including potentially oncogenic viruses at various steps of the production process.

Disposable versus steel fermenters
Driven by market needs and emergence of proven robust and reliable commercially available systems, several biotechnology facilities have been exploring the use of disposable production systems such as bioreactors for virus and cell propagation in small-scale production but also for up to 2500 L. In addition, systems are available for depth filtration with disposable filters (instead of disk stack centrifuges), media and buffer preparation, as intermediate product holding vessels, and even for small-scale ultrafiltration and diafiltration. For some of the production steps (e.g., ultracentrifugation) stainless steel equipment remains the only viable option. In the case of disposable bioreactors, the cultivation container is typically made from an approved plastic. A large number of mechanically or pneumatically driven bioreactor systems are available. They are said to offer greater flexibility, ease of handling, reduced incidence of cross-contamination, and savings in time for construction and operation. An assessment of the disposable bioreactors currently available confirms the popularity of mechanically driven, stirred bioreactor systems [45].

Modern bioreactors come with their own process parameters' measurement and control unit. Disposable systems offer several advantages and have been increasingly used in newly built or overhauled production facilities including those for influenza vaccine manufacturing. To avoid excessive waste that is subject to full decontamination, there is a preference for using disposable material in the "noninfectious" production steps (cell expansion, media and buffer preparation).

Production of live-attenuated influenza vaccines
Currently, two egg-derived LAIV are licensed: one in Russia [46] and one in several countries in the Americas, Europe, Asia, and the Middle East [47]. More than 100 million adults and children have been vaccinated with the Russian vaccine since its introduction more than 30 years ago. Both LAIV derived from attenuated donor strains that were adapted to grow well at a reduced temperature of 25°C, but have restricted growth at 37–39°C. Thus, replication of these vaccine strains occurs in the upper respiratory airways but not in the lower respiratory tracts. Donor strains for the Russian LAIV are A/Leningrad/134/17/57 (H2N2) and B/USSR/60/69); donor strains for the US LAIV are A/Ann Arbor/6/60 (H2N2) and B/Ann Arbor/1/66.

Manufacturing of a LAIV from continuous cell lines is particularly challenging. It is not possible at any of the production steps to introduce virus inactivation and/or incorporate some commonly used adventitious agent control measures such as orthogonal virus removal steps. Characterization of the cell substrate safety profile is therefore paramount. For the same reason, use of well-established cell lines without tumorigenic potential would be preferred.

The clinical advantages of LAIV including their ease of application (nasal), ability to induce a broader immune response as well as mucosal immunity are discussed in another chapter. In comparison with inactivated influenza vaccine, the manufacturing of LAIV is much simpler because of the abridged downstream process, thus requiring lower capital investment and operational costs. In addition, yield is 15- to 20-fold higher per egg without the inevitable antigen losses from inactivation and purification during downstream manufacturing of egg-derived vaccines. However, the prevention of extraneous agents including wild-type influenza viruses during the production process have to be addressed and biosafety levels at BSL 2 are required. In addition, SPF eggs are more expensive and supply may be more vulnerable than standard embryonated eggs. The concern of the potential for virus mutations during egg replication is being addressed by the requirement to test virus attenuation of each lot of vaccine before release.

Seed virus preparation

Producers of LAIV prepare their 6:2 HGR strains individually based on their backbone parent strain either by classic reassortment [46] or by reverse genetics (Medimmune). Preparation of seed lots and their testing and characterization is comparable with that of seed virus for inactivated vaccines. However, because removal or inactivation of microbial contaminants is not possible during the production process, the presence of any microbial agent in the seed lots of the attenuated parent strains and of the donor strain is not acceptable and respective testing is required for the release of seed lots [48,49]. Summary for United States see [50]. Use of reverse genetics may provide an added margin of safety with respect to extraneous microbial agents.

In addition, some regulators require that the seed virus is assessed for the maintenance of virus attenuation. This includes an attenuation assay in ferrets (detectable viral replication in the nasal turbinates; lack of detectable virus in the lung tissue), a phenotype assay (verification of the cold-adapted and temperature sensitivity of vaccine virus), and a genotype assay (vaccine virus contains proper genes from master donor virus and wild-type strains).

Upstream production process

Inoculation, virus propagation, and allantoic fluid harvesting is similar to inactivated vaccine production except that SPF eggs are used. However, because of higher yield per egg full-scale automation may not be required.

Downstream process including testing and release

Usually the harvested allantoic fluid is tested for sterility, identity, and absence of specific bacteria (e.g., mycoplasma). MedImmune's LAIV is purified by sucrose-density gradient. Subsequently, the three strains are blended to the required potency and a stabilizing buffer is added before filling. The allantoic fluid of the Russian LAIV is further processed by adding a stabilizer and subsequent microfiltration to remove cell detritus. After a final sterilizing filtration step, the bulk is diluted to the required potency and filled into special application devices (with a stabilizer) or ampules for lyophilization.

Cell cultures, bacteria, plants, and yeasts for the production of influenza viruses or derived recombinant proteins

Recent advances in microbiology offer the ability to express recombinant proteins, including from influenza viruses, in a variety of cells including from insects, bacteria, yeasts, and plants. The number of recombinant influenza candidate vaccines in preclinical or the early stage of development has exponentially increased in the last few years and several start-ups but also well-established companies have entered the field ([3,20]). Although very different approaches have been pursued, they all aim to express epitopes of the stem or the globular head of the HA (sometimes in combination with nucleoprotein or genetically fused to flaggelin for example) [51], monomeric HA or multiple, fully folded recombinant influenza proteins that self-assemble to virus-like particles (e.g., M, HA, NA).

Of the various cell-derived recombinant influenza vaccines that are in testing only one is in late stage development; one has been licensed in 2013. Both utilize insect cells (army worm, *Spodoptera frugiperda*) infected with an insect cell virus vector (baculovirus) that expresses selected virus proteins. This is now a well-accepted method for making vaccines; one of the licensed human papillomavirus vaccines is made using this general system [3]. The licensed cell-derived recombinant influenza vaccines contains single HA monomers instead of fully folded HA trimer proteins [52] and the other one, still in late stage, virus-like particles comprising complete HA, NA, and M proteins [53].

High expectations are placed on plant-derived expression systems [54]; two candidate vaccines that express full HA are currently in phase I and II, respectively. These candidate vaccines derived from genetically modified tobacco mosaic virus vectors [55] or plasmids [56] that are introduced into *Agrobacterium tumefaciens* which is vacuum infiltrated into Nicotania plants. After incubation for 3–7 days for target antigen expression and accumulation, plants are harvested and the target antigen extracted and purified.

The specific and product adapted downstream processes of protein expression systems (e.g., from cell systems, bacteria, plants, or yeasts) comprise harvesting and clarification steps to remove bulk contaminants such as particulates, carbohydrates, and oils followed by capturing and polishing steps that refine the feed stream until only the target product remains. A comprehensive and up-to-date overview on the downstream process in biomanufacturing can be found in [57].

References

1. Williams MS, Wood JM. A brief history of inactivated influenza virus vaccine. In: Hannoun C, Kendal AP, Klenk HD, Ruben FL, editors. Options for the Control of Influenza, Vol. 2. Amsterdam: Elsevier; 1993. p. 169–70.

2. Stöhr K, Bucher D, Colgate T, Wood J. Influenza virus surveillance, vaccine strain selection, and manufacture. In: Kawaoka J, Neumann G, editors. Influenza Virus: Methods and Protocols. Methods in molecular biology, Vol. 865. Humana Press; 2012. p. 147–62.

3. Shaw A. New technologies for new influenza vaccines. Vaccines. 2012;30(33):4927–33.

4. Centers for Disease Control and Prevention (CDC). Prevention and control of influenza with vaccines: recommendations of the Advisory Committee on Immunization Practices (ACIP) – United States, 2012–13 influenza season. MMWR. 2012;61(32):613–8.

5. Collin N, de Radiguès X. Vaccine production capacity for seasonal and pandemic (H1N1) 2009 influenza. Vaccine. 2009;27(38):5184–6.

6. UBS Investment Research, Q-Series®: Global Pharmaceuticals Amusa G, Goodman M, Zhang S. 2012:1–39.

7. Hickling J, E'Hondt E. A review of production technologies for influenza virus vaccines, and their suitability for deployment in developing countries for influenza pandemic preparedness. Geneva, Switzerland: World Health Organization; 2006. Available from: http://who.int/vaccine_research/diseases/influenza/Flu_vacc_manuf_tech_report.pdf (accessed 12 February 2013).

8. Belgharbi L. Regulatory Capacity Strengthening and Institutional Development Plans: Relevance to Influenza Vaccines. 5th International Partners Meeting Influenza Vaccines, 27–28 March 2012, Belgrade, Serbia. Available from: http://www.who.int/phi/Day1_Session5_Alfonso.pdf (accessed 12 February 2013).

9. Palache A. Seasonal influenza vaccine provision in 157 countries (2004–2009) and the potential influence of national public health policies. Vaccine. 2011;29(51):9459–66.

10. Zuber PL, El-Ziq I, Kaddar M, Ottosen AE, Rosenbaum K, Shirey M, et al. Sustaining GAVI-supported vaccine introductions in resource-poor countries. Vaccine. 2011;29(17):3149–54.

11. Report of the second WHO Consultation on the Global Action Plan for Influenza Vaccines (GAP), Geneva, Switzerland, 12–14 July 2011. Available from: http://whqlibdoc.who.int/publications/2012/9789241564410_eng.pdf (accessed 12 February 2013).

12. McKinsey & Company: Preliminary findings for the technical studies under resolution WHA63.1, 10 December 2010. Available from: http://apps.who.int/gb/pip/pdf_files/OEWG2/PIP_OEWG_Preliminary-findings-en.pdf (accessed 12 February 2013).

13. Kilbourne ED. Future influenza vaccines and the use of genetic recombinants. Bull World Health Organ. 1969;41(3):643–5.

14. Kilbourne ED, Schulman JL, Schild GC, Schloer G, Swanson J, Bucher D. Related studies of a recombinant influenza-virus vaccine. I. Derivation and characterization of virus and vaccine. J Infect Dis. 1971;124(5):449–62.

15. World Health Organization. Candidate vaccine viruses and potency testing reagents for influenza B. Available from: http://www.who.int/influenza/vaccines/virus/candidates_reagents/b/en/index.html (accessed 12 February 2013).

16. Le J, Manojkumar R, Pokorny BA, Silverman J, et al. Preparation of high growth reassortants by "classical" reassortment method. In: Kawaoka J, Neumann G, editors. Influenza Virus: Methods and Protocols. Methods in Molecular Biology. Humana Press; 2012. p. 153–7.

17. World Health Organization. WHO Collaborating Centres and Essential Laboratories. 2006. Available from: http://www.who.int/influenza/gisrs_laboratory/collaborating_centres/en/ (accessed 12 February 2013).

18. Wood JM, Dunleavy U. Reagents preparation for potency testing of influenza vaccines. In: Kawaoka J, Neumann G, editors. Influenza Virus: Methods and Protocols. Methods in molecular biology. Humana Press; 2012. p. 158–61.

19. Expert Committee on Biological Standardization, Geneva, 17–21 October 2011. Generic protocol for the calibration of seasonal/pandemic influenza antigen working reagents by WHO Essential Regulatory Laboratories. Geneva Switzerland: World Health Organization; 2012. Available from: http://www.who.int/biologicals/vaccines/INFLUENZA_Calibration_protocol_DB_CA_DB23_April.pdf (accessed 12 February 2013).

20. Bright R. Review of new vaccine platforms and vaccine pipeline. Second Consultation on the Global Action Plan for Influenza Vaccines (GAP-II). 12–14 July 2011. Geneva, Switzerland. Available from: http://www.who.int/influenza_vaccines_plan/resources/bright.pdf (accessed 12 February 2013).

21. Neuzil KM. Influenza vaccines: more options and more opportunities. J Infect Dis. 2012;205(5):700–1.

22. Influenza vaccine (surface antigen, inactivated); Influenza vaccine (split virion, inactivated). European Pharmacopoeia, 7th ed. 2012:788–90.

23. Matthews JT. Egg-based production of influenza vaccine: 30 years of commercial experience. Bridge. 2006;36:17–24.

24. WHO Expert Committee on Biological Standardization. Fifty-fourth report; Annex 3: Recommendations for the production and control of influenza vaccine (inactivated). WHO Technical Report Series, No. 927, 2005: 101–34.

25. Furminger IGS. Vaccine production. In: Nicholson KG, Webster RG, Hay AJ, editors. Textbook of Influenza. Oxford: Blackwell Science; 1998. p. 324–32.

26. Patriarca PA. Use of cell lines for the production of influenza virus vaccines: An appraisal of technical, manufacturing, and regulatory considerations. Initiative for Vaccine Research World Health Organization Geneva Switzerland. 10 April 2007. Available from: http://www.who.int/vaccine_research/diseases/influenza/WHO_Flu_Cell_Substrate_Version3.pdf (accessed 12 February 2013).

27. Perdue ML, Arnold F, Li S, Donabedian A, Cioce V, Warf T, et al. The future of cell culture-based influenza vaccine production. Expert Rev Vaccines. 2011;10(8): 1183–94.

28. Minor PD, Engelhardt OG, Wood JM, Roberson JS, Blayer S, Colegate T, et al. Current challenges in implementing cell-derived influenza vaccines: implications for production and regulation. Vaccine. 2009;27:2907–13.

29. Soons ZI, van den IJssel J, van der Pol LA, van Straten G. Scaling-up vaccine production: implementation aspects of a biomass growth observer and controller. Bioprocess Biosyst Eng. 2009;32(3):289–99.

30. Tree JA, Richardson C, Fooks AR, Clegg JC, Looby D. Comparison of large-scale mammalian cell culture systems with egg culture for the production of influenza virus A vaccine strains. Vaccine. 2001;19:3444–50.

31. Cell substrates for production of vaccines for human use. European Pharmacopoeia, 7.0: 5.2.3 2011:530–3.

32. US Department of Health and Human Services FDA. Guidance for industry: Characterization and qualification of cell substrates and other biological starting materials used in the production of viral vaccines for infectious disease indications. 2010. Available from: http://www.fda.gov/downloads/biologicsbloodvaccines/guidancecomplianceregulatoryinformation/guidances/vaccines/ucm202439.pdf (accessed 12 February 2013).

33. ICH Guidance Q5D: Derivation and characterization of cell substrates used for production of biotechnological/biological product. 63 FR 50244; 21 September 1998. Available from: http://www.ich.org/products/guidelines/quality/quality-single/article/derivation-and-characterisation-of-cell-substrates-used-for-production-of-biotechnologicalbiologica.html (accessed 12 February 2013).

34. Onions D, Egan W, Jarret R, Novicki D, Gregersen JP. Validation of the safety of MDCK cells as a substrate for the production of a cell-derived influenza vaccine. Biologicals. 2010;38(5):544–51.

35. Doroshenko A, Halperin SA. Trivalent MDCK cell culture derived influenza vaccine Optaflu (Novartis Vaccines). Expert Rev Vaccines. 2009 8;5:679–88.

36. Barrett PN, Mundt W, Kistner O, Howard MK. Vero cell platform in vaccine production: moving towards cell culture-based viral vaccines. Expert Rev Vaccines. 2009;8(5):607–18.

37. Gaydos CA, Gray GC. Adenovirus vaccine. In: Plotkin SA, Orenstein WA, Offit PA, editors. Vaccine, 5th edn. Elsevier; 2008. p. 1103–22.

38. Rappuoli R. Cell-culture-based vaccine production: technological options. Bridge. 2006;36:25–30.

39. Genzel Y, Reichl U. Continuous cell lines as a production system for influenza vaccines. Expert Rev Vaccines. 2009;8(12):1681–92.

40. Hu AYC, Tseng YF, Weng TC, Liao CC, Wu J, Chou AH, et al. Production of inactivated influenza H5N1 vaccines from MDCK cells in serum-free medium. PLoS ONE. 2011;6(1):e14578..

41. Sun LY, Lin SZ, Li YS, Harn HJ, Chiou TW. Functional cells cultured on microcarriers for use in regenerative medicine research. Cell Transplant. 2011;20(1):49–62.

42. Audsley JM, Tannock GA. Cell-based influenza vaccines: progress to date. Drugs. 2008;68(11):1483–91.

43. Gregersen JP. A quantitative risk assessment of exposure to adventitious agents in a cell culture-derived subunit influenza vaccine. Vaccine. 2008;26:3332–40.

44. Sheng-Fowler L, Lewis AM Jr, Peden K. Issues associated with residual cell-substrate DNA in viral vaccines. Biologicals. 2009;37:190–5.

45. Eibl R, Kaiser S, Lombriser R, Eibl D. Disposable bioreactors: the current state-of-the-art and recommended applications in biotechnology. Appl Microbiol Biotechnol. 2010;86(1):41–9.

46. Rudenko L. Live Attenuated Influenza Vaccine in Russia. 2nd WHO meeting on influenza vaccines that induce broad spectrum and long-lasting immune responses. 6–7 December 2005 Geneva. Available from: http://www.who.int/vaccine_research/diseases/influenza/Roudenko.pdf (accessed 12 February 2013).

47. Belshe RB, Edwards KM, Vesikari T, Black SV, et al. CAIV-T Comparative Efficacy Study Group, Live attenuated versus inactivated influenza vaccine in infants and young children. N Engl J Med. 2007;356:685–96.

48. EMEA; Committee for proprietary medicinal products (CHMP).Points to consider on the development of

live attenuated influenza vaccines. (EMEA/CPMP/BWP/2289/01): 2003. Available from: http://www.ema.europa.eu/docs/en_GB/document_library/Scientific_guideline/2009/09/WC500003899.pdf (accessed 12 February 2013).

49. WHO Expert Committee on Biological Standardization. WHO recommendations to assure the quality, safety, and efficacy of influenza vaccines (human, live attenuated) for intranasal Administration, Geneva, 19–23 October 2009. Available from: http://www.who.int/biologicals/areas/vaccines/influenza/Influenza_vaccines_final_14MAY_2010.pdf (accessed 12 February 2013).

50. Ye Z. Live attenuated influenza virus vaccine: Regulatory issues. WHO Consultation on Options for Live Attenuated Influenza Vaccines In the Control of Epidemic and Pandemic Influenza, Geneva, Switzerland, 12–13 June 2007. Available from: http://www.who.int/vaccine_research/diseases/influenza/Ye_Specific_reg_issues.pdf (accessed 12 February 2013).

51. Treanor JJ, Taylor DN, Tussey L, Hay C, Nolan C, Fitzgerald T, et al. Safety and immunogenicity of a recombinant hemagglutinin influenza-flagellin fusion vaccine (VAX125) in healthy young adults. Vaccine. 2010;28(52):8268–74.

52. Cox MM. Recombinant protein vaccines produced in insect cells. Vaccine. 2012;30(10):1759–66.

53. Bright RA, Carter DM, Daniluk S, Toapanta FR, Ahmad A, Gavrilov V, et al. Influenza virus-like particles elicit broader immune responses than whole virion inactivated influenza virus or recombinant hemagglutinin. Vaccine. 2007;25(19):3871–8.

54. Matoba N, Davis KR, Palmer KE. Recombinant Protein Expression in Nicotiana. Methods Mol Biol. 2011;701.

55. Yusibov V, Rabindran S. Recent progress in the development of plant derived vaccines. Expert Rev Vaccines. 2008;7(8):1173–83.

56. D'Aoust MA, Lavoie PO, Couture MM, Trépanier S, Guay JM, Dargis M, et al. Influenza virus-like particles produced by transient expression in Nicotiana benthamiana induce a protective immune response against a lethal viral challenge in mice. Plant Biotechnol J. 2008;6(9):930–40.

57. Gottschalk U. Overview of downstream processing in the biomanufacturing industry. In: Comprehensive Biotechnology, 2nd edn. Vol. 3: Industrial Biotechnology and Commodity Products. Elsevier. 2011. p. 669.

PART 7

Clinical aspects and antivirals

Section Editors: Robert G. Webster and Arnold S. Monto

24 Human influenza: Pathogenesis, clinical features, and management

Frederick G. Hayden[1] and Menno D. de Jong[2]

[1]University of Virginia School of Medicine, Charlottesville, VA, USA

[2]Department of Medical Microbiology, Academic Medical Center, University of Amsterdam, Amsterdam, The Netherlands

Introduction

Influenza virus infection causes an acute respiratory illness classically manifested by fever and prominent systemic symptoms early in its course. The spectrum of illness is broad and includes clinical syndromes affecting primarily the upper and lower respiratory tracts (common colds, pharyngitis, otitis media, sinusitis, tracheobronchitis, pneumonia) and less often other organ systems (Table 24.1) [1,2]. Most influenza patients make a full recovery, but they may require several weeks to return to usual functional status. While infections are typically self-limited and often subclinical, the outcomes depend on a variety of viral (strain, virulence, inoculum size and location), host (prior immunity, genetic predisposition, underlying conditions), and other factors (access to care, antiviral therapy). Some influenza viruses (e.g., avian A/H5N1, pandemic 1918 A/H1N1, and pandemic 2009 A/H1N1) have been associated with increased risk of severe complications, especially in children and young and middle-aged adults including pregnant women. The case fatality rate from seasonal influenza or pandemic 2009 A/H1N1 illness has been low (estimated 1–5 in 10^4), whereas that associated with proven avian A/H5N1 infections exceeds 50% [3,4]. Furthermore, while more than 85% of seasonal influenza-related deaths occur in persons older than 65 years, often related to deterioration in underlying conditions, most of deaths in the 1918 and 2009 pandemics occurred in persons less than 65 years of age and were linked to pneumonic complications [5]. Increased mortality in younger persons extending for 5–10 years during circulation of a pandemic virus and its subsequent seasonal progeny has been a consistent feature of recent pandemics.

Pathogenesis

Transmission and initial infection

Human influenza virus is transmitted from person to person by virus-laden respiratory secretions generated during coughing, sneezing, and perhaps talking. Influenza virus can be detected in both large and small particles from exhaled breaths and coughs. Depending on ambient conditions (temperature, humidity, air exchanges) and behaviors, spread of the virus to the upper and lower respiratory tract occurs by large droplets and small-particle aerosols, respectively, probably over short distances (1–2 m) [6]. In addition, hand contamination from fomites followed by self-inoculation into the nose, mouth, or perhaps eyes appears possible. The relative importance of different transmission routes may vary by setting (e.g., school, household, healthcare) and other factors. Human infection by avian or other animal influenza viruses

Textbook of Influenza, Second Edition. Edited by Robert G. Webster, Arnold S. Monto, Thomas J. Braciale, and Robert A. Lamb.
© 2013 John Wiley & Sons, Ltd. Published 2013 by John Wiley & Sons, Ltd.

Table 24.1. Proven and probable influenza-associated complications.

Upper respiratory tract

Acute otitis media; sinusitis
Supraglottitis

Lower respiratory tract

Acute bronchitis

Exacerbations of asthma, chronic bronchitis, cystic fibrosis, or other chronic obstructive airways disease

Bronchiolitis; laryngotracheobronchitis (croup)

Viral pneumonia

Bacterial pneumonia, empyema, lung abscess

Bacterial tracheitis

Aspergillosis

Pneumothorax

Pulmonary fibrosis, obliterative bronchiolitis

Central nervous system

Febrile seizures (children)

Encephalopathy, delirium, acute psychosis

Hemiballismus; Alice in Wonderland syndrome

Meningoencephalitis; acute necrotizing encephalopathy

Immune-mediated post-infectious encephalitis; posterior reversible encephalopathy syndrome

Guillain–Barré syndrome

Transverse myelitis; polyneuropathy

Bacterial meningitis; brain abscess

Transient ischemic attack, stroke

Reye's syndrome

Narcolepsy (uncertain)

Parkinson's disease (uncertain)

Cardiovascular

Electrocardiographic abnormalities

Exacerbation of congestive heart failure

Myocardial infarction, acute ischemia

Arrhythmias; atrioventricular block; sudden death

Myocarditis; pericarditis, cardiac tamponade

Fulminant heart failure

Musculoskeletal

Myositis

Rhabdomyolysis, myoglobinuria

Rectus abdominis muscle tear

Hematologic

Disseminated intravascular coagulopathy

Hemophagocytic syndrome

Transient hypogammaglobulinemia

Aplastic anemia (uncertain)

Renal

Renal failure from myoglobinuria, disseminated intravascular coagulopathy, hypotension, other causes
Hemolytic uremic syndrome

Exacerbation of nephrotic syndrome

Nephritis (uncertain)

Gastrointestinal

Reye's syndrome

Parotitis

Gastritis, duodenitis, hematemesis

Bowel ulceration

Maternal/fetal

Low birth weight

Fetal distress, spontaneous abortion, stillbirth

Preterm labor, premature delivery

Systemic/other

Hypotension, sepsis syndrome

Toxic shock syndrome

Poor diabetes control

Adrenal hemorrhage

Retinitis, choroiditis (uncertain)
Alopecia

Source: Adapted from Nicholson KG. Chapter 19, in Nicholson KG, Webster RG, and Hay AJ (Eds), *Textbook of Influenza*, Blackwell Sciences Ltd, 1998, pp. 219–264 [1] with permission from John Wiley & Sons, Inc.

can occur after direct contact with infected animals or their excreta through the respiratory route, sometimes by inoculation into the conjunctiva, and possibly through ingestion of undercooked food or contaminated water [3,4].

The initial site of infection is the respiratory mucosa but the location likely varies by virus. The $\alpha2,6$-linked sialic acid-bearing receptors, to which human influenza viruses preferentially bind, are abundant in the human upper and lower respiratory tract, particularly in tracheobronchial epithelium and type 1 pneumocytes. In contrast, the $\alpha2,3$-linked receptors preferred by avian viruses are present in the distal bronchioles, type 2 pneumocytes, alveolar macrophages, and conjunctiva. These differences in receptor distribution patterns may account in part for the high frequency of tracheobronchitis in human influenza, as well as the frequent occurrence of viral pneumonia and relative paucity of upper respiratory manifestations in those infected by avian A/H5N1 and A/H7N9 viruses and of conjunctivitis in some avian A/H7 infections. However, avian A/H5N1 viruses replicate in *ex vivo* organ cultures of the upper respiratory and high titers of virus are detectable in specimens of throat and tracheal aspirates from infected humans [3]. Although initial presentation with diarrheal symptoms has been documented, it remains unclear whether avian A/H5N1 or A/H7H9 virus can initiate infection in the gastrointestinal tract.

Viral replication patterns

Once the virus initiates infection of the respiratory tract epithelium, successive cycles of viral replication infect large numbers of cells and result in destruction of respiratory epithelium and sometimes pneumocytes through direct cytopathic effects or apoptosis. The incubation period averages 2 days and varies from about 1 to 4 days, but may be longer (up to 8–9 days) in infections caused by avian viruses.

The duration of viral replication depends on host age, immune status, underlying conditions, viral strain, and site of sampling. In uncomplicated seasonal influenza, viral detection in the upper respiratory tract begins about 1 day before illness onset, and nasal infectious viral titers peak within 1–3 days (typically 10^4 to 10^7 $TCID_{50}$ per mL). Pharyngeal viral titers are usually lower. Viral replication continues for about 3–5 days in outpatient adults and older children, but may last

for 1–3 weeks in infants and young children, particularly those lacking prior immunity. Replication may persist for weeks to months in highly immunocompromised hosts, including transplant recipients and AIDS patients, indicating the importance for viral clearance of intact cellular immunity. Prolonged viral replication is usually not observed in patients with hypo- or agamma-globulinemia although a possible association with IgG2 deficiency and severe pandemic 2009 A/H1N1 influenza has been described.

Hospitalized adults may shed infectious virus for a week or longer after illness onset. Major comorbidities and systemic corticosteroid use for asthma or chronic obstructive pulmonary disease exacerbations are associated with slower viral clearance [7]. In those with severe pandemic 2009 A/H1N1 and avian A/H5N1 or A/H7N9 illness, virus has been detected as late as 3 weeks after illness onset and sometimes longer, particularly in tracheal and lower respiratory tract samples of patients. In pneumonic cases viral titers are often higher and more sustained in the lower than upper respiratory tract [8]. Antiviral therapy has been associated with more rapid clearance from the upper than lower respiratory tract in such patients. In contrast to seasonal influenza, viral RNA levels may be higher in the throat than nose in avian A/H5N1 infections.

Viremia rarely occurs in uncomplicated influenza. Detection of viral RNA and very uncommonly infectious virus in blood, urine, and stool has been found in more seriously ill patients, possibly reflecting spill-over from the lung or presence in circulating leukocytes. However, isolation of virus from heart, liver, spleen, kidney, adrenals, muscle, placenta, and meninges in some fatal cases indicates the potential for extrapulmonary dissemination. In children with influenza-associated encephalopathy, detection of viral RNA in cerebrospinal fluid (CSF) has been reported inconsistently [9]. Viremia, gastrointestinal infection, and extrapulmonary dissemination, sometimes including the central nervous system (CNS), occur in some avian A/H5N1-infected patients, in whom detection of viral RNA in blood or feces is associated with worsened prognosis [10].

Histopathologic findings

Nasal and bronchial biopsy specimens from persons with uncomplicated influenza reveal degeneration and desquamation of the ciliated columnar epithelium with edema, hyperemia, and mononuclear cell infiltrates in the lamina propria. In fatal viral pneumonia, the lungs are typically airless, congested, and often hemorrhagic [11,12]. Necrotizing tracheobronchitis and bronchiolitis are usually present, with loss of ciliated epithelium, hyaline membrane formation, intra-alveolar exudate and hemorrhage, and interstitial edema, hemorrhage, and mononuclear cell infiltrates. Diffuse alveolar damage is characteristic but not specific. Depending on the time course, lymphohistiocytic alveolitis, metaplastic epithelial regeneration, and sometimes extensive fibrosis develop. Marked infiltration of neutrophils in alveolar airspaces and bronchioles typically occur with secondary bacterial infections. Direct viral cytopathic effects, virally induced apoptosis, and proinflammatory host immune responses contribute to the pathologic changes. Immune complex deposition and complement activation related to non-neutralizing antibodies have been found in some fatal cases and postulated to explain the age distribution of severe cases during some influenza pandemics [13].

Diffuse congestion and generalized swelling of the brain without inflammatory infiltration has been observed in fatal encephalopathy. Myocardial inflammation with interstitial edema and hemorrhage, myofibril necrosis, and lymphocytic infiltration have been described in endomyocardial biopsies from those with acute myocarditis and in about one-third of fatal influenza cases. Focal tubular necrosis and pigmented casts may be found in myoglobinuric renal failure. Bone marrow may show reactive histiocytosis and hemophagocytosis suggesting activation of macrophages by proinflammatory cytokines. In addition to pneumonic changes, the few autopsies of A/H5N1 cases have shown lymphocyte depletion, hemophagocytosis, myocyte degeneration, acute tubular necrosis, and hepatic necrosis [3].

Innate immune responses

Innate immune responses are essential in limiting early viral replication while adaptive immune responses are developing. The elaboration of cytokines and chemokines differ according to influenza severity, duration of illness, and the infecting virus. Peripheral blood gene expression profiles differ in experimentally infected volunteers with symptoms from those infected without symptoms or in uninfected subjects [14]. In uncomplicated seasonal influenza, interferon-α (IFN-α) levels increase in respiratory secretions and blood and peak about 1 day after the peak of virus replication. In contrast, deficient IFN-α responses have been found in those with severe viral pneumonia due to seasonal or pandemic 2009 influenza viruses [15], supporting the notion that interferon responses are central to early control of viral replication. Natural killer (NK) cell depletion and T-cell anergy have also been found in severe influenza.

Increased levels of a various cytokines and chemokines are observed in nasal lavage samples (IFN-α, IFN-γ, IL-6, TNF-α, IL-8, IL-1b, IL-10, MCP-10, and MIP-1α and MIP-1β) and blood during mild experimental or naturally occurring human influenza. In uncomplicated influenza, nasal IFN-γ levels correlate positively with decreases in viral titers, while nasal and plasma IL-6 levels correlate positively with measures of illness severity in outpatients.

Increased cytokine and chemokine levels are also observed in blood, particularly in hospitalized patients with complicated seasonal or pandemic influenza and less so in milder infections [16–19]. Hypercytokinemia appears to be sustained in influenza viral pneumonia and associated with a slower viral clearance. Higher expression of certain Toll-like receptors (TLR 3, 8, 9) on dendritic cells and macrophages at admission correlate with increased cytokine levels and lower nasopharyngeal viral loads [16]. Several of these mediators, including IL-6 and IL-8, correlate with length of stay, ICU admission, hypoxemia, and other severity measures. In hospitalized patients with pandemic 2009 influenza, high blood levels of IFN-γ and mediators involved in the development of T-helper 17 and T-helper 1 responses have been reported [18], although suppression of CXCL10/IP-10, CXCL9/MIG, and IL-17A has been found in severe pneumonia [17]. Particularly, IL-15, IL-12p70, and IL-6 appear to be robust markers of critical illness.

Experimental *in vitro* and animal studies indicate quantitative differences in innate responses to more pathogenic influenza strains such as 1918 A/H1N1 and avian A/H5N1 viruses, possibly due to dysregulation of cytokine responses by intrinsic viral properties. High plasma proinflammatory cytokine and chemokine responses have been found in patients with severe A/H5N1, in whom the highest levels were observed in fatal illness [10], and pandemic 2009 A/H1N1 infections. Dysregulated cytokine and chemokine responses may also contribute to the increased risk of severe influenza in obese and pregnant patients [20].

Disease pathogenesis

The direct damaging effects of influenza infection on respiratory tract epithelium likely accounts for much of the illness associated with influenza, particularly the high frequency of cough and tracheobronchitis. Even in uncomplicated influenza, bronchoscopy shows tracheobronchial inflammation and pulmonary function abnormalities, including restrictive and obstructive ventilatory defects, increased alveolar-arterial oxygen gradients, and decreased carbon monoxide diffusing capacity are commonly present. Airway hyperreactivity may persist for weeks to months after infection.

Constitutional symptoms during influenza likely result from elaboration of proinflammatory cytokines and chemokines by the involved respiratory epithelium and recruited inflammatory cells. Elevated levels of mediators like IFN-α, IL-6, and TNF-α occur in blood and respiratory secretions and probably contribute to systemic symptoms and fever. Early increases in nasal and blood levels of cytokines and chemokines correlate with illness measures in experimental and naturally acquired human influenza [16].

The quantity of virus in respiratory tract specimens generally correlates also with the severity of illness as well as with levels of inflammatory mediators. Upper respiratory tract viral loads in patients hospitalized with seasonal, pandemic 2009 A/H1N1 or avian A/H5N1 influenza generally correlate with plasma cytokine and chemokine levels [17]. Early antiviral intervention with neuraminidase inhibitors (NAIs) in experimental influenza markedly blunts these inflammatory responses and associated illness, supporting the importance of ongoing viral replication in driving these responses initially.

The precise extent to which host immunopathologic responses contribute to severe influenza illness and its complications remains largely unresolved. Certain viruses that are associated with severe lung injury, like the 1918 A/H1N1 and highly pathogenic avian A/H5N1 viruses, have been associated with dysregulated or excessive innate inflammatory responses [21]. In addition, elaboration of reactive oxygen species and other local inflammatory events contribute to tissue injury. Hypercytokinemia and injury to blood vessels or vascular endothelia are postulated to have roles in the pathogenesis of influenza-associated encephalopathy and other organ failure. Increases in blood and CSF mediators (e.g., IL-6, IL-8, TNF or sTNFR, MCP-1) have been found in influenza-associated encephalopathy. The acute phase reaction to influenza, which includes elevation of inflammatory markers like C-reactive protein (CRP), procalcitonin, serum amyloid A (SAA), and fibrinogen, likely contributes to the increased risks of cardiovascular events associated with influenza through increased platelet aggregation and perhaps endothelial dysfunction.

The risk of severe influenza and its complications is likely co-determined by host genetic factors, particularly those that modulate innate responses. Specific mutations in the gene encoding interferon-inducible transmembrane protein 3, which has a key role in controlling viral replication, have been found more often in hospitalized influenza patients than in community control subjects [22]. In fatal seasonal influenza cases, an increased risk for invasive methicillin-resistant *Staphyloccus aureus* (MRSA) disease has been observed in those with low-producing mannose binding lectin *(MBL2)* genotypes [23], and a possible association between IgG2 subclass deficiency and severe influenza has been suggested. Genetic predisposition to severe encephalopathy has been associated with mutations in carnitine palmitoyltransferase II leading to fever-associated abnormalities in mitochondrial metabolism and ATP production and in the nuclear pore protein Ran-binding protein 2.

Adaptive immune responses

Influenza infection elicits cell-mediated immune responses that are detectable before the appearance of humoral ones [2]. Cytotoxic T lymphocyte (CTL) responses develop by 1 week and peak by 14 days post infection in immunocompetent individuals. These are considered essential in terminating viral replication and modifying the risk of complications. Memory T-cell responses to previously encountered influenza viruses, particularly to conserved epitopes on the NP, M, and polymerase proteins, are thought to provide heterosubtypic protection and blunt the development of disease. In particular, pre-existing influenza-specific CD4+, although not CD8+, T cells correlate with reduced viral shedding and illness in experimentally infected sero-negative volunteers [24].

Table 24.2. General factors and specific examples contributing to bacterial infections following influenza.

1. Reduced bacterial clearance due to respiratory epithelial damage
   - Decreased tracheobronchial mucociliary clearance
   - Eustachian tube dysfunction
2. Enhanced bacterial adherence to respiratory epithelial cells
   - Increased pharyngeal colonization by bacterial pathogens
   - Viral NA activity exposes bacterial receptors thus promoting bacterial binding
   - Direct interaction between viral NA and the *Neisseria. meningitidis* capsule
3. Reduced bacterial clearance by immune effector cells
   - Decreased chemotaxis and bactericidal activity of alveolar macrophages and PMN leukocytes
   - Type I interferon inhibition of neutrophil recruitment and *Streptococcus pneumonie* killing by decreasing IL-17 production of γδ T cells
   - Interferon-gamma inhibition of bacterial clearance by alveolar macrophages
   - Decreased nitric oxide production in influenza-infected macrophages
   - Inhibition of PMN leukocyte chemotaxis and superoxide production by viral NP
   - Depressed mitogen-stimulated blastogenic responses and cutaneous anergy
   - Lymphopenia with decreases in both T and B-cell counts
   - Anergy of pathogen recognition receptors
4. Altered local environment promoting bacterial growth or inhibiting clearance
   - Increased inflammation due to expression of viral PB1-F2
5. Other viral and bacterial factors
   - Dysregulation of innate immune responses by viral NS1
   - Cleavage activation of influenza HA by bacterial proteases
   - Possible bacterial neuraminidase reduction of NAI effects on viral neuraminidase
   - Changes in viral receptor tropism

HA, hemagglutinin; NA, neuraminidase; NAI, neuraminidase inhibitor; PMN, polymorphonuclear.
Source: Adapted with permission from McCullers JA. Preventing and treating secondary bacterial infections with antiviral drugs. *Antiviral Therapy* 2011; 16:123–135. © 2012 International Medical Press. All rights reserved [25].

Neutralizing and other influenza-specific antibodies begin to appear in the sera of persons with primary influenza virus infection during the second week after infection and reach a peak by 4–7 weeks with slow declines thereafter. Adults often show earlier antibody rises. Secretory antibodies, predominantly of IgA antibodies, develop in the upper respiratory tract. The principal neutralizing antibody responses are strain-specific serum antibodies and nasal antibodies directed against HA. Non-neutralizing antibodies directed to other epitopes (e.g., M2e, NA) may facilitate viral clearance through opsonization, antibody-dependent cellular cytotoxicity, or inhibiting spread in the respiratory tract. Certain patient groups such as young infants and transplant patients often fail to develop protective humoral and cellular immune responses and are at risk for protracted infection and reinfection.

Secondary bacterial infections

Secondary bacterial infections are common following influenza. Multiple factors contribute to the increased risk of bacterial infection including increased bacterial cell adherence and tissue invasion due to damage to respiratory epithelium and depressed mucociliary clearance, decreased polymorphonuclear and alveolar macrophage chemotaxis and killing, accumulation of alveolar fluid, and suppression of other host immune responses (Table 24.2) [25]. Influenza neuraminidase activity can expose cellular receptors that enhance binding by *Streptococcus pneumoniae*, while the viral nucleoprotein inhibits polymorphonuclear leukocyte chemotaxis and superoxide production. The viral accessory protein PB1-F2, although non-functional in the 2009 A/H1N1 virus, appears to enhance inflammation and the severity of bacterial co-infection. Influenza commonly causes eustachian tube dysfunction that predisposes to inspissation of secretions in the middle ear and development of acute otitis media. Early antiviral therapy appears to diminish this risk.

Clinical manifestations

Influenza causes illness in the majority of those infected, although up to half of infections in adults may be subclinical. Infection may result in a variety of clinical syndromes ranging in severity from common colds to lethal viral pneumonia. Persons at higher risk for influenza-associated complications and hospitalization include infants and young children; the elderly; those with comorbidities, particularly asthma and other chronic cardiopulmonary diseases; pregnant women; morbidly obese patients; and immunosuppressed persons (Table 24.3). Hospitalization due to influenza can occur as result of severe respiratory tract infections and a variety of apparent extrapulmonary complications (Table 24.1). Overall mortality among

adults hospitalized with seasonal influenza has ranged 4–8%, although higher mortality (>10–15%) has been observed among the immunocompromised hosts and during pandemics in some age groups [26]. During the 2009 pandemic about 9–34% of hospitalized adults required ICU care and ventilation support, and 14–46% of such patients died.

Classic influenza syndrome

Sudden onset of systemic symptoms with feverishness, chills, headache, myalgia, malaise, and sometimes rigors and prostration is characteristic of influenza but occurs in only two-thirds or less of cases [1,2]. Fever usually rises rapidly to a peak of 38–40°C within the first day and is often continuous but may be intermittent, especially if antipyretics are taken. In adults with uncomplicated influenza, fever and systemic symptoms usually last about 3 days, ranging from 1 to 5 days. Respiratory symptoms, particularly dry cough and rhinorrhea, occur early in the illness and usually become more prominent as systemic complaints diminish. Nasal obstruction, sore throat, and

Table 24.3. Host factors and patient groups at increased risk for influenza complications.

Persons 65 years and older

Children aged 2 years and younger[a]

Residents of nursing homes and other chronic care facilities

Chronic pulmonary (including asthma) or cardiac disorder (except isolated hypertension)

Chronic metabolic (including diabetes), renal, hepatic, hematologic (including hemaglobinopathies) conditions

Neurologic or neuromuscular disorders, especially those that compromise respiratory function or increase aspiration risk (including cerebral palsy, epilepsy, muscular dystrophy, spinal cord injury, stroke)

Immunosuppression (including that caused by medications or human immunodeficiency virus infection)

Pregnant and early post-partum women (within 2 weeks of delivery)

Morbid obesity (body mass index ≥35–40)[b]

Indigenous peoples (e.g., American Indians or Alaska Natives)

Children and teens <19 years old receiving long-term aspirin

Genetic factors (e.g., persons with interferon-inducible transmembrane 3 protein allele)

Source: Adapted from Antiviral Agents for the Treatment and Chemoprophylaxis of Influenza: Recommendations of the Advisory Committee on Immunization Practices (ACIP) [38] with permission.

[a]Although all children aged <5 years are considered at higher risk for complications from influenza, the highest risk is for those aged <2 years, with the highest hospitalization and death rates among infants aged <6 months.

[b]Increased risk of complications relates to degree of obesity and appears to rise with body mass index ≥30.

hoarseness are common. Cough is the most frequent and troublesome respiratory symptom and may be accompanied by substernal discomfort or burning indicative of tracheobronchitis. Ocular complaints such as photophobia, tearing, burning, and painful eye movements occur in a minority.

Cough, lassitude, malaise, and reduced exercise tolerance may last several weeks. Apparently uncomplicated influenza is often accompanied by abnormal tracheobronchial clearance, airway hyperactivity, and dysfunction of small airways that may last for weeks. Illness may be more severe and convalescence prolonged in smokers and allergic patients.

Physical findings in uncomplicated influenza are nonspecific and limited. Early in the course of illness, the patient may appear acutely ill with flushed facies and hot, moist skin. Clear nasal discharge, hyperemic nasal and pharyngeal mucous membranes without exudate, and injection of the conjunctivae are common. Tracheal tenderness and small, tender cervical lymph nodes are often present. Transient scattered rhonchi or localized areas of rales are found in less than 20% of cases. Lymphopenia and mild neutrophilia occur early, often followed by neutropenia. Elevations of acute-phase proteins, SAA and CRP occur, especially in hospitalized elderly patients.

In hospitalized adults, cardinal findings like fever may be absent due to medication use (e.g., antipyretics, corticosteroids), immunocompromise, debilitation, or advanced age. Also, upper respiratory symptoms such as rhinorrhea and sore throat are reported in less than one-third of hospitalized adults [26].

The illnesses caused by human influenza A or B viruses are similar, although severity and complications risk have been generally greater with H3N2 than with B or seasonal H1N1 infections in adults. Pandemic 2009 A/H1N1 illness has been associated with relatively high frequencies of nausea, vomiting, and diarrhea [3]. In sporadic human infections with highly pathogenic avian A/H5N1 viruses, upper respiratory complaints are less predominant, diarrhea more common, and the risk of progressive viral pneumonia high [4]. Avian A/H7N9 cases also appear to be associated with few upper respiratory symptoms but high rates of pneumonic disease. The presence of rhinorrhea in children with A/H5N1 is associated with better prognosis. Conjunctivitis is a characteristic of human infections with avian A/H7 viruses, but has been infrequent in A/H7N9 or A/H5N1 cases.

Influenza C virus generally causes common colds or febrile bronchitis, usually in sporadic cases although outbreaks may occur in semi-closed populations including children's homes and the military.

Specific patient groups

Infants and young children

In infants with influenza, about 90% have fever, cough, and rhinitis, and up to 40% emesis or diarrhea. Otitis media and/or lower respiratory tract disease is observed in more than 25% of patients. While maternally derived antibodies provide some protection, lack of immunity and the small caliber of airways contribute to increased illness severity during the first year of life. Influenza is under-recognized in infants and young children, in whom unexplained fever or suspected sepsis, bronchiolitis, croup, gastrointestinal illness (poor feeding, vomiting, diarrhea), or neurologic signs including lethargy, apnea, seizures, and meningitis-like presentations, may lead to hospitalization. In children, maximum temperatures are often higher, cervical adenopathy more frequent, and nausea, vomiting, and abdominal pain are more common than in adults.

Pregnant women

The clinical presentation of influenza in pregnant women is similar to other patient groups, but increased morbidity and mortality have been observed during pandemics and seasonal influenza among pregnant women. Especially during the second or third trimester and early post-partum period, influenza has been associated with increased risk for complications, including severe maternal illness, spontaneous abortion, premature labor, fetal loss, low birth weight, and need for cesarean delivery [27]. The risks for viral pneumonia and maternal death have been much higher during pandemic disease, or in the presence of underlying valvular heart disease. Multiple immunologic and cardiopulmonary changes during pregnancy contribute to the increased risk of complications [20].

Transplacental spread of virus in humans has not been conclusively documented except during A/H5N1 infection. Possible associations between influenza and teratogenic effects, especially CNS abnormalities following first trimester infection, or an increased risk of childhood leukemia, schizophrenia, or Parkinson's disease remain uncertain.

Elderly

The risks for serious complications, hospitalization, and death from seasonal influenza are highest among the elderly particularly those with co-morbidities. Viral replication and illness duration are often more prolonged in elderly adults. Older adults, especially the infirm elderly, less frequently develop fever, myalgia, sore throat, and headache but more often have altered mental status and pulmonary complications. Lassitude, lethargy, confusion, anorexia, decreased activity level, cough, and/or low grade fever are often the main findings, although presentation with pneumonia or exacerbations of underlying cardiopulmonary conditions or other chronic comorbidities also occurs [26].

Immunocompromised hosts

Influenza in immunocompromised hosts, including hematopoietic stem cell transplant (HSCT) and solid organ transplant recipients, acute leukemia and oncology patients undergoing chemotherapy, and those with advanced HIV infection, is often more prolonged and associated with increased risks of complications, hospitalization, and death [28,29]. Immunocompromised hosts may present with apparently mild upper respiratory illness, few systemic complaints and often without fever, but then progress over days to severe pneumonia. Pediatric solid organ transplant recipients are substantially more likely to present with fever, rhinorrhea, sore throat, and headache than adult ones. Lymphopenia is a risk factor for protracted viral replication, progressive disease, and antiviral resistance emergence. Up to 50% of HSCT recipients, especially those infected pre-engraftment, develop lower respiratory tract disease and up to 20% die without antiviral therapy. Viral replication may continue for weeks to months in those with advanced immunodeficiency, representing a potential source for nosocomial transmission, including of drug-resistant virus. Infection in solid organ transplant patients has been linked with rejection episodes, including bronchiolitis obliterans syndrome in lung transplant recipients, and rarely graft loss.

Respiratory complications

Influenza A and B virus infections cause a wide range of respiratory complications affecting both the upper and lower respiratory tracts (Table 24.1). These include exacerbations of underlying airways disease (chronic bronchitis, asthma, or cystic fibrosis), croup and bronchiolitis in young children, and pneumonia. The most common complications are acute bronchitis in adults, which occurs in up to 20% of patients seeking care, and otitis media in children, especially those less than 3 years old. Exacerbations of underlying airways disease can be severe and are major causes of influenza-related hospitalizations. Allergic patients also have increased risk of pneumonia.

Influenza is associated with approximately 10% of community-acquired pneumonias in adults. Three pneumonic syndromes are usually distinguished: primary viral pneumonia, secondary bacterial pneumonia, and mixed viral–bacterial pneumonia. However, clinical presentations and courses overlap and most secondary bacterial pneumonias likely represent mixed infections. Similarly, otitis media and sinusitis may be due to primary viral, secondary bacterial, or mixed infection.

Primary influenza viral pneumonia

The spectrum of influenza viral pneumonia ranges in severity from relatively mild forms with patchy radiographic infiltrates, more common in children, to fulminant disease causing respiratory failure. The latter syndrome is uncommon during epidemics but has been the most common severe manifestation of pandemic 2009 A/H1N1 (approximately 50% of ICU admissions) and A/H5N1 or A/H7N9 illness [3,4]. It occurs predominantly in persons with underlying pulmonary or cardiac (congestive heart failure, rheumatic heart disease, classically mitral stenosis) disorders, pregnancy, or immunodeficiency conditions (malignancy, organ transplantation, corticosteroid or cytotoxic therapy). However, up to 40% of pandemic 2009 A/H1N1 cases and most patients with severe A/H5N1 infections have had no recognized underlying disease.

After a typical onset of influenza, progressive cough, dyspnea, and sometimes cyanosis develop over a period of 1–7 days. Persistent fever is usual but sometimes absent. Tachypnea, tachycardia, and sometimes hypotension with sepsis syndrome are present. Sputum is produced in about 50% and may be blood-tinged or frothy. Gram stain may show polymorphonuclear leukocytes but scant bacterial flora. Bilateral pulmonary infiltrates and impaired gas exchange with severe hypoxemia can evolve rapidly, culminating in acute respiratory distress syndrome (ARDS) and often

381

multiorgan failure. Lymphopenia is common and associated with poor prognosis, but either leukopenia or leukocytosis may occur. Thrombocytopenia and elevations in aminotransferases, lactate dehydrogenase, D-dimers, blood urea nitrogen, and creatinine are variably found. Sputum or endotracheal aspirates usually yield high titers of influenza virus by RNA detection or culture, while upper respiratory samples may be negative.

Severe cases usually require mechanical ventilation, often for extended periods. In contrast to other causes of ARDS, lung injury causing refractory hypoxemia has been the leading cause of death in those with influenza viral pneumonia. In patients progressing to respiratory failure, the mortality rate is approximately 25–50% but may be reduced by early antiviral therapy and ICU support. Bronchiolitis obliterans with organizing pneumonia (BOOP), pulmonary fibrosis, and/or chronic functional impairment sometimes develop in survivors.

Bacterial pneumonia

Bacterial pneumonias are common complications of seasonal influenza and were found in almost all reported pneumonia fatalities during the 1918 pandemic, about 70% of life-threatening pneumonia during the 1957 and 1968 pandemics, and about 20–40% of severe illnesses during the 2009 A/H1N1 pandemic. In patients with classic secondary bacterial infection, initial improvement is followed by recrudescent fever, worsening cough often with purulent sputum production, sometimes pleuritic chest pain, and consolidative changes on physical and radiologic examinations. In contrast to a biphasic illness course, rapid worsening of pneumonic symptoms may develop soon after illness onset when bacterial coinfection or early secondary infection occurs. Such illnesses may cause fatal outcomes within 1–4 days.

Secondary bacterial pneumonia is caused most commonly by *Streptococcus pneumoniae* and less often by *Staphylococcus aureus*, including community-acquired MRSA, *Haemophilus influenzae*, or *Streptococcus pyogenes*. Infections by *Neisseria meningitidis*, *Klebsiella pneumoniae*, and *Pseudomonas aeruginosa* may also occur, as rarely does invasive aspergillosis after influenza. Bacteremia and pleural space infections are relatively common. Severe invasive pneumococcal disease, including empyema and lung abscess,

may follow influenza in previously healthy children. Staphylococcal infections are often particularly virulent and may cause necrotizing pulmonary lesions with abscess formation, cavitation, and pneumatoceles. Increasing frequencies of influenza-associated community-acquired MRSA infections and associated deaths are being reported in children and adults, and empiric antimicrobic coverage should consider this possibility in seriously ill patients. A variety of nosocomial bacteria including MRSA and various, often multidrug-resistant gram-negative rods may cause ventilator-associated pneumonias in influenza patients.

Extrapulmonary complications

Influenza is associated with a wide variety of extrapulmonary complications (Table 24.1). Although most occur in temporal association with the acute respiratory illness, some develop before overt respiratory manifestations (e.g., acute cardiac events, encephalopathy), others be delayed in onset (e.g., stroke, Guillain–Barré syndrome), and many may manifest in absence of severe lower respiratory illness. Severe influenza may be associated with sepsis syndrome, acute renal insufficiency due to multiple causes, and multiorgan failure. Lymphopenia and thrombocytopenia are common in severe influenza, and the hemophagocytic syndrome can occur. Disseminated intravascular coagulation (DIC) develops rarely, but may be manifested by mucosal hemorrhage, purpura, renal failure, and jaundice. Diabetics are at increased risk of hospitalization due to poor diabetes control, as well as complications such as pneumonia and cardiovascular events. Of note, during the 2009 pandemic more fatalities in Japanese children were due to unexpected cardiopulmonary arrest or encephalopathy than to respiratory failure [30].

Invasive meningococcal infections, sometimes in clusters, are associated with influenza, possibly related to virus-induced mucosal damage, enhanced bacterial adherence to respiratory epithelium, or immunosuppressive effects (Table 24.2). Cases typically occur within several weeks following influenza and may develop shortly after symptom onset. Toxic shock syndrome caused by respiratory tract infection (pneumonia, tracheitis, sinusitis) or colonization with toxin-bearing *S. aureus* or *S. pyogenes* can develop, usually within a week of influenza onset.

Musculoskeletal complications

Myositis with tender leg muscles, impaired ambulation, and high serum creatine phosphokinase levels (up to 10 000 IU/mL) may develop, more often in children but also sometimes in adults and the elderly. Myopathy has been reported in 14–48% of children infected with influenza B virus, some of whom also manifest elevated levels of cardiac muscle creatine phosphokinase. Rhabdomyolysis can be severe and cause renal failure due to myoglobinuria; rarely, compartment syndromes develop. Virus has been recovered rarely from skeletal muscle.

Cardiovascular complications

Influenza infections have been associated with various arrhythmias, acute myocardial ischemia and infarction, exacerbation of congestive heart failure, and excess cardiovascular mortality [31]. A number of mechanisms may contribute, including fever, hypovolemia, hypoxia, proinflammatory cytokine elaboration, and procoagulant effects of acute phase reactants.

Subclinical electrocardiographic (EKG) changes, including T wave inversions and ST segment elevations, occur in many otherwise healthy adults with apparently uncomplicated influenza. These may last up to 4 weeks and are usually not associated with echocardiographic or cardiac enzyme abnormalities. Echocardiographic evidence of new or worsened left ventricular dysfunction has been found in approximately 5–15% of hospitalized influenza patients, and more often in those requiring intensive care. Myocarditis and pericarditis may present with dyspnea, chest pain, hypotension, elevated cardiac enzymes, abnormal EKG (low voltage, ST elevations, Q waves), pericardial effusion and rarely tamponade, or life-threatening arrhythmia [32]. Fulminant myocarditis with cardiogenic shock usually develops within 2 weeks of illness onset and may be an early presenting manifestation. High frequencies of myocardial injury and myocarditis have been found recently in fatal influenza B infections in children and also in critically ill patients with pandemic 2009 A/H1N1 infections. Myocardial dysfunction is often reversible within several weeks in surviving patients.

Myocyte damage may be due to a direct cytolytic effect of the virus or to host immune responses. Influenza RNA has been detected in the myocardium or blood in about 1–5% of all acute myopericarditis cases. Infection of myocardium with influenza A virus is associated with an increased expression of TNF-α and its receptors in the myocardium.

Nervous system complications

Acute uncomplicated influenza impairs psychomotor performance and slows reaction times. Febrile seizures occur in about 20% of hospitalized children less than 5 years of age. Lethargy, stupor, abnormal behavior, confusion, delirium, hallucinosis, and acute psychosis may be associated with influenza, particularly in children. Aseptic meningitis, transverse myelitis, encephalopathy, diffuse or focal encephalitis, and post-influenzal Guillain–Barré syndrome and presumably immune-mediated encephalitic syndromes have all been described. During the 2009 pandemic about 10–20% of those hospitalized with severe disease had neurologic manifestations and about 20% of these presented with primary neurologic syndromes. The estimated population-based frequency was approximately one neurologic case presentation in 10^5 pandemic H1N1 infections.

Acute influenza encephalopathy/encephalitis manifests most commonly in previously healthy children aged <6 years old but may occur across the age spectrum. About 5% of pediatric encephalopathy/encephalitis cases are associated with influenza infection. It usually develops on the first 2 days after illness onset, and is manifested by fever, altered consciousness, seizures, rapidly progressive coma, emesis, and sometimes focal neurologic signs [9,33]. Head computed tomography imaging may show edema and localized low density in the thalamus, brainstem, and parenchyma, and less commonly overt thalamic necrosis. Electroencephalograms (EEGs) usually show diffuse slowing consistent with encephalopathy, and occasionally an epileptogenic focus. Examination of CSF sometimes shows increased protein or pleocytosis, and uncommonly presence of viral RNA. Specific syndromes with different prognoses have been described, including acute encephalopathy, acute encephalopathy with biphasic seizures and late reduced diffusion (AESD), clinically mild encephalitis/encephalopathy with a reversible splenial lesion (MERS), acute necrotizing encephalopathy (ANE), and hemorrhagic shock and encephalopathy syndrome (HSES) [33]. Prognosis is worse in those with thrombocytopenia, multiorgan failure, and necrotizing changes.

Reye's syndrome is a well-recognized hepatic and CNS complication of influenza A and more often

383

influenza B virus infections in children, particularly those aged 5–14 years, that is closely associated with salicylate use. Increased aminotransferase levels, hyperammonemia, hypoglycemia, and fatty degeneration of the liver are characteristic. Its incidence has markedly decreased in association with reduced use of salicylates in children.

Post-influenza encephalitis begins 1–3 weeks after the illness with fever and decreased consciousness or coma and findings of lymphocytic pleocytosis and diffuse slowing on EEG. It may be caused by an autoimmune process with demyelination and vasculopathy. Influenza is associated with an increased risk of transient ischemic attack and stroke. Possible linkages of influenza to delayed onset encephalitis lethargica and post-encephalitic Parkinson's disease, most notably after the 1918 pandemic, remain to be proven.

Prognostic markers

The presence of underlying conditions that increase the risk of complications (Table 24.3) and of clinical manifestations like dyspnea, wheezing, hypoxemia, and radiographic infiltrates at presentation can be used to assess the likelihood of serious disease. Conversely, the absence of inspiratory crackles and presence of adequate oxygen saturation (>96%) provide strong evidence against pneumonia. Available prognostic scores for community-acquired pneumonia (e.g., CURB 65, PSI) appear to have low to moderate discriminatory value for identifying those requiring ICU admission or at risk of dying and have not been validated for use in influenza patients [34]. In pandemic 2009 A/H1N1 patients requiring ICU care, commonly used scoring systems such as the Acute Physiology and Chronic Health Evaluation II (APACHE II) for adults, the Pediatric Risk of Mortality III for children, and Sequential Organ Failure Assessment (SOFA), correlated with mortality.

In addition to lymphopenia, thrombocytopenia, and high aminotransferase levels, several laboratory markers indicate an increased risk of serious illness. Acute influenza is associated with elevations of SAA and CRP levels; higher levels are seen in patients requiring hospitalization, and especially in those requiring intensive care. Procalcitonin levels may help distinguish between viral and bacterial pneumonias. In ICU patients, high procalcitonin levels suggest the presence of bacterial infection, whereas low values,

particularly in conjunction with low CRP levels, indicate that bacterial infection is unlikely. In the future, gene expression profiles may prove useful in distinguishing those with influenza alone from those with bacterial infection [14].

Diagnosis

Clinical diagnosis

The term influenza-like illness (ILI), usually defined by the presence of fever >37.8°C or 100°F (or sometimes feverishness) and the presence of cough, sore throat, and sometimes other respiratory or systemic symptoms, is a useful epidemiologic tool. However, influenza virus infection cannot be distinguished from infection by many other respiratory viruses (e.g., respiratory syncytial virus, human metapneumovirus, and adenovirus) in an individual patient presenting with ILI, nor can influenza A and B virus be distinguished from one another. Conversely, when an epidemic of influenza A and B virus is occurring in a given community, an outpatient presenting with febrile respiratory illness is likely to have influenza virus infection. In ambulatory adults the presence of fever and cough has a positive predictive value of about 80% for laboratory-proven influenza during community outbreaks, but clinical diagnostic accuracy is substantially lower in children younger than 5 years and in hospitalized patients, or when influenza prevalence is low. The absence of fever, cough, or nasal congestion decreases the likelihood of influenza, as does the presence of sore throat without other respiratory symptoms. Because influenza vaccine effectiveness is incomplete, history of receipt does not exclude an influenza diagnosis.

As the clinical presentations of influenza are diverse and often complicated, the diagnosis is frequently not considered at time of hospitalization. In hospitalized influenza patients, the sensitivity and positive predictive value of ILI for diagnosis has been found to be only 21–43% and 23–50%, respectively [26]. Clinicians should consider influenza as the potential cause of compatible clinical syndromes (Table 24.1) or contributing factor to any hospitalization whenever influenza is circulating in the community. Evaluation of patients with unexplained respiratory illness, especially those with pneumonia or requiring hospitalization, should include a thorough history regarding possible exposures to human or animal influenza viruses (visiting or living in facilities or households where outbreaks are occurring; recent travel to places with outbreaks of influenza or to risk areas for infections with avian viruses (e.g., H5, H7, H9); exposure to persons on influenza antivirals; recent exposures to swine, birds, other ill animals; attendance at agricultural events).

Laboratory diagnosis

A variety of laboratory assays are available to support the diagnosis of influenza (Table 24.4) [35,36]. No single test result can reliably rule out influenza, and follow-up testing by sensitive methods is warranted if the results will affect clinical management. Priority circumstances for testing include patients with serious or progressive illness, including hospitalized patients, individuals with underlying conditions, suspected zoonotic infections, and institutional outbreaks. When clinical suspicion is high in seriously ill patients, repeated sampling over several days and preferably from the lower respiratory tract sites, should be performed for nucleic acid amplification testing (NAAT) and virus isolation. Detailed virologic studies in reference laboratories are indicated when there is suspicion for zoonotic infection or when influenza viruses or RNAs are found that are not typeable with standard reagents. A summary of tests available and their strengths and limitations is given in Table 24.4. These tests are discussed in detail in Chapter 15.

Management considerations

Antiviral therapy

The antiviral spectra, pharmacologic properties, safety and effectiveness of available antiviral agents are discussed in Chapter 25. Antiviral treatment is recommended as early as possible for any patient with confirmed or suspected influenza who is hospitalized or is presenting with severe, complicated, or progressive illness, regardless of prior vaccine receipt or underlying conditions [37,38]. In case of suspected influenza, therapy should be given empirically and not be delayed until laboratory confirmation. Empiric treatment should not be stopped if initial tests are negative, unless an alternative diagnosis has been made and influenza appears unlikely. While the great-est benefits are realized when antiviral treatment is started within 1–2 days of influenza illness onset, even later initiation reduces the risk of death in patients with severe or progressive illness, including those hospitalized and those with A/H5N1 infection [39,40]. Combined antibacterial and antiviral treatments are recommended for patients with community-acquired pneumonia if influenza is also suspected. While the precise role of viral replication in causing some influenza-associated nonrespiratory complications is uncertain (Table 24.1), antiviral therapy is appropriate in those with acute presentations.

Prompt antiviral treatment is also recommended for outpatients at increased risk for influenza complications (Table 24.3). Treatment decisions for these patients require good clinical judgment based on underlying conditions, disease severity, likelihood of influenza, and time since symptom onset. Antiviral treatment also can be considered for any otherwise healthy outpatient with uncomplicated confirmed or suspected influenza and without underlying conditions, if treatment can be initiated within 48 hours of illness onset.

Adamantanes

As currently circulating A/H3N2 and A/H1N1 strains, as well as many A/H5N1 and recent A/H7N9 viruses, show high-level resistance to adamantanes, these drugs are not recommended for routine use at present. However, an adamantane combined with oseltamivir could be considered for serious illness due to susceptible strains, like some clade 2 A/H5N1 viruses.

Neuraminidase inhibitors

The currently available NAIs, inhaled zanamivir and oral oseltamivir, are active against both influenza A and B viruses and are the current agents of choice in most countries. Oseltamivir has an advantage of ease of administration across the full spectrum of age and risk groups [41] but also higher risk of resistance development [42]. In part because of its systemic distribution, oseltamivir has been recommended as the preferred agent for treatment in pregnant women and those with lower respiratory tract or complicated illness. The optimal dosage and duration of treatment in seriously ill or immunocompromised hosts are uncertain. Higher than standard doses (i.e., 150 mg twice daily in adults) are not of proven value in outpatients or in hospitalized patients. However,

Table 24.4. Common laboratory diagnostic methods for influenza.

Assay method	Strengths	Limitations	Comment
Rapid antigen tests	Rapid (15–30 minutes) Simple specimen collection (nasal/throat swabs) Most differentiate influenza A vs B Point-of-care use	Do not distinguish influenza A subtypes Low sensitivities (<20–60%), especially in adults Variable specificities (generally >90%) More sensitive optical reader-based assay available	Negative test result does not exclude influenza Low positive predictive value outside season Useful in outbreak testing when other assays not available
Immunofluorescence	Higher sensitivity than RAT for seasonal influenza (70–85%) Excellent specificity Results available within 1–2 hours Ability to assess sample quality	Do not distinguish influenza A subtypes (unless HA-specific antibody) Less sensitive than culture or RT-PCR Requires intact epithelial cells (e.g., NPA, flocked swab) High laboratory expertise required	Potential to detect other respiratory viruses (other antibodies)
Viral culture	Higher sensitivity and specificity than RAT Applicable to all specimen types Proves presence of infectious virus	Less sensitive than RT-PCR Delays in reporting results (conventional: 3–10 days; shell-vial: 1–3 days) High technical expertise	Provides virus for subtyping, antigenic identification, and antiviral susceptibility testing Biosafety level 3 containment required for highly pathogenic viruses (e.g., H5N1)
RT-PCR, other NAATs	Highest sensitivity High specificity Results available within a few hours to next day Wide range of specimen types acceptable Can be configured to to distinguish virus subtypes and detect novel strains or antiviral resistance markers	False negative results if primer mismatches Unable to distinguish infectious from noninfectious virus Inhibitors in some samples Requires costly equipment and technical expertise	Both in-house and commercial assays Multiplex assays able to detect other respiratory viruses but sensitivity varies
Serology	Retrospective diagnosis Detects some infections missed by virus detection assays	Requirement for convalescent blood sample	Assess susceptibility to infection, subclinical infection or vaccine response

EIA, enzyme-linked immunosorbent assay; IF, immunofluorescence; HAI, hemagglutinin inhibition; NAAT, nucleic acid amplification test; NPA, nasopharyngeal aspirate; RAT, rapid antigen test; RT-PCR, reverse transcriptase polymerase chain reaction.

Source: Adapted with permission from Lee and Ison [26]. © 2012 International Medical Press. All rights reserved.

pre-clinical studies and other considerations suggest that higher oseltamivir doses may be reasonable in patients with anticipated high-level or protracted viral replication, such as in those with progressive viral pneumonia, immunocompromised status, or zoonotic infection, and in serious illness due to influenza B virus infection. Prolongation of therapy (e.g., 10 days) is appropriate in severe viral pneumonia or in immunocompromised hosts as viral replication and detectable viral RNA may persist in these patients. Monitoring of viral RNA load during therapy may prove useful in predicting outcomes in such patients.

Inhaled zanamivir is a reasonable option for treatment, especially if oseltamivir resistance is suspected or proven because most oseltamivir-resistant variant remain susceptible to zanamivir. However, its effectiveness in patients with serious lower respiratory tract involvement is uncertain. Inhaled zanamivir may be infrequently associated with bronchospasm, sometimes severe, particularly in influenza patients with pre-existing airways diseases. Use of the proprietary disk inhaler device is not possible in intubated patients, and nebulization of the lactose-containing commercial form is contraindicated in such patients.

Antiviral resistance testing should be considered for patients in priority risk groups, especially those with progressive disease despite therapy and immunocompromised hosts. Prolonged exposure to oseltamivir during sustained virus replication in such patients, suboptimal doses of oseltamivir (e.g., once daily prophylactic dosing in those with active influenza virus replication) or breaks in treatment while patients remain influenza positive appear to be risk factors for resistance development. Oseltamivir resistance should also be considered in those failing chemoprophylaxis or those developing illness after exposure to an oseltamivir-treated patient.

Intravenous formulations of zanamivir and peramivir provide rapid delivery of high NAI levels in seriously ill persons [4]. Whether these pharmacologic differences will result in greater antiviral activity, less frequent resistance emergence, and improved clinical outcomes compared with oral oseltamivir is currently under study. While extemporaneous oseltamivir given by nasogastric tube appears to be adequately absorbed in most intubated patients, intravenous NAI administration guarantees systemic drug delivery in those with critical illness and possible gastric paresis or other causes for poor oral absorption. Intravenous

zanamivir would be the current agent of choice for treating seriously ill patients with suspected or proven oseltamivir-resistant influenza [43,44]. Hyperimmune convalescent plasma added to NAI therapy appears to provide antiviral and clinical benefits [44]. Additional discussion of antiviral agents, including resistance, investigational agents, and combinations, is found in Chapter 25.

Supportive care

Symptom relief medications

Symptomatic measures often include antipyretic–analgesics and cough suppressants. Paracetamol (acetaminophen) and other non-steroidal anti-inflammatory drugs (NSAIDs), particularly ibuprofen, are used for treatment of fever and discomfort in many countries. Aspirin should not be used, especially in children younger than 19 years, because of its association with Reye's syndrome.

Maternal hyperthermia during the first trimester increases the risk of neural tube defects and possibly other birth defects like cleft palate and congenital heart defects, and maternal fever during labor has been shown to be a risk factor for adverse neonatal and developmental outcomes. Acetaminophen appears to be the best option for treatment of fever during pregnancy.

Increased mortality risk with aspirin and paracetamol, perhaps related to immunologic or anti-inflammatory effects, has been observed in some animal models of influenza [45]. Of note, since the use of diclofenac and mefenamic acid was restricted in children in Japan in 2000, the case fatality of influenza-associated encephalopathy has fallen.

Immunomodulators

Systemic corticosteroids have been given commonly to patients with influenza-associated pneumonia and ARDS. However, retrospective studies of patients with pandemic 2009 A/H1N1 or avian A/H5N1 infections indicate an association between corticosteroid use and increased risks of adverse effects, including nosocomial pneumonia, invasive fungal infections, and possibly increased mortality [46]. Corticosteroid therapy also prolongs viral replication [7]. Although sometimes needed for treating underlying reactive airways disease or suspected adrenal insufficiency, routine use of systemic corticosteroids should be avoided. Pulse methylprednisolone is part of the standard treatment regimen (combined with antivirals and intravenous immunoglublin) for treating influenza-associated encephalopathy in Japan.

A wide variety of immunomodulatory agents directed against proinflammatory host responses show benefits in animal models of influenza (e.g., gemfibrizol, pioglitazone, cyclo-oxygenase 2 inhibitors, pamidronate, erythromycin, resveratrol), but available clinical data are limited or absent. While several retrospective studies have reported mortality reductions in patients receiving statins (HMG-CoA reductase inhibitors) who were subsequently hospitalized for influenza or pneumonia [47], results are inconsistent across studies, and rosuvastatin was inactive in a murine model. Macrolides do not appear to improve outcomes in outpatients or critically ill patients treated with antivirals [48]. Further clinical studies are needed to determine the possible benefits and optimal timing of use for particular immunomodulatory agents.

Hospital-based care

Regular monitoring of vital signs and oxygen saturation are important in seriously ill patients with influenza, because rapid deterioration in status may occur. Supplemental oxygen to correct hypoxemia, fluids and sometimes vasopressors for hypotension, and treatment of bronchospasm are essential supportive measures.

Obstetric complications and/or refractory maternal hypoxemia may necessitate emergent cesarean delivery. In those with unexplained hypotension or arrhythmias, consideration should be given for echocardiogram, EKG, and cardiac enzymes.

Intensive care

Intubation and mechanical ventilatory support with positive end-expiratory airway pressures (PEEP) can be life-saving in patients with respiratory failure [49]. In general, noninvasive ventilation strategies have not been successful in those with influenza viral pneumonia and/or ARDS. Barotrauma may further complicate ARDS, and a low tidal-volume ventilation strategy is advisable. Other interventions including neuromuscular blockade, inhaled nitric oxide (NO), various ventilatory strategies (e.g., high-frequency oscillation, airway pressure release, prone position-

ing), and diuresis or fluid removal with continuous renal replacement therapy for treatment of interstitial pulmonary edema, have been used to help maintain oxygenation. Extracorporeal membrane oxygenation (ECMO) has been used with apparent success in some cases of severe ARDS. Ventilatory support or ECMO often need to be maintained for 2–3 weeks. Renal replacement therapy is frequently required. Those with fulminant myocarditis have been managed with use of inotropic agents, pacing as indicated, ECMO with cardiac bypass, intra-aortic balloon pump, and/or left ventricular assist devices (LVAD).

ICU complications, including pneumothorax, ventilator-associated pneumonia, and venous thromboembolism, are common but the risks can be decreased with preventive measures [49]. Secondary bacterial pneumonia should be treated with appropriate antibiotics.

Nosocomial precautions

Patients hospitalized with human influenza should be managed with standard and droplet precautions. Individual rooms are desirable, but cohorting of influenza patients may be necessary during high demand periods. Whether surgical masks are as effective as fit-tested respirators in protecting healthcare workers providing routine care for influenza patients remains to be clarified [50]. While surgical masks may provide some degree of protection against exposures with low infectious doses, compliance with a properly fitted N95-type respirator likely provides improved protection. The added value of eye protection (goggles or face shields) requires further study but is an easily implemented precaution. Source control by masking of suspected or proven influenza patients in healthcare settings (e.g., emergency department, during transport, in diagnostic facilities) likely reduces environmental contamination and the risk of nosocomial transmission. Visitors should be minimized in general and prohibited if ill.

Aerosol-generating procedures and devices (e.g., bronchoscopy, intubation, sputum induction, use of BiPAP machine) enhance the risk of nosocomial transmission and when feasible should be carried out in airborne infection isolation rooms (negative pressure, frequent air changes, HEPA filter exhaust). Use of N-95 respirators or equivalent (e.g., powered air purifying respirator) and face shields is recommended for healthcare workers under such circumstances. More stringent procedures are also required when patients are hospitalized with presumed A/H5N1 or other novel strains of concern. These situations warrant airborne, droplet, and contact precautions, including eye protection.

Clinicians should consider influenza virus infection as the possible cause of any febrile respiratory illness requiring hospitalization during influenza season and consider isolating the patient, testing for influenza, and starting empiric antiviral therapy. Similarly, when an unexplained febrile or respiratory illness develops in an inpatient, the possibility of nosocomial acquisition from other patients, staff, or visitors should be considered.

When influenza outbreaks develop in hospital wards or other institutional settings, stringent infection control measures and antiviral chemoprophylaxis (oseltamivir or zanamivir) all patients or residents regardless of vaccine receipt and for nonimmunized staff (or all staff in absence of an effective vaccine) is recommended for at least 10 days after illness onset in the last known case [38]. For post-exposure prophylaxis in immunocompromised hosts, standard treatment dose regimens (i.e., twice daily administration as contrasted with once daily) may reduce the risk of oseltamivir resistance emergence. If new cases develop despite oseltamivir prophylaxis, especially in care units containing immunocompromised patients or severely ill patients, the possible transmission of oseltamivir-resistant virus and switch to zanamivir for treatment and prophylaxis should be considered.

Specific guidance suggests that newborns born to mothers who have suspected or confirmed influenza illness should be separated temporarily from their mothers, although the length of separation has not been well defined and should be determined on a case-by-case basis. Women intending to breastfeed should express breast milk while separated from her newborn. Oseltamivir treatment of mothers is not a contraindication for use of breast milk.

Outpatient settings

In households, common sense tactics apply to reduce exposure of contacts to those with illness (i.e., hand hygiene, cough etiquette, social distancing). This includes minimizing visitors other than necessary caregivers for an ill person; washing and/or sanitizing hands frequently, including after every contact with a sick person; and maintaining ventilation in shared areas. Pregnant women should not provide care for ill persons, and sick family members should not care for infants. Visitors at increased risk for complications should maintain 6-foot distance. Compliance with masks and hand hygiene appears to reduce the risk of secondary infections in household contacts. Antiviral chemoprophylaxis is a consideration for persons, including pregnant women, at increased risk of complications when they are unimmunized or unlikely to respond to vaccine, or when the vaccine is poorly matched to circulating strains. Inhaled zanamivir would be the preferred prophylaxis agent for pregnant women.

References

1. Nicholson KG. Human influenza. In: Nicholson KG, Webster RG, Hay AJ, editors. Texbook of Influenza. Oxford, UK: Blackwell Science Ltd; 1998. p. 219–64.

2. Hayden FG, Palese P. Influenza virus. In: Clinical Virology, 3rd edn. Washington, DC: American Society for Microbiology Press; 2009. p. 943.

3. Writing Committee of the Second World Health Organization Consultation on Clinical Aspects of Human Infection with Avian Influenza A (H5N1) Virus. Human Influenza. N Engl J Med. 2008;358(3):261–73.

4. Writing Committee of the WHO Consultation on Clinical Aspects of Pandemic (H1N1) 2009 Influenza. Clinical aspects of pandemic 2009 influenza A (H1N1) virus infection. N Engl J Med. 2010;362(18):1708–19.

5. Shrestha SS, Swerdlow DL, Borse RH, Prabhu VS, Finelli L, Atkins CY, et al. Estimating the burden of 2009 pandemic influenza A (H1N1) in the United States (April 2009–April 2010). Clin Infect Dis. 2011;52(Suppl. 1):S75–82.

6. Brankston G, Gitterman L, Hirji Z, Lemieux C, Gardam M. Transmission of influenza A in human beings. Lancet Infect Dis. 2007;7(4):257–65.

7. Lee N, Chan PK, Hui DS, Rainer TH, Wong E, Choi KW, et al. Viral loads and duration of viral shedding in adult patients hospitalized with influenza. J Infect Dis. 2009;200(4):492–500.

8. Lee N, Chan PK, Wong CK, Wong KT, Choi KW, Joynt GM, et al. Viral clearance and inflammatory response patterns in adults hospitalized for pandemic 2009 influenza A(H1N1) virus pneumonia. Antivir Ther. 2011;16(2):237–47.

9. Amin R, Ford-Jones E, Richardson SE, MacGregor D, Tellier R, Heurter H, et al. Acute childhood encephalitis and encephalopathy associated with influenza: a pro-

spective 11-year review. Pediatr Infect Dis J. 2008;27(5): 390–5.

10. de Jong MD, Simmons CP, Thanh TT, Hien VM, Smith GJ, Chau TN, et al. Fatal outcome of human influenza A (H5N1) is associated with high viral load and hypercytokinemia. Nat Med. 2006;12(10):1203–7.

11. Shieh WJ, Blau DM, Denison AM, Deleon-Carnes M, Adem P, Bhatnagar J, et al. 2009 pandemic influenza A (H1N1): pathology and pathogenesis of 100 fatal cases in the United States. Am J Pathol. 2010;177(1): 166–75.

12. Sheng ZM, Chertow DS, Ambroggio X, McCall S, Przygodzki RM, Cunningham RE, et al. Autopsy series of 68 cases dying before and during the 1918 influenza pandemic peak. Proc Natl Acad Sci U S A. 2011;108(39): 16416–21.

13. Monsalvo AC, Batalle JP, Lopez MF, Krause JC, Klemenc J, Hernandez JZ, et al. Severe pandemic 2009 H1N1 influenza disease due to pathogenic immune complexes. Nat Med. 2011;17(2):195–9.

14. Zaas AK, Chen M, Varkey J, Veldman T, Hero AO III, Lucas J, et al. Gene expression signatures diagnose influenza and other symptomatic respiratory viral infections in humans. Cell Host Microbe. 2009;6(3):207–17.

15. Agrati C, Gioia C, Lalle E, Cimini E, Castilletti C, Armignacco O, et al. Association of profoundly impaired immune competence in H1N1v-infected patients with a severe or fatal clinical course. J Infect Dis. 2010;202(5):681–9.

16. Lee N, Wong CK, Hui DSC, Lee SKW, Wong RYK, Ngai KLK, et al. Role of human toll-like receptors in naturally occurring influenza A infections. Influenza and Other Respiratory Viruses. DOI: 10.1111/irv.12109; published online 2 April 2013.

17. Lee N, Wong CK, Chan PK, Chan MC, Wong RY, Lun SW, et al. Cytokine response patterns in severe pandemic 2009 H1N1 and seasonal influenza among hospitalized adults. PLoS ONE. 2011;6(10):e26050.

18. Bermejo-Martin JF, de Ortiz LR, Pumarola T, Rello J, Almansa R, Ramirez P, et al. Th1 and Th17 hypercytokinemia as early host response signature in severe pandemic influenza. Crit Care. 2009;13(6):R201.

19. To KK, Hung IF, Li IW, Lee KL, Koo CK, Yan WW, et al. Delayed clearance of viral load and marked cytokine activation in severe cases of pandemic H1N1 2009 influenza virus infection. Clin Infect Dis. 2010; 50(6):850–9.

20. Karlsson EA, Marcelin G, Webby RJ, Schultz-Cherry S. Review on the impact of pregnancy and obesity on influenza virus infection. Influenza Other Respi Viruses. 2012;6:449–60.

21. Howard WA, Peiris M, Hayden FG. Report of the "mechanisms of lung injury and immunomodulator interventions in influenza" workshop, 21 March 2010, Ventura, California, USA. Influenza Other Respi Viruses. 2011;5(6):453–75.

22. Everitt AR, Clare S, Pertel T, John SP, Wash RS, Smith SE, et al. IFITM3 restricts the morbidity and mortality associated with influenza. Nature. 2012;484(7395): 519–23.

23. Ferdinands JM, Denison AM, Dowling NF, Jost HA, Gwinn ML, Liu L, et al. A pilot study of host genetic variants associated with influenza-associated deaths among children and young adults. Emerg Infect Dis. 2011;17(12):2294–302.

24. Wilkinson TM, Li CK, Chui CS, Huang AK, Perkins M, Liebner JC, et al. Preexisting influenza-specific CD4+ T cells correlate with disease protection against influenza challenge in humans. Nat Med. 2012;18(2):274–80.

25. McCullers JA. Preventing and treating secondary bacterial infections with antiviral agents. Antivir Ther. 2011;16(2):123–35.

26. Lee N, Ison MG. Diagnosis, management and outcomes of adults hospitalized with influenza. Antivir Ther. 2012;17(1 Pt B):143–57.

27. Rasmussen SA, Jamieson DJ. Influenza and pregnancy in the United States: before, during, and after 2009 H1N1. Clin Obstet Gynecol. 2012;55(2):487–97.

28. Choi SM, Boudreault AA, Xie H, Englund JA, Corey L, Boeckh M. Differences in clinical outcomes after 2009 influenza A/H1N1 and seasonal influenza among hematopoietic cell transplant recipients. Blood. 2011; 117(19):5050–6.

29. Sheth AN, Althoff KN, Brooks JT. Influenza susceptibility, severity, and shedding in HIV-infected adults: a review of the literature. Clin Infect Dis. 2011;52(2): 219–27.

30. Okumura A, Nakagawa S, Kawashima H, Muguruma T, Saito O, Fujimoto J, et al. Deaths associated with pandemic (H1N1) 2009 among children, Japan, 2009–2010. Emerg Infect Dis. 2011;17(11):1993–2000.

31. Warren-Gash C, Smeeth L, Hayward AC. Influenza as a trigger for acute myocardial infarction or death from cardiovascular disease: a systematic review. Lancet Infect Dis. 2009;9(10):601–10.

32. Mamas MA, Fraser D, Neyses L. Cardiovascular manifestations associated with influenza virus infection. Int J Cardiol. 2008;130(3):304–9.

33. Hoshino A, Saitoh M, Oka A, Okumura A, Kubota M, Saito Y, et al. Epidemiology of acute encephalopathy in Japan, with emphasis on the association of viruses and syndromes. Brain & Development. 2012;34: 337–343.

34. Muller MP, McGeer AJ, Hassan K, Marshall J, Christian M. Evaluation of pneumonia severity and acute physiology scores to predict ICU admission and mortality in patients hospitalized for influenza. PLoS ONE. 2010;5(3):e9563.

35. Jernigan DB, Lindstrom SL, Johnson JR, Miller JD, Hoelscher M, Humes R, et al. Detecting 2009 pandemic influenza A (H1N1) virus infection: availability of diagnostic testing led to rapid pandemic response. Clin Infect Dis. 2011;52(Suppl. 1):S36–43.

36. Ginocchio CC, Zhang F, Manji R, Arora S, Bornfreund M, Falk L, et al. Evaluation of multiple test methods for the detection of the novel 2009 influenza A (H1N1) during the New York City outbreak. J Clin Virol. 2009;45(3):191–5.

37. WHO. World Health Organization guidelines for pharmacological management of pandemic influenza A (H1N1) 2009 and other influenza viruses. 2010. Available from: http://www.who.int/csr/resources/publications/swineflu/h1n1_guidelines_pharmaceutical_mngt.pdf (accessed 13 February 2013).

38. Antiviral agents for the treatment and chemoprophylaxis of influenza. Recommendations of the Advisory Committee on Immunization Practices (ACIP). MMWR. 2011;60(1):1–24. 2012.

39. Hsu J, Santesso N, Mustafa R, Brozek J, Chen YL, Hopkins JP, et al. Antivirals for treatment of influenza: a systematic review and meta-analysis of observational studies. Ann Intern Med. 2012;156(7):512–24.

40. Chan PKS, Lee N, Zaman M, Adisasmito W, Coker R, Hanshaoworakul W, et al. Determinants of antiviral effectiveness in influenza A subtype H5N1. J Infect Dis. 2012;206:1359–66.

41. Garg S, Fry AM, Patton M, Fiore AE, Finelli L. Antiviral treatment of influenza in children. Pediatr Infect Dis J. 2012;31(2):e43–51.

42. Hurt AC, Chotpitayasunondh T, Cox NJ, Daniels R, Fry AM, Gubareva LV, et al. Antiviral resistance during the 2009 influenza A H1N1 pandemic: public health, laboratory, and clinical perspectives. Lancet Infect Dis. 2012;12(3):240–8.

43. Hayden FG, de Jong M. Emerging influenza antiviral resistance threats. J Infect Dis. 2011;203(1):6–10.

44. Hung IFN, To KKW, Lee C-K, Lee K-L, Yan W_W, Chan K, et al. Hyperimmune Intravenous immunoglobulin treatment: A multicentre double-blind randomized controlled trial for patients with severe A(H1N1) pdm09. Infection. Chest. doi:10.1378/chest.12-2907; published online 28 February 2013.

45. Eyers S, Weatherall M, Shirtcliffe P, Perrin K, Beasley R. The effect on mortality of antipyretics in the treatment of influenza infection: systematic review and meta-analysis. J R Soc Med. 2010;103(10):403–11.

46. Brun-Buisson C, Richard JC, Mercat A, Thiebaut AC, Brochard L. Early corticosteroids in severe influenza A/H1N1 pneumonia and acute respiratory distress syndrome. Am J Respir Crit Care Med. 2011;183(9):1200–6.

47. Vandermeer ML, Thomas AR, Kamimoto L, Reingold A, Gershman K, Meek J, et al. Association between use of statins and mortality among patients hospitalized with laboratory-confirmed influenza virus infections: a multistate study. J Infect Dis. 2012;205(1):13–9.

48. Martın-Loeches I, Bermejo-Martin JF, Vallés J, Granada R, Vidaur L, Vergara-Serrano JC, et al. Macrolide-based regimens in absence of bacterial co-infection in critically ill H1N1 patients with primary viral pneumonia. Intensive Care Med. 2013;39:693–702.

49. Dellinger RP, Levy MM, Rhodes A, Annane D, Gerlach H, Opal SM, et al. Surviving sepsis campaign: international guidelines for management of severe sepsis and septic shock: 2012.Crit Care Med. 2013 Feb;41(2):580–637. doi:10.1097/CCM.0b013e3182.

50. MacIntyre CR, Wang Q, Seale H, Yang P, Shi W, Gao Z, et al. A randomised clinical trial of three options for N95 respirators and medical masks in health workers. Amer J Resp Crit Care Med. Published on February 14, 2013 as doi:10.1164/rccm.201207-1164OC.

391

25

Antivirals: Targets and use

Michael G. Ison[1] and Alan Hay[2]

[1]Divisions of Infectious Diseases and Organ Transplantation, Northwestern University Feinberg School of Medicine, Chicago, IL, USA

[2]Virology Division, MRC National Institute for Medical Research, London, UK

Introduction

The two principal classes of antivirals that have been widely licensed for use against influenza, targeted against the virus M2 proton channel and the virus neuraminidase (NA) (Table 25.1), were developed in contrasting ways. Amantadine was developed serendipitously in the 1960s and first licensed in 1966 for use against the contemporary influenza A (H2N2) [1] more than two decades before the target M2 protein and its function were identified [2]. Rimantadine, the α-methyl methylamine derivative, was subsequently developed in the former Soviet Union and has been licensed in many countries. Although other effective inhibitors (e.g., cyclo-nonylamine and spiroadamantane-pyrollidine) were studied, no others were fully developed and licensed, in part because they were ineffective against amantadine-resistant viruses and represented no advantage over the licensed products. These agents do not inhibit the analogous BM2 channel of influenza B viruses [3] and are as a consequence ineffective against influenza B, reflecting their high specificity. Their exclusive usefulness against susceptible influenza A viruses together with early concerns about side-effects and the emergence of resistance resulted in their limited but successful use initally against the novel A(H3N2) virus causing the 1968 pandemic. The current exclusive circulation

of amantadine-resistant viruses in the human population has largely abrogated their current usefulness.

In contrast, while attempts in the 1960s to develop effective inhibitors of the NA based on transition state anologs, for example 2,3 dehydro-2-deoxy-*N*-acetylneuraminic acid (DANA), were unsuccessful, zanamivir, a guanidino derivative of DANA was designed [4] following the determination of the three-dimensional structure of the NA by X-ray crystallography in the 1980s [5]. An inhaled formulation was licensed in 1999. Subsequently, oseltamivir, based on a different ring structure and active moiety, was developed and also licensed in 1999 as an orally available prodrug. The different mechanisms of interaction with the NA provide the basis for complementary resistance profiles of the two inhibitors. Two related neuraminidase inhibitors (NAIs) are also available. Peramivir, which possesses the active moieties of both zanamivir and oseltamivir [6], has been developed as an intravenous formulation, and licensed in Japan and South Korea in 2011, and has been available for emergency use during the 2009 pandemic in some other countries. Laninamivir, an octanoyl prodrug of 7-methoxyzanamivir, which has a long half-life in the respiratory tract [7], was licensed as a single dose inhaled formulation in Japan in 2011.

Arbidol, a broad-spectrum antiviral [8], was also developed empirically and initially licensed in Russia

Textbook of Influenza, Second Edition. Edited by Robert G. Webster, Arnold S. Monto, Thomas J. Braciale, and Robert A. Lamb.
© 2013 John Wiley & Sons, Ltd. Published 2013 by John Wiley & Sons, Ltd.

Table 25.1. (a) Dosing of commercially available M2 inhibitors (adamantanes) [23, 25].

Antiviral	Amantadine (Symmetrel)	Rimantadine (Flumadine)
Structure		
Prophylaxis dosing[a]	100 mg BID	100 mg BID
Treatment dosing[a]	100 mg BID	100 mg BID
Route of administration	Oral	Oral

[a]For normal renal function; see package insert for dosing with renal insufficiency. Reduce to four times daily dosing is recommended for adults ≥65 years of age for amantadine.

Table 25.1. (b) Dosing of commercially available neuraminidase inhibitors [30].

Antiviral	Laninamivir (Inavir)	Oseltamivir (Tamiflu)	Peramivir (Rapiacta, PeramiFlu)	Zanamivir (Relenza)
Structure				
Prophylaxis dosing[a]	Not indicated	≤15 kg 30 mg QD 15–23 kg 45 mg QD 23–40 kg 60 mg QD >40 kg 75 mg QD	Not indicated	10 mg QD for 10–28 days
Treatment dosing[a]	40 mg single dose	Birth–8 mo: 3 mg/kg BID 9 mo–11 mo: 3.5 m/kg BID Age ≥1 year: ≤15 kg 30 mg BID 15–23 kg 45 mg BID 23–40 kg 60 mg BID >40 kg 75 mg BID for 5 days	600 mg QD for 5–10 days	10 mg BID for 5 days
Route of administration	Inhaled	Oral[b]	Parenteral	Inhaled[b]

BID, twice daily; QD, four times daily.
[a]For normal renal function; see package insert for dosing with renal insufficiency.
[b]Parenteral formulations under development.

in 1990 for treatment and prophylaxis of influenza A and B [9], and subsequently in China in 2006 [10]. It represents a third class of antiviral which targets the fusion activity of the virus hemagglutinin (HA), although the basis of its clinical efficacy has not yet been established.

Mechanism of action and resistance

M2 inhibitors

The M2 protein is a minor component of the virus envelope which functions as a proton activated, proton-selective channel [11] during two stages of virus replication. During virus entry, via receptor-mediated endocytosis, passage of protons through M2 from the acidic environment of the endosome causes an acid-dissociation of the internal M1-RNP structure such that on fusion of the virus membrane with the endosomal membrane, mediated by the HA, the free RNP structure is released for transport to the nucleus to initiate replication. Inhibition of M2 by amantadine or rimantadine results in the M1-RNP complex being trapped in the cytoplasm. They also inhibit a function of M2 which reduces the acidity of the trans Golgi of virus-infected cells, which is necessary for the transport of native HA of highly pathogenic avian viruses to the plasma membrane [12].

The channel is formed by a homotetramer of 97 amino acid subunits which span the membrane, oriented with a short N-terminal domain external to the virus, a transmembrane domain comprising residues 25–43, and a C-terminal domain within the interior of the virus (described in detail in Chapter 6). Aminoadamantanes and related compounds inhibit M2 by interacting with a site within the N-terminal part of the transmembrane channel between residues 27 and 34, exterior to the His37-Trp41 structure which forms both the proton permeation mechanism and proton selectivity filter of the channel (Figure 25.1a; see also Figure 7.2 in Chapter 6). Resistance emerging *in vivo* (and *in vitro*) to amantadine and rimantadine, which exhibit strict cross-resistance (thus "amantadine resistance" and "rimantadine resistance" can, in general, be used interchangeably), is caused by single substitutions in residues 26, 27, 30, 31, or 34 [2] which line the interior of this region of the channel (Figure 25.1a) [13]. Similar amino acid substitutions have been responsible for resistance in human, swine, and

avian viruses of different subtypes: Leu26Phe, Val27Ala/Gly or Ileu27Ser/Thr, Ala30Val/Ser/Thr, Ser31Asn or Gly34Glu. pH-dependence of inhibition indicates that the inhibitor binds tightly and irreversibly to a neutral/high pH form of the channel. Nuclear magnetic resonance and X-ray crystallographic structural analyses have indicated that the large hydrophobic adamantane moiety of the inhibitor binds within a hydrophobic pocket formed by methyl side-chains of the four valine residues which form the "Val27 valve" (see Chapter 6) and the four alanine 30 residues, with the polar amino group oriented towards the C-terminal [13]. As a consequence, inhibition is principally by occlusion of the channel, the inhibitor excluding water molecules involved in the transfer of protons through the channel. Substitution of valine 27 by alanine (or glycine) causes an expansion of the site such that the affinity of the adamantane ring is substantially reduced; however, larger hydrophobic structures such as amino spiroadamantane inhibit the Val27Ala and Leu26Phe mutants with higher affinity than the wild-type protein. However, these molecules do not inhibit another common mutation, Ser31Asn, predominantly responsible for resistance among currently circulating human influenza A viruses. This substitution appears to cause a structural alteration in the channel such that, although the inhibitor can bind with reduced affinity, it no longer binds tightly to the neutral/high pH form [14]. Although these substitutions may influence channel activity, their emergence as features of currently circulating human, swine, and avian influenza viruses (Figure 25.1b) demonstrates that they do not impair, and may even enhance, the biologic properties of the viruses.

NA inhibitors

The catalytic activity of the NA removes the terminal sialic acid moiety from sialyl glycoprotein or glycolipid receptors to which the HA attaches. It functions in promoting release of virus from virus-infected cells and, by preventing aggregation of progeny virions, transmission of the virus. By removal of sialic acid from mucins and other potentially inhibitory molecules in the respiratory tract, NA also facilitates virus infection.

The guanidino group of zanamivir interacts with a pocket within the catalytic site formed by the acidic residues Glu119, Asp151, and Glu227, such that it

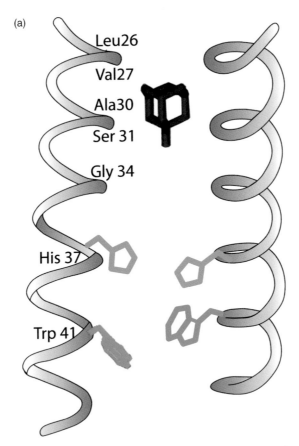

Figure 25.1. (a) Structure of the M2 channel showing the locations of residues substituted in amantadine-resistant viruses. (b) Phylogenetic comparison (using maximum parsimony) showing the relationships between the M genes of swine and human viruses and the emergence of amantadine resistance. Amantadine resistance, due to a Ser31Asn substitution in M2, emerged in the A/Wisconsin/67/2005-like viruses and has subsequently been maintained in human A(H3N2) viruses to date.

Amantadine resistance, also due to a Ser31Asn substitution in M2, which emerged in European swine viruses in the mid-1980s was maintained with the spread of the viruses in Eurasia and the subsequent incorporation of the M gene into the 2009 H1N1 pandemic virus. Influenza A(H1N1) viruses circulating in pigs in Ireland acquired a Ser31Asn mutation in the mid-1990s.

(b)

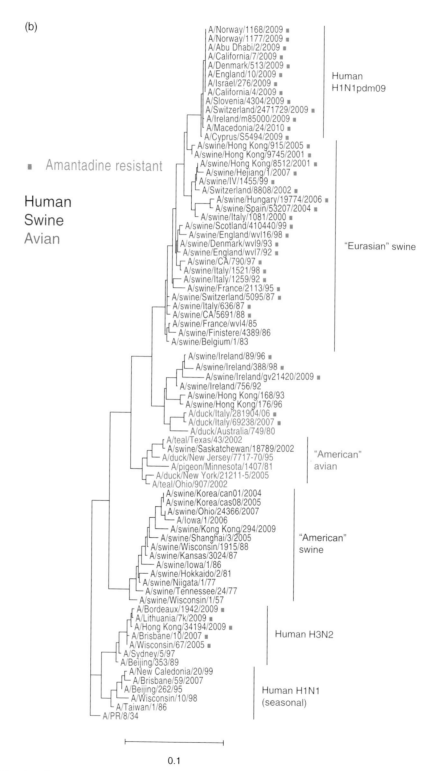

Figure 25.1. (*Continued*)

binds with more than a 1000-fold greater affinity than the substrate; dissociation constants for binding are in the nanomolar range compared with the micromolar range for the substrate. The pentyl ether moiety of oseltamivir binds to a different site, a hydrophobic pocket that is exposed by the reorientation of the side chain of Glu276 on interaction with the inhibitor, with a similar affinity of binding to that of zanamivir. The ethyl ester prodrug oseltamivir phosphate, with enhanced oral bioavailability, is converted by hepatic esterases to the active compound oseltamivir carboxylate. Peramivir, which possesses both the guanidino group of zanamivir and the hydrophobic pentyl group of oseltamivir, thus binds to the two sites. Because the structures of the NAs of influenza A and B viruses are similar, zanamivir exhibits similar activities against both virus types; however, oseltamivir has an IC_{50} some 10-fold greater against the NA of influenza B than influenza A, which may account for lower efficacy against influenza B [15]. The discovery of the 150-cavity adjacent to the catalytic site of group 1 NAs (Figure 25.2a, see Chapter 5) [16] has provided the basis for designing alternative inhibitors that target this site [17].

As zanamivir is structurally close to the transition-state analog of the sialic acid substrate, it has been rationalized that the potential for selection of resistance to zanamivir action, without compromising enzyme activity, would be low. Accordingly, few instances of zanamivir resistance have been associated with clinical use. Studies of resistance emergence in cell culture showed that this occurred much less readily than with amantadine or rimantadine and that in many instances mutations were initially selected in the HA, which caused a reduction in the affinity of receptor binding and as consequence a reduced requirement for NA activity; only on further passage were mutations in NA selected, directly reducing inhibition of the enzyme. *In vivo*, however, reduced susceptibility to NAIs has usually been associated with mutations in NA. Thus, in the absence of a robust cell-based assay for determining susceptibility of virus replication, an enzyme inhibition assay, using fluorescent or chemiluminescent substrates, is generally used to detect (and screen for) and analyze changes in NA, and hence virus, susceptibility to NAIs. As mixtures of viruses differing in NAI susceptibility may complicate interpretation of results, identification of mutations by sequencing the NA gene, or pyrosequencing

specific regions, is used to complement enzyme inhibition data. Selection of resistance to zanamivir of influenza A viruses in cell culture usually involved substitution of Glu119 of the NA by Gly or Ala, depending on the virus studied, which results in loss of interaction of the carboxylate with the guanidino group of the inhibitor, causing high resistance to both zanamivir and peramivir. However, such mutations decrease activity and/or stability of the enzyme and may abrogate their selection *in vivo*. An Arg152Lys substitution in the NA of an influenza B virus isolated from an immunocompromised child treated with zanamivir reduced susceptibility to all NAIs.

Considerably more is known about resistance to oseltamivir, which has emerged more readily *in vivo*, likely unrelated to its more widespread use. Subtype as well as type-specific differences in the principal oseltamivir resistance mutations reflect differences in the amino acid sequences of the viruses (Table 25.4). Resistance of H3N2 viruses, emerging in children treated with oseltamivir, due to amino acid substitutions Arg292Lys or Glu119Val in NA, correspond to those preferentially selected on passage of the subtype in the presence of oseltamivir in cell culture. In contrast to the substitution by Gly, the Glu119Val substitution confers resistance to oseltamivir alone and does not adversely affect properties of the enzyme or transmissibility of the virus in ferrets [18]. The Arg-292Lys substitution, which conferred high resistance to oseltamivir, caused an intermediate effect on susceptibility to peramivir, but little effect on susceptibility to zanamivir. Arg 292 is a highly conserved residue of the catalytic triad of the catalytic site and it is not surprising that substitution by Lys causes reduced enzyme activity and impaired virus infectivity and transmissibility in ferrets, possibly accounting in part for the lower frequency of detection of oseltamivir resistance among A(H3N2) viruses than A(H1N1) viruses. Resistance of N1-containing viruses (H1N1 and H5N1 subtypes) has been principally the result of the substitution His275Tyr (N1 numbering) which causes high resistance to oseltamivir and peramivir with little effect on susceptibility to zanamivir. An Asn294Ser (N2 numbering) mutation causing reduced susceptibility to oseltamivir, but a lesser effect on zanamivir susceptibility, has occurred in human isolates of both N1- and N2-containing viruses. In contrast, the incidence of reduced susceptibility of influenza B viruses to oseltamivir has been low and few of the mutations, Gly402Ser, Asp198Asn/Glu, or Ileu222Thr, have been associated with oseltamivir treatment. Substitutions in residue 222 (B NA numbering) have been associated with oseltamivir and zanamivir therapy and have been detected in influenza B and N1- and N2-containing A viruses. While alone they confer relatively low level reduced susceptibility to oseltamivir, zanamivir, and peramivir, they may act synergistically to markedly enhance resistance, for example due to the His275Tyr of double mutants. A number of other mutations (e.g., Ser 247Asn) have also recently been observed to have similar synergistic effects [19].

HA fusion inhibitors

In addition to binding to sialic acid receptors on the cell surface, the HA is responsible for promoting fusion between the virus and endosome membranes to effect entry of the virus genome (RNP) into the cell. The low pH in the endosome triggers an acid-induced conformational change in the HA which causes the membranes to fuse (see Chapter 5). A variety of small molecules have been identified that interact with the HA to increase its acid stability and decrease the pH of HA-mediated membrane fusion, and as a consequence inhibit genome entry and virus replication. Many of the inhibitors are group specific, for example tertiary butyl hydroquinone (TBHQ) only inhibits viruses with group 2 HAs, such as H3, while others, for example the quinolizidine-linked benzamide BMY 27709, inhibit viruses with H1 or H2 (group 1) but not H3 HA [20]. Arbidol (1-methyl-2-phenylthiomethyl-3-carbethoxy-4-dimethylaminomethyl-5-hydroxy-6-bromo-indole hydrochloride) was shown to inhibit the replication of all influenza A subtypes and influenza B viruses tested in cell culture with similar IC_{50} values, and to inhibit low pH-induced membrane fusion and virus entry [21]. Leneva *et al.* [22] confirmed that the determinant of susceptibility to arbidol was the HA and selected in cell culture arbidol-resistant mutants that mapped to the HA2 subunit, in a region similar to that occupied by other mutations which increased the pH of the conformational transition. The decrease in acid stability of the mutant HAs specifically abrogated the stabilizing effect of arbidol. Although viruses differ in their sensitivity to inhibition by arbidol, surveillance of susceptibility of human influenza viruses to arbidol has not identified the emergence of mutants with reduced susceptibility associated with its use. In the absence of such data and evidence that arbidol has immunomodulatory activity [9], the basis of its clinical efficacy is uncertain.

Approved agents

M2 inhibitors (aminoadamantanes)

There are currently two approved inhibitors of the influenza A M2 proton channel: amantadine (1-adamantanamine hydrochloride; Symmetrel®, Endo Pharmaceuticals Inc., PA and other generic equivalents) and rimantadine (α-methyl-1-adamantane-methylamine-hydrochloride; Flumadine®, Forest Pharmaceuticals Inc., Missouri and other generic equivalents) [23]. Both aminoadamantanes are symmetric tricyclic amines that specifically inhibit the replication of susceptible influenza A viruses at low concentrations (<1.0 µg/mL) [23]. Although these agents are approved for prevention and treatment of influenza A, widespread resistance among most currently circulating viruses preclude their use in most cases [24].

Amantadine

Pharmacokinetics/pharmacodynamics Amantadine is available as 100-mg tablets and capsules in addition to an oral solution and syrup (10 mg/mL); for dosing see Table 25.1 [23]. Available formulations are rapidly absorbed with 86–94% bioavailability and reach peak plasma levels (mean C_{max} 0.22 µg/mL, range 0.18–0.32 µg/mL after 100 mg; 0.51 µg/mL after 200 mg) within 4 h [23, 25, 26]. After a single 200-mg oral dose, mean nasal mucous concentrations were 0.15 ± 0.16, 0.28 ± 0.26, and 0.39 ± 0.34 µg/mL at 1, 4, and 8 hours, representing 31%, 59%, and 95% of plasma levels, respectively. Amantadine is predominately excreted unchanged in the urine by glomerular filtration and tubular secretion with a plasma elimination half-life of approximately 11–15 h in patients with normal renal function [25, 26]. Elimination is markedly prolonged in patients with renal impairment and the elderly, as a result of age-related reduction in renal function [25, 26]. Amantadine crosses the placenta and blood–brain barrier (levels in cerebrospinal fluid are around 75% of serum levels) as well as being present in breast milk. It has a plasma protein binding of about 67% [23, 25]. Amantadine is classified as a pregnancy class C drug; animal studies demonstrated teratogenicity and embryotoxicity with high doses, but not low doses, of amantadine in rats, but not in rabbits. Among susceptible H1N1, H2N2, and H3N2 subtypes of influenza A, the 50% effective concentration (EC_{50}) of amantadine in Madin–Darby canine kidney cells is in the range 0.15–0.4 μg/mL [27].

Adverse effects and drug interactions Most side effects of amantadine, including antimuscarinic effects, gastrointestinal upset, orthostatic hypotension, and congestive heart failure, occur in less than 10% of treated individuals. Central nervous system (CNS) side effects, include confusion, disorientation, mood alterations, memory disturbances, delusions, nightmares, ataxia, tremors, dizziness, anxiety, irritability, headache, slurred speech, visual disturbances, delirium, occulogyric episodes, and hallucinations, occur more frequently (15–30%), particularly in the elderly [23, 26, 28]. Seizures, coma, and acute psychosis are also observed in less than 1% of treated patients. Concomitant ingestion of antihistamines or anticholinergic drugs, co-trimoxazole, and the combination of triamterene and hydrochlorothiazide increases the CNS effects of amantadine [23, 26]. Quinine and quinidine also reduce the clearance of this drug. Co-administration of amantadine with monoamine oxidase inhibitors may precipitate life-threatening hypertension [26]. The drug does not appear to interact with the cytochrome P450 system.

Rimantadine

Pharmacokinetics/pharmacodynamics Rimantadine is available as 100-mg tablets and an oral syrup (10 mg/mL); for dosing see Table 25.1. Rimantadine has nearly complete oral bioavailability and achieves peak plasma concentration (mean C_{max} 74 ng/mL, range 45–138 ng/mL after 100 mg) 3–6 h after ingestion. Rimantadine undergoes extensive metabolism in the liver before being excreted in the urine resulting in a plasma half-life of 24–36 h. Only 25% of the parent drug is excreted unchanged in the urine. Patients with creatinine clearance ≤10 mL/min or serious hepatic dysfunction require dose reduction because of prolongation of the plasma half-life. Prolongation of the elimination half-life and associated higher plasma levels are also seen in elderly nursing home residents. Forty percent of the drug is bound by plasma proteins. Rimantadine is a pregnancy class C drug; animal studies demonstrated embryotoxicity with high doses of rimantadine in rats, but not in rabbits, although there was evidence of developmental abnormalities. Among susceptible H1N1, H2N2, and H3N2 subtypes of influenza A, the EC_{50} of rimantadine in Madin–Darby canine kidney cells is in the range 0.15–0.4 μg/mL [29].

Adverse effects and drug interactions The most common adverse effects of rimantadine include gastrointestinal disturbances such as nausea, vomiting and anorexia, and CNS effects such as headaches, insomnia, nightmares, nervousness, lightheadedness, and concentration difficulties, which occur in 1–3% of individuals [28]. Compared with amantadine, rimantadine causes significantly fewer CNS side effects in both young and elderly adults, with a 10-fold lower incidence of adverse effects in one study [28]. Although the histamine H2 receptor antagonist cimetidine increased plasma rimantadine concentrations by 15–20% and aspirin or acetaminophen reduced plasma levels by 10%, no dose adjustment is recommended. Co-administration of rimantadine with drugs affecting CNS function, such as antihistamines, antidepressants, and minor tranquilizers, should trigger close monitoring of the individual. No other significant drug interactions have been described.

Neuraminidase inhibitors

There are currently two NAIs approved in most countries, oseltamivir (GS4104; Tamiflu®, Genentech, South San Francisco, California and Chugai Pharmaceutical Co, Japan) and zanamivir (GG167; Relenza®, GlaxoSmithKline, Research Triangle Park, North Carolina), and two NAIs that are approved in more limited markets, laninamivir (CS08958; Inavir, Daiichi Sankyo, Japan and Biota Holdings Ltd, Australia; approved in Japan only) and peramivir (BCX-1812 and previously RWJ-270201; Rapiacta® in Japan and Peramiflu in South Korea, BioCryst Pharmaceuticals, Birmingham, Alabama) [30]. All four compounds inhibit the viral NA and thereby prevent destruction of sialic acid-bearing receptors that are recognized by influenza A and B virus HA. This prevents the virus from being released from infected calls and passing through respiratory secretions to initiate new cycles of replication, as the virions remain attached to the membrane of the infected cell and to each other; additionally, the NAIs may inhibit viral binding to cells.

Oseltamivir

Pharmacokinetics/pharmacodynamics Oseltamivir is available in 30, 45, and 75 mg oral capsules and an oral suspension (6 mg/mL); for dosing see Table 25.1. An intravenous formulation of oseltamivir is currently under development (see below). Oral oseltamivir phosphate is an ethyl ester prodrug that is readily absorbed by the gastrointestinal tract and converted by gastrointestinal tract, hepatic, and blood esterases to the active compound (oseltamivir carboxylate) resulting in an oral bioavailability of ranges of 79–93% [31, 32]. Oseltamivir carboxylate achieves a peak concentration 3–4 hours after oral administration and is widely distributed in the body [31]. Both the prodrug and the active metabolite are eliminated primarily unchanged through the kidney resulting in a plasma half-life of the carboxylate of 6–10 h [31]. The carboxylate undergoes both glomerular filtration and tubular secretion. The dose should be reduced by half for patients with a creatinine clearance of less than 30 mL/min and further reductions are indicated for a creatinine clearance of less than 10 mL/min after dialysis in patients on chronic renal replacement [31]. There are limited data on dosing of oseltamivir in patients on various forms of renal replacement therapy. In patients receiving standard hemodialysis, 30 mg given 1 hour after completion of dialysis provided plasma areas under the curve (AUCs) similar to healthy control subjects given 75 mg twice daily without significant accumulation over time [33]. Similarly, in patients receiving continuous ambulatory peritoneal dialysis

(CAPD), 30 mg doses of oseltamivir weekly provided similar exposure to healthy adults with standard dosing without accumulation [33]. There are more limited data in patients on continuous venovenous hemofiltration or hemodialysis; doses in such settings should be established based on dialysis perameters with careful collaboration between the treating nephrologist and pharmacist.

Although drug concentrations are 25% higher in the elderly at steady state, no dose adjustment is necessary. The AUC of oseltamivir carboxylate has been shown to be 30% lower in patients with cystic fibrosis than in healthy adults, so increased dosing is recommended for this population [34]. Bronchoalveolar lavage levels of oseltamivir carboxylate are similar to plasma levels in rats, and therapeutic concentrations of the active compound are attained in the lung, trachea, and nasal mucosa in humans [35]. Ethnicity does not affect the pharmacokinetics of the prodrug or the active metabolite. Drug levels in middle ear fluid and sinus aspirates are similar to those in blood [36]. Data in morbidly obese adults suggest that systemic exposure to oseltamivir carboxylate is similar to nonobese controls, therefore no dose adjustment appears to be needed in obese individuals [37]. Protein binding of oseltamivir and oseltamivir carboxylate are 42% and <3%, respectively [35]. In enzyme inhibition assays, the IC_{50} of oseltamivir for susceptible seasonal influenza A strains (0.01–2.24 nmol) is significantly lower than for influenza B strains (6.39–24.3 nmol); see Table 25.2 [38].

Although oseltamivir is a pregnancy class C drug, it is recommended and commonly used for the treatment of pregnant women [39]. Some studies suggest that oseltamivir carboxylate AUC may be lower and the clearance significantly higher during pregnancy, particularly during the third trimester [40–42]. As a result, increasing the dosage of oseltamivir during pregnancy may be necessary, particularly in the third trimester and in seriously ill pregnant women [42]. Further, transplacental transfer of the metabolite has been demonstrated to be low and accumulation minimal in an *ex vivo* human placental model [43]. Likewise, the incidence of adverse maternal or fetal outcomes after exposure to oseltamivir has generally not been higher than background rates [44].

Oseltamivir is approved for treatment in children 2 weeks of age and older. Several studies in neonates and young infants with influenza have found differ-

Table 25.2. (a) Inhibitory activity (IC_{50}) of laninamivir, oseltamivir, and zanamivir. Reprinted from Yamashita [7] with permission from International Medical Press.

Influenza subtype	Influenza strain	Laninamivir (nmol)	Oseltmivir (nmol)	Zanamivir (nmol)
A/H1N1	A/Yokohama/2006	3.03	2.28	2.70
	A/Yokohama/2006 (H275Y)	5.62	755.00	3.05
Pandemic H1N1	Wild-type (3 strains)	0.74	1.90	1.20
	H275Y (4 strains)	1.14	1146.00	1.04
A/H3N2	A/Kawasaki/2003	15.40	1.25	8.29
	A/Kawasaki/2003 (R292K)	10.60	10400.00	11.20
	A/Yokohama/2003	19.20	1.78	10.70
	A/Yokohama/2003 (E119V)	13.20	140.00	7.71
	A/Kawasaki/2002	13.40	1.18	7.82
	A/Kawasaki/2002 (N294S)	27.30	37.20	13.50
A/H5N1	A/Hanoi/2005	0.32	0.35	0.72
	A/Hanoi/2005 (H274Y)	1.10	430.00	0.68
	A/Hanoi/2004 (N294S)	1.60	1.60	0.57
	A/Vietnam/2004	0.28	0.31	0.15
	A/Vietnam/2004 (H274Y)	2.10	1100.00	0.22
	A/Vietnam/2004 (N294S)	1.40	28.00	0.48

(b) Inhibitory activity (IC_{50}) of oseltamivir, peramivir, and zanamivir. Reprinted from Sidwell and Smee [131] with permission of Informa Healthcare.

Compound	IC_{50} range (nM) of tested viruses				
	Influenza A/H1N1 (N = 5 viruses)	Influenza A/H2N2 (N = 1 virus)	Influenza A/H3N2 (N = 14 viruses)	Influenza A/H5N1 (N = 4 viruses)	Influenza B (N = 5 viruses)
Oseltamivir carboxylate	0.16–57	2.0	<0.01–0.8	0.10–0.27	0.7–2.0
Peramivir	0.9–8.9	0.4	<0.01–1.3	0.01–0.07	0.7–2.6
Zanamivir	0.14–60	0.9	<0.01–2.0	0.02–0.22	0.6–0.9

ences in drug disposition based on age and weight but have not identified safety problems. Studies have demonstrated that premature neonates treated with 1 mg/kg twice daily and term babies with 2 mg/kg twice daily should have expected average oseltamivir carboxylate concentrations of similar ranges to adults treated with 75 mg and older children receiving 3 mg/kg twice daily [45, 46].

Pharmacokinetics in critically ill patients is incompletely understood. Limited data suggest that the oral bioavailability of oseltamivir in severely ill children and adults when delivered by nasogastric tube is adequate in most, but not all, critically ill patients [47]. Alteration in gastrointestinal motility could have a significant impact on absorption.

Adverse effects and drug interactions Oral oseltamivir is generally well tolerated, and no serious end-organ toxicity has been found, even with doses of up to 450 mg twice daily [48]. Oral oseltamivir is associated with nausea, discomfort, and, less often, emesis in a minority of treated patients. Nausea and vomiting occur in approximately 3–19% of influenza-infected oseltamivir recipients [49]. Gastrointestinal complaints are usually mild in intensity, transient despite continued dosing, and ameliorated by administration with food. Side effects were similar in influenza-infected patients who received 75 or 150 mg doses twice daily (nausea: 17% and 19%, respectively, vs. 7.4% with placebo; vomiting 13.1% and 15.1%, respectively, vs. 3.4% with placebo) [49], but increased when doses of 225 and 450 mg twice daily were given to healthy control subjects (nausea: 25.8% and 31.3%, respectively; vomiting 7.2% and 16.2%, respectively) [48]. Treatment studies also demonstrated slightly more frequent insomnia and vertigo in patients who received oseltamivir. Rates of nausea and vomiting occur with a lower frequency in prophylaxis studies (7% and 2%, respectively, compared with 3% and 1%, respectively, in placebo treated patients). In addition, post-marketing experience has documented rare cases of anaphylaxis and serious skin reactions including toxic epidermal necrolysis, Stevens–Johnson syndrome, and erythema multiforme. There have also been post-marketing reports, mostly from Japan, of delirium and abnormal behavior leading to injury, and in some cases resulting in fatal outcomes; whether these are associated with the influenza or oseltamivir are unclear, but close monitoring of patients is recommended.

No clinically significant drug interactions have been recognized other than with probenecid, which blocks tubular secretion and doubles the half-life of the carboxylate [31]. No interactions with the cytochrome P450 enzymes occur *in vitro* or in clinical studies in transplant patients [50]. The drug may reduce the replication and immunogenicity of concurrently administered intranasal, live-attenuated vaccine.

Laninamivir

Pharmacokinetics/pharmacodynamics Laninamivir octanoate (CS-8958) is currently only licensed in Japan and is available as a 20-mg dry powder inhalation; for dosing see Table 25.1. Laninamivir octanoate (CS-8958) is a prodrug that is converted in the airway to laninamivir (R-125489), the active neuraminidase inhibitor. The exact mechanism by which laninamivir octanoate is retained in the target tissue is not well understood, but it appears to be retained in the target tissue with resultant prolonged exposure to laninamivir. Laninamivir concentrations in epithelial lining fluid, as assessed by serial bronchoalveolar lavage, exceed the IC_{50} for most influenza NAs through 240 hours (10 days) after a single inhalation of 40 mg laninamivir octanoate [7]. The plasma half-life of laninamivir octanoate is 2 hours but the plasma half-life of laninamivir is about 3 days [7]. The maximum concentration of laninamivir occurs within 4 hours [7]. Bioavailability is limited (15%), with significant protein binding of the octanoate (67%) but minimal protein binding (<0.1%) of laninamivir. As such, dose adjustment should not be necessary for renal or hepatic impairment [7]. Laninamivir has excellent *in vitro* activity against wild-type influenza A and B viruses currently circulating, including those H1N1 viruses containing H275Y mutations in the NA gene (Table 25.2) [7, 30].

Adverse effects and drug interactions Clinical studies in Asia found similar rates of nausea in laninamivir octanoate and oseltamivir treated patients, lower rates of vomiting in the laninamivir octanoate arm, and similar to or slightly higher rates of diarrhea in laninamivir octanoate arms [51, 52]. Dizziness was seen in 0.9–1.8% of laninamivir octanoate treated patients but not oseltamivir treated patients [51]. In a comparative study of inhaled laninamivir octanoate and inhaled zanamivir in children ≤15 years of age, there was no difference in adverse respiratory and systemic side effects; only 1 in 57 of the zanamivir and no laninamivir exposed children had asthmatic symptoms [53]. The tolerability of inhaled laninamivir octanoate in patients with underlying lung disease or reactive airways disease remains to be characterized. There are limited data on drug interactions with this compound, but its limited bioavailability may limit the impact of any drug interactions.

Peramivir

Pharmacokinetics/pharmacodynamics Peramivir is available in 150 and 300 mg solutions for intravenous use; for dosing see Table 25.1. It was initially developed as an oral agent, but low bioavailability limited its efficacy [54]. Studies of the drug delivered intramuscularly provided inconsistent results, likely due to delivery issues. An intravenous formulation is approved in Japan and South Korea and is under study in other countries [55]. The median peak plasma concentration of peramivir after 300 and 600 mg IV doses in hospitalized patients in Asia was 25 500 ng/mL (range 15 600–26 200 ng/mL) and 51 500 ng/mL (range 37 300–78 900 ng/mL), while median trough levels were 45.7 ng/mL (range 7.37–139 ng/mL) and 86.7 ng/mL (range 22.7–435 ng/mL), respectively [56]. Peramivir is not extensively metabolized in humans and is predominately eliminated unchanged by renal excretion with a plasma half-life of 12–25 hours [57, 58]. Plasma protein binding is low (<30%) [58]. The IC_{50} of peramivir was comparable to or lower than oseltamivir carboxylate and zanamivir for influenza A (0.09–1.39, 0.01–2.24, and 0.30–2.32 nmol, respectively) and influenza B strains (0.60–10.8, 6.39–24.3, and 1.53–17.0 nmol, respectively); (Table 25.2) [38]. Peramivir differs structurally from the other NAIs by having two active substituents that result in multiple binding interactions with the active site and allows the antiviral to be active against some viruses that are resistant to other antivirals [6].

Adverse effects and drug interactions Recognized adverse events associated with the administration of peramivir are diarrhea, nausea, vomiting, and decreased neutrophil count; other less common adverse events observed in studies to date include dizziness, headache, somnolence, nervousness, insomnia, feeling agitated, depression, nightmares, hyperglycemia, hyperbilirubinemia, elevated blood pressure, cystitis, ECG abnormalities (prolonged QTc interval observed in one patient in a phase 1 trial), anorexia, and proteinuria. There are no recognized drug interactions with peramivir [58].

Zanamivir

Pharmacokinetics/pharmacodynamics Zanamivir is available pre-packaged in the Diskhaler inhalation device, with four blisters, each containing 5 mg zanamivir and 20 mg lactose; for dosing see Table 25.1. The proprietary inhaler device for delivering zanamivir is breath actuated and requires a cooperative patient [59]. Following inhalation of the dry powder, approximately 15% is deposited in the lower respiratory tract and the remainder in the oropharynx; the oral bioavailability of zanamivir is low, but can range 4–17% [58]. Peak serum concentrations range 17–142 ng/mL within 2 hours following a 10-mg inhaled dose. Plasma protein binding is below 10% [58]. Median zanamivir concentrations are above 1 μg/mL in the sputum 6h after inhalation and remain detectable up to 24 h [60]. An intravenous formulation is under development and available on compassionate use basis for treatment of serious infections, especially those resulting from suspected oseltamivir-resistant viruses. The IC_{50} of zanamivir for susceptible influenza A and B viruses is 0.30–2.32 and 1.53–17.0 nmol, respectively; (Table 25.2) [38].

Adverse effects and drug interactions Generally, inhaled zanamivir has been well tolerated, although it may cause cough, a reversible decrease in pulmonary function, or fatal bronchospasm in some patients, particularly those with underlying pulmonary disease [61]. Zanamivir is not recommended for treatment or prophylaxis of influenza in individuals with underlying airways disease, such as asthma or chronic obstructive pulmonary disease. Additionally, the commercial inhaled formulation contains a lactose carrier and may be associated with ventilator failure due to filter blockade, and death if nebulized for patients on ventilators [62]. Because bioavailability of zanamivir is low, the circulating levels of the drug are low and no clinically significant drug interactions have been recognized. *In vitro* studies suggest that zanamivir does not inhibit or induce cytochrome P450 enzymes [30].

Investigational agents in clinical development

Neuraminidase inhibitors

Oseltamivir is being developed as a prodrug for intravenous administration, with the dose selection focused on demonstrating bioequivalence with oral oseltamivir and clinical efficacy as a secondary outcome [63]. Intravenous zanamivir is also being developed clinically [63]. Early studies demonstrated clinical and virologic efficacy, while recent published experience has suggested efficacy against oseltamivir-resistant strains [64, 65]. Additionally, intravenous peramivir and inhaled laninamivir are undergoing development for approval of use outside Asia [63]. Pharmacokinetics and adverse effects of these four agents are generally as described above, from available published data [55, 58, 64, 65].

Polymerase inhibitors

Viral polymerase inhibitors have a novel mechanism of action and are typically active against viruses with mutations conferring resistance to M2 and/or NAIs and against both influenza A and B. Ribavirin, approved for oral treatment of chronic hepatitis C and aerosol treatment of respiratory syncytial virus, has been studied for treatment of influenza when delivered by aerosol, oral, and intravenous routes. *In vitro* studies show inhibition against most strains of influenza at 3–5 ug/mL concentrations, while clinical studies assessing the activity of ribavirin have generally been small observational studies with significant limitations [66, 67]. Insufficient data have been developed to prove clinical efficacy. A randomized study found that 1 gm/day ribavirin for 5 days resulted in no difference in clinical signs, symptoms, or viral shedding compared with placebo [68], while another small study found that higher doses (1200 mg three times a day) may provide clinical benefit [69]. Side effects include hemolytic anemia and potential risk of teratogenicity [66, 67].

Favipiravir (T-705, Toyama Chemical Co, Ltd, Japan and MediVector, Boston, Masschusetts) is a novel viral polymerase inhibitor that is active against all influenza virus types (A, B, and C) [70]. After ribosylation and then phosphorylation, T-705 functions like a nucleoside [70]. It is active in murine models of lethal influenza, including H5N1 virus infection, and shows synergistic interactions with oseltamivir [71]. Initial unpublished human pharmacology data suggest excellent oral absorption and tolerability, and efficacy studies in Japan are ongoing [72]. Antiviral effects comparable to oseltamivir were found in a randomized trial in Japan [73]. There is a phase I study in adults with hepatic impairment (Clin-

icalTrials.gov identifier: NCT01419457) and a phase II, dose-ranging, placebo-controlled study of influenza in adults currently enrolling outside of Japan (ClinicalTrials.gov identifier: NCT01068912).

Sialidase

DAS181 (FluDase, NexBio, San Diego, California) is a recombinant fusion protein linking the *Actinomyces viscosus* sialidase to a human epithelium-anchoring domain, which increases the activity of the compound 5- to 30-fold. The sialidase component cleaves cell surface α2,6-sialic acid and α2,3-sialic acid linked receptors to which influenza virus HAs bind [74]. Due to its novel mechanism of action, the agent inhibits both influenza and parainfluenza viral replication, including viruses that are resistant to existing classes of antivirals [75]. Experiments utilizing serial passage of B/Maryland/1/59 and A/Victoria/3/75 (H3N2) demonstrated that resistance to DAS181 can be selected and that resistant variants phenotypically exhibit reduced fitness [75]. Resistance likely emerges due to mutations in the HA and/or NA which alter their function [75]. Phase I and II studies are ongoing.

Investigational agents in preclinical development

A number of agents and potential mechanisms of action have been investigated as part of preclinical development of antiviral agents. Small molecules such as nitazoxanide which inhibits the maturation of the HA glycoprotein, or the 101 amino acid protein cyanovirin-N, which inhibits its activity by binding to high-mannose oligosaccharides, are undergoing further studies [76, 77]. The wealth of information on the structures of potential targets is being used to assist the design and development of promising lead compounds. Structures of complexes between broadly neutralizing antibodies and a conserved epitope in the stem of the HA (see Figure 5.11) have been used to design computationally a 51-residue protein that inhibits the acid-induced fusion activity and broadly neutralizes group 1 HAs, as a promising lead for next generation anti-influenza therapeutics. The structures of different functional domains of the RNA polymerase have renewed enthusiasm for developing inhibitors of the endonuclease activity of the PA component [78, 79], the cap-binding function of the PB2 component [78, 80], and the transcriptase activity of PB1 [81]. Nucleozin represents another class of inhibitors which interact with different sites on the nucleoprotein, causing aggregation of the protein and inhibition of virus replication [82, 83]. Inhibition of both host and viral genes through siRNA show promise as well [84–86]. Immunomodulators, such as cyclo-oxygenase inhibitors, peroxisome proliferator-activated receptor agonists, and 3-hydroxy-3-methyl-glutaryl-CoA (HMGCoA) reductase inhibitors have been studied and likewise show promise, but require further clinical investigation [87–89].

Combination therapy

Experience with other RNA viruses has demonstrated the theoretical reasons for considering combination therapy for influenza: improved efficacy, reduced risk of resistance emergence, and potentially reduced toxicity [90]. A small study conducted when most circulating strains were susceptible to M2 inhibitors found encouraging trends in clinical outcomes with combination therapy with oral rimantadine plus nebulized zanamivir and no M2 inhibitor resistance emergence compared with rimantadine monotherapy [91]. More recent data suggest that a triple combination of amantadine, ribavirin, and oseltamivir (TCAD) is highly active and synergistic against both drug susceptible and resistant influenza virus strains [92]. A retrospective cohort study in 245 critically ill patients with pandemic A(H1N1)pdm2009 infection found adequate tolerance and trends towards reduced mortality in the TCAD group at 14 days (17% vs. 35%; $P = 0.08$) and at 90 days (46% vs. 59%; $P = 0.23$) [93]. A clinical trial comparing the triple combination with oral oseltamivir for the treatment of influenza in adults at high risk of complications is currently recruiting subjects (ClinicalTrials.gov identifier: NCT01227967).

Caution must be used when selecting combinations to use clinically as not all combinations have been shown to be beneficial. Some combinations of NAIs show antagonistic interactions *in vitro*, and the combination of oral oseltamivir and inhaled zanamivir appeared less effective virologically and clinically

than oseltamivir monotherapy and not significantly more effective than zanamivir monotherapy in uncomplicated seasonal influenza [94].

Efficacy and use

Prophylaxis

Both the M2 and NAIs have been studied and approved for the prevention of influenza. When the circulating strains are susceptible, amantadine has been found to be 61% effective in preventing influenza in studies of seasonal prophylaxis [28]. Rimantadine was found to be effective in preventing influenza in only two (34–85% efficacy) of three studies published to date [28]. Comparative effectiveness studies between the two agents suggest similar efficacy [28]. Post-exposure prophylaxis also appears to be effective with these agents for susceptible strains, but not when the index case is also given treatment because of the transmission of M2 inhibitor-resistant variants [95]. One comparative prophylaxis study in nursing homes found that inhaled zanamivir was superior to oral rimantadine because of frequent M2 inhibitor resistance emergence [28].

Both oseltamivir and zanamivir have been shown to be 68–90% effective in preventing influenza-proven illness after exposure for close contacts, such as household members, or as seasonal prophylaxis in the community for otherwise healthy adults and children [61, 96, 97]. Efficacy is enhanced in exposure settings when treatment of the index case is combined with prophylaxis of the exposed individuals. Oseltamivir prophylaxis in high-risk patients, such as elderly in residential homes (92% reduction of laboratory-confirmed influenza) and immunocompromised patients (80% reduction of PCR-confirmed and 89% culture-confirmed influenza) [98, 99]. Inhaled zanamivir prophylaxis has also shown high levels of protection in nursing home outbreaks and in at-risk patients (83% efficacy) [100]. The existing data suggest benefit in addition to vaccination, because response may be limited in these populations. During the pandemic, NAIs were utilized for prevention of influenza. Although post-exposure prophylaxis, mostly with oseltamivir, was associated with a reduced rate of infection during outbreaks of pandemic influenza, asymptomatic infections during prophylaxis did occur. Furthermore, there were individuals who developed oseltamivir-resistant influenza after post-exposure prophylaxis [101]. As a result, post-exposure prophylaxis is not generally recommended; early therapy is instead preferred.

Therapy

Both M2 and NAIs have been studied and approved for the treatment of influenza. To date, most randomized clinical studies have been conducted in otherwise healthy ambulatory adults and children. Existing data for the management of specialized populations, including the hospitalized, pregnant, and immunocompromised patient populations have been derived from observational studies. One feature consistently true of treatment data for M2 and NAIs to date is that efficacy, whether judged clinically or virologically, is maximized by instituting therapy as early as possible. For example, in uncomplicated influenza, oseltamivir initiated within 6 hours, 6–12 hours, and 24–36 hours of symptom onset resulted in a 4.1, 3.1, and 2.2 day reduction of illness, respectively, compared with treatment starting at 36–48 hours [102]. In more seriously ill patients, this means instituting empiric therapy as soon as possible and not waiting for laboratory test results.

M2 inhibitors
In placebo controlled studies, amantadine and rimantadine treatment is able to shorten the duration of fever by about 1 day [28]. Treatment is also associated with more rapid symptom resolution, functional recovery, and, in some studies, resolution of small airways functional abnormalities [25]. Controlled studies of the M2 inhibitors in severely ill, hospitalized patients or immunocompromised patients are limited. Emergence of resistant variants develops quickly and at higher rates in immunocompromised patients and may be shed for a prolonged period of time [103]. Retrospective analysis of 83 immunocompetent adults hospitalized for influenza found no significant difference in duration of fever or of hospitalization between the amantadine-treated and untreated patients [28]. M2 inhibitors are associated with decreased progression to pneumonia and death in hematopoietic stem cell transplant patients [104].

Available data suggest that the M2 inhibitors are safe and efficacious in reducing length of fever and illness in children older than 2 years of age, but data are far more limited in younger children [25].

Neuraminidase inhibitors
In otherwise healthy, ambulatory adults and children, oseltamivir is associated with a significant reduction (0.5–4.1 days) in the length of illness as long as the medication is started within 48 h after symptom onset [39, 61]. The impact is greatest with early onset initiation of therapy [102]. Oseltamivir is also associated with a significant reduction in the use of antibiotic therapy for lower respiratory tract complications and/or otitis media [57, 105, 106]. Inhaled zanamivir generally results in a 1–2 day reduction in the duration of influenza illness when started within 48 h of symptom onset in otherwise healthy adults and children [39, 61]. A comparative study in adults with uncomplicated seasonal influenza found a somewhat faster time to illness alleviation with oseltamivir than zanamivir. Additionally, there are more recent studies involving intravenous peramivir and inhaled laninamivir. Compared with oseltamivir, a single inhalation of laninamivir was associated with similar to improved time to allivation of influenza illness in otherwise healthy adults and children with influenza [30]. Similarly, a single infusion of peramivir was associated with more rapid time to alleviation of influenza symptoms and resumption of usual activity than placebo and was non-inferior compared with oseltamivir in otherwise healthy ambulatory adults [30]. Five days of intravenous peramivir was associated with similar clinical and antiviral efficacy in adults hospitalized with influenza [30]. Further studies of these last two agents are ongoing to study their antiviral efficacy.

Data in specialized populations, including hospitalized, immunocompromised, and pregnant patients, has generally been derived from small single center case series or retrospective cohort studies. The greatest body of data in hospitalized patients involves the use of oseltamvir, particularly from the 2009 H1N1 pandemic, although published experience with newer NAIs is increasing [47]. Available data on NAIs in hospitalized patients with seasonal, pandemic, or avian H5N1 influenza suggests that early therapy is associated with improved clinical outcomes and reduced mortality; many of the studies have documented positive effects on prescriptions for antibacterial agents, in terms of either total duration or use, as well as reduced duration of hospitalization [47, 107]. Additionally, some of the studies have demonstrated a more rapid reduction in virus shedding [47, 108]. Available evidence suggests that clinical and virologic benefit is obtained even if started up to, and perhaps beyond, 4 days after symptom onset [47]. Significant gaps in our understanding of treatment of hospitalized patients with influenza still exist, including optimal dose, duration, and delivery method [109]. Enterally delivered oseltamivir results in adequate systemic exposure in most patients [110–112]. As such, the role for parenterally administered NAIs is still being evaluated; parenteral routes could be considered when oral absorption may be altered or is documented.

Despite uncertainty as to the optimal dose and duration of therapy in influenza-infected immunocompromised patients (solid organ transplant, hematopoietic stem cell transplant, and oncology patients undergoing chemotherapy), antiviral therapy has consistently demonstrated clinical benefit [113–117]. Early antiviral therapy, generally with oseltamivir, is associated with clinical benefit with reduced mortality, progression to pneumonia, and hospitalization [111, 113–117]. Therapy initiated beyond 48 h after symptom onset is probably beneficial and, because of prolonged virus shedding, therapy beyond 5 days is likely necessary.

Despite oseltamivir and zanamivir being listed as pregnancy category C agents, data clearly demonstrate that early antiviral therapy is associated with overall improvement in mother and fetal outcomes compared with late or no therapy [118, 119]. As such, early antiviral therapy is recommended for all pregnant or early post-partum women with proven or suspected influenza.

Recommendations for use by national and international organizations

Given rapid changes in circulating viruses, available antivirals, and resistance emergence, several national and international bodies provide regularly updated guidance on the optimal use of antivirals for the prevention and treatment of influenza. For current guidance see Table 25.3.

Table 25.3. Available national and international guidelines for the use of antivirals for the prevention and treatment of influenza.

Country or entity	Website
US Centers for Disease Control	http://www.cdc.gov/flu/antivirals/index.htm
United Kingdom	http://www.hpa.org.uk/Topics/InfectiousDiseases/InfectionsAZ/SeasonalInfluenza/InformationForHealthProfessionals/
World Health Organization	http://www.who.int/influenza/patient_care/antivirals/en/

Emergence of resistance

Although the emergence of antiviral resistance is generally associated with drug treatment, due to drug pressure, it may emerge coincidentally during virus evolution when mutations are either neutral or confer an evolutionary advantage on the (epidemic) virus variant, and are maintained in the absence of drug pressure, as recently observed for both amantadine/rimantadine and oseltamivir.

M2 inhibitors

As the genetic basis of resistance to amantadine and rimantadine is well established and there is a consistent correlation between resistance and the presence of a substitution in one or more of the five residues in M2 detailed above, surveillance of resistance is generally by screening for these resistance mutations by sequencing the M gene. The consequent high level resistance can also be readily monitored by lack of inhibition of virus replication in ELISA assays; plaque reduction assays have proved to be less reliable [120]. Contrary to the situation today, prior to the 1980s there was little evidence of amantadine resistance among naturally circulating influenza A viruses,

407

although resistance was observed to emerge frequently in the presence of the antiviral in cell culture and in experimental animals. However, in the mid-1980s, the swine A(H1N1) and A(H3N2) viruses, which shared the internal genes of the "avian-like" H1N1 viruses which had emerged in pigs in Europe in the late 1970s, acquired the Ser31Asn amantadine resistance mutation, apparently in the absence of any use of the antiviral (Figure 25.1b). This characteristic was subsequently maintained and passed on to the 2009 pandemic H1N1 virus (Figure 25.1b), fulfilling an earlier concern of the potential transmission of this phenotype to human viruses by genetic reassortment. The acquisition of a similar resistance mutation by a distinct lineage of "avian-like" A(H1N1) viruses in

pigs in Ireland, shortly after their detection in 1991 (Figure 25.1b), suggests that the amino acid substitution represents an adaptive mutation. Whereas the highly pathogenic avian A(H5N1) viruses which caused human infections in Hong Kong in 1997 were sensitive to amantadine, the clade 1 highly pathogenic avian A(H5N1) viruses which emerged in 2003 in South-East Asia possessed the Ser31Asn mutation [121]. While other A(H5N1) clades causing human infection were initially sensitive to amantadine, resistance mutations have either subsequently become predominant, as for the clade 2.1 viruses circulating in Indonesia due to a Val27Ala M2 substitution, or have been observed sporadically (e.g., in clade 2.2 viruses) [121].

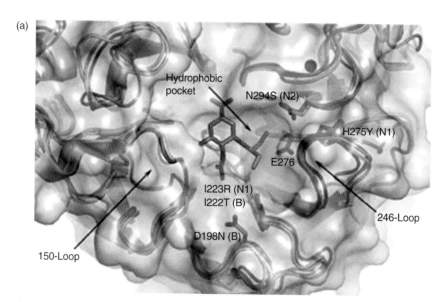

(a)

Figure 25.2. (a) Locations of amino acid changes in neuraminidase (NA) (numbered according to N1, N2, or B NA sequence, as indicated) which reduce sensitivity to oseltamivir (shown) by interfering with its interaction with the hydrophobic pocket. The structures of the open and closed forms of N1 in gold and green, respectively, N2 in yellow and B NA in blue are superimposed. A deletion (residues 244–247) in the 246 loop of N2 is in red. (b) Phylogenetic comparison (using maximum parsimony) of the NA genes of seasonal A(H1N1) viruses showing the

amino acid changes associated with and preceding acquisition of oseltamivir resistance due to the His275Tyr substitution. Sequences with Tyr275 are shown in red; prototype vaccine viruses are in blue. The principal amino acid differences between the NAs of clade 2A, 2B, and 2C viruses are indicated. The M2 proteins of clade 2C viruses were amantadine-resistant, due to a Ser31Asn substitution. (c) Locations of the amino acid substitutions in the NA structure showing their proximity to His275Tyr and the interaction of oseltamivir with the catalytic site.

(b)

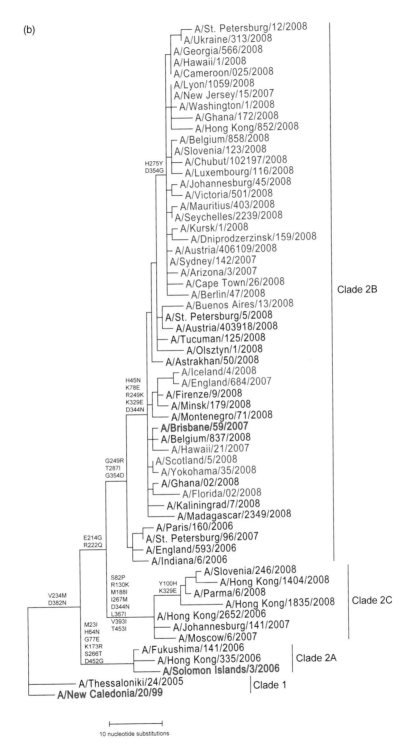

Figure 25.2. (*Continued*)

(c)

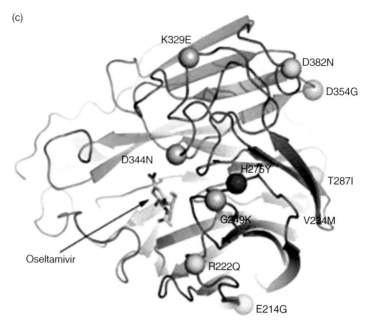

Figure 25.2. (*Continued*)

Clinical studies of rimantadine effectiveness [120] and use of amantadine to control influenza in institutions, such as nursing homes [25], revealed that amantadine-resistant viruses were shed with high frequency and could spread between individuals; however, prior to 2000 there was little evidence of their spread to the wider community. Between 2002 and 2004 saw the emergence of amantadine-resistant A(H3N2) viruses in South-East Asia and the subsequent worldwide spread of amantadine-resistant A/Wiscosin/67/2005(H3N2)-like viruses during 2005–2006 and retention of the resistance phenotype in subsequent epidemic A(H3N2) viruses to date [122]. Among seasonal A(H1N1) viruses, amantadine resistance was a characteristic phenotype of clade 2C viruses (Figure 25.2b) which were prominent in 2006–2008, but not of the clade 2B viruses which co-circulated, and subsequently acquired oseltamivir resistance (see below). Amantadine resistance of the A(H1N1)pdm2009 virus which caused the 2009 pandemic was a characteristic phenotype of the M gene, which was derived from the Eurasian lineage of swine influenza viruses. Thus, the two influenza A subtypes currently circulating in the human population are

resistant to this class of antiviral, which consequently is no longer recommended for use. Furthermore, irrespective of the origin of amantadine resistance in the different instances, it is readily apparent that the phenotype is maintained in the absence of drug, that the mutations do not have an adverse effect on viruses of different subtypes and may even be selected for their beneficial effects on virus fitness.

Neuraminidase inhibitors

Few instances of zanamivir resistance associated with clinical use were reported during clinical trials, and few have subsequently been associated with zanamivir therapy (Table 25.4). On the contrary, not only has resistance been more frequently associated with oseltamivir therapy, but oseltamivir-resistant seasonal influenza A(H1N1) viruses emerged to become the predominant epidemic A(H1N1) virus in 2008–2009. Although in early clinical trials during development of oseltamivir resistance detection was relatively low, at less than 1% in adults, but about 4% in children [123], in subsequent clinical studies of oseltamivir therapy in children in Japan, infected with A(H1N1)

Table 25.4. Mutations in the neuraminidase (NA) of viruses, isolated during antiviral treatment or during surveillance, which reduce susceptibility to NA inhibitors.

Amino acid substitution[a]	Virus type/subtype	Oseltamivir[b]	Zanamivir	Peramivir
V116A	H5N1	M	M	L
I117V + I131V	H5N1	M	S	S
E119V	H3N2	M	S	S
E119I	H3N2	H	M	L
E119A	B	H	H	H
Q136L	H5N1	M	H	–
Q136K	H1N1	S	H	H
	H3N2	S	M	–
V149A	H5N1	L	L	–
D151V/D	H3N2	L	H	–
R152K	B	H	H	H
Y155H	H1N1	M	H	H
D198Y	B	M	M	–
D198N	B	L	L	L
D198E	B	M	L	M
I222R	H1N1pdm	L	M	L
I222K	H1N1pdm	M	L	S
I222V/I	B	L	S	L
I222T	B	L	S	–
S246N	H1N1pdm	L	L	S
	H5N1	M	S	–
S246G	H1N1	L	S	–
H274Y	H1N1	H	S	H
	H1N1pdm	H	S	H
	H5N1	H	S	H
	B	L	S	S
R292K	H3N2	H	M	H
N294S	H3N2	H	M	M
	H5N1	M	M	M
	B	M	S	–
Q313K + I427T	H1N1pdm	M	M	L
R371K	B	H	M	–
G402S	B	L	L	–

[a]N2 numbering.
[b]Estimation of degree of resistance/reduced susceptibility based on increase in IC$_{50}$ of mutant relative to sensitive wild-type: L, <10-fold increase; M, 10- to 50-fold increase; H, >50-fold increase; S, sensitive – equivalent to wild-type. The locations of several of the residues in the structure of the NA are indicated in Figure 5.2 and in Figure 5.6 in Chapter 5. A more comprehensive list of resistance mutations generated *in vivo* and *in vitro* can be found in the literature [131].

or A(H3N2) viruses, the incidence of resistance was 16–18% [124]. Oseltamivir resistance was also observed in 25% (2/8) of patients receiving oseltamivir therapy for highly pathogenic A(H5N1) virus infection [125].

Earlier perceptions that the His275Tyr resistance mutation, which caused high level resistance in N1 viruses, was deleterious to the virus were overturned by the emergence of resistance due to that mutation in seasonal A(H1N1) viruses in late 2007 [126]. Whether or not initially associated with antiviral treatment, the resistance phenotype was maintained in the absence of drug pressure and oseltamivir-resistant viruses emerged as the predominant epidemic strain during 2008. Co-circulation of oseltamivir-resistant clade 2B viruses and amantadine-resistant clade 2C viruses (Figure 25.2b) provided the opportunity for the occurrence of reassortant viruses with dual resistance against the two classes of antivirals, although these viruses did not become prevalent [127]. Since there were few changes in other genes of these viruses that might be associated with the acquisition of the His275Tyr mutation, it appears that changes in the NAs of preceding viruses may have predisposed them to the selection of the His275Tyr substitution. On the one hand, it has been suggested the Asp344Asn substitution, which increased enzyme activity [128], compensated for the reduced activity due to the His275Tyr mutation. On the other hand, a combination of Arg222Gln and Val234Met which increased cell surface expression, and thus activity of NA [129], may have been instrumental. In any case it is apparent that the His275Tyr substitution in NA was an adaptive mutation, which coincidentally caused oseltamivir resistance.

Intensive monitoring of oseltamivir resistance following the emergence of the 2009 A(H1N1) pandemic and the more widespread use of the antivirals revealed less than 1.5% of viruses tested over the following 2 years were resistant to oseltamivir [19]. Although most resistant viruses were associated with antiviral use, particularly among immunosuppressed patients, a significant proportion (14%) of patients had not been exposed to the antiviral, with evidence for nosocomial and community transmission of resistant virus to close contacts. Studies in animals which showed that transmission of the resistant virus was not reduced relative to sensitive virus were rein-

forced by the detection of a cluster of oseltamivir-resistant A(H1N1)pdm 2009 viruses (15% of viruses tested) from 29 patients, only one of whom had received oseltamivir, in the Hunter New England community in Australia between May and September 2011 [130]. The emergence and spread of oseltamivir resistance among A(H1N1) viruses with two quite different N1 NAs illustrates its potential impact on the usefulness of oseltamivir, and emphasizes the importance of developing other effective agents against different viral targets and the application of antiviral combinations to reduce emergence of resistance.

References

1. Hayden FG. Antivirals for influenza: historical perspectives and lessons learned. Antiviral Res. 2006;71(2–3):372–8.
2. Hay AJ, Wolstenholme AJ, Skehel JJ, Smith MH. The molecular-basis of the specific anti-influenza action of amantadine. EMBO J. 1985;4(11):3021–4.
3. Mould JA, Paterson RG, Takeda M, Ohigashi Y, Venkataraman P, Lamb RA, et al. Influenza B virus BM2 protein has ion channel activity that conducts protons across membranes. Dev Cell. 2003;5(1):175–84.
4. von Itzstein M, Wu WY, Kok GB, Pegg MS, Dyason JC, Jin B, et al. Rational design of potent sialidase-based inhibitors of influenza virus replication. Nature. 1993;363(6428):418–23.
5. Colman PM, Varghese JN, Laver WG. Structure of the catalytic and antigenic sites in influenza virus neuraminidase. Nature. 1983;303(5912):41–4.
6. Babu YS, Chand P, Bantia S, Kotian P, Dehghani A, El-Kattan Y, et al. BCX-1812 (RWJ-270201): discovery of a novel, highly potent, orally active, and selective influenza neuraminidase inhibitor through structure-based drug design. J Med Chem. 2000;43(19):3482–6.
7. Yamashita M. Laninamivir and its prodrug, CS-8958: long-acting neuraminidase inhibitors for the treatment of influenza. Antivir Chem Chemother. 2010;21(2):71–84.
8. Boriskin YS, Leneva IA, Pecheur EI, Polyak SJ. Arbidol: a broad-spectrum antiviral compound that blocks viral fusion. Curr Med Chem. 2008;15(10):997–1005.
9. Glushkov RG. Arbidol: antiviral immunostimulant interferon inducer. Drugs Future. 1992;17(12):1079–81.
10. Liu M-Y, Wang S, Yao W-F, Wu H-Z, Meng S-N, Wei M-J. Pharmacokinetic properties and bioequivalence of two formulations of arbidol: an open-label, single-

dose, randomized-sequence, two-period crossover study in healthy Chinese male volunteers. Clin Ther. 2009;31(4):784–92.

11. Chizhmakov IV, Geraghty FM, Ogden DC, Hayhurst A, Antoniou M, Hay AJ. Selective proton permeability and pH regulation of the influenza virus M2 channel expressed in mouse erythroleukaemia cells. J Physiol. 1996;494(2):329–36.

12. Steinhauer DA, Wharton SA, Skehel JJ, Wiley DC, Hay AJ. Amantadine selection of a mutant influenza virus containing an acid-stable hemagglutinin glycoprotein – evidence for virus-specific regulation of the pH of glycoprotein transport vesicles. Proc Natl Acad Sci U S A. 1991;88(24):11525–9.

13. Cady SD, Wang J, Wu Y, DeGrado WF, Hong M. Specific binding of adamantane drugs and direction of their polar amines in the pore of the influenza M2 transmembrane domain in lipid bilayers and dodecylphosphocholine micelles determined by NMR spectroscopy. J Am Chem Soc. 2011;133(12):4274–84.

14. Pielak RM, Oxenoid K, Chou JJ. Structural investigation of rimantadine inhibition of the AM2-BM2 chimera channel of influenza viruses. Structure. 2011;19(11):1655–63.

15. Sugaya N, Mitamura K, Yamazaki M, Tamura D, Ichikawa M, Kimura K, et al. Lower clinical effectiveness of oseltamivir against influenza B contrasted with influenza A infection in children. Clin Infect Dis. 2007;44(2):197–202.

16. Russell RJ, Haire LF, Stevens DJ, Collins PJ, Lin YP, Blackburn GM, et al. The structure of H5N1 avian influenza neuraminidase suggests new opportunities for drug design. Nature. 2006;443(7107):45–9.

17. Rudrawar S, Dyason JC, Rameix-Welti M-A, Rose FJ, Kerry PS, Russell RJM, et al. Novel sialic acid derivatives lock open the 150-loop of an influenza A virus group-1 sialidase. Nat Commun. 2010;1:113.

18. Yen HL, Herlocher LM, Hoffmann E, Matrosovich MN, Monto AS, Webster RG, et al. Neuraminidase inhibitor-resistant influenza viruses may differ substantially in fitness and transmissibility. Antimicrob Agents Chemother. 2005;49(10):4075–84.

19. Hurt AC, Chotpitayasunondh T, Cox NJ, Daniels R, Fry AM, Gubareva LV, et al. Antiviral resistance during the 2009 influenza A H1N1 pandemic: public health, laboratory, and clinical perspectives. Lancet Infect Dis. 2012;12(3):240–8.

20. Luo GX, Torri A, Harte WE, Danetz S, Cianci C, Tiley L, et al. Molecular mechanism underlying the action of a novel fusion inhibitor of influenza A virus. J Virol. 1997;71(5):4062–70.

21. Glushkov RG, Fadeyeva NI, Leneva IA, Gerasina SF, Budanova LI, Sokolova ND, et al. Molecular biological features of the action of arbidol, a new antiviral drug. Khimiko-Farmatsevticheskii Zhurnal. 1992;26(2):8–15.

22. Leneva IA, Russell RJ, Boriskin YS, Hay AJ. Characteristics of arbidol-resistant mutants of influenza virus: implications for the mechanism of anti-influenza action of arbidol. Antiviral Res. 2009;81(2):132–40.

23. Ison MG, Hayden FG. Therapeutic options for the management of influenza. Curr Opin Pharmacol. 2001;1(5):482–90.

24. Deyde VM, Xu X, Bright RA, Shaw M, Smith CB, Zhang Y, et al. Surveillance of resistance to adamantanes among influenza A(H3N2) and A(H1N1) viruses isolated worldwide. J Infect Dis. 2007;196(2):249–57.

25. Hayden FG, Aoki FY. Amantadine, rimantadine, and related agents. In: Yu VL, Marigan TCJ, Barriere SL, editors. Antimicrobial Therapy and Vaccines. Baltimore, Maryland: Williams & Wilkins; 1999. p. 1344–65.

26. Aoki FY, Sitar DS. Clinical pharmacokinetics of amantadine hydrochloride. Clin Pharmacokinet. 1988;14(1):35–51.

27. Browne MJ, Moss MY, Boyd MR. Comparative activity of amantadine and ribavirin against influenza virus in vitro: possible clinical relevance. Antimicrob Agents Chemother. 1983;23(3):503–5.

28. Jefferson T, Demicheli V, Di Pietrantonj C, Rivetti D. Amantadine and rimantadine for influenza A in adults. Cochrane Database Syst Rev. 2006;(2): CD001169.

29. Bukrinskaya AG, Vorkunova NK, Kornilayeva GV. Narmanbetova RA, Vorkunova GK. Influenza virus uncoating in infected cells and effect of rimantadine. J Gen Virol. 1982;60(Pt 1):49–59.

30. Ison MG. Antivirals and resistance: influenza virus. Curr Opin Virol. 2011;1(6):563–73.

31. Davies BE. Pharmacokinetics of oseltamivir: an oral antiviral for the treatment and prophylaxis of influenza in diverse populations. J Antimicrob Chemother. 2010;65(Suppl. 2):ii5–10.

32. Wattanagoon Y, Stepniewska K, Lindegardh N, Pukrittayakamee S, Silachamroon U, Piyaphanee W, et al. Pharmacokinetics of high-dose oseltamivir in healthy volunteers. Antimicrob Agents Chemother. 2009;53(3):945–52.

33. Robson R, Buttimore A, Lynn K, Brewster M, Ward P. The pharmacokinetics and tolerability of oseltamivir suspension in patients on haemodialysis and continuous ambulatory peritoneal dialysis. Nephrol Dial Transplant. 2006;21(9):2556–62.

34. Jullien V, Hubert D, Launay O, Babany G, Lortholary O, Sermet I. Pharmacokinetics and diffusion into sputum of oseltamivir and oseltamivir carboxylate in adults with cystic fibrosis. Antimicrob Agents Chemother. 2011;55(9):4183–7.

35. He G, Massarella J, Ward P. Clinical pharmacokinetics of the prodrug oseltamivir and its active metabolite Ro 64-0802. Clin Pharmacokinet. 1999;37(6):471–84.

36. Kurowski M, Oo C, Wiltshire H, Barrett J. Oseltamivir distributes to influenza virus replication sites in the middle ear and sinuses. Clin Drug Investig. 2004;24(1): 49–53.

37. Thorne-Humphrey LM, Goralski KB, Slayter KL, Hatchette TF, Johnston BL, McNeil SA. Oseltamivir pharmacokinetics in morbid obesity (OPTIMO trial). J Antimicrob Chemother. 2011;66(9):2083–91.

38. Bantia S, Parker CD, Ananth SL, Horn LL, Andries K, Chand P, et al. Comparison of the anti-influenza virus activity of RWJ-270201 with those of oseltamivir and zanamivir. Antimicrob Agents Chemother. 2001;45(4): 1162–7.

39. Fiore AE, Fry A, Shay D, Gubareva L, Bresee JS, Uyeki TM. Antiviral agents for the treatment and chemo-prophylaxis of influenza – recommendations of the Advisory Committee on Immunization Practices (ACIP). MMWR Recomm Rep. 2011;60(1):1–24.

40. Greer LG, Leff RD, Rogers VL, Roberts SW, McCracken GH Jr, Wendel GD Jr, et al. Pharmacoki-netics of oseltamivir according to trimester of preg-nancy. Am J Obstet Gynecol. 2011;204(6 Suppl. 1):S89–93.

41. Greer LG, Leff RD, Rogers VL, Roberts SW, McCracken GH Jr, Wendel GD Jr, et al. Pharmacokinetics of osel-tamivir in breast milk and maternal plasma. Am J Obstet Gynecol. 2011;204(6):524 e1–4.

42. Beigi RH, Han K, Venkataramanan R, Hankins GD, Clark S, Hebert MF, et al. Pharmacokinetics of oseltamivir among pregnant and nonpregnant women. Am J Obstet Gynecol. 2011;204(6 Suppl. 1): S84–8.

43. Berveiller P, Mir O, Vinot C, Bonati C, Duchene P, Giraud C, et al. Transplacental transfer of oseltamivir and its metabolite using the human perfused placental cotyledon model. Am J Obstet Gynecol. 2012;206(1): 92 e1–6.

44. Svensson T, Granath F, Stephansson O, Kieler H. Birth outcomes among women exposed to neuraminidase inhibitors during pregnancy. Pharmacoepidemiol Drug Saf. 2011;20(10):1030–4.

45. Maltezou HC, Drakoulis N, Siahanidou T, Karalis V, Zervaki E, Dotsikas Y, et al. Safety and pharmacoki-netics of oseltamivir for prophylaxis of neonates exposed to influenza H1N1. Pediatr Infect Dis J. 2012;31(5):527–9.

46. Acosta EP, Jester P, Gal P, Wimmer J, Wade J, Whitley RJ, et al. Oseltamivir dosing for influenza infection in premature neonates. J Infect Dis. 2010;202(4): 563–6.

47. Lee N, Ison MG. Diagnosis, management and out-comes of adults hospitalized with influenza. Antivir Ther. 2012;17(1 Pt B):143–57.

48. Dutkowski R, Smith JR, Davies BE. Safety and pharmacokinetics of oseltamivir at standard and high dosages. Int J Antimicrob Agents. 2010;35(5): 461–7.

49. Treanor JJ, Hayden FG, Vrooman PS, Barbarash R, Bettis R, Riff D, et al. Efficacy and safety of the oral neuraminidase inhibitor oseltamivir in treating acute influenza: a randomized controlled trial. US Oral Neuraminidase Study Group. JAMA. 2000;283(8): 1016–24.

50. Lam H, Jeffery J, Sitar DS, Aoki FY. Oseltamivir, an influenza neuraminidase inhibitor drug, does not affect the steady-state pharmacokinetic characteristics of cyclosporine, mycophenolate, or tacrolimus in adult renal transplant patients. Ther Drug Monit. 2011;33 (6):699–704.

51. Watanabe A, Chang SC, Kim MJ, Chu DW, Ohashi Y. Long-acting neuraminidase inhibitor laninamivir octanoate versus oseltamivir for treatment of influ-enza: a double-blind, randomized, noninferiority clini-cal trial. Clin Infect Dis. 2010;51(10):1167–75.

52. Sugaya N, Ohashi Y. Long-acting neuraminidase inhibitor laninamivir octanoate (CS-8958) versus osel-tamivir as treatment for children with influenza virus infection. Antimicrob Agents Chemother. 2010;54(6): 2575–82.

53. Katsumi Y, Otabe O, Matsui F, Kidowaki S, Mibayashi A, Tsuma Y, et al. Effect of a Single Inhalation of Laninamivir Octanoate in Children With Influenza. Pediatrics. 2012;129:e1431–6.

54. Barroso L, Treanor J, Gubareva L, Hayden FG. Effi-cacy and tolerability of the oral neuraminidase inhibi-tor peramivir in experimental human influenza: randomized, controlled trials for prophylaxis and treatment. Antivir Ther. 2005;10(8):901–10.

55. Hernandez JE, Adiga R, Armstrong R, Bazan J, Bonilla H, Bradley J, et al. Clinical experience in adults and children treated with intravenous peramivir for 2009 influenza A (H1N1) under an Emergency IND program in the United States. Clin Infect Dis. 2011;52(6): 695–706.

56. Kohno S, Kida H, Mizuguchi M, Hirotsu N, Ishida T, Kadota J, et al. Intravenous peramivir for treatment of influenza A and B virus infection in high-risk patients. Antimicrob Agents Chemother. 2011;55(6): 2803–12.

57. Whitley RJ, Hayden FG, Reisinger KS, Young N, Dutkowski R, Ipe D, et al. Oral oseltamivir treatment of influenza in children. Pediatr Infect Dis J. 2001;20(2): 127–33.

58. Chairat K, Tarning J, White NJ, Lindegardh N. Pharmacokinetic properties of Anti-influenza neuraminidase inhibitors. J Clin Pharmacol. 2013;53:119–139

59. Diggory P, Fernandez C, Humphrey A, Jones V, Murphy M. Comparison of elderly people's technique in using two dry powder inhalers to deliver zanamivir: randomised controlled trial. BMJ. 2001;322(7286):577–9.

60. Peng AW, Milleri S, Stein DS. Direct measurement of the anti-influenza agent zanamivir in the respiratory tract following inhalation. Antimicrob Agents Chemother. 2000;44(7):1974–6.

61. Moscona A. Neuraminidase inhibitors for influenza. N Engl J Med. 2005;353(13):1363–73.

62. Kiatboonsri S, Kiatboonsri C, Theerawit P. Fatal respiratory events caused by zanamivir nebulization. Clin Infect Dis. 2010;50(4):620.

63. Hayden F. Developing new antiviral agents for influenza treatment: what does the future hold? Clin Infect Dis. 2009;48(Suppl. 1):S3–13.

64. Dulek DE, Williams JV, Creech CB, Schulert AK, Frangoul HA, Domm J, et al. Use of intravenous zanamivir after development of oseltamivir resistance in a critically Ill immunosuppressed child infected with 2009 pandemic influenza A (H1N1) virus. Clin Infect Dis. 2010;50(11):1493–6.

65. Elbahlawan L, Gaur AH, Furman W, Jeha S, Woods T, Norris A, et al. Severe H1N1-associated acute respiratory failure in immunocompromised children. Pediatr Blood Cancer. 2011;57(4):625–8.

66. Chan-Tack KM, Murray JS, Birnkrant DB. Use of ribavirin to treat influenza. N Engl J Med. 2009;361(17):1713–4.

67. Riner A, Chan-Tack KM, Murray JS. Original research: intravenous ribavirin–review of the FDA's Emergency Investigational New Drug Database (1997–2008) and literature review. Postgrad Med. 2009;121(3):139–46.

68. Smith CB, Charette RP, Fox JP, Cooney MK, Hall CE. Lack of effect of oral ribavirin in naturally occurring influenza A virus (H1N1) infection. J Infect Dis. 1980;141(5):548–54.

69. Stein DS, Creticos CM, Jackson GG, Bernstein JM, Hayden FG, Schiff GM, et al. Oral ribavirin treatment of influenza A and B. Antimicrob Agents Chemother. 1987;31(8):1285–7.

70. Furuta Y, Takahashi K, Shiraki K, Sakamoto K, Smee DF, Barnard DL, et al. T-705 (favipiravir) and related compounds: novel broad-spectrum inhibitors of RNA viral infections. Antiviral Res. 2009;82(3):95–102.

71. Kiso M, Takahashi K, Sakai-Tagawa Y, Shinya K, Sakabe S, Le QM, et al. T-705 (favipiravir) activity

72. Boltz DA, Aldridge JR Jr, Webster RG, Govorkova EA. Drugs in development for influenza. Drugs. 2010;70(11):1349–62.

73. Kobayashi T, Kashiwagi S, Iwamoto A. Clinical effectiveness and safety of favipiravir: a novel anti-influenza drug with a selective inhibition activity against viral RNA polymerase. 51st Intersience Conference on Antimicrobial Agents and Chemotherapy; Chicago, Illinois, 2011. p. V-405.

74. Malakhov MP, Aschenbrenner LM, Smee DF, Wandersee MK, Sidwell RW, Gubareva LV, et al. Sialidase fusion protein as a novel broad-spectrum inhibitor of influenza virus infection. Antimicrob Agents Chemother. 2006;50(4):1470–9.

75. Triana-Baltzer GB, Sanders RL, Hedlund M, Jensen KA, Aschenbrenner LM, Larson JL, et al. Phenotypic and genotypic characterization of influenza virus mutants selected with the sialidase fusion protein DAS181. J Antimicrob Chemother. 2011;66(1):15–28.

76. Smee DF, Bailey KW, Wong MH, O'Keefe BR, Gustafson KR, Mishin VP, et al. Treatment of influenza A (H1N1) virus infections in mice and ferrets with cyanovirin-N. Antiviral Res. 2008;80(3):266–71.

77. Rossignol JF, La Frazia S, Chiappa L, Ciucci A, Santoro MG. Thiazolides, a new class of anti-influenza molecules targeting viral hemagglutinin at the post-translational level. J Biol Chem. 2009;284(43):29798–808.

78. Baughman BM, Jake Slavish P, Dubois RM, Boyd VA, White SW, Webb TR. Identification of influenza endonuclease inhibitors using a novel fluorescence polarization assay. ACS Chem Biol. 2012;7(3):526–34.

79. Hastings JC, Selnick H, Wolanski B, Tomassini JE. Anti-influenza virus activities of 4-substituted 2,4-dioxobutanoic acid inhibitors. Antimicrob Agents Chemother. 1996;40(5):1304–7.

80. Hsu JT, Yeh JY, Lin TJ, Li ML, Wu MS, Hsieh CF, et al. Identification of BPR3P0128 as an inhibitor of cap-snatching activities of influenza virus. Antimicrob Agents Chemother. 2012;56(2):647–57.

81. Su CY, Cheng TJ, Lin MI, Wang SY, Huang WI, Lin-Chu SY, et al. High-throughput identification of compounds targeting influenza RNA-dependent RNA polymerase activity. Proc Natl Acad Sci U S A. 2010;107(45):19151–6.

82. Kao RY, Yang D, Lau LS, Tsui WH, Hu L, Dai J, et al. Identification of influenza A nucleoprotein as an antiviral target. Nat Biotechnol. 2010;28(6):600–5.

83. Gerritz SW, Cianci C, Kim S, Pearce BC, Deminie C, Discotto L, et al. Inhibition of influenza virus replication via small molecules that induce the formation of

against lethal H5N1 influenza A viruses. Proc Natl Acad Sci U S A. 2010;107(2):882–7.

higher-order nucleoprotein oligomers. Proc Natl Acad Sci U S A. 2011;108(37):15366–71.

84. Zhang W, Wang CY, Yang ST, Qin C, Hu JL, Xia XZ. Inhibition of highly pathogenic avian influenza virus H5N1 replication by the small interfering RNA targeting polymerase A gene. Biochem Biophys Res Commun. 2009;390(3):421–6.

85. Zhou H, Jin M, Yu Z, Xu X, Peng Y, Wu H, et al. Effective small interfering RNAs targeting matrix and nucleocapsid protein gene inhibit influenza A virus replication in cells and mice. Antiviral Res. 2007;76(2): 186–93.

86. Karlas A, Machuy N, Shin Y, Pleissner KP, Artarini A, Heuer D, et al. Genome-wide RNAi screen identifies human host factors crucial for influenza virus replication. Nature. 2010;463(7282):818–22.

87. Budd A, Alleva L, Alsharifi M, Koskinen A, Smythe V, Mullbacher A, et al. Increased survival after gemfibrozil treatment of severe mouse influenza. Antimicrob Agents Chemother. 2007;51(8):2965–8.

88. Carey MA, Bradbury JA, Seubert JM, Langenbach R, Zeldin DC, Germolec DR. Contrasting effects of cyclooxygenase-1 (COX-1) and COX-2 deficiency on the host response to influenza A viral infection. J Immunol. 2005;175(10):6878–84.

89. Brett SJ, Myles P, Lim WS, Enstone JE, Bannister B, Semple MG, et al. Pre-admission statin use and in-hospital severity of 2009 pandemic influenza A(H1N1) disease. PLoS ONE. 2011;6(4):e18120.

90. Perelson AS, Rong L, Hayden FG. Combination antiviral therapy for influenza: predictions from modeling of human infections. J Infect Dis. 2012;205(11): 1642–5.

91. Ison MG, Gnann JW Jr, Nagy-Agren S, Treannor J, Paya C, Steigbigel R, et al. Safety and efficacy of nebulized zanamivir in hospitalized patients with serious influenza. Antivir Ther. 2003;8(3):183–90.

92. Nguyen JT, Smee DF, Barnard DL, Julander JG, Gross M, de Jong MD, et al. Efficacy of combined therapy with amantadine, oseltamivir, and ribavirin in vivo against susceptible and amantadine-resistant influenza A viruses. PLoS ONE. 2012;7(1):e31006.

93. Kim WY, Young Suh G, Huh JW, Kim SH, Kim MJ, Kim YS, et al. Triple-combination antiviral drug for pandemic H1N1 influenza virus infection in critically ill patients on mechanical ventilation. Antimicrob Agents Chemother. 2011;55(12):5703–9.

94. Duval X, van der Werf S, Blanchon T, Mosnier A, Bouscambert-Duchamp M, Tibi A, et al. Efficacy of oseltamivir-zanamivir combination compared to each monotherapy for seasonal influenza: a randomized placebo-controlled trial. PLoS Med. 2010;7(11): e1000362.

95. Hayden FG, Sperber SJ, Belshe RB, Clover RD, Hay AJ, Pyke S. Recovery of drug-resistant influenza A virus during therapeutic use of rimantadine. Antimicrob Agents Chemother. 1991;35(9):1741–7.

96. Hayden FG, Belshe R, Villanueva C, Lanno R, Hughes C, Small I, et al. Management of influenza in households: a prospective, randomized comparison of oseltamivir treatment with or without postexposure prophylaxis. J Infect Dis. 2004;189(3):440–9.

97. Hayden FG, Gubareva LV, Monto AS, Klein TC, Elliot MJ, Hammond JM, et al. Inhaled zanamivir for the prevention of influenza in families. Zanamivir Family Study Group. N Engl J Med. 2000;343(18): 1282–9.

98. Peters PH Jr, Gravenstein S, Norwood P, De Bock V, Van Couter A, Gibbens M, et al. Long-term use of oseltamivir for the prophylaxis of influenza in a vaccinated frail older population. J Am Geriatr Soc. 2001;49(8):1025–31.

99. Ison MG, Szakaly P, Shapira MY, Krivan G, Nist A, Dutkowski R. Efficacy and safety of oral oseltamivir for influenza prophylaxis in transplant recipients. Antivir Ther. 2012;17(6):955–64.

100. LaForce C, Man CY, Henderson FW, McElhaney JE, Hampel FC Jr, Bettis R, et al. Efficacy and safety of inhaled zanamivir in the prevention of influenza in community-dwelling, high-risk adult and adolescent subjects: a 28-day, multicenter, randomized, double-blind, placebo-controlled trial. Clin Ther. 2007;29(8): 1579–90; discussion 7–8.

101. Baz M, Abed Y, Papenburg J, Bouhy X, Hamelin ME, Boivin G. Emergence of oseltamivir-resistant pandemic H1N1 virus during prophylaxis. N Engl J Med. 2009;361(23):2296–7.

102. Aoki FY, Macleod MD, Paggiaro P, Carewicz O, El Sawy A, Wat C, et al. Early administration of oral oseltamivir increases the benefits of influenza treatment. J Antimicrob Chemother. 2003;51(1): 123–9.

103. Englund JA, Champlin RE, Wyde PR, Kantarjian H, Atmar RL, Tarrand J, et al. Common emergence of amantadine- and rimantadine-resistant influenza A viruses in symptomatic immunocompromised adults. Clin Infect Dis. 1998;26(6):1418–24.

104. Ison MG. Epidemiology, prevention, and management of influenza in patients with hematologic malignancy. Infect Disord Drug Targets. 2011;11(1): 34–9.

105. Kaiser L, Keene ON, Hammond JM, Elliott M, Hayden FG. Impact of zanamivir on antibiotic use for respiratory events following acute influenza in adolescents and adults. Arch Intern Med. 2000;160(21): 3234–40.

106. Kaiser L, Wat C, Mills T, Mahoney P, Ward P, Hayden F. Impact of oseltamivir treatment on influenza-related lower respiratory tract complications and hospitalizations. Arch Intern Med. 2003;163(14):1667–72.

107. Adisasmito W, Chan PK, Lee N, Oner AF, Gasimov V, Zaman M, et al. Strengthening observational evidence for antiviral effectiveness in influenza A (H5N1). J Infect Dis. 2011;204(5):810–1.

108. Louie JK, Yang S, Acosta M, Yen C, Samuel MC, Schechter R, Guevara H, Uyeki, TM. Treatment with neuraminidase inhibitors for critically ill patients with influenza A (H1N1)pdm09. Clin Infect Dis. 2012;55:1198–1204.

109. Ison MG, de Jong MD, Gilligan KJ, Higgs ES, Pavia AT, Pierson J, et al. End points for testing influenza antiviral treatments for patients at high risk of severe and life-threatening disease. J Infect Dis. 2010;201(11): 1654–62.

110. Giraud C, Manceau S, Oualha M, Chappuy H, Mogenet A, Duchene P, et al. High levels and safety of oseltamivir carboxylate plasma concentrations after nasogastric administration in critically ill children in a pediatric intensive care unit. Antimicrob Agents Chemother. 2011;55(1):433–5.

111. Taylor WR, Thinh BN, Anh GT, Horby P, Wertheim H, Lindegardh N, et al. Oseltamivir is adequately absorbed following nasogastric administration to adult patients with severe H5N1 influenza. PLoS ONE. 2008;3(10):e3410.

112. Wildschut ED, de Hoog M, Ahsman MJ, Tibboel D, Osterhaus AD, Fraaij PL. Plasma concentrations of oseltamivir and oseltamivir carboxylate in critically ill children on extracorporeal membrane oxygenation support. PLoS ONE. 2010;5(6):e10938.

113. Ison MG, Sharma A, Shepard JA, Wain JC, Ginns LC. Outcome of influenza infection managed with oseltamivir in lung transplant recipients. J Heart Lung Transplant. 2008;27(3):282–8.

114. Khanna N, Steffen I, Studt JD, Schreiber A, Lehmann T, Weisser M, et al. Outcome of influenza infections in outpatients after allogeneic hematopoietic stem cell transplantation. Transpl Infect Dis. 2009;11(2): 100–5.

115. Kumar D, Michaels MG, Morris MI, Green M, Avery RK, Liu C, et al. Outcomes from pandemic influenza A H1N1 infection in recipients of solid-organ transplants: a multicentre cohort study. Lancet Infect Dis. 2010;10(8):521–6.

116. Ljungman P, de la Camara R, Perez-Bercoff L, Abecasis M, Nieto Campuzano JB, Cannata-Ortiz MJ, et al. Outcome of pandemic H1N1 infections in hematopoietic stem cell transplant recipients. Haematologica. 2011;96(8):1231–5.

117. Ng BJ, Glanville AR, Snell G, Musk M, Holmes M, Chambers DC, et al. The impact of pandemic influenza A H1N1 2009 on Australian lung transplant recipients. Am J Transplant. 2011;11(3):568–74.

118. Dubar G, Azria E, Tesniere A, Dupont H, Le Ray C, Baugnon T, et al. French experience of 2009 A/H1N1v influenza in pregnant women. PLoS ONE. 2010;5(10): e13112..

119. Siston AM, Rasmussen SA, Honein MA, Fry AM, Seib K, Callaghan WM, et al. Pandemic 2009 influenza A(H1N1) virus illness among pregnant women in the United States. JAMA. 2010;303(15): 1517–25.

120. Belshe RB, Smith MH, Hall CB, Betts R, Hay AJ. Genetic basis of resistance to rimantadine emerging during treatment of influenza virus infection. J Virol. 1988;62(5):1508–12.

121. Cheung CL, Rayner JM, Smith GJD, Wang P, Naipospos TSP, Zhang JX, et al. Distribution of amantadine-resistant H5N1 avian influenza variants in Asia. J Infect Dis. 2006;193(12):1626–9.

122. Deyde V, Garten R, Sheu T, Smith C, Myrick A, Barnes J, et al. Genomic events underlying the changes in adamantane resistance among influenza A(H3N2) viruses during 2006–2008. Influenza Other Respi Viruses. 2009;3(6):297–314.

123. Ward P, Small I, Smith J, Suter P, Dutkowski R. Oseltamivir (Tamiflu (R)) and its potential for use in the event of an influenza pandemic. J Antimicrob Chemother. 2005;55:5–21.

124. Kiso M, Mitamura K, Sakai-Tagawa Y, Shiraishi K, Kawakami C, Kimura K, et al. Resistant influenza A viruses in children treated with oseltamivir: descriptive study. Lancet. 2004;364(9436):759–65.

125. de Jong MD, Thanh TT, Khanh TH, Hien VM, Smith GJD, Chau NV, et al. Brief report – Oseltamivir resistance during treatment of influenza A (H5N1) infection. N Engl J Med. 2005;353(25):2667–72.

126. Lackenby A, Hungnes O, Dudman SG, Meijer A, Paget WJ, Hay AJ, et al. Emergence of resistance to oseltamivir among influenza A(H1N1) viruses in Europe. Euro Surveill. 2008;13(5).

127. Cheng PKC, To APC, Leung TWC, Leung PCK, Lee CWC, Lim WWL. Oseltamivir- and Amantadine-Resistant Influenza Virus A (H1N1). Emerg Infect Dis. 2010;16(1):155–6.

128. Collins PJ, Haire LF, Lin YP, Liu J, Russell RJ, Walker PA, et al. Structural basis for oseltamivir resistance of influenza viruses. Vaccine. 2009;27(45): 6317–23.

129. Bloom JD, Gong LI, Baltimore D. Permissive secondary mutations enable the evolution of influenza

oseltamivir resistance. Science. 2010;328(5983): 1272–5.

130. Hurt AC, Hardie K, Wilson NJ, Deng YM, Osbourn M, Gehrig N, et al. Community transmission of oseltamivir-resistant A(H1N1)pdm09 influenza. N Engl J Med. 2011;365(26):2541–2.

131. Sidwell RW, Smee DF. Peramivir (BCX-1812, RWJ-270201): potential new therapy for influenza. Expert Opin Investig Drugs. 2002;11(6):859–69.

132. Nguyen HT, Fry AM, Gubareva LV. Neuraminidase inhibitor resistance in influenza viruses and laboratory testing methods. Antivir Ther. 2012;17(1 Pt B):159–73.

26 The control of influenza and cost-effectiveness of interventions

Carolyn B. Bridges,[1] Samuel K. Peasah[2] and Martin I. Meltzer[3]

[1]Immunization Services Division, National Center for Immunizations and Respiratory Diseases, Centers for Disease Control and Prevention (CDC), Atlanta, GA, USA

[2]Epidemiology and Prevention Branch, Influenza Division/NCIRD/Centers for Disease Control and Prevention, Atlanta, GA, USA

[3]Health Economics and Modeling Unit (HEMU), Division of Preparedness and Emerging Infections, National Center for Emerging and Zoonotic Infectious Diseases, Centers for Disease Control and Prevention (CDC), Atlanta, GA, USA

Introduction

Influenza poses an annual threat of seasonal influenza and the risk of sporadic, unpredictable pandemics. Neither the severity of pandemics nor seasonal influenza outbreaks can be predicted in advance. Because of the reservoir of influenza viruses among birds, pigs, and other animals and the occurrence of interspecies transmission, eradication of influenza is not possible [1]. Evidence supports transmission of influenza viruses from person to person through multiple modes of transmission, including droplet, droplet nuclei, and contact transmission. In any given year, influenza infection rates can be as high as 30% or more in susceptible subpopulations, such as children under 5 years of age or nursing home residents. Transmission from person to person is rapid, with a short incubation period of only 1–4 days, with an average of 2 days [2,3]. The ability of influenza viruses to spread rapidly was recently documented during the 2009 H1N1 pandemic when the virus was confirmed in 74 countries within 8 weeks of initial identification [4].

In addition to rapid spread, the control of influenza is further complicated by the wide range of clinical presentations, making initial recognition of influenza illness challenging. Infections can cause a range of health outcomes, from asymptomatic infection to classic symptoms of body aches, fever, and cough to nonfebrile illnesses with worsening of underlying chronic health conditions, such as congestive heart failure. Infected individuals can shed influenza virus beginning the day before illness onset through 5–7 days after illness onset in otherwise healthy adults and older children and longer in young children, those with more severe illness, and immune compromised persons [2,3,5,6]. Challenges in early recognition of influenza illness and prolonged viral shedding make reliance on the identification and isolation of infected persons a likely unsuccessful strategy for preventing the spread of influenza in the general population [7].

Other environmental, host, and virologic factors may impact the transmission of influenza viruses (Figure 26.1). For example, periods of lower temperature and humidity appear to be strong predictors of the timing of peak influenza transmission in temperate climates [8]. Other environmental factors such as air exchange and airflow, person density, distance from infected and susceptible persons, and duration of exposure can also impact transmission [9–11].

Influenza vaccination is the primary tool for the prevention and control of influenza. Other tools used to decrease influenza transmission and reduce morbidity and mortality include the use of antiviral medications for treatment and prophylaxis, social

Textbook of Influenza, Second Edition. Edited by Robert G. Webster, Arnold S. Monto, Thomas J. Braciale, and Robert A. Lamb.
© 2013 John Wiley & Sons, Ltd. Published 2013 by John Wiley & Sons, Ltd.

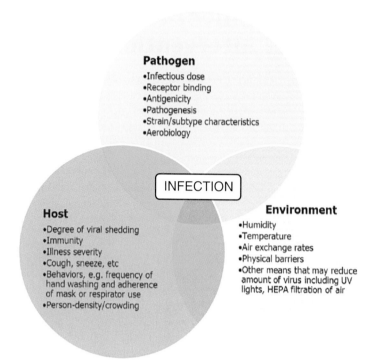

Pathogen
- Infectious dose
- Receptor binding
- Antigenicity
- Pathogenesis
- Strain/subtype characteristics
- Aerobiology

INFECTION

Host
- Degree of viral shedding
- Immunity
- Illness severity
- Cough, sneeze, etc
- Behaviors, e.g. frequency of hand washing and adherence of mask or respirator use
- Person-density/crowding

Environment
- Humidity
- Temperature
- Air exchange rates
- Physical barriers
- Other means that may reduce amount of virus including UV lights, HEPA filtration of air

Figure 26.1. Factors impacting the transmission and infection from influenza include pathogen, host, and environmental factors.

distancing, hand hygiene, surgical mask use, respirators, and other measures to prevent the spread of influenza.

In this chapter, we review the tools available for the prevention and control of influenza and application of these measures in outbreak settings. In addition, we review information on the cost-effectiveness of these interventions, with an emphasis on influenza vaccination.

Tools for the prevention and control of influenza

Influenza vaccine

Influenza vaccination is the primary means to reduce the risk of influenza illness in individuals and to increase population immunity. The effectiveness of influenza vaccination has been demonstrated in young children, healthy adults, healthcare workers (HCW), pregnant women, the elderly, nursing home residents, and persons with high-risk conditions, although randomized trial data are strongest for children and healthy younger adults and least robust for elderly persons [12–14]. Outcomes that can be prevented through influenza vaccination include infection, respiratory illness, hospitalization, and death [12]. In the United States and in Ontario, Canada, all persons 6 months of age and older are recommended for annual vaccination. Many other countries recommend annual vaccination for specific populations at increased risk of influenza-related complications such as pregnant women, older adults, and/or persons with chronic medical conditions, such as chronic heart or lung disease, that increase the risk of influenza-related complications [15].

Increasing population immunity through influenza vaccination has a number of advantages for prevention, most notably decreasing the number of people susceptible to influenza in the community, which can reduce both the rate of spread and the peak incidence of illness requiring medical care. Influenza vaccination also causes relatively little social disruption compared to other interventions such as social distancing. In addition, influenza vaccines are well tolerated and severe adverse reactions are rare. However, because influenza vaccination is imperfect, and notable portions of the population remain susceptible to infection even after vaccination, other interventions should be used in concert with vaccination. The use of other influenza prevention strategies may also be needed due to lack of vaccine availability early in a pandemic. Nonvaccination strategies may also be especially important when a very poor antigenic match between the vaccine and circulating influenza virus strains occurs, such as during the 1997–1998 influenza season [16].

Influenza vaccination has been demonstrated to reduce not only infection in vaccinated persons, but also to decrease the risk of influenza among nonvaccinated persons in the community. Studies demonstrating the benefit of vaccination of schoolchildren in preventing influenza in nonvaccinated community members have been conducted. A study conducted during the 1968 pandemic compared two Michigan communities: one in which 85% of schoolchildren were vaccinated and one in which children remained unvaccinated. Reductions in illness among unvaccinated adults in the vaccinated community were demonstrated [17]. A study conducted during the 2009 H1N1 pandemic demonstrated that teachers had moderately lower risk of absenteeism at schools with higher vaccination rates among the children, who were the primary target of vaccination efforts [18]. The only other study conducted during a seasonal influenza outbreak, measuring the impact of vaccinating school-aged children on the rate of illness in nonvaccinated community members, was a cluster randomized trial among Hutterite communities in Canada [19]. Over 80% vaccination coverage among schoolchildren was achieved in communities randomized to influenza vaccination. Among nonvaccine recipients in these communities, compared with communities in which schoolchildren were not vaccinated, there was a 61% reduction in laboratory-confirmed influenza illness. Illnesses among unvaccinated persons, however, would not be eliminated by only vaccinating schoolchildren; therefore, direct vaccination of children and adults at increased risk of influenza-related complications remains an important strategy for preventing severe influenza illnesses [17,19].

Elderly persons are at highest risk of influenza-related mortality from seasonal influenza, but have suboptimal protection from influenza vaccination [13,20,21]. Even though influenza vaccine effectiveness is reduced in elderly persons, influenza vaccination of 80% or more of nursing home residents has been found to decrease the risk of influenza outbreaks in these settings [22,23]. Studies have also demonstrated that vaccination of HCW can reduce deaths in nursing home residents, even at a relatively modest HCW vaccination rate [23–25].

Vaccination of pregnant women can reduce the risk of influenza in the women themselves and also decrease the risk of influenza illness and hospitalization in their infants during the first 6 months of life, during which infants are at highest risk of influenza-related complications but are too young for influenza vaccination [26,27]. See Chapter 20 for more information on influenza vaccines.

Influenza antiviral medications

Influenza antiviral medications are especially useful for the prevention of influenza illness among persons at high risk of influenza-related complications with recent exposure to infection, or for treating those with recent onset of influenza illness, as well as for treating individuals with severe influenza. Antiviral medications are a key intervention for influenza outbreak control in confined populations at increased risk of severe illness and death from influenza, such as during influenza outbreaks in nursing homes (Figure 26.2). Judicious use of such drugs is advised, however, as the widespread use of such medications increases the risk of the emergence and spread of antiviral-resistant influenza viruses.

There are two classes of antiviral medications for the treatment and prevention of influenza: the adamantanes and the neuraminidase inhibitors. The adamantanes (amantadine and rimatadine) are M2 proton inhibitors with activity against influenza A viruses only, while the neuraminidase inhibitors (oseltamivir and zanamivir) are effective against both influenza A and B viruses. The use of adamantanes is currently not recommended, however, because of high levels of resistance to these drugs among currently circulating influenza A viruses. More information on antiviral medications can be found in Chapter 25.

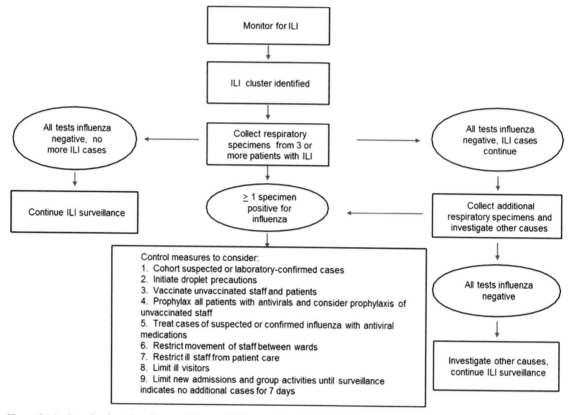

Figure 26.2. Sample algorithm for surveillance of influenza-like illness (ILI) and initiation of antiviral treatment and prophylaxis in long-term care facilities to reduce severe morbidity and mortality during influenza outbreaks.

Use of antiviral medications for outbreak control

Use of antivirals has been demonstrated to reduce transmission and control outbreaks in nursing homes (Figure 26.2), summer camps (Figure 26.3), cruise ships, and households [7,28,29]. For example, Bowles et al. [30] reported oseltamivir was associated with effective termination of influenza outbreaks in eight nursing homes in Ontario, Canada. Miller et al. [7] also reported that rimantadine given during influenza outbreaks among cruise ship passengers and crew between August and September 1997 appeared to have interrupted transmission between passengers and crew after cohorting and quarantine of ill persons was ineffective in controlling the outbreak. Similarly, in a summer camp outbreak, initial cohorting of ill campers and staff did not reduce the course of the

outbreak, but cases dropped rapidly in the 2 days after rimantadine was initiated camp-wide (Figure 26.3; Neil Pascoe, Texas Department of Health, unpublished data, 2000).

A major concern is the potential for emergence and rapid spread of antiviral-resistant influenza viruses, particularly given that only one of the two classes of antivirals is effective against currently circulating influenza virus strains. Because antiviral resistance may emerge when the drugs are being used for the treatment and prevention of influenza, cases of influenza that occur 3 days or more after starting antiviral prophylaxis should be tested for influenza and antiviral resistance. Ideally, contact between ill persons and non-ill persons taking antiviral medications should be limited to reduce the potential for transmission of resistant viruses.

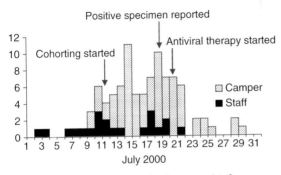

Figure 26.3. Epidemic curve of influenza and influenza-like illnesses reported among campers and staff, and control measures initiated during an influenza A (H1N1) outbreak at a summer camp, Texas, United States, July 2000. Previously unpublished data, reported by permission of Neil Pascoe, Texas Department of Health.

Hand hygiene

Several studies have documented the persistence of viable influenza viruses on surfaces and the potential for self-inoculation after touching infected surfaces and then touching the mucous membranes. Influenza viruses can remain viable on nonporous surfaces for more than 24 hours, and for as long as 7 days [31,32]. Influenza viruses have increased duration of viability in lower temperatures and drier, less humid conditions [33].

Hand hygiene has been demonstrated in clinic trials to prevent a number of important infectious diseases and syndromes, including gastroenteritis, conjunctivitis, and overall respiratory illness [34,35]. Data demonstrating the benefits of hand hygiene alone to prevent influenza illness are limited. Only one randomized study has shown a reduction in laboratory-confirmed influenza based solely on improvements in hand hygiene [35], while other randomized trials have not shown that hand hygiene prevents influenza in the absence of concurrent use of other interventions such as face masks [36]. A challenge for many studies of hand hygiene and influenza has been the difficulty in achieving substantial differences in hand hygiene practices between study arms. The one study that showed a difference in influenza illness between treatment arms was conducted in Egyptian children; the study population did not have a culture of routine frequent hand washing in school, enabling achieve-

ment of substantial differences in hand washing behaviors between control and intervention groups [35]. Additional studies in developing countries are underway.

Even if hand hygiene does not provide substantial protection against influenza illness, this practice can reduce the risk of other illnesses that may have syndromes similar to influenza and can reduce the overall burden of infectious diseases. This may be especially important in a severe influenza pandemic to reduce demands on overburdened medical care systems. Hand hygiene is a critical component of infection control for respiratory illnesses in general.

Preventing spread of influenza through the air

Face masks are designed and approved for medical use to block large-droplet splashes and sprays from reaching the wearer's mouth and nose; they are not tested for fit. Respirators, many of which require fit testing to assure a tight seal on the face, are designed and approved to prevent the wearer's inhalation of small airborne particles. The role of face masks versus respirators for preventing transmission of influenza was an area of major controversy during the 2009 H1N1 pandemic, in part due to limited understanding about the relative contribution of different modes of influenza transmission and limited data on the relative effectiveness of each [37]. Most observational studies suggest increased person-to-person transmission with prolonged exposure and at relatively short distances between exposed and infected patients [10,11]. These data support the role in transmission of both large droplets and droplet-nuclei (i.e., airborne) transmission. Other studies point to the potential for spread by droplet-nuclei over greater distances in the setting of suboptimal airflow conditions, as occurred in a hospital ward [9]. Studies have confirmed the presence of influenza virus in particles small enough to be inhaled (i.e., droplet-nuclei particles of respirable size) collected from the cough-producing aerosol of influenza-infected individuals as well as in emergency department air samples during influenza season [38]. Also suggesting a role of droplet-nuclei was an observational study by McLean [39] during the 1957 pandemic. He found that patients housed in a hospital ward with upper-room ultraviolet germicidal irradiation (UVGI) had an influenza infection rate of only 1.9% compared with

423

a rate of 18.9% among patients on wards without UVGI. A study by McDevitt et al. [40] demonstrated the sensitivity of influenza viruses to UVGI, supporting the biologic plausibility of McLean's observations. More data are needed to determine the effectiveness of UVGI in preventing transmission.

Supporting the contribution to transmission of large droplets, clinical evidence has found some benefit associated with the use of face masks when they are used consistently and within the first 36 hours of exposure to an influenza-infected person in the household [36,37,41], and when used by HCW [42]. Among studies that have directly compared the effectiveness of face masks with respirators, one study found a possible benefit of respirators over face masks but the difference was not statistically significant [37,43,44]. Infection control guidelines for seasonal influenza recommend both standard contact and droplet precautions, including use of face masks, and also the use of airborne precautions and respirators by HCW during aerosol-generating procedures.

Prevention of transmission of influenza through the air also relies on appropriate use of environmental and engineering control measures. These include installing air handling and air exchange systems that can reduce the spread of potentially contaminated air, adherence to infection control practices (ideally initiated before first contact with potentially infectious persons), and limiting the number of persons who come in contact with ill persons. Such contact can be limited by discouraging ill persons from attending work or school, and limiting the number of persons caring for those who are ill. Placing a face mask on the ill person when in contact with others may also help to reduce transmission [45].

Social distancing

Social distancing can slow the spread of pandemic influenza by reducing transmission via limiting the number of contacts between infected and susceptible individuals. Such measures may include school closure, canceling mass gatherings (e.g., large sports events, community celebrations), limiting travel, and other means to reduce the number of contacts between people. Social distancing may be the primary means to reduce the rate of spread of influenza during a pandemic before appropriate vaccines are available. When applied very early in outbreaks for sustained periods, school closures and other types of social distancing were associated with lower peak incidence of severe outcomes including mortality during the 1918–1919 pandemic and also appeared to reduce the number of ill individuals during the 2009 pandemic [46]. Closure of schools in Hong Kong in 2009 was estimated to reduce transmission of pandemic influenza by approximately 25% [47]. Based on data from seasonal influenza and holiday school closures, Cauchemez et al. [46] estimated a 20–29% reduction in respiratory illness rates in children during holidays in France, but predicted less impact on illness rates in other age groups. However, social distancing can generate substantial disruptions in routine activities; school closures alone can increase work absenteeism as parents may miss work to care for children out of school. Social distancing may be even less useful in controlling seasonal influenza because of the significant economic and social costs involved. Further, school closure during nonpandemic situations is often implemented as a reaction to already high absenteeism, after most students have likely been exposed [46,48].

Combined approaches for the control of influenza outbreaks

Approaches to reduce the health impact of influenza differ based on the overall susceptibility, risk of severe illness and death, and relative isolation of the affected community or group. For seasonal influenza, the primary means to reduce the impact of influenza is through widespread vaccination. However, additional measures to control influenza may be employed in certain circumstances, such as in the control of influenza outbreaks in nursing homes (Figure 26.2).

Depending on its severity, influenza control may involve a combination of measures, including social distancing, use of antiviral medications, cough and respiratory hygiene, voluntary isolation of ill persons and quarantine of their contacts, and use of face masks and respirators where available. Patterns of viral shedding of influenza, high levels of susceptibility to a new virus, and the initial difficulty in accurately diagnosing patients (due to wide range of influenza clinical syndromes) make the complete prevention of pandemic influenza impossible. Preventing the introduction of influenza may only be possible for geographically isolated communities able to endure a prolonged period without any mixing with other populations, as occurred in American Samoa during the 1918–1919 pandemic [49,50].

Control of outbreaks in closed populations

Surveillance and early recognition of outbreaks are essential to limiting the health impact of influenza outbreaks in nursing homes and other settings. HCW should be trained to recognize and report new acute respiratory illnesses and plans should be in place to allow for timely collection and testing of respiratory specimens for influenza. Because elderly patients often present with atypical symptoms, the identification of a single case of laboratory-confirmed influenza in a nursing home or occurrence of two or more suspected cases within 72 hours should trigger prompt action including the following:

• Isolating ill persons in a private room, when possible, and treating suspected influenza cases with antiviral medications for 5 days.
• Implementing droplet and standard infection control precautions, including use of face masks, gloves, and hand hygiene, for 7 days after illness onset or until 24 hours after the resolution of fever and respiratory symptoms, whichever is longer.
• Ensuring other environmental engineering controls are in place and properly functioning.
• Initiating a 2-week course of antiviral prophylaxis for non-ill residents.
• Considering initiation of antiviral prophylaxis of nonvaccinated staff.
• Limiting or cancelling group events.
• Limiting new admissions and visitors and prohibiting visitations by ill persons.
• Having ill employees stay at home and not return until at least 24 hours after resolution of fever.
• Ensuring unvaccinated staff and residents are vaccinated promptly and initiating antiviral prophylaxis for 2 weeks after initial vaccination, the time to reach peak antibody response after vaccination.
• Notifying the local health department of the outbreak.

Prompt initiation of antiviral administration can be greatly facilitated through the use of standing orders obtained from clinicians in advance of influenza outbreaks. Antiviral medications should not be withheld pending laboratory confirmation because the greatest clinical benefit is associated with early antiviral treatment. When initial results of a rapid antigen test are negative for influenza virus antigen, additional specimens should be collected for more sensitive confirmatory tests including polymerase chain reaction (PCR) and viral culture. However, antiviral prophylaxis should continue pending final results of confirmatory testing. During confirmed or suspected influenza outbreaks, all residents in the facility should be given antivirals for treatment or prophylaxis regardless of their vaccination status. Given the likelihood of influenza spreading between areas of the facility by infected HCW, patients, visitors, even patients not on wards or floors with known cases, should be given antiviral prophylaxis. Patients on antiviral treatment should be separated from those on antiviral prophylaxis to reduce the potential for spreading of antiviral-resistant viruses which may emerge during treatment of patients infected with influenza.

Prophylaxis of non-ill residents should continue for a minimum of 2 weeks or until at least 1 week after the onset of illness in the last case in the facility, whichever is longer. Surveillance should continue during this time to identify cases that start after initiation of antiviral prophylaxis. Such cases should raise concern that an antiviral-resistant strain is circulating among the affected population and should trigger additional respiratory specimen collection to test for antiviral resistance [51].

Introduction to applied health economics

The economics of controlling and preventing influenza are most typically assessed using either cost-effectiveness or cost–benefit analyses. The general formula for cost-effectiveness is as follows:

Cost per unit health outcome averted due to intervention = (Costs of intervention − savings from health outcomes prevented)/Number of health outcomes prevented.

Examples of common health outcomes are illnesses, hospitalizations, or premature deaths prevented. Cost–benefit analyses require that every input and output (e.g., health outcome) is assigned a monetary valuation. The analytic outcome is then either net cost or net savings resulting from the intervention. While it may be easy to interpret and compare net savings or costs, the difficulty is in assigning monetary values to some inputs, particularly death.

Other cost-effectiveness methodologies attempt to overcome this drawback by valuing outcomes in terms of impact on quality of life – such as quality-adjusted life-years (QALYs). QALYs attempt to measure the health status of an individual on a scale of 0 (death) to 1 (perfect health). An example of a method used to measure QALYs is the time tradeoff method where respondents are asked how they value the tradeoff between experiencing a specific disease or condition, and how much of their life they would surrender to avoid such an experience.

Key factors in the economics of influenza vaccination

The economics (i.e., cost-effectiveness) of influenza vaccination is primarily influenced by:
1. The influenza clinical attack rate (i.e., the percentage of persons who become clinically ill).
2. The proportion of the population with comorbidities (e.g., emphysema, asthma, pregnancy[1]) that place them at increased risk of needing a physician visit, being hospitalized, or dying from influenza. In the United States, approximately 9% of persons <18 years, 17% of those aged 18–64 years, and 48% of those >64 years have pre-existing medical conditions. Those with high-risk medical conditions have a 2–10 times greater risk of having a physician visit, hospitalization, or premature death related to influenza.
3. The effectiveness of influenza vaccination which can vary from year to year based on the match between the circulating viruses and vaccine strains,

and based on the age and immune competence of the vaccinated person.
4. The cost of influenza-related medical care (Table 26.1).
5. Value of influenza-related deaths in the economic analysis.

Figure 26.4 illustrates the relative importance of the parameters used in a cost-effectiveness analysis of vaccination in children [52]. In this example, the rate of excess deaths is the most influential factor in both high-risk and non-high-risk children.

Evidence of cost-effectiveness of vaccination

Researchers have evaluated the cost-effectiveness of vaccinating different target groups as well as universal vaccination. Vaccinating those at highest risk of influenza-related complications and/or death is generally cost-saving, except when vaccine effectiveness is very low and/or during years with little influenza activity [12].

Mullooly [53] assessed the cost-effectiveness of vaccinating elderly persons in a health maintenance organization from the payer's perspective and found that vaccinating high-risk elderly persons saved the organization an estimated $6.11 per vaccination; vaccinating all elderly persons irrespective of risk saved an estimated $1.10 per vaccination. In contrast, from a health systems perspective, Scuffham and West [54] used 1998–1999 data to estimate that vaccination of the elderly cost €0.6 in England, €5.2 in France, and €9.2 in Germany per day of morbidity (including deaths) saved.

Maciosek et al. [55], using the societal perspective in the United States, found vaccination of those aged 65 years and older cost an estimated $980/QALY saved and vaccination of 50- to 64-year-olds cost an estimated $28 000/QALY saved (in 2000 $). They further estimated that when patient time and travel time are ignored, the cost-effectiveness ratio for vaccination of 50- to 64-year-olds was $7200/QALY saved. When ignoring time and travel costs, vaccinating those aged 65 and older saves $17 per person vaccinated. Similarly, Aballea et al. [56], using both third-party payer and societal perspectives in Brazil, France, Germany, and Italy, found vaccination of 50- to 64-year-olds to be R$4000, €13 200, €31

[1]High risk conditions for influenza-related complications for adults include: diabetes, emphysema, coronary heart disease, angina, heart attack, or other heart conditions; a diagnosis of cancer during the preceding 12 months (excluding non-melanoma skin cancer); chronic bronchitis; weak or failing kidneys; having had an asthma episode or attack during the preceding 12 months. For children aged <18 years, high-risk conditions include diabetes, cystic fibrosis, sickle cell anemia, congenital heart disease, other heart disease, or neuromuscular conditions (seizures, cerebral palsy, and muscular dystrophy), or having an asthma episode or attack during the preceding 12 months. Source: Fiore et al. [12].

Table 26.1. Mean direct medical cost of cases of influenza by age group in the United States ($2003).

Age (years)	Hospitalized		Outpatient	
	Average cost *(std. dev.)*		Average cost *(std. dev.)*	
	Non-risk patients[a]	High-risk patients[a]	Non-risk patients[a]	High-risk patients[a]
<5	$10 880 *(36 189)*	$81 596 *(123 626)*	$167 *(307)*	$574 *(1266)*
5–17	$15 014 *(86 804)*	$41 918 *(50 393)*	$95 *(258)*	$649 *(1492)*
18–49	$19 012 *(44 636)*	$47 722 *(85 644)*	$125 *(438)*	$725 *(1717)*
50–64	$22 304 *(95 727)*	$41 948 *(74 798)*	$150 *(766)*	$733 *(1307)*
65+	$11 451 *(23 128)*	$16 750 *(32 091)*	$242 *(1544)*	$476 *(1131)*

std. dev. = standard deviations in dollars.

[a]Influenza patients are divided into high-risk and non-high-risk groups depending on the presence of pre-existing medical conditions: asthma, neurologic and neurodevelopmental conditions, chronic lung disease, heart disease, disorders of the blood disorders, endocrine system, kidneys, liver, and metabolic system, weakened immune system, younger than 19 years and receiving long-term aspirin therapy, and people who are morbidly obese (see: http://www.cdc.gov/flu/about/disease/high_risk .htm) Upon contracting a clinical case of influenza, those with pre-existing medical conditions have a 2–10 times greater risk of needing a physician visit, being hospitalized, or premature death than those without such conditions.

Source: Adapted from Molinari et al. [67] with permission from Elsevier.

400, and €15 700 per QALY, respectively. Table 26.2 summarizes several other studies of influenza vaccination among the 50–64 year age group with their incremental cost-effectiveness ratios, showing differences between societal and healthcare system perspectives [57].

Another target group with extensive evidence of the cost-effectiveness of influenza vaccination is children, especially those below 5 years old. In the United States, vaccination of high-risk children 6–24 months old was found to be cost-saving [52,58]. While a study in Italy estimating the cost-effectiveness of vaccinating all healthy children 6–60 months of age with an adjuvanted influenza vaccine from a societal perspective found that universal vaccination of 3 million children saved €63 million and averted 1 million clinical influenza episodes. From the Italian healthcare system perspective, they estimated a cost-effectiveness ratio of €10 000/QALY saved [59].

Another high-risk group benefiting from influenza vaccination is pregnant women. Skedgel et al. [60] compared universal vaccination of all pregnant women in Nova Scotia, Canada, with vaccinating only high-risk pregnant women. They found vaccinat-

ing only high-risk pregnant women to be cost-saving, whereas universal vaccination of all pregnant women cost $40 000/QALY if given as part of a routine family practitioner or a public health clinic visit. Jit et al. [61] estimated vaccination of pregnant women in England and Wales to have a cost-effectiveness ratio of £23 000/QALY if infants are assumed to be protected and £28 000/QALY if infants are assumed to be unprotected.

Bridges et al. [16] studied the impact of influenza vaccination among healthy adults aged 18–64 years in a US manufacturing company in a double-blind randomized control trial from 1997 to 1999. With a good match between vaccine and circulating virus strains, they estimated a net societal cost of $11.17 per person vaccinated, with a 42% reduction in physician visits, and a 34% reduction in cases of influenza-like illness, and 32% reduction in lost work days. In a year with a poor match, the net societal cost increased to $65.59/person. Gatwood et al. [62] reviewed a number of economic studies of influenza vaccination in healthy working adults, and found results that ranged from cost savings to a net cost of about $85.92 per person vaccinated. Two of the

(a) Non high risk: $60 per vaccine dose administered

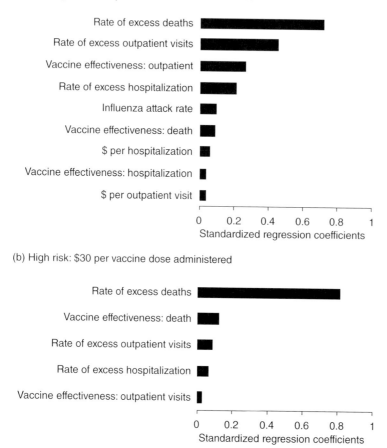

Figure 26.4. Relative importance of the input probability distributions: age group 6–59 months, clinical attack rate of influenza modeled as a uniform distribution with a range of 20–30%. The relative importance of various factors impacting the cost–benefit analysis of vaccinating children aged 6–59 months, for (a) non-high-risk children and (b) high-risk children. Longer bars indicate more influential factors. In these results, the rate of excess influenza-related death was the most influential parameter. The rate of outpatient visits was the next most influential parameter; however, the cost per outpatient visit was the least influential. Variables with coefficients of 0.3 or less can be considered to be of relative minor consequence. Source: Adapted from Meltzer et al. [52] with permission from Elsevier.

reviewed studies reported cost-effectiveness ratios that ranged $26 565–50 512/QALY.

Few studies have compared the cost-effectiveness of universal vaccination with that of targeted vaccination. In 2000, Ontario Province in Canada implemented a free universal vaccination program. Sander et al. [63] evaluated the cost-effectiveness of this program from the healthcare system perspective. Using 1997–2004 data (pre- and post-implementation), they estimated a 61% reduction in influenza cases, a 28% reduction in mortality rates, and a 52% reduction in related healthcare costs. It costs the province about twice as much for the universal vaccination program than for the previous targeted vaccination. The incremental cost-effectiveness ratio was CAN$10 797 per additional QALY saved due to switching from a targeted to universal vaccination program.

The cost-effectiveness of vaccination in different settings has also been studied. Prosser et al. [64] estimated that vaccination in pharmacies had the lowest cost ($11.57) per vaccination, less than both mass vaccination clinic settings ($17.04) and vaccination during a traditional scheduled physician visit ($28.67). They found using a nontraditional setting for both healthy adults aged 50 years and older and all high-risk adults to be cost-saving. Additionally, vaccinating healthy adults aged 18–49 years in the pharmacy setting cost $90 per clinical case of influenza prevented compared with $210 in mass vaccination settings and $870 in scheduled physician office visits.

Table 26.2. Summary of influenza vaccination cost-effectiveness ratios for adults aged 50–64 years.

Study	Country	Model	Perspectives[d]	Type of sensitivity analysis	Primary outcome	Quality-of-life loss	Discount rate (QALY/future earnings)	Cost-effectiveness ratios $US/QALY saved (2005 value): by perspective[d]	
								Societal	Healthcare system
Aballea et al. [56]	Brazil, France, Germany, Italy	Decision tree	1. Societal 2. Healthcare system	PSA	QALY	Only from death	3% (varied by country)	Brazil: 1040 per QALY gained France: 9753 per QALY gained Germany: cost-saving Italy: cost-saving	Brazil: 1151 per QALY gained France: 16060 per QALY gained Germany: 38316 per QALY gained Itlay: 19108 per QALY gained
Maciosek et al. [55]	US	Incremental analysis	1. Societal	Univariate/multivariate	QALY	2.1 QALD per case	3%	31805 per QALY gained	NA
Newall et al. [57]	Australia	Decision tree	1. Societal 2. Healthcare payer 3. Governmental	PSA	QALY	Only from death	5%	6348 per QALY gained	6782 per QALY gained[a]
Prosser et al. [64]	US	Decision tree	1. Societal	PSA	Case prevented	NA	NR (3%[b])	Cost-saving in non-traditional settings[c] (but not when targeting healthy adults in traditional settings)	NA
Turner et al. [65]	UK	Decision tree	1. Societal 2. Healthcare system	PSA	QALY	4.27 QALD per case	NR (1.5%[b])	17912 per QALY gained	10272 per QALY gained

NA = not applicable; NR = not reported; PSA = probabilistic analysis; QALY = quality-adjusted life-years; QALD = quality-adjusted life-days.

[a]Healthcare payer perspective, governmental perspective = 17060 per QALY gained.

[b]Unpublished rate obtained from authors.

[c]Nontraditional settings are pharmacies and mass vaccination sites); traditional settings are healthcare provider offices/clinics with individually scheduled patient visits.

[d]Perspective identifies who pays and who benefits from an intervention, and thus determines what is included in a particular cost-effectiveness calculation. See main text for further explanation.

Source: Adapted from Newall et al. [57] with permission from Springer Science+Business Media.

Evidence of cost-effectiveness of antiviral prophylaxis or treatment

Less information is available on the cost-effectiveness of antivirals and other means for controlling the spread of influenza. A systematic review by Turner et al. [65] estimated that using neuraminidase inhibitors to treat persons with influenza illness cost $6117–30825 per QALY saved in children, $5057–21781 per QALY saved in elderly residents in residential care, $6190–31529 per QALY saved in healthy adults, and $4535–22502 per QALY saved in high-risk patients. Lee et al. [66] did not find antiviral prophylaxis in pregnant women to be cost-saving in seasonal influenza, but found prophylaxis to be cost-saving during a pandemic when attack rates are 20% or greater.

Conclusions

The control of influenza remains a formidable challenge given multiple routes of transmission, wide range of clinical symptoms, and potential for rapid spread. Surveillance and early identification of outbreaks and emerging novel influenza viruses are essential for prompt initiation of intervention measures. Influenza vaccination is the primary means to reduce the impact of influenza. However, other measures, most notably antiviral medications in conjunction with other control measures, can have an important role in reducing the morbidity and mortality of influenza. To improve evidence-based guidance for the control of seasonal and pandemic influenza, more information is needed on the best use of face masks and respirators to prevent infection and transmission and on the cost-effectiveness of other mitigation strategies.

Acknowledgments

Any views expressed in the Work by contributors employed by the United States government at the time of writing do not necessarily represent the views of the United States government, and the contributor's contribution to the Work is not meant to serve as an official endorsement of any statement to the extent that such statement may conflict with any official position of the United States government.

References

1. Kasowski EJ, Garten RJ, Bridges CB. Influenza pandemic epidemiology and virologic diversity: reminding ourselves of the possibilities. Clin Infect Dis. 2011;52(Suppl. 1):S44–9.

2. Carrat F, Vergu E, Ferguson NM, Lemaitre M, Cauchemez S, Leach S, et al. Time lines of infection and disease in human influenza: a review of volunteer challenge studies. Am J Epidemiol. 2008;167:775–85.

3. Lau LL, Nishiura H, Kelly H, Ip DK, Leung GM, Cowling BJ.. Household transmission of 2009 pandemic influenza A (H1N1): a systematic review and meta-analysis. Epidemiology. 2012;23:531–42.

4. WHO. New influenza A (H1N1) virus: global epidemiological situation, June 2009. Wkly Epidemiol Rec. 2009;25:249–57.

5. Lee N, Chan PK, Hui DS, Rainer TH, Wong E, Choi KW, et al. Viral loads and duration of viral shedding in adult patients hospitalized with influenza. J Infect Dis. 2009;200(4):492–500.

6. Esposito S, Daleno C, Baldanti F, Scala A, Campanini G, Taroni F, et al. Viral shedding in children infected by pandemic A/H1N1/2009 influenza virus. Virol J. 2011;8:349.

7. Miller J, Tam T, Afif C, Maloney S, Cetron M, Fukata K, et al. Influenza A outbreak on a cruise ship. Can Commun Dis Rep. 1998;24(2):9–11.

8. Shaman J, Kohn M. Absolute humidity modulates influenza survival, transmission, and seasonality. Proc Natl Acad Sci. 2009;106:3243–8.

9. Wong BC, Lee N, Li Y, Chan PK, Qiu H, Luo Z, et al. Possible role of aerosol transmission in a hospital outbreak of influenza. Clin Infect Dis. 2010;51(10):1176–83.

10. Gregg MB. The epidemiology of influenza in humans. Ann N Y Acad Sci. 1980;353:45–53.

11. Han K, Zhu X, He F, Liu L, Zhang L, Ma H, et al. Lack of airborne transmission during outbreak of pandemic (H1N1) 2009 among tour group members, China, June 2009. Emerg Infect Dis. 2009;15(10):1578–81.

12. Fiore AE, Bridges CB, Katz JM, Cox NJ. Inactivated influenza vaccines. In: Plotkin SA, Orenstein WA, Offit PA, editors. Vaccines, 6th edn 2013, China: Sanders Elsevier, Inc.; p. 257–93..

13. Fiore AE, Uyeki TM, Broder K, Finelli L, Euler GL, Singleton JA, et al. Prevention and control of influenza with vaccines: recommendations of the Advisory Committee on Immunization Practices (ACIP), 2010. MMWR Recomm Rep. 2010;59(RR–8):1–62.

14. Manzoli L, Ioannidis JPA, Flacco ME, De Vito C, Villari P. Effectiveness and harms of seasonal and pandemic

influenza vaccines in children, adults and elderly: a critical review and re-analysis of 15 meta-analyses. Hum Vaccin Immunother. 2012;8(7):851–62.

15. Palache A. Seasonal influenza vaccine provision in 157 countries (2004–2009) and the potential influence of national public health policies. Vaccine. 2011;29(51): 9459–66.

16. Bridges CB, Thompson WW, Meltzer MI, Reeve GR, Talamonti WJ, Cox NJ, et al. Effectiveness and cost-benefit of influenza vaccination of healthy working adults. JAMA. 2000;284:1655–63.

17. Monto AS, Davenport FM, Napier JA, Francis T Jr. Modification of an outbreak of influenza in Tecumseh, Michigan by vaccination of schoolchildren. J Infect Dis. 1970;122:16–25.

18. Graitcer S, Dube NL, Basurto-Davila R, Smith PF, Ferdinands J, Thompson M, et al. Effects of immunizing school children with 2009 influenza A (H1N1) monovalent vaccine on absenteeism among students and teachers in Maine. Vaccine. 2012;30:4835–41.

19. Loeb M, Russell ML, Moss L, Fonseca K, Fox J, Earn DJ, et al. Effect of influenza vaccination of children on infection rates in Hutterite communities: a randomized trial. JAMA. 2010;303(10):943–50.

20. Thompson WW, Moore MR, Weintraub E, Cheng PY, Jin X, Bridges CB, et al. Estimating influenza-associated deaths in the United States. Am J Public Health. 2009;99(S2):S225–30.

21. Monto AS, Hornbuckle K, Ohmit SE. Influenza vaccine effectiveness among elderly nursing home residents: a cohort study. Am J Epidemiol. 2001;154:155–60.

22. Patriarca PA, Weber JA, Parker RA, Hall WN, Kendal AP, Bregman DJ, et al. Efficacy of influenza vaccine in nursing homes. Reduction in illness and complications during an influenza A (H3N2) epidemic. JAMA. 1985; 253:1136–9.

23. Oshitani H, Saito R, Seki N, Tanabe N, Yamazaki O, Hayashi S, et al. Influenza vaccination levels and influenza-like illness in long-term-care facilities for elderly people in Niigata, Japan, during an influenza A (H3N2) epidemic. Infect Control Hosp Epidemiol. 2000;21:728–30.

24. Hayward AC, Harling R, Wetten S, Johnson AM, Munro S, Smedley J, et al. Effectiveness of an influenza vaccine programme for care home staff to prevent death, morbidity, and health service use among residents: cluster randomized controlled trial. BMJ. 2006; 333:1241.

25. Lemaitre M, Meret T, Rothan-Tondeur M, Belmin J, Lejonc JL, Luquel L, et al. Effect of influenza vaccination of nursing home staff on mortality of residents: a cluster-randomized trial. J Am Geriatr Soc. 2009;57: 1580–6.

26. Zaman K, Roy E, Arifeen SE, Rahman M, Raqib R, Wilson E, et al. Effectiveness of maternal influenza immunization in mothers and infants. N Engl J Med. 2008;359:1555–64.

27. Poehling KA, Szilagyi PG, Staat MA, Snively BM, Payne DC, Bridges CB, et al. Impact of maternal immunization on influenza hospitalizations in infants. Am J Obstet Gynecol. 2011;204(6 Suppl 1):S141–8.

28. van Boven M, Donker T, van der Lubben M, van Gageldonk-Lafeber RB, te Beest DE, Koopmans M, et al. Transmission of novel influenza A (H1N1) in households with post-exposure antiviral prophylaxis. PLoS ONE. 2010;5(7):e11442.

29. Monto AS, Pichichero ME, Blanckenberg SJ, Ruuskanen O, Cooper C, Fleming DM, et al. Zanamivir prophylaxis: an effective strategy for the prevention of influenza types A and B within households. J Infect Dis. 2002;186(11):1582–8.

30. Bowles SK, Lee W, Simor AE, Vearncombe M, Loeb M, Tamblyn S, et al. Use of oseltamivir during influenza outbreaks in Ontario nursing homes, 1999–2000. J Am Geriatr Soc. 2000;50(4):608–16.

31. Dublineau A, Batejat C, Pinon A, Burguière AM, Leclercq I, Manuguerra JC, et al. Persistence of the 2009 pandemic influenza A (H1N1) virus in water and on non-porous surface. PLoS ONE. 2011;6(11):e28043.

32. Bean B, Moore BM, Sterner B, Peterson LR, Gerding DN, Balfour HH Jr. Survival of influenza viruses on environmental surfaces. J Infect Dis. 1982;146:47–51.

33. McDevitt J, Rudnick S, First M, Spengler J. Role of absolute humidity in the inactivation of influenza viruses on stainless steel surfaces at elevated temperatures. Appl Environ Microbiol. 2010;76(12):3943–7.

34. Ryan MA, Christian RS, Wohlrabe J. Handwashing and respiratory illness among young adults in military training. Am J Prev Med. 2001;21:79–83.

35. Talaat M, Afifi S, Dueger E, El-Ashry N, Marfin A, Kandeel A, et al. Effects of hand hygiene campaigns on incidence of laboratory-confirmed influenza and absenteeism in schoolchildren, Cairo, Egypt. Emerg Infect Dis. 2011;17(4):619–25.

36. Aiello AE, Coulborn RM, Aragon TJ, Baker MG, Burrus BB, Cowling BJ, et al. Research findings from nonpharmaceutical intervention studies for pandemic influenza and current gaps in the research. Am J Infect Control. 2010;38(4):251–8.

37. Bin-Reza F, Lopez Chavarrias V, Nicoll A, Chamberland ME.. The use of masks and respirators to prevent transmission of influenza: a systematic review of the scientific evidence. Influenza Other Respi Viruses. 2012;6(4): 257–67.

38. Lindsley WG, Pearce TA, Hudnall JB, Davis KA, Davis SM, Fisher MA, et al. Quantity and size distribution of

cough-generated aerosol particles produced by influenza patients during and after illness. J Occup Environ Hyg. 2012;9(7):443–9.

39. McLean RL. Discussion after paper: the mechanism of spread of Asian influenza. Am Rev Respir Dis. 1961;83: 36–8.

40. McDevitt J, Rudnick SN, Radonovich LJ. Aerosol susceptibility of influenza virus to UV-C light. Am Soc Microbiol. 2012;78(6):1666–9.

41. Suess T, Remschmidt C, Schink SB, Schweiger B, Nitsche A, Schroeder K, et al. The role of facemasks and hand hygiene in the prevention of influenza transmission in households: results from a cluster randomised trial; Berlin, Germany, 2009–2011. BMC Infect Dis. 2012; 12:26.

42. Apisarnthanarak A, Mundy LM. Factors associated with health care–associated 2009 influenza A (H1N1) virus infection among Thai health care workers. Clin Infect Dis. 2010;51(3):368–9.

43. Loeb M, Dafoe N, Mahony J, John M, Sarabia A, Glavin V, et al. Surgical mask vs N95 respirator for preventing influenza among health care workers: a randomized trial. JAMA. 2009;302(17):1865–71.

44. MacIntyre CR, Wang Q, Cauchemez S, Seale H, Dwyer DE, Yang P, et al. A cluster randomized clinical trial comparing fit-tested and non-fit-tested N95 respirators to medical masks to prevent respiratory virus infection in health care workers. Influenza Other Respi Viruses. 2011;5(3):170–9.

45. Johnson DF, Druce JD, Birch C, Grayson ML. A quantitative assessment of the efficacy of surgical and N95 masks to filter influenza virus in patients with acute influenza infection. Clin Infect Dis. 2009;49(2):275–7.

46. Cauchemez S, Ferguson NM, Wachtel C, Tegnell A, Saour G, Duncan B, et al. Closure of schools during an influenza pandemic. Lancet Infect Dis. 2009;9(8): 473–81.

47. Wu JT. School closure and mitigation of pandemic (H1N1) 2009, Hong Kong. Emerg Infect Dis. 2010;16 (3):538–41.

48. Johnson AJ, Moore ZS, Edelson PJ, Kinnane L, Davies M, Shay DK, et al. Household responses to school closure resulting from outbreak of influenza B, North Carolina. Emerg Infect Dis. 2008;14(7):1024–30.

49. Shanks GD, Brundage JF. Pacific islands which escaped the 1918–1919 influenza pandemic and their subsequent mortality experiences. Epidemiol Infect. 2013;141: 353–6.

50. Finnie TJ, Hall IM, Leach S. Behaviour and control of influenza in institutions and small societies. J R Soc Med. 2012;105:66–73.

51. Centers for Disease Control and Prevention (CDC). Interim guidance for influenza outbreak management in long-term care facilities. 2011. Available from: http://www.cdc.gov/flu/professionals/infectioncontrol/ltc-facility-guidance.htm (accessed 15 february 2013).

52. Meltzer MI, Neuzil KM, Griffin MR, Fukuda K. An economic analysis of annual influenza vaccination of children. Vaccine. 2005;23(8):1004–14.

53. Mullooly JP. Influenza vaccination programs for elderly persons: cost-effectiveness in a health maintenance organization. Am J Intern Med. 1994;121(12):947–52.

54. Scuffham PA, West PA. Economic evaluation of strategies for the control and management of influenza in Europe. Vaccine. 2002;20(19–20):2562–78.

55. Maciosek MV, Solberg LI, Coffield AB, Edwards NM, Goodman MJ. Influenza vaccination: health impact and cost-effectiveness among adults aged 50 to 64 and 65 and older. Am J Prev Med. 2006;31(1):72–9.

56. Aballea S, Chancellor J, Martin M, Wutzler P, Carrat F, Gasparini R, et al. The cost-effectiveness of influenza vaccination for people aged 50 to 64 years: an international model. Value Health. 2007;10:98–116.

57. Newall AT, Kelly H, Harsley S, Scuffham PA. Cost effectiveness of influenza vaccination in older adults: a critical review of economic evaluation for the 50- to 64 year age group. Pharmacoeconomics. 2009;27(6): 439–50.

58. Prosser LA, Bridges CB, Uyeki TM, Hinrichsen VL, Meltzer MI, Molinari NA, et al. Health benefits, risks, and cost-effectiveness of influenza vaccination of children. Emerg Infect Dis. 2006;12(10):1548–58.

59. Marchetti M, Kuhnel UM, Colombo GL, Esposito S, Principi N. Cost-effectiveness of adjuvanted influenza vaccination of healthy children 6 to 60 months of age. Hum Vaccin. 2007;3(1):14–22.

60. Skedgel C, Langley JM, MacDonald NE, Scott J, McNeil S. An incremental economic evaluation of targeted and universal influenza vaccination in pregnant women. Can J Public Health. 2011;102(6):445–50.

61. Jit M, Cromer D, Baquelin M, Stowe J, Andrews N, Miller E. The cost-effectiveness of vaccinating pregnant women against seasonal influenza in England and Wales. Vaccine. 2010;29(1):115–22.

62. Gatwood J, Meltzer MI, Messonnier M, Ortega-Sanchez IR, Balkrishnan R, Prosser LA. Seasonal influenza vaccination of healthy working-age adults. Drugs. 2012;72 (1):35–48.

63. Sander B, Kwong JC, Bauch CT, Maetzel A, McGeer A, Raboud JM, et al. Economic appraisal of Ontario's universal influenza immunization program: a cost utility analysis. PLoS Med. 2010;7(4):e1000256.

64. Prosser LA, O'Brien MA, Molinari NM, Hohman KH, Nichol KL, Messonnier ML, et al. Non-traditional settings for influenza vaccination of adults: costs and cost effectiveness. Pharmacoeconomics. 2008;26(2):163–78.

65. Turner D, Wailoo A, Nicholson K, Cooper N, Sutton A, Abrams K. Systematic review and economic decision modeling for the prevention and treatment of influenza A and B. Health Technol Assess. 2003;7(35):3–13.

66. Lee BY, Bailey RR, Wiringa AE, Assi TM, Beigi RH. Antiviral medications for pregnant women for pan-demic and seasonal: an economic computer model. Obstet Gynecol. 2009;114(5):971–80.

67. Molinari NA, Ortega-Sanchez IR, Messonnier ML, Thompson WW, Wortley PM, Weintraub E, et al. The annual impact of seasonal influenza in the US: measuring disease burden and costs. Vaccine. 2007;25:5086–96.

27 Applications of quantitative modeling to influenza virus transmission dynamics, antigenic and genetic evolution, and molecular structure

Marc Lipsitch[1] and Derek Smith[2]

[1]Center for Communicable Disease Dynamics and Department of Epidemiology, Harvard School of Public Health, Boston, MA, USA

[2]Centre for Pathogen Evolution, WHO Collaborating Centre for Modeling Evolution and Control of Emerging Infectious Diseases, Department of Zoology, University of Cambridge, UK

Introduction

Quantitative modeling techniques have become essential to understanding influenza population genetics and evolution, antigenic change, and transmission dynamics, and are of growing importance to understand virus structure. Notably, a number of important advances in computational technique, analysis of antigenic change, and the nascent field of "phylodynamics" (the integration of transmission dynamics and pathogen evolution) have been driven by the need to answer important questions about seasonal influenza and to guide preparation for responses to pandemic influenza. In this chapter, we describe these quantitative modeling approaches and their main conclusions, while providing references to allow the reader to learn more about the technical details of the methods themselves.

We begin with transmission dynamic models applied to seasonal and pandemic influenza, both for scientific purposes – to understand the determinants of transmission dynamics – and for the purposes of policy guidance. We discuss models of the antigenic evolution of the virus and then turn to evolutionary and population genetic models to describe change over time in the virus sequence, with obvious ties both to antigenic evolution (which drives much of the genetic change) and transmission dynamics (which provides the ecologic context for virus evolution). Finally, we conclude by discussing structural modeling of the virus and its potential to bridge the observed patterns in antigenic and genetic evolution, and understand changes in receptor binding.

Transmission dynamic models

While transmission dynamic models differ in their details, they have several fundamental properties that should be understood before attempting to evaluate their findings. All such models consider transmission as a process of encounters between infectious individuals and individuals susceptible to becoming infected; following infection, individuals may recover and become immune, or (in some models) may die. For influenza models considering timescales longer than a year or so, immune individuals may become susceptible again; this process may be modeled as a

Textbook of Influenza, Second Edition. Edited by Robert G. Webster, Arnold S. Monto, Thomas J. Braciale, and Robert A. Lamb.
© 2013 John Wiley & Sons, Ltd. Published 2013 by John Wiley & Sons, Ltd.

simple gradual loss of immunity, or may explicitly consider changes in the circulating strains that lead to escape from existing immune responses. Such models are often called "SIR" or "SIRS" models to indicate this progression from *susceptible* to *infected/ infectious* to *recovered* and possibly back to susceptible. On top of these common features, different models specify varying amounts of detail about the natural history of infection, symptoms, and infectiousness; about the particular venues and groups where contact between susceptible and infectious people occur; about the sources of variation in contact and transmission opportunities (e.g., seasonality, individuals' ages and occupations, location and long-distance travel); about the evolutionary dynamics of circulating viral strains; and about the possible effects of antiviral drugs, vaccines, and nonpharmaceutical interventions.

In all such models, a key summary of the dynamics of infection in a modeled population is the *effective reproductive number* at a given time, written variously R or R_E or $R(t)$, the last to denote that the quantity changes over time. $R(t)$ is defined as the mean number of secondary infectious cases directly infected by a typical infectious case who becomes infected at time t. This quantity depends on the patterns of contact in the population, the proportion of susceptible individuals in the population (because only contacts with susceptible individuals can result in transmission) and the probability that a contact from an infectious to a susceptible individual will result in transmission. When $R(t) > 1$, the number of infectious cases grows, because each case more than replaces itself; when $R(t) < 1$, the size of the epidemic shrinks, because each case fails to replace itself on average. This perspective makes clear that control of transmission does not require preventing every transmission event, but rather requires that enough transmission is prevented so that $R(t)$ is maintained below 1. Much attention in the literature is focused on estimation of the *basic reproductive number*, written R_0, which is in some sense the maximum possible value of the effective reproductive number, namely its value in a fully susceptible population and in the absence of interventions. Seen in this light, the goal of interventions to control transmission is to bring the effective reproductive number from its maximum value, R_0, to a value below 1, so that the number of cases must decline. This may be achieved temporarily by

behavioral changes or social measures such as school closure; it may occur naturally by changes in environmental factors (e.g., increasing absolute humidity, see below) to become less favorable for transmission; or long-term reductions in the effective reproductive number may be achieved by vaccination (which removes susceptible individuals from the population, at least as long as the vaccine remains effective). Likewise, the natural dynamics of an epidemic lead to a reduction of susceptible people (as individuals become infected and recover, gaining immunity); the natural "bell-shaped" epidemic in the absence of interventions results from declining numbers of those who are susceptible, with the peak occurring as the effective reproductive number reaches 1, with each case just replacing itself.

The need for better models of influenza has sparked many of the important methodologic developments in the field of transmission dynamic modeling, from the early development of models incorporating household structure [1] and global travel [2] to more recent, computationally intensive, "agent-based" models that maintain information on the demographic, geographic, social, and infection status of many millions of virtual individuals [3–8]. These models are used together with simpler, more mathematically tractable models to assess the impact of various transmission scenarios and interventions.

Many models suggest that control of pandemic influenza by a combination of measures may be feasible if at the start of the pandemic the infection has a value of R_E below 1.8, but infeasible at higher values. An important use of transmission models in setting the stage for the work described below was to estimate the value of R_E at the start of the fall wave of the 1918 pandemic. The finding that this value was near that threshold in many US cities ([9], later adjusted downwards using improved estimates of the generation interval, or time from infection to infection [3]), set the stage for efforts to model interventions.

Models of interpandemic influenza: Seasonality and geography

A central feature of interpandemic influenza is the winter seasonality observed in temperate regions, with weaker and sometimes multi-peaked epidemics observed closer to the equator. As with many other infections, disentangling the contributions of host behavior, host physiology, and pathogen survival to seasonal variation in incidence is difficult with influenza, because these vary seasonally. Almost certainly, the accumulation of susceptible children in schools during the fall, winter, and spring facilitates influenza transmission; one model estimates a 20–29% reduction in transmission among children during school vacations [10]. However, several lines of evidence suggest this is unlikely to be the sole driver of winter seasonality [11]. Building on laboratory data suggesting that ambient absolute humidity is a strong determinant of influenza virus survival and transmission between laboratory animals [12], a simple transmission dynamic model showed that seasonal variation in absolute humidity could predict the shape of interpandemic influenza epidemics in the United States [13], and that periods of unseasonably low absolute humidity tend to precede the onset of influenza transmission in the winter. The same authors subsequently used a similar model to test a competing hypothesis – that winter declines in immune function resulting from declines in serum vitamin D could drive the winter seasonality of influenza. They found that the vitamin D driven model fit the data less well than the absolute humidity driven model and concluded that variation in vitamin D is not a strong candidate for explaining influenza's winter seasonality [14]. Additional work is needed to understand the quantitative contributions of school terms and environmental factors in driving seasonality of transmission.

In contrast to temperate regions, the seasonal pattern of influenza in the subtropics and tropics is less pronounced and more variable [15]. Moreover, experimental studies of absolute humidity and influenza transmission and/or survival suggest that the sensitivity of the virus to fluctuations in absolute humidity is smaller in the range of high-humidity conditions present in these regions, indicating that some other driver is more likely important in these regions [12,13]. More work is needed to understand what drives the epidemic behavior of influenza in the tropics and subtropics. An even more basic question is: if summer conditions in temperate countries are so unfavorable that transmission of influenza nearly ceases during the summer, how can transmission persist at detectable levels in tropical areas that maintain such weather conditions nearly year-round? Mathematical models of transmission suggest that

this observation is not as paradoxical as it might seem. Summertime conditions in temperate areas do not make influenza impossible, as evidenced by the transmission of pandemic influenza even in summer in some temperate regions [11]. Rather, it is believed that extensive summer transmission in temperate regions is precluded by a combination of unfavorable conditions in the summer with a reduced number of susceptible hosts following a winter epidemic (Figure 27.1a). In regions that have less pronounced winter epidemics, the proportion of susceptible hosts will not decline so much, transmission may be possible for more of the year, despite less favorable environmental conditions. This process may be enhanced by transmission between tropical sites, especially in Asia, as described later.

Earlier work addressed the subtler question within the United States of what determines geographic patterns of the timing of influenza seasonality. A transmission dynamic model tested various possible explanations for two observations: that certain parts of the country tend to get influenza ahead of others each season, and that the asynchrony across the country is greatest in years of low transmission. The study found that geographic spread of influenza is best explained by the amount of work-related travel between locations, tending toward later seasons in areas with less work-related travel, and that such a mechanism was consistent with the observed increase in synchrony in high-transmission seasons [16].

Planning models

Nonvaccine interventions for pandemics

Transmission dynamic models have been applied to many of the key public health decision and planning problems for pandemic influenza: detection of an emergent pandemic, feasibility of early containment, mitigation of a pandemic once it has become widespread, and the threat of antiviral resistance.

As a novel zoonotic strain of influenza infects humans, it may occasionally cause secondary transmission. A pandemic becomes possible if such secondary transmission occurs frequently enough to allow human-to-human transmission to sustain a growing epidemic, that is, if the effective reproductive number exceeds 1. Early sporadic clusters of transmission present an analytical challenge, because effective reproductive numbers below 1 can create

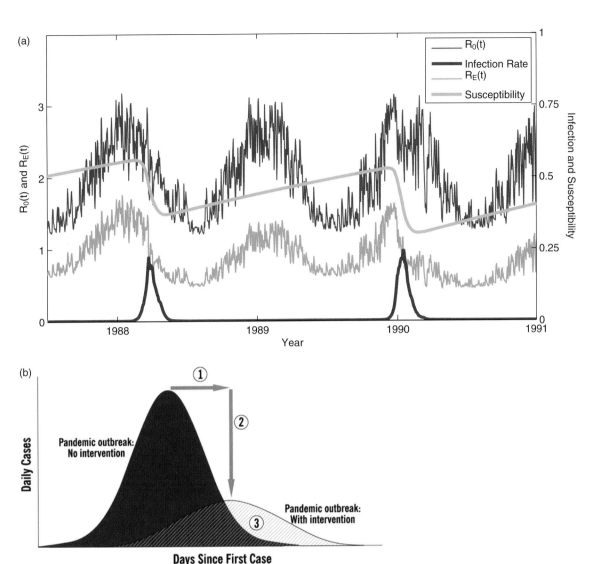

Figure 27.1. Transmission dynamic models. (a) Interplay between the availability of susceptible hosts (depleted during seasonal epidemics) and variation in the intrinsic transmissibility of influenza (R_0, jagged black curve), here modeled as a function of daily measured absolute humidity, determines the ability of influenza cases to spread (R_E, jagged gray curve). Seasonal epidemics (smooth black curve) start when conditions become sufficiently favorable to allow spread given the limited number of susceptible hosts ($R_E > 1$), and decline when depletion of susceptibles (smooth gray curve) and/or less favorable environmental conditions bring R_E below 1Reproduced from Shaman et al. [11] with permission from Oxford University Press. (b) Interventions during an influenza pandemic may delay the peak of the epidemic [1], reduce the peak demand on health services [2], and reduce the total number infected (3, the area under the incidence curve). Reproduced from US Department of Health and Human Services [83] with permission. (c) An early and important application of transmission dynamic ideas in the 2009 pandemic was to suggest that estimates of severity based on counting deaths and confirmed cases in Mexico were much higher than true severity. The approach was to estimate incidence of influenza in travelers who had gone to Mexico based on numbers of cases ascertained in the home countries of these travelers. Assuming comparable incidence in Mexicans and in foreign travelers to Mexico, the incidence in Mexico was estimated to be much higher than reported, indicating that severity was lower. Reprinted from Fraser et al. [34] with permission from American Association for the Advancement of Science.

(c)

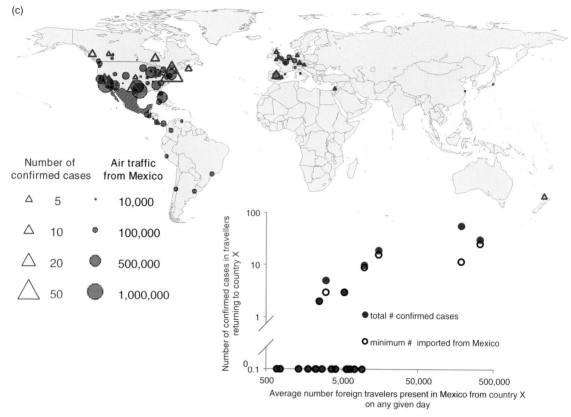

Figure 27.1. (*Continued*)

clusters of cases (though these will eventually die out), while conversely, it is possible for a strain with an effective reproductive number >1 to make sporadic, small clusters of human-to-human transmitted cases that die out by chance. Ferguson et al. [17] showed how the distribution of human-to-human cluster sizes could be used to make estimates of the effective reproductive number of an emerging strain, and emphasized that the sizes of the largest clusters, in particular, gives a better measure of the risk of pandemic emergence than the raw number of cases (which is a mix of animal-to-human and human-to-human transmission).

With growing concern about the possibility of a highly virulent pandemic with a strain like the A/H5N1 circulating in birds for the last decade, there has been significant policy and modeling attention to the possibility of containing such a pandemic at the source. The idea here is to detect the first self-sustaining human-to-human transmission early, while it is geographically limited, and to use mass antiviral treatment and prophylaxis to prevent its further spread. Two modeling studies, which used detailed accounts of the movement and possible transmission behavior in rural Thailand (then seen as a likely source for an H5N1 pandemic emergence), suggested that such an approach might be feasible if several conditions were met, including: the presence of adequate antiviral stockpiles; highly sensitive, timely and specific case detection and compliance with prophylaxis and/or treatment; sufficiently high coverage of cases with treatment and geographic regions around the cases with prophylaxis; and the good fortune to have the emergence event occur far enough from an urban center so that there was time to respond before the infection reached the city [3,7]. These models indicated that if the effective reproductive number at the point of emergence was below 1.6–1.8, source containment would be more likely to succeed, while if it was much larger than 2, source containment would fail in most scenarios. While there was much debate about whether the preconditions identified by these models would ever be met in practice, and a subsequent analysis noted the possibility of multiple introductions of human-to-human transmissible strains that would compound the challenge of containment [18], these models served the important function of quantifying the requirements for source containment to succeed. To improve the scientific basis of a debate that had relied mainly on opinion, these models suggested that there were specific quantities – population compliance, antiviral stockpile size, etc. – that should be considered in assessing the feasibility of source containment.

A few models assessed how well international border controls could do in delaying the global spread of pandemic influenza. These models universally suggest that the delay would be modest (order of 1–3 weeks) [4,19,20], mainly because even a 90% effective border control would be equivalent to delaying the introduction until the number of incoming cases was 10 times as high, a matter of a few weeks during an influenza pandemic [20].

Additional modeling efforts addressed the question of how pharmaceutical and nonpharmaceutical measures could be used to mitigate a pandemic once human-to-human transmission is widespread. Using agent-based models of the United States or part thereof, parameterized based on data on where individuals live, how far they travel for work and other purposes, and how much time they spend in various venues (school, work, home, and elsewhere), several groups attempted to quantify the impact of various interventions individually and together [4–6]. Common findings of these studies about interventions other than vaccination included:

• One or more interventions could measurably reduce the total size of the epidemic if the basic reproductive number were less than 1.8–2.0; beyond that range, interventions tended to have more modest effects unless many different ones were combined and sustained for a long period.

• The major challenge to the effectiveness of nonvaccine interventions by themselves is scale: by themselves, they can substantially reduce the overall epidemic size only if they can be sustained over a long period, requiring substantial social costs (e.g., keeping schools closed for months until a vaccine is ready) or unrealistically large supplies of antivirals (if used for prophylaxis and treatment).

• Despite these major barriers to the use of nonvaccine interventions to prevent an epidemic, they can be useful in delaying the peak (thus "buying time" for vaccine production), lowering the peak (thus reducing demand on stretched health services), and somewhat reducing the size of the epidemic (partly by reducing "epidemic overshoot" (Figure 27.1b) [21,22]). In some cases, these goals can be achieved by rather short-term interventions, such as closing schools near the peak of epidemic activity [4].

• Multiple interventions implemented together can have substantially greater effects than individual interventions.

• For interventions that can be sustained for a long period, early implementation (well before the illness attack rate hits 10%) of control measures dramatically improves their effectiveness, consistent with findings from historical studies of the 1918 pandemic in the United States [23,24].

Several details of the model predictions varied, and these variations could be traced to the differing assumptions of the different models. Subsequently, several models addressed how well widespread antiviral use could work, given the risk of resistance emerging and spreading under the unprecedented selection pressure provided by the level of use likely in a pandemic. These models suggest that – if the pandemic in a population is started by a drug-susceptible strain – substantial benefits can be achieved by treatment and prophylaxis even though resistance will begin to spread during the course of the epidemic in that population. This occurs because the susceptible strain will likely have a significant "head start," having infected many people before the resistant strain begins to increase to appreciable frequencies; not until the epidemic is near or past its peak is the fraction of resistant cases likely to be so high as to reduce the efficacy of continued antiviral use [22,25]. This impact could be extended by a policy of using a second drug, sequentially or in combination with the primary stockpiled drug, to postpone the appearance of resistance [26,27].

Vaccines for pandemic and seasonal influenza

In models, as in reality, vaccines merit special consideration, as they are the only control measure that can provide lasting protection against infection and transmission; other measures (nonpharmaceutical measures to reduce contact, and use of antiviral treatment and prophylaxis) have population-level effects only as long as they are in place. Indeed, perhaps the best way to think of most other interventions is as ways of "buying time" for the manufacture of a vaccine. In general, vaccines have two effects. They *directly* protect those who receive them, by reducing recipients' risk of infection and of illness. Also, by preventing infection or reducing infectiousness of those who are infected, they reduce transmission, thereby *indirectly* protecting others, even those who are not vaccinated.

In designing influenza vaccine strategy (seasonal or pandemic), there is a tradeoff between these two types of protection: children are typically the most important group for transmission, but in both seasonal and pandemic influenza, children over 2 years of age are at quite low risk for severe outcomes. High risk groups for severe outcomes, such as adults (pandemics), the elderly (seasonal influenza), and individuals with particular underlying conditions, may not have such an important role in transmission. Thus, a direct protection strategy may favor vaccinating those at high risk, while an indirect protection strategy favors vaccinating the major transmitters, typically school-age children. Only in the case of having enough vaccine to bring the reproductive number below 1 (stop the growth of the epidemic) is the same strategy beneficial for both objectives [28].

Models have helped to clarify how the choice of strategy may best be made. The key point is that when transmissibility is low, vaccine supply is plentiful, and vaccines are available early in the epidemic, it is beneficial to concentrate on indirect protection, because adequate vaccines can be delivered to strongly depress transmission and efficiently protect those at highest risk. When vaccine availability is limited, or delayed, focus on the high-risk groups is more practical because modest reductions in transmission from focusing on children will offer little protection to the high-risk individuals [29]. A nonmodeling considera-

tion is that, of course, vaccinating the high-risk group can work only if the vaccine is effective in this group, a premise that has been questioned in the case of seasonal influenza and the elderly [30]. With detailed knowledge of who transmits to whom, finer optimization of vaccine targeting can be achieved [31,32]. Since such detailed data are not always available for emerging diseases, a method has been developed by which the best group to vaccinate to achieve *indirect* benefits (reduced transmission) can be identified as that with the highest incidence rate; this group is typically children early in a pandemic, but incidence becomes flatter across age groups as the pandemic progresses, depleting the supply of susceptible children [33].

Real-time and retrospective use of models during a pandemic

Given the model-based predictions described above that intervention effectiveness will depend strongly on the value of the reproductive number, an obvious priority in the early phases of a new pandemic is to estimate this quantity. The first estimates of the reproductive number for the 2009 pandemic were obtained by fitting a transmission dynamic model to an outbreak of a respiratory virus in La Gloria, Mexico, and confirmed by independent estimates based on coalescent methods applied to genome sequences [34] (see below), and by other methods based on epidemic curves; all methods gave point estimates in the range 1.2–1.6. An analysis of the US Centers of Disease Control and prevention (CDC) line list, which obtained reproductive number estimates around 1.7–1.8, emphasized that such estimates are highly sensitive to changes in reporting and other statistical artifacts; efforts to correct such artifacts can change the estimates by 30% or more. Given the imperfect nature of such corrections and the inevitable changes in reporting that will occur in the early stages of a pandemic, the authors concluded that such estimates must be interpreted cautiously. Specifically, the uncertainty surrounding such estimates is more than the statistical uncertainty expressed by confidence bounds; it also should include uncertainty about the assumptions (e.g., about changing case reporting) that go into the estimate [35]. The consistency of most estimates across settings reinforces the approximate accuracy of the earliest estimates, though some variation by geography and time (due to seasonality) is expected. As the pandemic progressed, changes in the estimates of $R(t)$ were used to examine the impact of particular interventions, notably school closure, on transmission [36].

Another key quantity of interest to decision makers in a pandemic is severity, most simply measured by the case:fatality ratio, the probability that infection results in death. While not itself a topic for transmission dynamic modeling, accurate estimation of this ratio depends on estimating both numerator (deaths) and denominator (cases) accurately. The early assessment of the 2009 pandemic borrowed ideas from transmission modeling to estimate the "force of infection" in Mexico based on that experienced by travelers to the United States, Spain, and other countries (in whom milder cases were more readily ascertained), and suggested that the number of symptomatic cases in Mexico must have been considerably higher than the number reported. This provided some reassurance that early estimates of severity (case fatality ratios of up to several per cent) were overstated, because they were based on under-reported denominators (Figure 27.1c) [34]. Later, detailed fits of transmission dynamic models to data on serologic evidence of infection, as well as reported cases of influenza-like illness, were used to estimate severity with greater precision in Hong Kong [37] and elsewhere, reinforcing that severity was indeed lower than initially feared.

Unprecedented efforts were made during the 2009 pandemic to fit models to data in real time for "nowcasting" (estimation of the current state of the epidemic, including cumulative number infected by age) and forecasting of its future course and the possible impact of vaccination. Because of the computational demands of agent-based models and the large number of parameters required for such models, these types of models were little used for real-time investigations; more common was the fitting of age-structured, differential-equation based models to data. The remarkably fast work of several groups (including [38,39]) showed that such models could be fit in real time, but emphasized that when fitting to time series on case reporting (e.g., influenza-like illness consultations), a major uncertainty was the appropriate, population- and age-specific "multiplier" to determine how many infections were represented by each reported case. Without knowing such

a multiplier, forecasting is difficult because the dynamics of the epidemic depend on the number of susceptible people remaining. Once the epidemic peaks, the multiplier can be estimated from the fit of the model, but this may be too late for many forecasting purposes [38,39]. Modelers have called for ongoing serosurveillance to facilitate estimates of the numbers infected [40] in real time.

Antigenic analyses

The antigenic variation of influenza viruses is the reason why the viruses can reinfect humans multiple times during their lifetimes, why vaccinating both humans and birds against avian H5 influenza virus is difficult, and what necessitates the enormous worldwide effort to track the evolution of influenza viruses so as to repeatedly update the strains in the influenza virus vaccines to track the latest variants. Thus, antigenic variation is a root cause of the substantial public and animal health burden of influenza, and also one of the things that makes influenza so fascinating from a scientific perspective.

Antigenic differences among influenza viruses are routinely measured using the hemagglutination inhibition (HAI) assay. The HAI assay is a binding assay based on the ability of hemagglutinin (HA), a surface glycoprotein of the influenza virus, to agglutinate red blood cells, and the complementary ability of antisera raised against the same or related strains to block this agglutination [41]. Thus, an HAI titer gives information about the affinity of an antiserum for a virus strain.

Tables of HAI data, comprising titers of multiple antigens measured against multiple sera, are notoriously difficult to interpret quantitatively due to paradoxes and irregularities in the data. Difficulties include some antisera being able to see differences between two antigens while other antisera cannot, and heterologous titers sometimes being higher than homologous titers. Consequently, the accuracy of HAI data was thought to be such that only a fourfold difference in titer was considered reliable.

Despite these difficulties, the vaccine strain selection process for the influenza virus vaccine has been an effective process for many years. However, to address scientific questions that require a quantitative measure of antigenic difference, a higher resolution

441

than a fourfold dilution in titer, to potentially optimize vaccine strain selection, and to be free from the uncertainties associated with the paradoxes in the tables of HAI data, there has been a substantial need for an understanding of the paradoxes of binding assay data in general, and HAI data in particular.

Early methods to analyze antigenic data quantitatively [42–44] have mostly been based on the methods of, or equivalent to, numerical taxonomy [45]. However, these methods do not have an accurate way to interpret data below the sensitivity threshold of the assay, they approximate antigenic distances in indirect ways, and perhaps most importantly, do not resolve the paradoxes and irregularities of HAI data mentioned above and are thus sensitive to the problems of these paradoxes.

Antigenic cartography is a direct way to interpret HAI data, resolves the paradoxes in HAI data, and correctly handles data below the sensitivity of the assay [46,47]. Antigenic cartography uses mathematical, computational, and statistical techniques to create a geometric representation binding assay data. Thus, in the case of influenza, cartography allows HAI titers to be used to construct "antigenic maps." These maps provide a spatial layout of antigens and antisera, with distances and direction among the antigens and antisera representing antigenic differences. Such maps give a visualization of the underlying data and, more importantly, they provide a concrete mathematical foundation for the quantitative analysis of antigenic data.

In an antigenic map, the distance between antiserum point S and antigen point A corresponds to the difference between the $\log_2$ of the maximum titer observed for antiserum S against any antigen and the $\log_2$ of the titer for antiserum S against antigen A. Each titer in an HAI table can thus be thought of as specifying a target distance for the points in an antigenic map. Modified multi-dimensional scaling methods [48] are used to arrange the antigen and antiserum points in an antigenic map to best satisfy the target distances specified by the HAI data. Because antisera are tested against multiple antigens, and antigens are tested against multiple antisera, many measurements can be used to determine the position of the antigen and antiserum points. Thus, points in the map can be triangulated more accurately than the accuracy of a single HAI measurement, and the maps can have increased resolution compared to the raw HAI data.

Because of this direct relationship between each HAI titer and a distance in the antigenic map, the accuracy of the map can be tested by measuring the difference between table and map distances, and furthermore the underlying model and its assumptions, tested by cross-validation tests in which maps are made from a subset of the tabular data and the left-out data predicted from the resulting antigenic map, and by blind prediction experiments in which maps are made from data in which some titers have never been measured, those titers predicted from the maps, and then measured in the laboratory. Cross-validation and blind prediction experiments show that with well-triangulated data, the accuracy of the data is on average 0.8 of a twofold difference in HAI titer. Importantly, the accuracy of such predictions is the same for both nonparadoxical titers and titers that were previously considered paradoxical such as higher than homologous titers.

Antigenic maps can be constructed in any number of dimensions; for example, in one, two, or three dimensions, and higher dimensions. Surprisingly, the HAI data for human influenza A(H3N2) viruses allow accurate placement of strains and antisera in 2D – thus, substantially facilitating the analyses of such data.

Antigenic cartography is not specific to the HAI assay, it is applicable to any binding assay data. Within influenza they have also been used to show the evolution of a CTL epitope [49], and the discordant antigenic drift of the HA and neuraminidase (NA) [50]. Here, however, we focus on the antigenic evolution of the HA.

Figure 27.2(a) shows an antigenic map of 35 years of antigenic evolution of influenza A (H3N2) virus, from its emergence in humans in 1968 until 2003. Virus strains are shown as colored shapes, and antisera as open shapes. The map reveals both high-level and detailed features of the antigenic evolution of the virus. The strains tend to group in clusters, like an archipelago of islands, rather than forming a continuous antigenic lineage. Within most clusters there is little antigenic evolution, with strains from each season scattered throughout the cluster, until there are jumps to the next antigenic cluster – the antigenic evolution proceeding in this punctuated fashion from cluster to cluster. Each cluster is approximately the same size, and the distances between clusters are large enough to warrant an update of the strain used in the

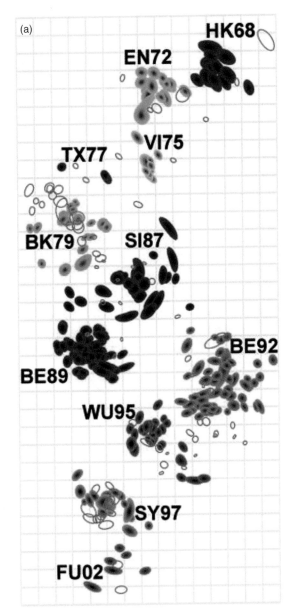

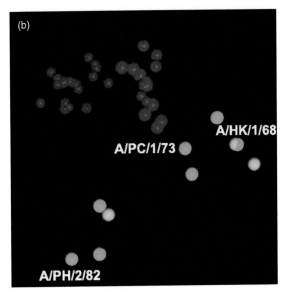

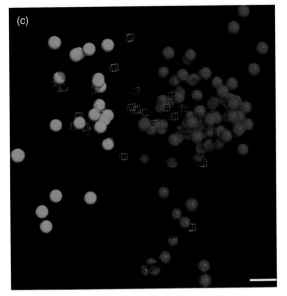

Figure 27.2. (a) Two-dimensional antigenic map of human influenza A (H3N2) virus from 1968 to 2003. The relative positions of strains (colored shapes) and antisera (uncolored open shapes) were adjusted such that the distances between strains and antisera in the map represent corresponding hemagglutination inhibition (HAI) measurements with the least error. Strain color represents the antigenic cluster to which the strain belongs. The name of each cluster indicates the first vaccine strain in the cluster. The vertical and horizontal axes both represent antigenic distance, and, because only the relative positions of antigens and antisera can be determined, the orientation of the map within these axes is free. The spacing between grid lines is 1 unit of antigenic distance – corresponding to a twofold dilution of antiserum in the HAI assay. Source: Smith et al. [46] , with permission from AAAS. (b) Three-dimensional antigenic map of swine influenza A (H3N2) virus from 1984 to 1999. Swine strains from 1984 are blue, from 1999 are red, and the in-between years on a color scale between blue and red. Green strains are human viruses. Yellow strains swine strains not of the PC/1/73 lineage. The antisera are not shown. Source: de Jong et al. [51] (c) American Society of Microbiology. (c) Three-dimensional antigenic map of equine influenza A (H3N8) influenza viruses from 1968 to 2007. Strain color represents the antigenic cluster to which the strain belongs. Scale bar represents 1 unit of antigenic distance. Source: Lewis et al. [54] (c) American Society of Microbiology.

vaccine. The rate of antigenic evolution has been approximately the same throughout the 35 years of H3 evolution shown. The antigenic evolution of the other seasonal human influenza viruses, A (H1N1), B-Victoria, and B-Yamagata, is similarly clustered, with clusters size and cluster gaps approximately the same as those for A (H3N2).

The order of clusters is mostly chronological, from the original Hong Kong 1968 cluster to the Fujian 2002 cluster – indeed, order of the clusters is somewhat one-dimensional, but with some two-dimensional structure. The low dimensionality of this map is a surprise given the complexity of the virus, and indicates that the virus is under strong selection pressure to evolve away from prior immunity. The null model for escaping immunity most efficiently is evolution in straight line – in one dimension. The two-dimensional structure of the map, together with some repeated amino acid substitutions after evolutionary dead ends [46], suggests that there are constraints on the evolution. The existence of strong selection pressure, constraints, and a surprisingly simple structure to the antigenic evolution, raise the possibility that this evolution might be predictable.

Though the antigenic evolution of influenza A (H3N2) virus is clustered, the genetic evolution of the virus is gradual and continuous, suggesting that most amino acid substitutions have little antigenic effect. Analyses of the amino acid substitutions that define antigenic clusters indicate that a minority of amino acid substitutions contribute disproportionately to antigenic change [46].

Figure 27.2b shows the antigenic evolution of swine A (H3N2) influenza viruses in Europe from 1984 to 1999 [51]. In contrast to the antigenic evolution of influenza viruses in humans, the antigenic evolution in swine is substantially slower [51–53]. However, the genetic evolution of swine and human A (H3N2) viruses are very similar, both in terms of the rate of fixation of nucleotide and amino acid substitutions, and the structure of the phylogenetic trees [51]. Thus, compared with human A (H3N2) viruses, swine A (H3N2) influenza viruses have accumulated many more nucleotide and amino acid substitutions in HA1 that had little effect on the antigenic properties of the virus.

The substantial difference between the antigenic evolution of influenza viruses in swine and humans is likely because the majority of swine are slaughtered at 6–9 months of age, thus the driving force of antigenic drift of influenza viruses in humans – escaping immunity – is substantially less in the swine population. The human virus requires antigenic change to ensure a sufficiently large pool of immunologically susceptible hosts, whereas the susceptible swine population is continuously renewed, thus limiting the build-up of immune pressure and consequently putting less selective pressure on swine influenza viruses to evolve antigenically.

In birds there has been limited antigenic evolution from the first isolations of avian influenza viruses in the 1950s through to the present, apart from the A (H5N1) viruses since 1997 in which there been a similar amount of antigenic evolution as has been seen in the human A (H3N2) viruses over the same period. This antigenic evolution of the recent A (H5N1) viruses is potentially due to immune selection pressure introduced by large-scale vaccination of poultry. The size of antigenic clusters, and the gaps among clusters, is similar to that in humans, but clusters are spread out in two dimensions, rather than the mostly sequential ordering of the human virus antigenic clusters, and the clusters circulate concurrently, mostly in separate geographic locations.

The antigenic evolution of influenza viruses in horses from 1968 to 2007 is shown in Figure 27.2(c) [54]. The antigenic clusters and antigenic distance of gaps between clusters is approximately the same size as those of human influenza viruses. Also similarly to human influenza viruses there is continuous genetic evolution, little antigenic evolution within most clusters, and punctuated jumps to new antigenic clusters. These antigenic jumps are mediated by single amino acid substitutions, indicating, as with humans, that most amino acid substitutions have little antigenic effect, and that only a small number have a large, and epidemiologically significant antigenic effect [54]. Similarly to A (H5N1) viruses in birds, and in contrast to A (H3N2) in the human influenza viruses, multiple antigenic clusters circulate concomitantly. In contrast to the situation in birds, however, viruses from different antigenic clusters co-circulate in the same region.

It is remarkable that the antigenic evolution of influenza viruses has common features such as the size of clusters and gaps between clusters across substantially different host species. Despite these similarities, there are substantial differences of epidemiologic significance such as the rate of antigenic evolution and thus the number of clusters over a period of time, the relative positions of these clusters with respect to each other, and whether new clusters replace old ones or whether they co-circulate.

Genetic and evolutionary models

The analysis of phylogenetic data is pervasive across much of biology and virology, and is increasingly ubiquitous and important as sequencing becomes faster and cheaper [55]. Phylogenetic analyses are deeply rooted in theory, and there is a large community of scientists who continue to develop and extend the methods. Today phylogeny is much more than making a tree to visualize similarity and determine ancestry. Phylogenetic reconstruction and analysis of the sequences within a phylogenetic framework permits researchers to estimate the timing of lineage divergence, determine rates of evolution, estimate the geographic spread of particular influenza lineages and the rates of growth of these lineages, identify sites within the genome that are subject to positive or negative selection, compare selective pressures across genes, and detect reassortment events. Here we provide an overview of these methods and some of the findings that have resulted from their application to the study of influenza viruses.

Because of the importance of the HA in the antigenic evolution of influenza viruses, and that influenza vaccination is directed at raising antibodies to the HA protein, it is the antigenic domain of the HA, the HA1, that has been sequenced most extensively to date. The phylogenetic tree of the HA1 of human influenza viruses has a distinctive ladder-like appearance, indicating the sequential accumulation of substitutions along the trunk of the tree, together with relatively short branches off the trunk. Epidemiologically, this indicates high rates of strain turnover (replacement) on a global scale, such that each of the short branches has a relatively short life of several years. Surveillance has now reached a density such that there are usually multiple strains on the trunk of the tree, and at the nodes of the internal branches. This level of coverage enables a mostly straightforward accurate visual interpretation of relationships and ancestry, and the sort of detailed further analyses described below.

Genetic analyses of all eight gene segments indicate that there is substantial reassortment of gene segments, over both short and long timescales. Over short timescales, a combination of surveillance data [56] and full-genome sequencing and analysis projects [57,58] have shown that there are a substantial number of reassortment events, both within HA antigenic clusters of A/H3N2 viruses and associated with A/H3N2 virus HA antigenic cluster transitions. It is yet to be determined whether the reassortments are the cause of cluster transitions, hitchhike (facilitated by the evolutionary bottleneck) along with the transition, or are compensatory after a cluster transition. Nevertheless, it is clear that intrapandemic reassortment can result in changes of various properties of the virus including its pathogenicity [59].

Over longer timescales, influenza pandemics are caused by the circulation of a new HA in humans. Such pandemic events also typically result from the reassortment of other segments between human and animal viruses. For example, the provenance of the segments of the 2009 swine-origin human influenza pandemic [52,60] illustrated in Figure 27.3(a) shows substantial reassortment and persistence of segments over multiple years and species.

Though surveillance of influenza viruses in swine has been substantially less than that in humans, the coverage was substantial enough such that, within days of the detection of the first cases of the 2009 human influenza pandemic in the United States, a straightforward interpretation of the combined all-species phylogenetic trees for each gene segment allowed the determination of the gene segment constellation of the human 2009 pandemic, the swine-origin of the virus, and a detailed genetic analysis of the early isolates [52,60].

The use of coalescent theory to estimate the timing of the most recent common ancestor (MRCA) of a lineage of strains is an increasingly powerful method of genetic analysis [61]. The MRCA is dated as the time at which the earliest branching point within a lineage occurs in a phylogenetic tree. An effective way to visualize these results is a tree format in which branch length represents time. In such a tree, the horizontal axis thus represents time, and the timing of branch points is directly interpretable, together with confidence intervals on the estimates.

MRCA analysis was put to rapid use during the early weeks of the 2009 influenza pandemic to

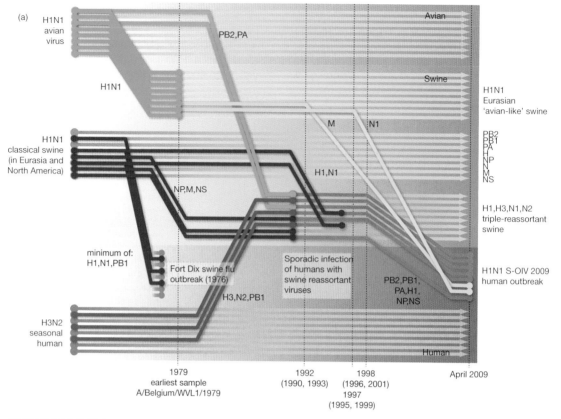

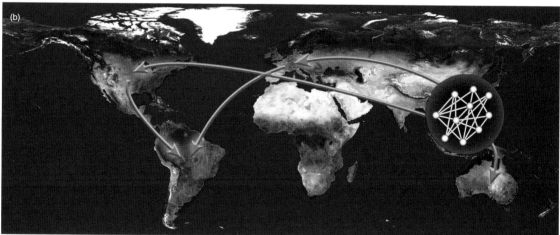

Figure 27.3. (a) Reassortment events leading up to the emergence of the 2009 pandemic influenza virus. Shaded boxes represent host species; avian (green), swine (red), and human (blue). Colored lines represent interspecies transmission pathways of influenza genes. The eight genomic segments are represented as parallel lines in descending order of size. Dates marked with dashed vertical lines on "elbows" indicate the mean time of divergence of the 2009 pandemic virus from corresponding virus lineages.

Reassortment events not involved with the emergence of human disease are omitted. The first triple-reassortment swine viruses were detected in 1998, but to improve clarity the origin of this lineage is placed earlier. Reproduced from Smith et al. [60] with permission from Nature Publishing Group. (b) Schematic of the dominant seeding hierarchy of seasonal influenza A (H3N2) viruses. The structure of the network within East–South-East Asia is unknown. Source: Russell et al. [68].

estimate the time when the virus first started circulating in humans by inferring the date of the most recent common ancestor of the swine and human viruses. The MRCA analysis dated the emergence in humans to be several months before the recognition of the outbreak [60]. Related analyses were done on the 1918 pandemic, potentially showing that the constellation of gene segments that led to the emergence in humans in 1918 had likely been coming together in swine over many years [62]. However, because there is only a small number of sequences on which these inferences can be made, the confidence intervals on the dates are substantially larger than for analyses of modern events such as the 2009 pandemic, and passage history issues might also confound such analyses.

Coalescent-based methods can be used to estimate the exponential growth rate of the virus population early in an epidemic; with assumptions, this growth rate can be converted into an estimate of R, the effective reproductive number in the early part of the epidemic. In the 2009 pandemic, this method gave results similar to the lower end of estimates using more classic epidemiologic methods [34]. A number of technical issues remain to be resolved with this specialized application, which should improve the accuracy of the estimates obtained.

Phylodynamics is the combined study of evolutionary genetics and epidemiology [63], and coalescent-based and other phylogenetic methods provide a powerful toolkit for such analyses across multiple pathogens, including influenza. Such work has shown how different influenza gene segments are more or less associated with each other during interpandemic periods, and the how the genetic diversity, and thus effective population size, changes during the evolution [64]. Related work combing genetic and epidemiologic models is beginning to address questions about the evolutionary dynamics of seasonal influenza viruses such as the role of neutral networks [65], and other mechanisms that inhibit the branching of the genetic evolution and that would give the ladder-like structure of the HA phylogenetic tree such as short-term broadly acting immunity being the only mechanism that gave such a structure in the model [66].

Global migration

The depth and mostly global nature of the sampling to date has in addition made it possible to carry out detailed investigations of the global migration of human A (H3N2) viruses. A major step on the global migration work came from the analysis of full genome data from New York State [67], from which it was determined that influenza A (H3N2) viruses do not persist locally from year to year, but that there are multiple seeding events each influenza season. Subsequently it was determined that these viruses are sourced from one region of the world and spread to other regions each season [64,68], and that this source region is most often East–South-East Asia (Figure 27.3b) [68]. Even in the source East–South-East Asian region, the viruses do not persist in any single population from season to season, but instead persist as a metapopulation by passing from country to country in a circulation network – a process enabled by the substantial travel among the countries in the region and by the countries having their influenza seasons at different times of the year (often associated with rainy seasons), meaning there can always be an influenza epidemic going on in one country in the region at any time of the year.

The increased sampling, and increasing global coverage, the increasing speed and reduction of the cost of sequencing, deep-sequencing technology to now sequence beyond consensus [69], and the continued development of phylogenetic techniques are such that we expect substantial further increases in knowledge, and utility for public and animal health, in the years to come.

Computational structural analyses

The crystallization of the influenza HA [70] and NA [71] were tremendously important events in influenza virology, and together with more than 100 further HA and NA crystal structures have led to important wide-ranging insights including the structural basis of receptor binding, antigenic variation, virus neutralization, fusion, and antiviral design, mechanism, and escape.

Because of the importance of understanding the structural basis of many aspects of influenza virology there is a need for even more structures to be able to address, for example, questions related to the underlying mechanisms that govern the evolution of seasonal influenza viruses and the receptor binding changes as pandemic-potential viruses continue to evolve. One approach is the continued improvement of the generation and resolution of crystal structures. Another complementary approach is the prediction of derivative structures, from related crystal structures by computational methods. Advances in such computational methods are resulting in increased impact in many areas of biology, including a molecular basis of Gaucher's disease [72], drug targets against *Trypanosoma brucei* [73], and determining the structure of Mason–Pfizer monkey virus [74].

Two widely used computational methods are comparative modeling [75] and molecular dynamics [76]. Comparative modeling is based on the concept of homology (proteins that are evolutionarily related) and the observation that many changes in the sequence of a protein cause only a small change in the structure of the folded protein. Therefore, if there is a protein with a known crystal structure, amino acid substitutions are placed into it and, using the physics of biomolecules, the structure of the mutated protein is relaxed into a predicted structure for the protein. Molecular dynamics uses the same process but in addition to the physical forces that relax the model in comparative modeling Newton's equations of motion are iteratively solved, incorporating both time and heat components. These simulations allow for movement and the flexibility of the protein to be modeled. Such dynamics simulations have great potential, if accurate, for systems in which the dynamics of molecular interactions are important.

Much of the effort of computational structural biology in influenza has been directed to the HA and NA proteins. These molecules, though large, are tantalizingly tractable for computational modeling because of the availability of excellent crystal structures from which to build, and because of the small number of insertions and deletions in their genomes which simplifies the comparative modeling step and improves accuracy. Here we describe two examples of computational analyses whose predictions have been confirmed by experimental work.

Fleishman et al. [77] set out to design proteins targeting the conserved stem of influenza HA. Their computational protein design strategy first docked individual amino acids on to the surface of the stem region of HA. They identified three "hot-spots" that were able to form high affinity interactions which were complementary to the surface of HA. Initial protein scaffolds were then identified by searching a database of protein structures for peptides that were able to maintain the position of either two or three of the disembodied hot-spot residues and were complementary in shape to the stem region. A total of 51 peptides containing two of the hot-spots and 37 containing all three were selected for further verification. These peptides were synthesized, expressed in yeast, and the binding HA was measured by flow cytometry. Two designs showed reproducible binding activity toward the HA stem region, albeit with low to medium Kd values (200 and 5000 nM). An experimental affinity maturation process using error prone polymerase chain reaction (PCR) was then used in an attempt to improve the affinity of these designs. The resulting proteins bound HA with low nanomolar affinity (3 and 4 nM, respectively). The binding surface of one design that was subsequently crystallized in complex with HA was nearly identical to that predicted by the computational design model.

Genetic analyses of the viruses in the first cases of the 2009 influenza pandemic revealed that the DG222 substitution in HA might induce a highly pathogenic phenotype as some fatal cases had this substitution (it later found that there was no strong association). This same substitution had also been observed in the alteration of the binding profile of the 1918 pandemic [78] and thus potentially contributing to the highly pathogenic phenotype. At this stage of the pandemic, no 2009 strain crystal structure was available, and thus, to determine the effect of this substitution on receptor binding in the 2009 pandemic strains, comparative models were built from the crystal structure of a 1918 strain followed by molecular dynamics simulations. The models agreed with the glycan array analysis by Stevens et al. [78] that DG222 would substantially reduce binding to 2,6-linked glycans by the 1918 virus, but predicted, contrary to expectation, that DG222 would have little effect on the binding to 2,6-linked glycans by the 2009 virus. The predicted mechanism for this stability was specific amino acids forming a network of interactions in the protein and with the ligand [79]. Despite the 72 amino acids difference between the HA of the 1918 and 2009 viruses, 10 of which are close to the receptor binding site, the computational predictions proved to be accurate: both the prediction of maintenance of 2,6-binding of the 2009 virus matched carbohydrate microarray analyses [80] and glycan arrays [81], and the predicted network of interactions was confirmed in the crystal structure [82].

Today, computational structural biology can give accurate results for some questions, but is not yet broadly and routinely accurate, and the results must be particularly carefully examined before use. Further understanding of the physics and statistics of biomolecules, such as the treatment of solvent, quantum effects, and entropy, together with advances in computer processing power, will undoubtedly improve the accuracy of computational structural biology over time. At some point, it is difficult to predict when, computational methods will be able to routinely predict highly accurate structures from somewhat homologous crystals, and be able to determine the dynamics of those structures. At this point, such computational methods will provide a broadly powerful complement to existing crystallization methods of the type we are beginning to see the first signs of today.

Conclusions

We have described the application of quantitative modeling to key questions across a wide range of influenza research and public health. Such models have had substantial impact on scientific understanding, on the evidence base for decision making about pandemic preparedness and response, and on vaccine strain selection. Increasing availability of genomic sequence data, antigenic data, and, in some cases, population-based serologic data will be essential raw materials for the next generation of models, which in turn will rely on newly developed quantitative techniques, some still in their early stages, for integrating these forms of data into analyses. Careful attention to the source, interpretation, and limitations of input data, assumptions of the model, and interpretation of the results – together with collaborative, multidisciplinary teams including virologists, immunologists, computational and mathematical modelers, and classic epidemiologists – are often the hallmark of the most useful models.

References

1. Elveback LR, Fox JP, Ackerman E, Langworthy A, Boyd M, Gatewood L. An influenza simulation model for immunization studies. Am J Epidemiol. 1976;103(2): 152–65.

2. Rvachev L, Longini IM Jr. A mathematical model for the global spread of influenza. Math Biosci. 1985;75: 3–22.

3. Ferguson NM, Cummings DA, Cauchemez S, Fraser C, Riley S, Meeyai A, et al. Strategies for containing an emerging influenza pandemic in Southeast Asia. Nature. 2005;437:209–14.

4. Ferguson NM, Cummings DA, Fraser C, Cajka JC, Cooley PC, Burke DS. Strategies for mitigating an influenza pandemic. Nature. 2006;442(7101):448–52.

5. Germann TC, Kadau K, Longini IM Jr, Macken CA. Mitigation strategies for pandemic influenza in the United States. Proc Natl Acad Sci U S A. 2006;103(15): 5935–40.

6. Halloran ME, Ferguson NM, Eubank S, Longini IM Jr, Cummings DA, Lewis B, et al. Modeling targeted layered containment of an influenza pandemic in the United States. Proc Natl Acad Sci U S A. 2008;105(12): 4639–44.

7. Longini IM Jr, Nizam A, Xu S, Ungchusak K, Hanshaoworakul W, Cummings DA, et al. Containing pandemic influenza at the source. Science. 2005;309(5737): 1083–7.

8. Yang Y, Sugimoto JD, Halloran ME, Basta NE, Chao DL, Matrajt L, et al. The transmissibility and control of pandemic influenza A (H1N1) virus. Science. 2009;326 (5953):729–33.

9. Mills CE, Robins JM, Lipsitch M. Transmissibility of 1918 pandemic influenza. Nature. 2004;432(7019): 904–6.

10. Cauchemez S, Valleron AJ, Boelle PY, Flahault A, Ferguson NM. Estimating the impact of school closure on influenza transmission from Sentinel data. Nature. 2008;452(7188):750–4.

11. Shaman J, Goldstein E, Lipsitch M. Absolute humdity and pandemic versus epidemic influenza. Am J Epidemiol. 2011;173:127–35.

12. Shaman J, Kohn M. Absolute humidity modulates influenza survival, transmission and seasonality. Proc Natl Acad Sci U S A. 2009;106:3243–8.

13. Shaman J, Pitzer VE, Viboud C, Grenfell BT, Lipsitch M. Absolute humidity and the seasonal onset of influenza in the continental United States. PLoS Biol. 2010; 8(2):e1000316.

14. Shaman J, Jeon CY, Giovannucci E, Lipsitch M. Shortcomings of vitamin D-based model simulations of seasonal influenza. PLoS ONE. 2011;6(6):e20743.

15. Viboud C, Alonso WJ, Simonsen L. Influenza in tropical regions. PLoS Med. 2006;3(4):e89.

16. Viboud C, Bjornstad ON, Smith DL, Simonsen L, Miller MA, Grenfell BT. Synchrony, waves, and spatial

hierarchies in the spread of influenza. Science. 2006;312 (5772):447–51.

17. Ferguson NM, Fraser C, Donnelly CA, Ghani AC, Anderson RM. Public health. Public health risk from the avian H5N1 influenza epidemic. Science. 2004;304 (5673):968–9.

18. Mills CE, Robins JM, Bergstrom CT, Lipsitch M. Pandemic Influenza: risk of Multiple Introductions and the Need to Prepare for Them. PLoS Med. 2006;3(6):e135.

19. Cooper BS, Pitman RJ, Edmunds WJ, Gay NJ. Delaying the international spread of pandemic influenza. PLoS Med. 2006;3(6):e212.

20. Scalia Tomba G, Wallinga J. A simple explanation for the low impact of border control as a countermeasure to the spread of an infectious disease. Math Biosci. 2008;214(1–2):70–2.

21. Handel A, Longini IM Jr, Antia R. What is the best control strategy for multiple infectious disease outbreaks? Proc Biol Sci. 2007;274(1611):833–7.

22. Lipsitch M, Cohen T, Murray M, Levin BR. Antiviral resistance and the control of pandemic influenza. PLoS Med. 2007;4(1):e15.

23. Bootsma MC, Ferguson NM. The effect of public health measures on the 1918 influenza pandemic in U.S. cities. Proc Natl Acad Sci U S A. 2007;104(18):7588–93.

24. Hatchett RJ, Mecher CE, Lipsitch M. Public health interventions and epidemic intensity during the 1918 influenza pandemic. Proc Natl Acad Sci U S A. 2007;104(18):7582–7.

25. Handel A, Longini IM Jr, Antia R. Antiviral resistance and the control of pandemic influenza: the roles of stochasticity, evolution and model details. J Theor Biol. 2009;256(1):117–25.

26. McCaw JM, Wood JG, McCaw CT, McVernon J. Impact of emerging antiviral drug resistance on influenza containment and spread: influence of subclinical infection and strategic use of a stockpile containing one or two drugs. PLoS ONE. 2008;3(6):e2362.

27. Wu JT, Leung GM, Lipsitch M, Cooper BS, Riley S. Hedging against antiviral resistance during the next influenza pandemic using small stockpiles of an alternative chemotherapy. PLoS Med. 2009;6(5):e1000085.

28. Medlock J, Galvani AP. Optimizing influenza vaccine distribution. Science. 2009;325(5948):1705–8.

29. Dushoff J, Plotkin JB, Viboud C, Simonsen L, Miller M, Loeb M, et al. Vaccinating to protect a vulnerable subpopulation. PLoS Med. 2007;4(5):e174.

30. Simonsen L, Taylor RJ, Viboud C, Miller MA, Jackson LA. Mortality benefits of influenza vaccination in elderly people: an ongoing controversy. Lancet Infect Dis. 2007;7(10):658–66.

31. Goldstein E, Apolloni A, Lewis B, Miller JC, Macauley M, Eubank S, et al. Distribution of vaccine/antivirals and the "least spread line" in a stratified population. J R Soc Interface. 2010;7(46):755–64.

32. Patel R, Longini IM Jr, Halloran ME. Finding optimal vaccination strategies for pandemic influenza using genetic algorithms. J Theor Biol. 2005;234(2):201–12.

33. Wallinga J, van Boven M, Lipsitch M. Optimizing infectious disease interventions during an emerging epidemic. Proc Natl Acad Sci U S A. 2010;107(2):923–8.

34. Fraser C, Donnelly CA, Cauchemez S, Hanage WP, Van Kerkhove MD, Hollingsworth TD, et al. Pandemic potential of a strain of influenza A (H1N1): early findings. Science. 2009;324(5934):1557–61.

35. White LF, Wallinga J, Finelli L, Reed C, Riley S, Lipsitch M, et al. Estimation of the reproductive number and the serial interval in early phase of the 2009 influenza A/H1N1 pandemic in the USA. Influenza Other Respi Viruses. 2009;3(6):267–76.

36. Wu JT, Cowling BJ, Lau EH, Ip DK, Ho LM, Tsang T, et al. School closure and mitigation of pandemic (H1N1) 2009, Hong Kong. Emerg Infect Dis. 2010;16(3):538–41.

37. Wu JT, Ma ES, Lee CK, Chu DK, Ho PL, Shen AL, et al. The infection attack rate and severity of 2009 pandemic H1N1 influenza in Hong Kong. Clin Infect Dis. 2010;51(10):1184–91.

38. Baguelin M, Hoek AJ, Jit M, Flasche S, White PJ, Edmunds WJ. Vaccination against pandemic influenza A/H1N1v in England: a real-time economic evaluation. Vaccine. 2010;28(12):2370–84.

39. Ong JB, Chen MI, Cook AR, Lee HC, Lee VJ, Lin RT, et al. Real-time epidemic monitoring and forecasting of H1N1-2009 using influenza-like illness from general practice and family doctor clinics in Singapore. PLoS ONE. 2010;5(4):e10036.

40. Van Kerkhove MD, Asikainen T, Becker NG, Bjorge S, Desenclos JC, dos Santos T, et al. Studies needed to address public health challenges of the 2009 H1N1 influenza pandemic: insights from modeling. PLoS Med. 2010;7(6):e1000275.

41. Hirst GK. Studies of antigenic differences among strains of influenza a by means of red cell agglutination. J Exp Med. 1943;78(5):407–23.

42. Weijers TF, Osterhaus AD, Beyer WE, van Asten JA, de Ronde-Verloop FM, Bijlsma K, et al. Analysis of antigenic relationships among influenza virus strains using a taxonomic cluster procedure. Comparison of three kinds of antibody preparations. J Virol Methods. 1985;10(3):241–50.

43. Dekker A, Wensvoort G, Terpstra C. Six antigenic groups within the genus pestivirus as identified by cross neutralization assays. Vet Microbiol. 1995;47(3–4):317–29.

44. Alexander FE, Chan LC, Lam TH, Yuen P, Leung NK, Ha SY, et al. Clustering of childhood leukaemia in Hong

Kong: association with the childhood peak and common acute lymphoblastic leukaemia and with population mixing. Avian Pathol. 1997;26:399

45. Sneath PHA, Sokal RR. Numerical Taxonomy: The Principles and Practice of Numerical Classification. San Francisco: W.H. Freeman; 1973.

46. Smith DJ, Lapedes AS, de Jong JC, Bestebroer TM, Rimmelzwaan GF, Osterhaus AD, et al. Mapping the antigenic and genetic evolution of influenza virus. Science. 2004;305(5682):371–6.

47. Lapedes A, Farber R. The geometry of shape space: application to influenza. J Theor Biol. 2001;212(1): 57–69.

48. Borg I, Groenen PJF. Modern Multidimensional Scaling. New York: Springer; 2005.

49. Boon ACM, de Mutsert G, van Baarle D, Smith DJ, Lapedes AS, Fouchier RAM, et al. Recognition of homo- and heterosubtypic variants of influenza A viruses by human CD8(+) T lymphocytes. J Immunol. 2004;172(4):2453–60.

50. Sandbulte MR, Westgeest KB, Gao J, Xu XY, Klimov AI, Russell CA, et al. Discordant antigenic drift of neuraminidase and hemagglutinin in H1N1 and H3N2 influenza viruses. Proc Natl Acad Sci U S A. 2011;108 (51):20748–53.

51. de Jong JC, Smith DJ, Lapedes AS, Donatelli I, Campitelli L, Barigazzi G, et al. Antigenic and genetic evolution of swine influenza A (H3N2) viruses in Europe. J Virol. 2007;81(8):4315–22.

52. Garten RJ, Davis CT, Russell CA, Shu B, Lindstrom S, Balish A, et al. Antigenic and genetic characteristics of swine-origin 2009 A(H1N1) influenza viruses circulating in humans. Science. 2009;325(5937):197–201.

53. Lorusso A, Vincent AL, Harland ML, Alt D, Bayles DO, Swenson SL, et al. Genetic and antigenic characterization of H1 influenza viruses from United States swine from 2008. J Gen Virol. 2011;92(Pt 4):919–30.

54. Lewis NS, Daly JM, Russell CA, Horton DL, Skepner E, Bryant NA, et al. Antigenic and genetic evolution of equine influenza A (H3N8) virus from 1968 to 2007. J Virol. 2011;85(23):12742–9.

55. Holmes EC. The Evolution and Emergence of RNA Viruses. Oxford, UK: Oxford University Press; 2009.

56. Barr IG, Komadina N, Hurt A, Shaw R, Durrant C, Iannello P, et al. Reassortants in recent human influenza A and B isolates from South East Asia and Oceania. Virus Res. 2003;98(1):35–44.

57. Ghedin E, Sengamalay NA, Shumway M, Zaborsky J, Feldblyum T, Subbu V, et al. Large-scale sequencing of human influenza reveals the dynamic nature of viral genome evolution. Nature. 2005;437(7062):1162–6.

58. Holmes EC, Ghedin E, Miller N, Taylor J, Bao Y, St George K, et al. Whole-genome analysis of human influenza A virus reveals multiple persistent lineages and reassortment among recent H3N2 viruses. PLoS Biol. 2005;3(9):e300.

59. Memoli MJ, Jagger BW, Dugan VG, Qi L, Jackson JP, Taubenberger JK. Recent human influenza A/H3N2 virus evolution driven by novel selection factors in addition to antigenic drift. J Infect Dis. 2009;200(8):1232–41.

60. Smith GJ, Vijaykrishna D, Bahl J, Lycett SJ, Worobey M, Pybus OG, et al. Origins and evolutionary genomics of the 2009 swine-origin H1N1 influenza A epidemic. Nature. 2009;459(7250):1122–5.

61. Drummond AJ, Ho SY, Phillips MJ, Rambaut A. Relaxed phylogenetics and dating with confidence. PLoS Biol. 2006;4(5):e88.

62. Smith GJD, Bahl J, Vijaykrishna D, Zhang JX, Poon LLM, Chen HL, et al. Dating the emergence of pandemic influenza viruses. Proc Natl Acad Sci U S A. 2009;106(28):11709–12.

63. Grenfell BT, Pybus OG, Gog JR, Wood JLN, Daly JM, Mumford JA, et al. Unifying the epidemiological and evolutionary dynamics of pathogens. Science. 2004;303 (5656):327–32.

64. Rambaut A, Pybus OG, Nelson MI, Viboud C, Taubenberger JK, Holmes EC. The genomic and epidemiological dynamics of human influenza A virus. Nature. 2008; 453(7195):615–U2.

65. Koelle K, Cobey S, Grenfell B, Pascual M. Epochal evolution shapes the phylodynamics of interpandemic influenza A (H3N2) in humans. Science. 2006;314(5807): 1898–903.

66. Ferguson NM, Galvani AP, Bush RM. Ecological and immunological determinants of influenza evolution. Nature. 2003;422(6930):428–33.

67. Nelson MI, Simonsen L, Viboud C, Miller MA, Taylor J, George KS, et al. Stochastic processes are key determinants of short-term evolution in influenza a virus. PLoS Pathog. 2006;2(12):e125.

68. Russell CA, Jones TC, Barr IG, Cox NJ, Garten RJ, Gregory V, et al. The global circulation of seasonal influenza A (H3N2) viruses. Science. 2008;320(5874): 340–6.

69. Murcia PR, Baillie GJ, Daly J, Elton D, Jervis C, Mumford JA, et al. Intra- and interhost evolutionary dynamics of equine influenza virus. J Virol. 2010;84(14): 6943–54.

70. Wilson IA, Skehel JJ, Wiley DC. Structure of the haemagglutinin membrane glycoprotein of influenza virus at 3 A resolution. Nature. 1981;289(5796):366–73.

71. Varghese JN, Laver WG, Colman PM. Structure of the influenza virus glycoprotein antigen neuraminidase at 2.9 A resolution. Nature. 1983;303(5912):35–40.

72. Offman MN, Krol M, Silman I, Sussman JL, Futerman AH. Molecular basis of reduced glucosylceramidase

activity in the most common Gaucher disease mutant, N370S. J Biol Chem. 2010;285(53):42105–14.

73. Amaro RE, Schnaufer A, Interthal H, Hol W, Stuart KD, McCammon JA. Discovery of drug-like inhibitors of an essential RNA-editing ligase in Trypanosoma brucei. Proc Natl Acad Sci U S A. 2008;105(45):17278–83.

74. Khatib F, DiMaio F, Cooper S, Kazmierczyk M, Gilski M, Krzywda S, et al. Crystal structure of a monomeric retroviral protease solved by protein folding game players. Nat Struct Mol Biol. 2011;18(10):1175–7.

75. Marti-Renom MA, Stuart AC, Fiser A, Sanchez R, Melo F, Sali A. Comparative protein structure modeling of genes and genomes. Annu Rev Biophys Biomol Struct. 2000;29:291–325.

76. Karplus M, McCammon JA. Molecular dynamics simulations of biomolecules. Nat Struct Biol. 2002;9(9):646–52.

77. Fleishman SJ, Whitehead TA, Ekiert DC, Dreyfus C, Corn JE, Strauch EM, et al. Computational design of proteins targeting the conserved stem region of influenza hemagglutinin. Science. 2011;332(6031):816–21.

78. Stevens J, Blixt O, Glaser L, Taubenberger JK, Palese P, Paulson JC, et al. Glycan microarray analysis of the hemagglutinins from modern and pandemic influenza viruses reveals different receptor specificities. J Mol Biol. 2006;355(5):1143–55.

79. Chutinimitkul S, Herfst S, Steel J, Lowen AC, Ye J, van Riel D, et al. Virulence-associated substitution D222G in the hemagglutinin of 2009 pandemic influenza A(H1N1) virus affects receptor binding. J Virol. 2010;84 (22):11802–13.

80. Belser JA, Jayaraman A, Raman R, Pappas C, Zeng H, Cox NJ, et al. Effect of D222G mutation in the hemagglutinin protein on receptor binding, pathogenesis and transmissibility of the 2009 pandemic H1N1 influenza virus. PLoS ONE. 2011;6(9):e25091.

81. Liu Y, Childs RA, Matrosovich T, Wharton S, Palma AS, Chai W, et al. Altered receptor specificity and cell tropism of D222G hemagglutinin mutants isolated from fatal cases of pandemic A(H1N1) 2009 influenza virus. J Virol. 2010;84(22):12069–74.

82. Xu R, McBride R, Nycholat CM, Paulson JC, Wilson IA. Structural characterization of the hemagglutinin receptor specificity from the 2009 H1N1 influenza pandemic. J Virol. 2012;86(2):982–90.

83. US Department of Health and Human Services. Interim pre-pandemic planning guidance: community strategy for pandemic influenza mitigation in the United States – Early targeted layered use of nonpharmaceutical interventions. In: Services HH, editor. Washington, DC. 2007.

28 Pandemic preparedness and response

Jonathan S. Nguyen-Van-Tam[1] and Joseph Bresee[2]

[1]Health Protection and Influenza Research Group, University of Nottingham Medical School, City Hospital, Nottingham, UK

[2]Epidemiology and Prevention Branch, Influenza Division, Centers for Disease Control and Prevention, Atlanta, GA, USA

Historical context of health emergency planning and response

Ancient history

Early historical accounts of outbreaks of infectious diseases have not only described the clinical and pathologic features in humans, but also the complex interactions between such outbreaks and human society. The etiology of the Plague of Athens, 430–427 BC, is unknown, but the historian and writer Thucydides clearly describes the breakdown of social order, disruption of military operations, spontaneous social distancing, abandonment of normal burial rites in the face of massive population mortality, person-to-person transmission (often associated with care of the sick), excess mortality among physicians, and spread to neighboring territories; from which we can conclude that there was no organized response to this severe epidemic [1]. Nevertheless, the acquisition of immunity after recovery from infection is clearly documented, along with the observation that such individuals could safely care for the sick without risk of personal harm, suggesting early insight into how an organized response could prove advantageous.

The re-emergence of bubonic plague (*Yersinia pestis*) or "Black Death" in Europe in 1345 produced the first notions that the impact of infectious diseases could be mitigated through organized response. The city of Venice implemented quarantine measures in 1374 by holding ships offshore for 40 days and through the isolation of affected families [2].

Local and national coordination

Possibly the first recognition that there should be an overall coordinated response to outbreaks or epidemics of infectious diseases came in 1493 when the Italian city of Florence established a board of officials charged with responding to such incidents. Under its auspices, public gatherings were at one point banned to prevent spread the spread of plague from Rome. During the sixteenth century permanent health committees were established in many European cities, whose purpose was to monitor and control the spread of infectious diseases [3].

Supra-national coordination

Besides the need for an organized local response to infectious diseases, clear recognition of the need for a coordinated supra-national response resulted in the first International Sanitary Conference in Paris, 1851, the objective of which was to harmonize quarantine regulations across European nations. Subsequently, an Office for International Public Hygiene (OIHP) was established in 1907; but it was in the aftermath of World War II that the World Health Organization (WHO) was founded in 1948.

Textbook of Influenza, Second Edition. Edited by Robert G. Webster, Arnold S. Monto, Thomas J. Braciale, and Robert A. Lamb.
© 2013 John Wiley & Sons, Ltd. Published 2013 by John Wiley & Sons, Ltd.

Preparedness and response to pandemics of the twentieth century

During the 1918 pandemic, well-organized responses were seen throughout the world, mainly coordinated at national (governmental) level. In almost all jurisdictions the focus was on public health measures such as respiratory etiquette, case isolation, quarantining of contacts, school closures, limitation or prohibition of public gatherings, and border closures; most of these with limited evidence of effectiveness [4]. This emphasis may have arisen in part due to the absence of antiviral drugs and antibiotics and lack of understanding about the etiology of influenza, forcing a reliance on simple preventive measures.

By 1957, influenza vaccines had been available for more than a decade and the focus in national responses, especially in the United States and United Kingdom had switched towards vaccination, with healthcare and "essential" workers prioritized in both countries. However, vaccine arrived too late to be maximally effective and was in short supply compared to population size [5]. None whatsoever was available in resource-poor countries. The same principles were followed in 1968 although vaccine was slightly more widely available.

Although it is not possible to comment in detail on the A(H1N1) swine influenza incident at Fort Dix, United States, in 1976 (see Chapter 2), this was a pandemic "false alarm" that resulted in a massive vaccination campaign during which 25% of the US population was vaccinated (>40 million persons), before the program was halted due to an excess of cases of Guillain–Barré syndrome temporally associated with the vaccine. The program did, however, adhere to the important principle of early vaccine intervention, although the pandemic threat never finally materialized. Unfortunately, it also did much to undermine public confidence in the organized governmental response to influenza threats.

Modern day pandemic preparedness

Emergence of pandemic preparedness activities

In 1997 an outbreak of highly pathogenic avian influenza A(H5N1) in humans in Hong Kong resulted in 18 cases of whom six died [6]. The incident served as a clear reminder that the last pandemic virus had emerged almost 30 years previously and of the enduring threat to humans from the avian influenza reservoir in wild birds [7]. While efficient spread of A(H5N1) infection from person-to-person has not occurred to date, the emergence of a different novel zoonosis, severe acute respiratory syndrome (SARS) in late 2002, provided a different perspective, with efficient person-to-person transmission and rapid international spread via the medium of air travel [8]. When influenza A(H5N1) re-emerged in South-East Asia in 2003 [9], and the virus became endemic in poultry flocks in several, mainly South-East Asian, countries it became clear that substantial efforts were needed to improve global influenza pandemic preparedness.

Although little pandemic preparedness had been undertaken anywhere in the world prior to 2004, a few countries had developed pandemic preparedness plans earlier; for example, the United Kingdom's first national plan was published in 1997, and the first WHO pandemic plan came out in 1999. However, the now familiar, whole-of-society, multisectoral approach was most clearly established upon publication of the second WHO pandemic plan and its associated checklist in 2005 [10,11].

Pandemic preparedness principles and assumptions prior to 2009

Pandemic preparedness is predicated on the emergence of an influenza virus that is sufficiently novel that large sections of the global population have no pre-existing immunity. In addition, the virus must be readily transmissible from person-to-person and cause clinical illness. Based on the experience in 1918 when the case–fatality rate due to the pandemic A(H1N1) virus was about 2.5%, and the 63% case–fatality rate observed due to A(H5N1) between 2003 and 2008, it was assumed by many authorities that a pandemic virus would be more virulent than seasonal influenza. However, the pandemic viruses of 1957 and 1968 inflicted a far lower case fatality of around 0.1% [12], leaving a wide range of uncertainty for planners. The data on clinical attack rates in the pandemics of the twentieth century offered more consistent estimates around 25–30% [13]. Similarly, the literature on geographic spread of past pandemics revealed that in both 1957 and 1968 effective global spread from an epicenter in South-East Asia occurred in under 6 months [13]. However, in 2003 SARS spread from Hong Kong to Vietnam, Singapore, and Canada in just 3 weeks, illustrating the potential for modern day air passenger movement to accelerate substantially international spread of a novel respiratory infection (Table 28.1).

The purpose of pandemic preparedness is to plan, organize, and coordinate activities that will be necessary to respond to all aspects of a pandemic. A national pandemic plan should serve as an overarching strategy, beneath which sub-national and local

operational plans can be established and tested. Although widely different formats and approaches may be pursued, all require firm political support and dedicated financial resources. As countries are heterogeneous in terms of how they are organized administratively (e.g., centralized versus federal systems, including health services and the extent to which these lie in the private or public sectors), many different approaches to pandemic preparedness exist but all are underpinned by specific common elements described below.

Specific elements of pandemic preparedness

Planning for epidemiologic monitoring and surveillance of a pandemic

Table 28.1. Basic epidemiologic and virologic assumptions in pandemic preparedness prior to 2009.

Epicenter

- Unknown
- On basis of loci of 1957 and 1968 pandemics and endemicity of A(H5N1) in poultry, considered most likely to be South-East Asia

Subtype

- Unknown
- Most worrisome possibility: A(H5N1) due to high case–fatality rate of sporadic human cases
- Other possibilities: A(H7N7), A(H7N2), A(H9N2), A(H2N2)

Case–fatality rate

- Unknown
- Planning ranges from 2.5% (1918-like) to 0.1% (1968-like)
- CFR for avian influenza A(H5N1) noted to be circa 60% – assumption this would fall if virus became transmissible between humans

Attack rates

- Clinical attack rate 25–35% (cumulative)
- Serologic attack rates roughly twofold higher
- Highest attack rates in younger age groups

Transmissibility and spread

- Global spread within 6 months of emergence
- International travel restrictions unlikely to slow spread
- Reproductive number R_0: 1.2–2.0
- Up to three separate pandemic waves over 18-month period

A fundamental requirement for an effective pandemic response is the ability to conduct appropriate disease and viral surveillance, and to gather additional data required for decision-making from targeted field investigations. The establishment of the WHO World Influenza Center in 1947 (now the Global Influenza Surveillance and Response System; GISRS), was a response to concerns that new pandemic strains be detected as quickly as possible [14,15]. The 1957 A(H2N2) pandemic was the first in which both virus and disease were identified and monitored during its global spread [5]. Since that time, ensuring robust surveillance systems has been a centerpiece of all pandemic plans [16].

Even so, the global capacity to conduct viral and disease surveillance capable of detecting and monitoring an emergent pandemic remained limited during the decades following the A(H2N2) pandemic. During this period, the primary goal shaping expansion of global influenza surveillance was to gather and characterize influenza viruses in support of seasonal vaccine production [15]. National surveillance systems that produced data on risk groups, seasonality, and disease burden were mostly confined to high-income countries in Asia, Europe, Oceania, and North America. For most countries, laboratory capacity to detect potential pandemic viruses, and the ability to detect and investigate clusters of respiratory illnesses remained inadequate [17]. Interest in influenza surveillance for pandemic readiness increased

455

following the 1997 avian influenza A(H5N1) outbreak among humans in Hong Kong and was further galvanized by the SARS outbreak and re-emergence of A(H5N1) in 2003.

While all pandemic plans contain substantially similar surveillance goals, the specific objectives of surveillance (or uses of surveillance data) will vary between countries and potentially change during the course of a pandemic [16,18]. During the interpandemic period, surveillance systems must be sufficiently sensitive and comprehensive to identify the emergence of a pandemic strain as early as possible, thereby triggering a public health response. Countries also must be able to test reliably for influenza and have access to laboratories that can characterize potentially novel influenza A strains. During the last decade, growth of WHO's global laboratory surveillance network, GISRS, which now includes 123 countries, and the expansion of reverse transcriptase polymerase chain reaction (RT-PCR) testing in clinical and public laboratories, has dramatically improved the speed with which a future pandemic strain will be detected and confirmed. Interpandemic surveillance is also used to establish baselines against which pandemic influenza can be compared (for instance, to assess severity). Once a pandemic virus has emerged, disease surveillance must be sufficiently robust to monitor the geographic spread, changes in epidemiologic features, severity or impact in a community, and the effect of public health interventions [19]. Viral surveillance systems should monitor changes in the virus that may make medical interventions less effective (e.g., mutations that confer antiviral resistance) or would guide vaccine and diagnostic test development.

Strong seasonal influenza surveillance systems are critical as foundations for pandemic surveillance. The stress on human and health resources during a pandemic mainly precludes development of new systems or enrollment of new surveillance sites once a pandemic has started. Rather, modification of seasonal surveillance systems to provide more timely data (e.g., daily rather than weekly) or more information (e.g., finer age strata, additional clinical data) is preferred. Even so, some information needed for a pandemic response is not likely to be available from routine seasonal surveillance. For instance, systems that monitor healthcare delivery or hospital bed availability may be important for surge planning. Advance identification of these specific data needs, and designing and exercising plans to collect them are crucial.

International health regulations

In 2005, all WHO Member States agreed to become legally bound to a group of regulations intended to ensure that the international community would detect, respond, and share information on acute public health events posing an international health risk and which might require a coordinated international response [20]. These regulations, the International Health Regulations (IHR) (2005) came into effect in June 2007. Human influenza caused by a new subtype is specifically listed as a disease that must be reported under the IHR agreement. IHR (2005) has served as a powerful catalyst for improved surveillance and response particularly relevant to countries at higher risk for A(H5N1) outbreaks [21]. Countries are now required to be able to detect influenza viruses, and refer suspicious isolates to WHO collaborating laboratories for further characterization. Countries also responded by improving processes to investigate outbreaks and communicate the results to WHO. Following the implementation of IHR (2005) there was a marked increase in data and isolates sent to GISRS. The ability of countries worldwide to detect first cases of A(H1N1)pdm09 and to share epidemiologic data and laboratory samples with WHO was, in part, the result of IHR implementation [21].

Planning for use of antivirals

The use of antiviral drugs remains a cornerstone of many countries' pandemic plans. Because of the time required to create and distribute a pandemic vaccine, antivirals that can treat or prevent influenza are attractive tools to limit disease complications, and perhaps influenza transmission during a pandemic. Pandemic antiviral strategies have been based on profiles of the available medications, models of potential effects of various approaches, programmatic requirements, and resources available.

Currently, two classes of antivirals are licensed for treatment or prophylaxis of influenza A: the M2 channel blockers (or adamantanes) and the neuraminidase inhibitors (NAIs). While two adamantanes are currently licensed, the propensity of influenza A viruses to develop rapid resistance to these agents has limited enthusiasm for including them in pandemic plans [22]. Most plans have focused on use of NAIs, of which two are widely available – oseltamivir and zanamavir. NAIs have been incorporated into national, international, and private stockpiles and were used widely during the 2009 pandemic [23]. Zanamavir use has been more limited than oseltamivir because of its narrower age indication, contraindication for use among persons with some respiratory conditions, and relative complexity of administration. While oseltamivir resistance was observed in A(H1N1) viruses circulating before the 2009 pandemic, resistance among currently circulating viruses (including A(H1N1) pdm09) and A(H5N1) remains uncommon [24]. Even so, the reliance of pandemic plans on NAIs, together with the threat of rapidly developing resistance during a pandemic or the emergence of a resistant pandemic strain, highlight the importance of additional antiviral choices. In addition, the difficulty of administering oral or inhaled medications to severely ill persons has led to increased testing and emergency use of intravenous NAIs. The anticipated worldwide licensure of second generation NAIs should offer options for intravenous administration to severely ill patients and "once only" dosing (Table 28.2).

Because NAIs are effective in both treating and preventing influenza, a variety of pandemic approaches has been proposed. While strategies that emphasize prophylaxis could produce reductions in overall illness rates [25], and better preserve critical infrastructures (e.g., prophylaxis of healthcare workers), they require far larger stockpiles for effective implementation than do treatment-based approaches. Most countries' plans, therefore, focus on treatment of ill persons, with prophylaxis reserved for specific, limited circumstances (e.g., high-risk household members) [18,26]. In some high-income countries, such as the United Kingdom and United States, with large stockpiles, all persons suspected of having a pandemic illness were recommended to be treated. Other countries with more limited stockpiles have chosen to target specific groups, either to maximize reduction of severe disease (e.g., persons at high risk for severe influenza) or safeguard critical national infrastructure (CNI) resiliency. Because decisions on the use of scarce resources have public, political, scientific, and ethical implications, these deliberations should be systematic and transparent.

Programs to deliver antivirals during a pandemic are complex given the dispersed geographic nature of pandemic illness (compared with delivery of antibiotics following a point-source anthrax exposure, for instance). Planners should exercise distribution and administration in advance of a pandemic. In addition, because effective treatment requires early administration after illness onset, strategies to ensure easy access to treatment in all localities within a country are critical. Antiviral stockpiling and use during a pandemic is complex and expensive, but can result in substantial public health benefits [27]. A global consideration continues to be the equitable distribution of antivirals.

Planning for use of pandemic vaccines

While vaccines are the best tool for the prevention of influenza, they will not be available early in a pandemic unless production techniques are vastly improved or a "universal" vaccine is developed. The current steps in producing influenza vaccines, whether live, attenuated, or inactivated, require several months, and cannot be initiated until a suitable pandemic vaccine seed strain is produced following the emergence of a novel virus. Because it is unlikely that seasonal vaccines will provide adequate protection against a newly emergent pandemic strain, planning for pandemic vaccines has taken two approaches: the creation of vaccines based on the pandemic virus once detected; and creation and stockpiling of "pre-pandemic" vaccines based on assumptions about future pandemic strains [28].

The optimal antigenic match between a pandemic strain and vaccine will be achieved by creating vaccines specifically against the new pandemic strain. This approach is taken in the production of seasonal vaccine and has been used in each pandemic since 1957, but requires several months to progress from strain characterization to vaccine delivery [29]. As a result, vaccination is not currently a viable strategy for mitigating spread or limiting disease at the start of a pandemic.

An approach to reduce the time from pandemic detection to vaccine delivery is to produce and stockpile pre-pandemic vaccines during the interpandemic period, designed to protect against strains thought to represent a pandemic risk. Many countries and WHO undertook the creation of vaccine stockpiles

457

Table 28.2. Summary of characteristics of drugs licensed for use against influenza.

Class	M2 channel blockers (adamantanes)		Neuraminidase inhibitors (NAIs)			
Agent	Amantadine	Rimantadine	Zanamivir	Oseltamivir	Peramivir	Laninamivir
Trade name(s)	Lysovir®, Symadine®	Flumadine®	Relenza®	Tamiflu®	Rapiacta® Peramiflu®	Inavir®
Influenza activity	A viruses only	A viruses only	A and B viruses	A and B viruses	A and B viruses	A and B viruses
Route of administration	Oral	Oral	Oral inhalation (dry powder)	Oral	Intravenous	Oral inhalation (dry powder)
Use for treatment	Yes	Yes	Yes	Yes	Yes[a]	Yes
Use for prophylaxis	Yes	Yes	Yes	Yes	No	No[b]
Pandemic application	Unreliable choices for pandemic application due to propensity for rapid emergence of resistance Adverse event profile for amantadine unfavorable compared with NAIs		Highly suitable provided patient can operate delivery device and make sufficient inspiratory effort to inhale dry powder Twice daily dosing (treatment) necessitates good compliance Large pack size increases warehousing space for stockpiles	Highly suitable general choice; available in capsules and pediatric suspension Twice daily dosing (treatment) necessitates good compliance Risk of resistance emergence (H275Y mutation) in viruses of N1 moiety	Unsuitable for use in ambulatory care Most suitable and possibly "best choice" in severely ill (ventilated) patients who cannot be given zanamivir and who can only be given oseltamivir by nasogastric instillation	Similar use issues as for zanamivir Once and only dosing offers "fire and forget" simplicity; may be useful in low compliance populations (e.g., homeless) or situations where facilities or living conditions are basic (military, refugee settings, etc.)

[a]Intravenous route of administration makes it most suitable for use in hospital for severely ill patients.
[b]Not yet licensed for prophylaxis (April 2012); theoretically likely to be effective for post-exposure prophylaxis.
Source: Adapted with permission from Van-Tam J, Lim WS. Pharmaceutical interventions. In: *Pandemic Influenza*, 2nd edn. J. Van-Tam and C. Sellwood, editors. 2012, Wallingford: CABI, p. 123.

and conducted extensive testing of avian influenza A(H5N1) vaccines in the last decade for this purpose [30]. Stockpiles of monovalent A(H5N1) vaccines (some adjuvanted) against clades 1, 2.1, 2.2, and 2.3 viruses were created and are maintained by several countries. Use of stockpiled vaccines has been promoted to limit disease or delay spread among the first countries affected, or to provide early vaccination of high-risk groups. However, stockpiling of vaccines in advance of a pandemic carries the inherent risk that the pandemic strain will be antigenically different from stockpiled vaccines, limiting their usefulness. Even so, the prospect of early prevention through vaccination, particularly in a severe pandemic, has maintained interest in this approach.

A challenge to pandemic vaccination is to ensure sufficient quantity to meet demand, particularly if protection were to require two doses or high antigen content per dose. This challenge has been addressed in two ways. Several adjuvanted vaccines have been developed, both for pandemic use (e.g., A(H5N1) and A(H1N1) monovalent vaccines) and in seasonal campaigns (trivalent) (see Chapter 20) [29]. Adjuvants enhance immune responses in recipients, and can generate greater heterotypic protection against drifted strains. Adjuvant can also be stockpiled to be mixed with pandemic antigen. A second approach to ensure adequate pandemic vaccine supply is to increase global production capacity [31]. Because most vaccine stockpiles and manufacturing capacity exist in high-income countries, concerns about the equitable access to vaccines during a pandemic has led to a concerted program to increase global vaccine supply and production capacity. The WHO Global Action Plan for Influenza Vaccines is designed to help ensure greater global availability of pandemic vaccines by increasing the number of manufacturers in mid- and low-income countries. As a result of the program, which began in 2005, global vaccine production has risen from 350 million doses in 2006 to more than 900 million doses in 2009. Eleven manufacturers in non-high-income settings are developing or producing vaccines [32].

Finally, consideration has been given to vaccinating with stockpiled vaccines before the emergence of a pandemic [28]. This approach would ensure that a person receives a vaccine prior to exposure, and would be primed for later boosting with a pandemic vaccine when available. Such a strategy would also allow for use of stockpiled vaccines before loss of potency. The drawbacks of the approach are several. First, because a person would receive a vaccine designed well before the identification of a pandemic strain, the risk that the pandemic strain will be antigenically different is relatively high; so, reduced protection or priming might be conferred. Second, the ethical implications of exposing a person to a vaccine for which there is currently minimal risk of wild-type virus exposure must be resolved. Finally, policies for the use of these vaccines, such as target groups, must be settled. While some countries have licensed A(H5N1) vaccines that could be used for such purposes, no pre-pandemic vaccination program has so far been implemented.

Planning for use of antibiotics and pneumococcal vaccines

Although antiviral drugs and influenza vaccines dominate the pharmaceutical responses to pandemic influenza, there is a strong temporal association between influenza activity and bacterial pneumonia, the most common pathogens being (in numerical order) *Streptococcus pneumoniae* (the pneumococcus), *Haemophilus influenzae* and *Staphylococcus aureus*. It has been estimated that 15–20% of pandemic influenza cases develop secondary bacterial pneumonia [33], therefore, given an influenza clinical attack rate of 25–50%, planning for antibiotic stockpiles to cover up to 10% of the population seems reasonable [34]. The precise choice of agents should be driven by local and national surveillance data on antimicrobial resistance. However, there should be a planning assumption around the need to cover the three major etiologic organisms named above using empirical therapy, because demand for laboratory diagnostic services is likely to exceed supply and the emphasis will be on timely intervention. Because antibiotics are used year round in large numbers, true stockpiling may not be necessary if buffer stocks are introduced into the routine supply chain (Figure 28.1); this approach allows for gradual variations in the types and proportions of antibiotics held in response to changes in patterns of resistance [35].

It has also been suggested that pneumococcal polysaccharide vaccines (PPV) and pneumococcal conjugate vaccines (PncCV) may form part of a coherent pandemic response strategy, most likely achieved through routine immunization programs

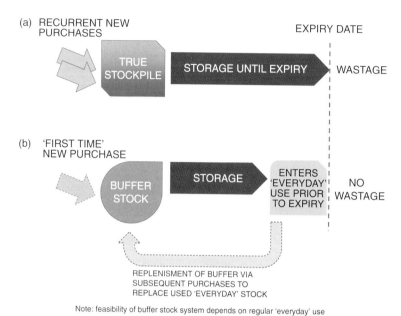

Figure 28.1. Conceptual illustration of differences between (a) true stockpiling and (b) buffer stock method. (Originally drawn by Wei Shen Lim and Jonathan Van-Tam and reproduced with permission from *Pandemic Influenza*, 2nd edn. CABI: Wallingford, 2012, p. 136.)

and pre-pandemic usage. PPV offers moderate protection in adults against invasive pneumococcal disease (IPD) and the introduction of PncCV into childhood immunization schedules has substantially reduced IPD in children by direct effect, and in adults through its impact on pneumococcal carriage in children. It seems highly likely that such a strategy would avert deaths and hospitalizations in a pandemic situation where secondary pneumococcal disease was a prominent feature [36].

Public health measures

A significant part of pandemic planning before the 2009 pandemic was focused on a variety of nonpharmaceutical public health interventions that could be employed to reduce or delay the spread of a pandemic. The principle of all such interventions is to limit exposure of ill persons to susceptible persons. Even if overall disease rates are not reduced, application of public health measures might slow the progress of a pandemic, "flatten" the epidemic curve and in doing so reduce surge pressure on health systems and other components of CNI [37]. Plans to use such strategies were based on the assumption that influenza-specific interventions, vaccines and antivi-

rals, would be available late or in short supply during a pandemic. The utility of these measures to mitigate the impact of pandemic influenza was based on experience from past pandemics and mathematical models [38,39].

The variety of nonpharmaceutical mitigation measures can be divided into those that are employed at country or community levels (e.g., school closures, cancellation of mass gatherings, travel restrictions) and those employed by individuals (e.g., use of face masks, handwashing, isolation from others while ill). Each measure has potential benefits and costs. For those measures for which an individual is responsible, the real and opportunity costs are likely to be minimal, and offer the advantage of empowering the person to act to protect themselves. However, data on the effectiveness of individual measures is often lacking [40,41]. Furthermore, effectiveness likely suffers because of challenges in maintaining compliance during prolonged community transmission. Conversely, the costs of community-level measures are often quite large, both in terms of real and opportunity costs. For instance, border screening or closures require substantial manpower and, even then are unlikely to be effective; during a pandemic, critical personnel may be more usefully deployed in other parts of the response. Like individual measures, high quality data on the effectiveness of community interventions are sparse. Because of the difficulty with estimating the true value and costs of the interventions, developing consensus on which and when to implement them has proved challenging.

Planning must also account for changing needs during a pandemic [16,26,37]. For instance, while handwashing and cough etiquette are equally reasonable at any time, the value of other mitigation measures is likely to change over time. A good example of this time dependency relates to school closures. School closures are intended to mitigate local community spread early in a local outbreak but work best when schools are closed before the introduction of the virus into the school-aged population [42].

Another principle is that the actual tools employed will depend on the severity and the epidemiologic features of the pandemic [4,26]. Because of the high costs and disruption caused by some interventions, they might be relegated to the most severe pandemics, while others would be used in even mild pandemics, where the cost–benefit is more favorable. Similarly, features of a pandemic such as age-specific attack rate or complication rate might result in targeting measures to the affected age groups. Finally, pandemic models have repeatedly demonstrated that public health measures should be used in combination to be maximally effective [37,38]. WHO and national governments have developed plans for "targeted," "layered" containment and mitigation strategies. As each measure, along with the use of vaccines and antivirals, is imperfect, plans rely on the additive effects of employing several at any time.

Health sector preparedness issues

In its 2005 plan and checklist, WHO drew specific attention to the fact that health services will be at the forefront of any national response to pandemic influenza from the earliest stages when first human cases are recognized through to the peak of disease activity in a given country, and thereafter into the decline and recovery phases of the response [10,11]. The important underpinning requirement is to plan for responding to four interrelated threats:

1. The need to provide surge capacity as the number of patients requiring care for pandemic influenza rises

then falls, perhaps repeatedly over one to three separate waves as in 1918–1919.

2. The need to mount such a response with potentially lower staff availability due to sickness absence, mortality, and potentially refusal to work during a severe pandemic threat.

3. The requirement to maintain care provision in "mission critical" noninfluenza areas, for example the handling of trauma cases, severe bacterial infections, emergency surgery, obstetric services, and coronary care.

4. To minimize the risk that healthcare becomes part of the problem (as opposed to part of the solution) through nosocomial spread of pandemic influenza.

The impact on healthcare demand during a pandemic will depend upon the clinical attack rate and the propensity of the novel virus to cause severe infection that cannot be managed through self-care (or informal care provided by family members) and over-the-counter remedies, that is the requirements for ambulatory (primary) care, hospital admission, and critical care (ventilatory support). Sensible ranges for such indices can be estimated from previous pandemics but cannot be accurately predicted, emphasizing the need for adequate surveillance data that also cover secondary and tertiary care settings. Modeling data support the fact that the impact on healthcare during a pandemic is likely to be concentrated into a typical epidemic wave of about 12 weeks, during which almost one-quarter of total associated healthcare demand might fall in a single concentrated 1-week period at the peak [43]. Therefore, the ability of interventions such as the early use of antiviral drugs and public health measures to "flatten" the peak of healthcare demand (even if this broadens the period of time affected) would be an important factor [38]. Supply issues focus principally on availability and planned usage of antiviral drugs alongside other "pandemic consumables," notably antibiotics for the treatment of secondary bacterial pneumonias [33], oxygen, and personal protective equipment for healthcare workers. It is clear from a recent meta-analysis that healthcare workers are at increased risk of influenza infection compared with nonhealth workers [44], emphasizing the need for well-planned and rehearsed infection control procedures that reduce the risks of nosocomial spread and protect staff. In this area one critical defect remains the inadequacy of understanding about modes of influenza transmission [45,46] and the effectiveness of specific interventions such as face masks and respirators [47].

Business continuity and preservation of critical national infrastructures

Besides the likely impact on healthcare systems, it is clear that the mortality and morbidity of a severe pandemic would have a major macroeconomic and societal impact justifying a whole-of-society multisectoral response. In addition, it seems likely that the disease effects such as workplace absenteeism, supply chain disruption, and threats to social order might be compounded by intervention effects of public health measures related to travel restrictions, social distancing measures, and school closures whether implemented formally by governments or informally by private citizens [48,49]. In light of such considerations, planning for the maintenance of business functions and preservation and maintenance of CNI has become an integral part of pandemic preparedness; however, not all national pandemic plans offer the same degree of emphasis on this point. While the emergency planning movement has been driven to a large extent by the threat posed by "big-bang" incidents such as terrorist attacks and sudden impact natural disasters (e.g., earthquakes) where the duration is generally short (days to weeks) and mutual aid is possible, a pandemic represents a "rising tide" incident that will last for an extended period (months). In addition, their global nature makes it far less likely that mutual aid will be available, locally, nationally or internationally (Table 28.3).

Exercises, simulations, and drills

Although there is a long history of using exercises, simulations, and drills to maintain and improve operational efficiency in the military, their use in civilian settings has been largely confined to police, fire, rescue, and ambulance services. However, events such as the 9/11 terrorist attack, anthrax letters in 2001, the SARS outbreak in 2003, and the 7/7 London bombings in 2005 have highlighted the benefits of rehearsing a wider mobilization of the healthcare system to address an emergency situation. The objectives of pandemic healthcare exercises are: to develop multiagency links with relevant nonhealthcare organizations; clarify roles and responsibilities between

Table 28.3. Civilian organizations for consideration under pandemic planning arrangements for Critical National Infrastructure (CNI).

Emergency services[a]

- Police and security forces
- Fire authorities
- Ambulance services
- Maritime and Coastguard Agencies

Local and regional government tiers

- Principal local, municipal, and regional authorities
- Port Health Authorities

Health bodies

- Primary care providers
- Hospitals
- Public health and environmental authorities
- Burial services

Utilities

- Electricity distributors and transmitters
- Gas distributors
- Water and sewage services
- Telephone service providers (fixed and mobile)

Transport

- Rail networks and operating companies (passenger and freight)
- Urban mass transportation systems
- Airport operators
- Harbor authorities
- Public highways agencies
- Food distributors
- Fuel distributors

[a]Military personnel may feature as part of national pandemic arrangements but are usually subject to their own contingency plans.

agencies and between tiers within organizations (e.g., primary and secondary care) and rehearse interaction at critical interfaces; to identify lessons and gaps in capability which can then be rectified; to reinforce training and identify training gaps [50]. Both desktop and command post exercise formats have been used for pandemic preparedness. In the former, players from participating agencies assemble in one place for a typical period of 1–2 days and play out in theory what might happen in practice, using specially designed scenarios and "compressed time"; in the latter, players participate from their normal place of duty which is especially useful for testing communication between agencies and facilities. Examples of complex exercises that took place before the 2009–2010 pandemic include Exercise Common Ground (2006) in the European Union, Exercise Cumpston (2006) in Australia, and Exercise Winter Willow (2007) in the United Kingdom.

Ethical and legal challenges

It has long been recognized that a severe influenza pandemic will apply stress to the whole of society, especially healthcare systems, and that under such extraordinary pressures ethical issues will emerge. However, the first of these relates to pandemic preparedness itself. While it is relatively easy for high-income countries to undertake such activities (e.g., improving influenza surveillance and stockpiling antiviral drugs), in low-income countries with large and immediate unresolved health challenges (e.g., sanitation, childhood vaccination, and maternal mortality), the decision to divert scarce resources into planning for an event whose future timing is uncertain raises ethical issues [51]. Nevertheless, under Article 12 of the United Nations International Covenant on Economic, Social and Cultural Rights (1966) and the International Health Regulations (2005), a duty of international cooperation and assistance has been established in the context of the prevention, treatment, and control of epidemic diseases and the WHO has a prominent role in coordinating international pandemic preparedness.

It is also recognized that many of the public health measures that are proposed for a severe pandemic may infringe personal liberty; for example, restrictions on domestic and international movement, restriction on social and mass gatherings, workplace and school closures, quarantine arrangements and isolation. These might be enacted voluntarily, but if enforced by the state then the ethical dimensions of such decisions (which may not necessarily be wrong) will require consideration [51].

In the area of healthcare, many issues are potentially raised such as the obligation of healthcare workers to provide care during a time of increased danger to themselves, the principle of reciprocity in terms of the employer's duty to provide personal protective equipment, antiviral drugs and vaccine (when available) to frontline healthcare workers, and many circumstances related to potential rationing or prioritization of healthcare [51]. In the 2009–2010 pandemic, few ethical issues were raised because the A(H1N1)pdm09 virus was of generally low severity; however, it is clear that the unexpectedly high demand for intensive care beds that ensued would have created ethical issues over the allocation of scarce resources had the pandemic virus been even slightly more severe. WHO and several individual countries (France, New Zealand, Switzerland, United Kingdom) have recognized the ethical issues that might be raised by pandemic preparedness and response. In the United Kingdom a Committee of Ethical Aspects of Pandemic Influenza (CEAPI) was formed and met regularly from 2006 to 2009.

Communications

The 2009–2010 pandemic highlighted the importance of communication in pandemic response activities. Although some issues were well anticipated, for example the use of antiviral drugs and vaccines, several others such as the mildness of the A(H1N1)pdm09 virus, the fact that it was not A(H5N1), the epicenter (Mexico), and lack of clarity about severity in the early stages placed authorities "on the back foot."

Communication between the authorities, the public, and other stakeholders such as frontline healthcare workers should be planned for and the role of the media anticipated. Abraham and Pople [52] suggest that principles of the approach should be:

1. Building and maintenance of trust between authorities and the public – this depends on establishing the authorities as knowledgeable, competent and fair with transparent, early communication of facts. Once trust is lost, the management of an outbreak becomes difficult.

2. Early release of information – even if this is bad news or there is uncertainty. In the latter case, the public also needs to be prepared for the fact that the situation and the response might change as more information becomes available.

3. Transparency – sharing dilemmas and challenges with the public and communicating the rationale for decisions, even if these change over time.

4. Listening to the public and maintaining media relations – communication during a health crisis should not be seen as a one-way flow of information.

463

In modern societies the media is powerful and there should be investment in planning how to communicate with them, how to answer queries and rebut false information.

During the 2009–2010 pandemic it became clear that social media networks (e.g., Facebook® and Twitter®) are potentially important in terms of both reaching new audiences with public health information and the rapid promulgation of rumors and misinformation. The power of these tools was not fully appreciated prior to 2009 but needs to be fully taken account of in future pandemic preparedness activities.

The 2009–2010 pandemic response

In spring 2009, a novel A(H1N1)pdm09 strain emerged that was of swine origin and had a collection of genes not identified previously in humans or animals [53]. During the few weeks following the initial detection, the virus spread rapidly worldwide, causing the first influenza pandemic since the emergence of A(H3N2) in 1968. The response to the 2009–2010 pandemic at local, national, and international levels highlighted the benefits and shortcomings of the pandemic preparedness activities reviewed in the previous sections.

Most reviews have pointed to epidemiologic and virologic surveillance and dissemination of data as a success during the pandemic, although early information was imprecise with high variability. Some keys to successes in this area are informative. First, the presence of existing surveillance structures that monitored seasonal influenza incorporated into pandemic planning allowed for a fairly seamless transition from seasonal to pandemic monitoring [9,54]. The response benefited from recent efforts to strengthen global surveillance, and led to further expansion of surveillance capacity; 138 National Influenza Centers now participate in global data sharing, and increasing numbers of countries report epidemiologic data along with viral data [55]. An additional WHO Collaborating Center in China has been added which will make viral characterization and pandemic confirmation more timely and representative, and further expansion is planned. On 11 June, only weeks after the first identification of the virus, 74 countries had confirmed illness using laboratory tests in their country and shared the information with WHO, enabling the official declaration of a pandemic [56]. The expanded global laboratory capacity also produced timely data on antigenic and genetic viral characteristics which informed treatment and vaccine policies. Finally, the ability to confirm the virus quickly and report through the IHR and GISRS mechanisms provided situational awareness to the public, health systems, public health officials, media, and politicians which informed the response and fostered trust among stakeholders [21]. Another notable product of enhanced surveillance was the rapid understanding developed regarding risk groups and age distribution [57]. These data led to policies that targeted these groups for prevention and control strategies [58]. The pandemic also highlighted the value of data on severely ill persons, which has accelerated countries' adoption of surveillance systems focusing on severe acute respiratory illness (SARI). SARI surveillance provides countries with limited resources data on disease occurrence, severity, and provides a platform for virus and clinical data collection to inform control policies [58].

However, some aspects related to the collection and communication of epidemiologic data were problematic [19]. First, use of the data to understand and articulate the severity of the pandemic was difficult and led to some confusion among public partners. In the United States, the Pandemic Severity Index (PSI) which was developed in 2006 to assess and communicate severity was quickly abandoned after the start of the pandemic [37]. The PSI was difficult to calculate with sufficient precision given the data available early in the pandemic, and mortality alone did not capture the potential impact of the pandemic [53]. WHO developed a plan based on comparison of the pandemic to past pandemics, while many individual countries had poorly developed severity and risk assessment frameworks and instead relied on WHO assessments [19]. Another source of confusion was that the ability to track laboratory-confirmed cases early in the pandemic led to an expectation that public health authorities would provide the same regular disease counts throughout the pandemic. When countries transitioned to aggregate reporting, more general statements regarding the levels of disease, or modeled estimates, confusion among public and political leaders ensued [54,59].

The pandemic response did provide opportunities to employ and study the effects of nonpharmaceutical mitigation and containment efforts. However, because the pandemic virus lacked the severity of 1918, the full range of mitigation and containment tools was not employed or employed in limited fashion. For instance, the countries initially affected – Mexico, United States and Canada – almost immediately abandoned "containment"-style interventions in favor of community mitigation strategies [19]. So, the quenching strategy conceived of in pre-pandemic planning phases was not possible. Communities focused on early case treatment with antiviral drugs, reducing transmission through voluntarily decreasing exposures (e.g., requesting ill persons to stay home, voluntary school closures), rather than contact tracing and enforced isolation or quarantine. The United Kingdom, Australia, and many other countries employed "delaying" strategies which included active case finding and treatment with antiviral drugs, border restrictions, voluntary quarantine or close follow-up of contacts, and household post-exposure prophylaxis (United Kingdom) [19,25,60]. Most countries abandoned these approaches once transmission was confirmed within the country because of the high costs of manpower to administer the programs compared with the diminishing value once that point was reached. The appreciation that the pandemic was not a severe 1918-like scenario, which was planned for by most countries, meant that most national responses principally involved the health sector rather than requiring a broad whole-of-government approach. When responses did involve institutions outside of the health sector, public and political acceptance was often low. An example was the difficulty encountered when school closures were recommended as a community mitigation measure in the United States [54].

Because of the emergence of an A(H1N1) pandemic virus, rather than an A(H5N1) virus, pre-pandemic vaccine stockpiles were not put to use in the response. Even so, the rapid production and approval of pandemic vaccines was a notable success in the public health response [61]. The vast experience in making seasonal vaccines, together with substantial amount of planning involving public and private partners, was critical to this success. After the production, building on infrastructure used in seasonal campaigns to evaluate the effectiveness and safety of the vaccines and monitor coverage allowed for rapid and reliable data. However, the inherent time constraints in making influenza vaccines resulted in vaccine delivered too late for the first peaks of disease in many countries, limiting the demand for the vaccine in some places, and value of the vaccine in general. Countries that had used seasonal influenza vaccines routinely had fewer problems with delayed delivery and distribution. Low-income countries where influenza vaccine programs were not routine relied more heavily on donations of vaccine, and had little vaccine before January 2010 [61]. While some countries reached target vaccine coverage goals, vaccine uptake in most was less than expected due to some skepticism about the need for vaccine in a "mild" pandemic and concerns over its safety. Improving the vaccine response for the next pandemic will build upon the lessons learned in 2009–2010. Building pandemic vaccine production, delivery and monitoring on solid seasonal vaccine programs is critical, but reaching low and middle-income countries to a greater extent will require expansion of seasonal programs to more countries and increasing global production capacity [31,32].

The absence of significant antiviral resistance of the pandemic strain to NAIs enabled governments and healthcare systems to employ antivirals according to their pandemic plans. Most responses used antivirals for treatment and focused on methods to ensure early treatment of ill persons, such as by removing the requirement for laboratory confirmation and by allowing the dispensing of drug via telephone triage, obviating the delay caused by a clinic visit. Where antivirals were used as prophylaxis, it was often in subsets of high-risk persons with likely exposure or in early community outbreaks as a delaying tactic [49,60]. The scarcity of antivirals feared in the planning stages was not a significant factor that shaped the response in countries with stockpiles, although many resource-poor countries had little access to antivirals drugs. In the United States, while the national stockpile was deployed, antivirals were widely available and often obtained through the usual healthcare delivery systems. Despite the general availability of antiviral drugs and absence of widespread shortages, the need for licensed intravenous preparations for the treatment of severely ill persons was a clear lesson from the pandemic. While some preparations were available, they generally required special approvals which delayed treatment.

In general, pandemic planning and exercises conducted in the years before the emergence of the

H1N1pdm09 virus resulted in real benefits to communities affected. Areas of the pandemic response that built on systems used in interpandemic periods, such as surveillance, communications, and vaccine programs, generally fared well during the pandemic. Activities that were initiated during the pandemic or were difficult to exercise were often less effective. The importance of exercising the response components of national plans cannot be overstated; countries with true operational plans generally fared better than those with strategic plans that had not been tested operationally. While an international group of experts that reviewed WHO's response to the pandemic was generally complementary, it noted that the world remained ill-prepared for a severe pandemic [21].

The future of pandemic preparedness

The experiences of 2009–2010 have served to remind public health authorities and the public that influenza pandemics remain totally unpredictable in terms of their timing, origin, epicenter, and severity. Although these facts were well understood long before, the natural tendency was to plan for the possible emergence of an A(H5N1) related pandemic threat, potentially of avian origin and indeed few experts would have bet against that scenario. It is therefore hardly surprising that although pandemic preparedness activity had generally proven useful, there was a widespread acknowledgment that pre-2009 plans lacked flexibility for dealing with less severe scenarios, which now needs to be addressed [63]. Nevertheless, although the 2009–2010 pandemic was not of mainly avian origin, not of the A(H5) hemagglutinin subtype, did not emerge in South-East Asia, and was generally mild, the degree of difficulty experienced in the response related mainly to communications, vaccine logistics, and intensive care capacity reinforces the worth of pandemic preparedness activity [62] and the potential for massive disruption in a severe pandemic. However, many nonhealth components of the national plans were not tested in 2009. Most experts agree that the pandemic threat posed by influenza viruses in the animal kingdom, notably A(H5N1), A(H7N7), A(H7N2), A(H9N2), and A(H2N2), has neither increased nor decreased since 2008. Thus, although it is clear that planning prior to 2009 lacked flexibility to deal with a range of milder scenarios [63], severe scenarios remain equally valid.

Although political support for pandemic preparedness and the eventual response in 2009–2010 had been strong in many countries, there was a degree of pandemic fatigue by mid-2010 when the WHO declared the pandemic over and perhaps a sense among the unwary that pandemics are easy to cope with. Subsequently, the continuing global financial crisis has focused political attention on pressures to control or reduce public spending which, in turn, has somewhat dampened enthusiasm for investment in activities such as pre-pandemic vaccination (where skeptics can argue the choice of vaccine–A(H5N1) – turned out to be wrong) and the establishment or replenishment of antiviral drug stockpiles. However, this attitude is not universal; for example, the UK Cabinet Office continues to rank pandemic influenza as its highest civil emergency threat due to natural events in terms of both likelihood (at some point) and potential impact [63].

Aside from political issues the biggest "forward lesson" from the 2009–2010 pandemic undoubtedly relates to vaccination. The considerable manufacturing success of producing pandemic vaccines within 6 months of the first signs of a pandemic crisis did not alter the fact that in epidemiologic terms, this was too late to be of maximum benefit and reinforces the pressing need for improved cross-reactive vaccines that can be produced and administered in advance of a crisis [29]. Sadly, the global vaccination response to A(H1N1)pdm09 also highlighted inequities in both the distribution and timing of delivery of vaccines that remain to be addressed.

Acknowledgments

Any views expressed in the Work by contributors employed by the United States government at the time of writing do not necessarily represent the views of the United States government, and the contributor's contribution to the Work is not meant to serve as an official endorsement of any statement to the extent that such statement may conflict with any official position of the United States government.

References

1. Thucydides. The Peloponnesian War (Introduction by Finley MI; Translation by Warner R.). London: Penguin Books; 1972.

2. Simpson WJ. A Treatise on Plague Dealing with the Historical, Epidemiological, Clinical, Therapeutic and Preventive Aspects of the Disease. Cambridge: Cambridge University Press; 1905.

3. Cipolla CM. Cristofano and the Plague: A Study in the History of Public Health in the Age of Galileo. Berkeley: University of California Press; 1973.

4. Bell DM, G. World Health Organization Writing. Non-pharmaceutical interventions for pandemic influenza, national and community measures. Emerg Infect Dis. 2006;12(1):88–94.

5. Henderson DA, Courtney B, Inglesby TV, Toner E, Nuzzo JB. Public health and medical responses to the 1957–58 influenza pandemic. Biosecur Bioterror. 2009;7(3):265–73.

6. Tam JS. Influenza A (H5N1) in Hong Kong: an overview. Vaccine. 2002;20(Suppl. 2):S77–81.

7. Horimoto T, Kawaoka Y. Pandemic threat posed by avian influenza A viruses. Clin Microbiol Rev. 2001;14(1):129–49.

8. Abdullah AS, Tomlinson B, Cockram CS, Thomas GN. Lessons from the severe acute respiratory syndrome outbreak in Hong Kong. Emerg Infect Dis. 2003;9(9): 1042–5.

9. Peiris JS, Yu WC, Leung CW, Cheung CY, Ng WF, Nicholls JM, et al. Re-emergence of fatal human influenza A subtype H5N1 disease. Lancet. 2004;363(9409): 617–9.

10. World Health Organization. WHO global influenza preparedness plan. The role of WHO and recommendations for national measures before and during pandemics. 2005. Available from: http://www.who.int/csr/resources/publications/influenza/WHO_CDS_CSR_GIP_2005_5.pdf (accessed 19 February 2013).

11. World Health Organization. WHO checklist for influenza pandmeic preparedness. 2005. Available from: http://www.who.int/csr/resources/publications/influenza/WHO_CDS_CSR_GIP_2005_4/en/ (accessed 19 February 2013).

12. Taubenberger JK, Morens DM. 1918 Influenza: the mother of all pandemics. Emerg Infect Dis. 2006; 12(1):15–22.

13. Nguyen-Van-Tam JS, Hampson AW. The epidemiology and clinical impact of pandemic influenza. Vaccine. 2003;21(16):1762–8.

14. Payne AM. The influenza programme of WHO. Bull World Health Organ. 1953;8(5–6):755–74.

15. Hampson AW. Surveillance for pandemic influenza. J Infect Dis. 1997;176(Suppl. 1):S8–13.

16. World Health Organization. Pandemic Influenza Preparedness and Response. WHO Publication, 2009. p. 1–58.

17. Oshitani H, Kamigaki T, Suzuki A. Major issues and challenges of influenza pandemic preparedness in developing countries. Emerg Infect Dis. 2008;14(6):875–80.

18. US Department of Health and Human Services. HHS Pandemic Influenza Plan. 2005. Available from: http://www.flu.gov/planning-preparedness/federal/hhspandemicinfluenzaplan.pdf (accessed 19 February 2013).

19. Nicoll A, Ammon A, Amato Gauci A, Ciancio B, Zucs P, Devaux I, et al. Experience and lessons from surveillance and studies of the 2009 pandemic in Europe. Public Health. 2010;124(1):14–23.

20. World Health Organization. International Health Regulations: (2005). 2nd ed. Lyon, France: World Health Organization; 2008. p. 1.

21. World Health Organization. Implementation of the International Health Regulations (2005): Report of the Review Committee on the Functioning of the International Health Regulations (2005) in relation to Pandemic (H1N1) 2009. Geneva, Switzerland: World Health Organization; 2011. p. 1. Available from: http://apps.who.int/gb/ebwha/pdf_files/WHA64/A64_10-en.pdf (accessed 25 February 2013).

22. Monto AS. Vaccines and antiviral drugs in pandemic preparedness. Emerg Infect Dis. 2006;12(1):55–60.

23. Greene SK, Shay DK, Yin R, McCarthy NL, Baxter R, Jackson ML, et al. Patterns in influenza antiviral medication use before and during the 2009 H1N1 pandemic, Vaccine Safety Datalink Project, 2000–2010. Influenza Other Respi Viruses. 2012;6:143–51.

24. Hurt AC, Hardie K, Wilson NJ, Deng YM, Osbourn M, Gehrig N, et al. Community transmission of oseltamivir-resistant A(H1N1)pdm09 influenza. N Engl J Med. 2011;365(26):2541–2.

25. Pebody RG, Harris R, Kafatos G, Chamberland M, Campbell C, Nguyen-Van-Tam JS, et al. Use of antiviral drugs to reduce household transmission of pandemic (H1N1) 2009, United Kingdom. Emerg Infect Dis. 2011;17(6):990–9.

26. Department of Health Pandemic Influenza Preparedness Team. UK Influenza Pandemic Preparedness Strategy. 2011. London, UK. p. 1–70. Available from: http://www.dh.gov.uk/prod_consum_dh/groups/dh_digitalassets/documents/digitalasset/dh_131040.pdf (accessed 19 February 2013).

27. Muthuri SG, Myles PR, Venkatesan S, Leonardi-Bee J, Nguyen-Van-Tam JS. Impact of neuraminidase inhibitor treatment on outcomes of public health importance during the 2009–2010 influenza A(H1N1) pandemic: a

28. Jennings LC, Monto AS, Chan PK, Szucs TD, Nicholson KG. Stockpiling prepandemic influenza vaccines: a new cornerstone of pandemic preparedness plans. Lancet Infect Dis. 2008;8(10):650–8.

29. Carrasco P, Leroux-Roels G. Pandemic vaccines. In: Van-Tam J, Sellwood C, editors. Pandemic Influenza, 2nd edn. Wallingford: CABI; 2012. p. 139–51.

30. El Sahly HM, Keitel WA. Pandemic H5N1 influenza vaccine development: an update. Expert Rev Vaccines. 2008;7(2):241–7.

31. World Health Organization. Global pandemic influenza action plan to increase vaccine supply. WHO Publication, 2006. Available from: http://www.who.int/csr/resources/publications/influenza/WHO_CDS_EPR_GIP_2006_1/en/index.html (accessed 25 February 2013).

32. Friede M, Palkonyay L, Alfonso C, Pervikov Y, Torelli G, Wood D, et al. WHO initiative to increase global and equitable access to influenza vaccine in the event of a pandemic: supporting developing country production capacity through technology transfer. Vaccine. 2011;29 (Suppl. 1):A2–7.

33. Brundage JF. Interactions between influenza and bacterial respiratory pathogens: implications for pandemic preparedness. Lancet Infect Dis. 2006;6:303–12.

34. Gupta RK, George R, Nguyen-Van-Tam JS. Bacterial pneumonia and pandemic influenza planning. Emerg Infect Dis. 2008;14(8):1187–92.

35. Van-Tam J, Lim WS. Pharmaceutical interventions. In: Van-Tam J, Sellwood C, editors. Pandemic Influenza, 2nd edn. Wallingford: CABI; 2012. p. 122–38.

36. Crowe S, Utley M, Walker G, Grove P, Pagel C. A model to evaluate mass vaccination against pneumococcus as a countermeasure against pandemic influenza. Vaccine. 2011;29(31):5065–77.

37. Centers for Disease Control and Prevention (CDC). Interim Pre-pandemic Planning Guidance: Community Strategy for Pandemic Influenza Mitigation in the United States – Early, Targeted, Layered Use of Nonpharmaceutical Interventions, US Department of Health and Human Services. 2007. p. 1–97.

38. Ferguson NM, Cummings DA, Fraser C, Cajka JC, Cooley PC, Burke DS. Strategies for mitigating an influenza pandemic. Nature. 2006;442(7101):448–52.

39. Markel H, Lipman HB, Navarro JA, Sloan A, Michalsen JR, Stern AM, et al. Nonpharmaceutical interventions implemented by US cities during the 1918–1919 influenza pandemic. JAMA. 2007;298(6):644–54.

40. Cowling BJ, Zhou Y, Ip DK, Leung GM, Aiello AE. Face masks to prevent transmission of influenza virus: a systematic review. Epidemiol Infect. 2010;138(4):449–56.

41. Aledort JE, Lurie N, Wasserman J, Bozzette SA. Non-pharmaceutical public health interventions for pandemic influenza: an evaluation of the evidence base. BMC Public Health. 2007;7:208.

42. Cauchemez S, Ferguson NM, Wachtel C, Tegnell A, Saour G, Duncan B, et al. Closure of schools during an influenza pandemic. Lancet Infect Dis. 2009;9(8):473–81.

43. Department of Health. Pandemic flu: a national framework for responding to an influenza pandemic. 2007. Available from: http://www.dh.gov.uk/en/Publicationsandstatistics/Publications/PublicationsPolicyAndGuidance/DH_080734 (accessed 19 February2013).

44. Kuster SP, Shah PS, Coleman BL, Lam PP, Tong A, Wormsbecker A, et al. Incidence of influenza in healthy adults and healthcare workers: a systematic review and meta-analysis. PLoS ONE. 2011;6(10):e26239.

45. Brankston G, Gitterman L, Hirji Z, Lemieux C, Gardam M. Transmission of influenza A in human beings. Lancet Infect Dis. 2007;7(4):257–65.

46. Tellier R. Review of aerosol transmission of influenza A virus. Emerg Infect Dis. 2006;12(11):1657–62.

47. Bin-Reza F, Lopez Chavarrias V, Nicoll A, Chamberland ME. The use of masks and respirators to prevent transmission of influenza: a systematic review of the scientific evidence. Influenza Other Respi Viruses. 2012;6(4):257–67.

48. Blank PR, Szucs TD. Socio-economic impact. In: Van-Tam J, Sellwood C, editors. Pandemic Influenza, 2nd edn. Wallingford: CABI; 2012. p. 173–80.

49. Nicoll A, Lopez Chavarrias V. National and international public health measures. In: Van-Tam J, Sellwood C, editors. Pandemic Influenza, 2nd edn. Wallingford: CABI; 2012. p. 152–63.

50. Simpson J. The role of exercises in pandemic preparedness. In: Van-Tam J, Sellwood C, editors. Pandemic Influenza, 2nd edn. Wallingford: CABI; 2012. p. 97–103.

51. Gadd EM. Ethical issues related to pandemic preparedness and response. In: Van-Tam J, Sellwood C, editors. Pandemic Influenza, 2nd edn. Wallingford: CABI; 2012. p. 181–8.

52. Abraham T, Pople D. Pandemic communications. In: Van-Tam J, Sellwood C, editors. Pandemic Influenza, 2nd edn. Wallingford: CABI; 2012. p. 189–97.

53. Centers for Disease Control and Prevention (CDC). Swine influenza A (H1N1) infection in two children – Southern California, March–April 2009. Morb Mortal Wkly Rep. 2009;58:400–2.

54. Presidential Advisors on Science and Technology. Report to the President on US preparations for 2009-H1N1 influenza, Executive Office of the President. 2009. p. 1–86.

55. World Health Organization. Global Influenza Surveillance and Response System (GISRS). 2012. Available

The first partial entry at top left:

systematic review and meta-analysis in hospitalized patients. J Infect Dis. 2013;207(4):553–63.

from: http://www.who.int/influenza/gisrs_laboratory/en/ (accessed 19 February 2013).

56. World Health Organization. World now at the start of 2009 influenza pandemic. 2009. Available from: http://www.who.int/mediacentre/news/statements/2009/h1n1_pandemic_phase6_20090611/en/index.html (accessed 19 February 2013).

57. Van Kerkhove MD, Vandemaele KA, Shinde V, Jaramillo-Gutierrez G, Koukounari A, Donnelly CA, et al. Risk factors for severe outcomes following 2009 influenza A (H1N1) infection: a global pooled analysis. PLoS Med. 2011;8(7):e1001053.

58. Centers for Disease Control and Prevention. Interim results: influenza A (H1N1) 2009 monovalent and seasonal influenza vaccination coverage among health-care personnel – United States, August 2009–January 2010. MMWR Morb Mortal Wkly Rep. 2010;59(12): 357–62.

59. World Health Organization. WHO global technical consultation: global standards and tools for influenza surveillance. 2011. Available from: http://www.who.int/influenza/resources/documents/technical_consultation/en/index.html (accessed 19 February 2013).

60. Australia Government, Department of Health and Ageing. Review of Australia's Health Sector Response to Pandemic (H1N1) 2009: Lessons Identified. 2011: Canberra. Available from: http://www.flupandemic.gov.au/internet/panflu/publishing.nsf/Content/review-2011/$File/lessons%20identified-oct11.pdf (accessed 19 February 2013).

61. Partridge J, Kieny MP; World Health Organization H1N1 influenza vaccine Task Force. Global production of seasonal and pandemic (H1N1) influenza vaccines in 2009–2010 and comparison with previous estimates and global action plan targets. Vaccine. 2010;28(30): 4709–12.

62. Hashim A, Jean-Gilles L, Hegermann-Lindencrone M, Shaw I, Brown C, Nguyen-Van-Tam J. Did pandemic preparedness aid the response to pandemic (H1N1) 2009? A qualitative analysis in seven countries within the WHO European Region. J Infect Public Health. 2012;5:286–96.

63. Cabinet Office. National Risk Register of Civil Emergencies 2012 edition. 2012. Available from: http://www.cabinetoffice.gov.uk/resource-library/national-risk-register (accessed 19 February 2013).

29 Influenza: The future

Thomas J. Braciale

Carter Immunology Center, University of Virginia School of Medicine, Charlottesville, VA, USA

Whence come we?
What are we?
Whither go we?

Paul Gauguin (1897)

When he looked and saw the traveler in the city square the old man asked, "Where are you going? Where did you come from?"

Judges 19:17

What can we predict about the encounter between influenza virus and humanity in the future? One answer to this question comes, not from this textbook, but from the history books. Influenza has likely been a fellow traveler with the human race throughout recorded history. The historical record contains descriptions of outbreaks of respiratory illness whose symptoms are characteristic of pandemic influenza – most notably the classic description of such an outbreak in 1658 by the Oxford physician and neuroanatomist, Thomas Willis [1]. Similarly, there is evidence suggesting periodic outbreaks of pandemic influenza infection in the eighteenth and nineteenth centuries [2]. The implication of history is that influenza virus will be with us in the future and that pandemic outbreaks will occur, again and again in the future, without effective intervention.

This textbook is designed to provide the reader with the full spectrum of current knowledge of influenza virus, ranging from basic molecular virology to the epidemiology and economic impact of influenza infection. Along with the knowledge comes controversy and uncertainty, the potential implications of which bear on our ability to predict future influenza outbreaks, as well as to prevent, treat, and monitor influenza infection. In this chapter, we address several controversial topics that directly impact on our encounter with influenza in the future.

The next influenza pandemic

There is general agreement that influenza is an avian virus which has in the past adapted to replicate and transmit in mammals, most notably humans, and continues to adapt and infect humans. As discussed elsewhere in this textbook (see Chapter 2), we have incontrovertible evidence for at least four influenza A pandemics over the last century. These pandemics were produced by viruses of the H1N1, H2N2, and H3N2 subtypes [3]. However, because of the large number of distinct influenza A subtypes within avian species, it was possible that one or more of these avian influenza subtypes could acquire the ability to

Textbook of Influenza, Second Edition. Edited by Robert G. Webster, Arnold S. Monto, Thomas J. Braciale, and Robert A. Lamb.
© 2013 John Wiley & Sons, Ltd. Published 2013 by John Wiley & Sons, Ltd.

infect and transmit in humans, thereby representing the next pandemic threat.

Following the outbreak in domestic poultry of highly pathogenic avian H5N1 infection with sporadic infection of humans in Hong Kong in 1996, there has been great concern among public health officials, influenza virologists, and government officials that this highly virulent H5N1 subtype virus could adapt to infect and, equally importantly, transmit efficiently from human to human, resulting in the next human influenza A pandemic.

Consequently, the outbreak of pandemic influenza A H1N1 infection in 2009 was in some respects unanticipated. Influenza A H1N1 viruses had been co-circulating with the dominant H3N2 subtype epidemic virus strains since 1977; one would anticipate that there would be sufficient herd immunity to limit the transmission of any new H1N1 epidemic strain introduced into the human population from a zoonotic source (e.g., pigs or birds). This 2009 H1N1 pandemic points out our lack of real insight and knowledge into the process of adaptation of avian viruses for efficient replication in the mammalian respiratory epithelium, the genetic changes in the virus that allow efficient person-to-person transmission, and the limitations in our understanding of the human immune response to the virus whose job is to limit virus replication and spread.

So, researchers (as well as public health officials and government officials) are at a crossroads. Should efforts be focused on understanding the mechanism(s) by which highly pathogenic avian H5N1 viruses produce disease in humans, defining the virus genetic signature(s) that will result in efficient person-to-person transmission of avian H5N1 virus and stockpiling of vaccine for administration following an outbreak of virus transmissible in humans?

On the other hand, while there is no definitive evidence for a prior influenza pandemic produced by H5N1 viruses, we can say with absolute certainty that a virus of the H2N2 subtype produced an influenza pandemic in 1957 and variants of this influenza A subtype persisted and circulated through the human population until 1968 when it was replaced by the outbreak of pandemic H3N2 subtype infection in 1968. Should our efforts be focused on preparing for the inevitable re-emergence of the human H2N2 subtype virus in the future? Individuals aged 45 or under have not experienced infection with viruses of

the H2N2 subtype and infection of this demographic with an H2N2 pandemic virus with the pathogenicity of the 1918 pandemic virus would have dire social and economic consequences.

Highly pathogenic avian H5N1 subtype viruses have spread via waterfowl through a large portion of the globe over the past 15 years. These viruses, in principle, have had ample opportunity to "jump" into the human population, but there is no definitive evidence for the evolution of these viruses toward efficient human-to-human transmission. This could reflect effective surveillance measures and aggressive measures to prevent infection of domestic poultry (and livestock). Alternatively, maybe H5N1 is not the next "big one." That is, maybe H5N1 subtype viruses and, in particular, the H5 hemagglutinnin cannot mutate to transmissibility in humans and retain the high pathogenicity of H5N1 subtype strains. Are we prepared to accept the risk and possible consequences of adhering to this alternative viewpoint? If there are only three influenza A virus subtypes (H1N1, H2N2, and H3N2) capable of efficiently infecting and transmitting within the human population, should our resources and efforts be focused on preventing or at least monitoring the re-emergence of a pandemic H2N2 subtype virus?

Genetic engineering, influenza, and dual-use research of concern

The development of genetic techniques to reverse engineer influenza virus (see Chapter 9) along with advances in high throughput viral genome sequencing have revolutionized the study of influenza virus biology in areas as diverse as virus surveillance, viral pathogenesis, and vaccine design. Particularly exciting is the possibility of employing reverse genetics techniques to identify the viral genes, or more precisely clusters of genes, that confer the ability of the virus to infect and replicate efficiently to high titer in the human upper and lower respiratory tracts and which confer transmissibility from human to human.

While the application of elegant techniques like reverse genetics to address fundamental questions in influenza biology and pathogenesis is both exciting and elegant, the application of this technology to address such fundamental questions can have unintended consequences. Recently, two laboratories applied this technology to determine if highly pathogenic avian H5N1 virus can be engineered to transmit efficiently by the aerosol route in mammals. The findings from these laboratories, which demonstrated the ability of avian H5N1 virus to be engineered for transmissibility in mammals, raised important issues of biosafety and bioterrorism resulting in the embargo from publication of these findings for approximately 6 months [4,5] and considerable debate (e.g., *Science*, volume 336, 22 June 2012) as to the justification and merits of carrying out research which could be of value and importance for human health, but, at the same time, could lead to the development of an agent of mass destruction. Such research goes by the acronym DURC (dual-use research of concern). The many issues raised by this research led to a call for a moratorium on research to adapt H5N1 virus into a highly transmissible virus with the potential for pandemic spread.

The DURC issue goes well beyond the study of influenza and impacts on fundamental principles ranging from the free dissemination of ideas and scientific integrity to national security. In considering the research on highly pathogenic avian H5N1 virus, a strong case can be made that defining the genetic changes associated with the virulence and transmissibility in humans is key, both for surveillance in the field as these viruses evolve in nature and for understanding influenza pathogenesis. Can we risk the potential for an accidental release from the research laboratory into the environment of a genetically engineered highly pathogenic and readily transmissible virus as a byproduct of influenza research? Is it legitimate to withhold information on the construction and properties of such viruses as a deterrent to bioterrorism? Do we compromise our ability to understand the biology of influenza virus by carrying out experiments exclusively aimed at loss of function (i.e., loss of virulence and/or transmissibility)? Should there be a permanent moratorium on research dealing with gain of function (e.g., enhanced transmissibility) when dealing with highly pathogenic organisms like avian H5N1 virus? What should be the role of government and the private sector in this decision-making? These are some of the questions and challenges that face influenza research in the future.

Public health: Harnessing the social network

Among the many lessons of the influenza A pandemic of 2009 (see Chapter 2) is the realization that, because of modern transportation, in particular air travel, a newly emergent lethal influenza strain with pandemic potential (efficient transmissibility and high virulence) could circumnavigate the globe in a matter of days if not hours. A stylized, but not completely inaccurate description of such an outbreak is found in Steven Soderbergh's 2011 film *Contagion*. The combination of high-speed global travel, population growth, and urbanization conspire to facilitate the spread of a virus with pandemic potential. This reality poses profound, and some might say, insurmountable challenges for the public health community, for governments, and ultimately for the social order. Conventional approaches to monitoring the spread of infection and therefore our ability to control the spread of disease will likely be inadequate in the face of this new reality.

Is there a way out of this conundrum? Can the technologic advances that gave us the possibility of engineering influenza viruses also allow us to deal effectively with the public health threat posed by high-speed travel and urbanization? One potential solution is posited by the instantaneous speed and connectivity of social network sites (e.g., Facebook and Twitter). Can we harness the social network to allow us to determine in real-time the extent and rapidity of spread of an influenza pandemic? While this concept may appear to be far-fetched, Christakis and Fowler [6] have recently reported evidence to suggest the importance of a social network as a potential tool in the early detection and spread of an influenza pandemic. These investigators demonstrated that, by monitoring of the friends of randomly selected university undergraduate students for the onset and duration of symptoms during the 2009 H1N1 influenza pandemic, they were able to detect the onset, progression, and peak of the outbreak well in advance of the population as a whole.

Christakis and Fowler lay out strategies that could be employed to monitor the health of the defined population (e.g., university students or even a nation) employing a social network. Clearly, the ability to monitor in real-time the onset and spread of an influenza outbreak would allow us to utilize vaccination and, perhaps more importantly, antiviral treatment and prophylaxis strategies in the most optimal way – particularly as observed in the 2009 influenza pandemic when vaccine and antiviral drugs were in limited supply.

New drug targets

Advances in molecular and in particular structural biology, along with comparable advances in synthetic chemistry, have allowed researchers to identify microbial gene products that can serve as targets for therapeutic intervention with drugs. Striking examples of the success of "rational drug design" are the drug combinations directed to several distinct gene products employed in the control of HIV infection and of course the neuraminidase inhibitors used to treat influenza infection. As discussed in this textbook (see Chapters 24 and 25), research is ongoing to identify additional drug targets among the constellation of influenza gene products (e.g., the polymerase–transcriptase complex). As new targets within the influenza genome are identified, we can imagine a time when a cocktail of inhibitory drugs directed to different influenza targets will be routinely employed in influenza therapeutics. Whether this strategy of combination chemotherapy will eliminate the emergence of resistance variants, as observed for current influenza drug therapies, remains to be determined.

An emerging area of research is to identify and target for drug therapy host cell machinery supporting virus replication (e.g. [7,8]). This is a challenging area for obvious reasons; because inhibition of essential functions simultaneously utilized by the virus and the host could result in a cellular dysfunction or even cell death. Cellular machinery involved in the uptake of virus or virion assemblies are potential targets for drug development. An attractive feature of this approach is the potential for a "one-size-fits-all" drug. That is, for viruses like influenza which enter and uncoat in the endosome, a drug that blocks a critical step in that process would, in principle, be useful in the treatment of infection with several different classes of viruses. More realistically, different class of viruses using the same pathway of entry (e.g., endosome) and assembly (e.g., viral constituent assembly at the plasma membrane) are likely to have nuanced differences in their utilization of cellular constituents. Consequently, if critical cellular targets for drug therapy can be identified, the targets, and therefore the drugs, would most likely be virus specific.

Prospects for the "universal vaccine"

The best defense against influenza infection is not to get infected. More realistically, if someone is exposed to and infected by influenza, the preferred outcome is that the infection is subclinical. That is, virus replication should be minimal, resulting in an asymptomatic infection with no human-to-human transmission. In principle, an effective influenza vaccine should result in minimal virus replication and no spread.

The Holy Grail of influenza vaccinology is a vaccine that can protect against any influenza strain independent of type or subtype, shift or drift. A vaccine targets the adaptive immune system (B and T lymphocytes) because this component of the host immune response has the "memory" to respond rapidly and robustly to infection following prior vaccination.

A universal vaccine tailored to B lymphocytes would most likely stimulate neutralizing antibodies directed towards the hemagglutinin. In this textbook, the response of B lymphocytes to influenza virus has been discussed both from a mechanistic standpoint (see Chapter 18) and from the perspective of the antibody response of humans to influenza vaccine (see Chapter 20), as well as novel vaccination strategies that could produce antibodies to the influenza hemagglutinin capable of neutralizing influenza A strains across multiple subtypes (see Chapter 21). These vaccination strategies are based on insights obtained through the application of modern molecular and structural biology. They relied on the identification of influenza A specific antisera and, more importantly, monoclonal antibodies isolated from humans and experimental animals which neutralized influenza A strains of more than one hemagglutinnin subtype. The availability of these reagents allowed investigators to identify the site(s) on the hemagglutinnin recognized by these heterosubtypic monoclonal antibodies.

If conserved sites displayed on multiple hemagglutinin subtypes are immunogenic, why does not the majority of the population, either by vaccination or infection, produce these antibodies in abundance, which would then make them resistant to pandemic (or seasonal) influenza? There is no clear-cut answer to this question. One possibility is that these conserved hemagglutinnin epitopes are normally not displayed efficiently or presented efficiently to B lymphocytes with the appropriate immunoglobulin receptor. Such an explanation means that a vaccine that displays the conserved hemagglutinin site in the proper conformation and in appropriate abundance would work effectively as a universal vaccine. Another possibility is that the majority of the population lacks B lymphocytes capable of efficiently recognizing the conserved region(s) of the hemagglutinin. In this case, the prospects for a universal vaccine become more problematic.

In contrast to B lymphocytes, it was demonstrated more than 30 years ago that T lymphocytes can recognize conserved epitopes shared by influenza A strains across multiple subtypes. These T lymphocytes are directed primarily to conserved sites on influenza internal virion proteins (i.e., the NP, M, and polymerase proteins). The existence of these heterosubtypic T cells raises the question: why is no protection from pandemic (or indeed even seasonal) influenza afforded by these cross-reactive T cells? As discussed in this textbook (see Chapter 19), T lymphocytes circulate as quiescent primary or memory small lymphocytes which must be activated for the T cells to exhibit their effector activity. As the activation of these memory small lymphocytes can take from 2–5 days following infection of a vaccinated individual, infection is established and virus is potentially transmitted prior to the action of these activated effector T lymphocytes to control virus replication in the respiratory tract. This fact does not preclude an important role for these heterosubtypic effector T lymphocytes in controlling the replication and ultimately facilitating the elimination of seasonal or pandemic influenza virus. Presumably, to utilize these cross-reactive T lymphocytes effectively, a universal vaccine facilitates the persist-

ence of these heterosubtypic effector T cells continuously in the respiratory tract following vaccination. Whether such an approach is feasible without unintended pathologic consequences to the vaccine is unclear.

Is the end in sight?

Can we realistically foresee the end to human influenza infection in the twenty-first century? In principle, yes. Vaccinologists point to the success of the polio and smallpox vaccine programs, with the elimination of polio from the Western Hemisphere and the complete eradication of smallpox worldwide as glowing examples of the possibility of control of virus infection and even elimination. Undoubtedly, the most effective way to control and prevent influenza infection is by vaccination.

The success of "ring vaccination" following smallpox outbreaks in containing infection and therefore in the ultimate eradication of this pathogen was in part predicated upon the relatively slow replication and transmission of the virus. By contrast, influenza replicates rapidly and is not only transmitted by fomites and contact, but also by the aerosol route. Ring vaccination is consequently unrealistic and the best hope of containing a new pandemic outbreak (assuming that surveillance could detect the emergence of the new pandemic strain early enough in its progression) would be "ring prophylaxis" with antiviral drugs.

The remarkable success of the live-attenuated oral polio vaccine in controlling polio was based on the ability of the vaccine to stimulate the potent local mucosal immune response and the capacity of the passively shed live virus to infect and thereby immunize individuals not actively vaccinated. The live-attenuated influenza vaccine can stimulate local humoral and cellular immune responses, but the developments of a vaccine strain capable of transmitting from individual to individual would pose the very unlikely but still unacceptable risk of mutation to virulence.

The prospects for a universal vaccine were greatly strengthened by the finding that heterosubtype-specific antibodies against the hemagglutinin were demonstrable in the human and the conserved sites recognized by the antibodies identifiable. The challenge now is to engineer these conserved sites into a vaccine platform which will expand the range of individuals capable of producing heterosubtype-specific antibodies following vaccination. It is to be hoped that in the future these advances in adjuvant development will deal with the problems of vaccine efficacy in very young children and in the elderly – two of the most vulnerable segments of the population to severe influenza disease. Both successful engineering of conserved influenza hemagglutinin epitopes and the advances in adjuvant efficacy will require a deeper understanding of the basic mechanism of the innate and adaptive immune responses.

An obvious concern for the prospect of a universal vaccine is whether the virus will mutate under the selective pressure of antibody produced in response to the universal vaccine and generate escaped variants with alterations in these otherwise highly conserved regions of the hemagglutinin. Further experimentation will be necessary to address this important issue.

What will be the future if a vaccine (or antiviral drug) strategy is devised that successfully eliminates influenza infection in the human population? Will it also be necessary to vaccinate domestic poultry and livestock? Will that lead to the elimination of influenza as has been demonstrated with smallpox? Unlike smallpox (or polio), influenza is a zoonotic virus, and the reservoir of virus present in the wild bird populations of the world will represent the continuing potential threat to human population, thus requiring continued vigilance in the form of surveillance and prophylactic vaccination for the foreseeable future.

References

1. Thompson ES. Influenza, Or Epidemic Catarrhal Fever: an Historical Survey of Past Epidemics in Great Britain from 1510 to 1890. London: Percival and Co.; 1890.
2. Potter CW. A history of influenza. J Appl Microbiol. 2001;91(4):572–9.
3. Flahault A, Zylberman P. Influenza pandemics: past, present and future challenges. Public Health Rev. 2010; 32:319–40.
4. Imai M, Watanabe T, Hatta M, Das SC, Ozawa M, Shinya K, et al. Experimental adaptation of an influenza H5 HA confers respiratory droplet transmission to a reassortant H5 HA/H1N1 virus in ferrets. Nature. 2012;486(7403):420–8.
5. Herfst S, Schrauwen EJ, Linster M, Chutinimitkul S, de Wit E, Munster VJ, et al. Airborne transmission of influenza A/H5N1 virus between ferrets. Science. 2012; 336(6088):1534–41.
6. Christakis NA, Fowler JH. Social network sensors for early detection of contagious outbreaks. PLoS ONE. 2010;5(9):e12948.
7. Lingappa VR, Hurt CR, Garvey E. Capsid assembly as a point of intervention for novel anti-viral therapeutics. Curr Pharm Biotechnol. 2012 Mar 20. [Epub ahead of print].
8. Meliopoulos VA, Andersen LE, Birrer KF, Simpson KJ, Lowenthal JW, Bean AG, et al. Host gene targets for novel influenza therapies elucidated by high-throughput RNA interference screens. FASEB J. 2012;26(4): 1372–86.

PART 8

The outbreak of H7N9

30 Appendix

Thomas J. Braciale[1] and Robert G. Webster[2]

[1]Carter Immunology Center, University of Virginia School of Medicine, Charlottesville, VA, USA

[2]Department of Infectious Diseases, Division of Virology, St. Jude Children's Research Hospital, Memphis, TN, USA

An outbreak of influenza H7N9 in China: Implications for influenza evolution and pandemic preparedness

Influenza is an emerging disease which requires constant vigilance on the part of the public health and medical community as well as effective and aggressive pandemic preparedness procedures in place. At the time of final preparation of the first edition of this *Textbook of Influenza* in 1997 an outbreak of infection of domestic poultry with highly pathogenic avian influenza (HPAI) H5N1 occurred in Hong Kong in 1997 which was transmissible to humans with close contact to infected poultry flocks and resulted in high mortality in infected humans. The initial phase of this outbreak of HPAI influenza A virus (H5N1) infection was the subject of an Appendix to the first edition of this Textbook and the response to and implications of this initial H5N1 outbreak and subsequent outbreaks are discussed throughout this second edition of the Textbook.

As the galley proofs of the Chapters for the second edition of the *Textbook of Influenza* are in final preparation, in an ironic twist of fate, we are experiencing another outbreak of avian influenza infection transmissible to humans in China, in this instance, infection with a novel avian influenza A H7N9 virus. At

the time that this appendix Chapter is being finalized, documented infections of humans with the H7N9 virus have been recognized for less than two months. Consequently, vital information on the sequence of the H7N9 virus genome (isolated from humans, domestic poultry and in the preliminary stages of analyses in experimental mammalian hosts undergoing infection with this virus), the possibility of efficient human to human transmission of the virus as well as the extent to which the virus has infected poultry within China (and potentially elsewhere) is limited or as yet unavailable. Thus, in this Chapter, we will focus on known or likely properties of the virus, the pattern of human infection and the similarities and differences apparent between this avian influenza A and outbreaks with other Influenza A viruses with pandemic potential, for example, influenza A virus H5N1.

The cases of human infection

On April 1, 2013, the World Health Organization (WHO) reported three cases of human infection with a novel influenza A H7N9 virus in China. The WHO was notified by the China National Health and Family Planning Commission following the confirmation by

---

Textbook of Influenza, Second Edition. Edited by Robert G. Webster, Arnold S. Monto, Thomas J. Braciale, and Robert A. Lamb.

the Chinese Center for Disease Control and Prevention of two fatal cases of Influenza A H7N9 in late February and early March 2013 [1–3]. These initial cases were localized to Shanghai but by April 2, seven people from Shanghai and the eastern Chinese provinces of Jiangsu and Anhui were infected. While Shanghai and the East Central Chinese provinces along the Yangtze River have been the major sites where human infections have been documented, more recently several cases have been reported in Beijing and Northeast China. At present, there have been no cases reported in southern China. The number of cases increased to 24 by the end of the first week of April. As of April 21, 2013 there have been 108 documented cases of human H7N9 infection with 21 fatalities directly attributed to the infection. This is a case fatality rate (~20%–25%) slightly lower than that observed for documented human HPAI H5N1 infections (~50%–60%) but considerably greater than that observed in the 2009 H1N1 pandemic.

Since influenza A H7N9 virus is a low pathogenic virus in domestic poultry, morbidity and mortality in poultry flocks is not an indicator of H7N9 infected poultry as it is for infection of gallinaceous poultry by H5N1. While the majority of those with documented H7N9 have had direct contact with infected poultry, for example, in poultry markets or farms, up to 40% of infected individuals report no direct contact with poultry. For example, in the first two cases reported there was no contact with poultry (or domesticated birds) but contact with pigs was noted [1,2]. The percentage human infections with direct contact with poultry or poultry products will likely increase when more detailed and rigorous epidemiologic assessment of exposure to this virus is obtained. There is one report (not as yet independently verified) from Beijing of the isolation of the H7N9 virus from an asymptomatic young child who appeared to have no direct exposure to domestic poultry but whose older sibling was hospitalized for H7N9 infection. Nevertheless, there is no direct epidemiological evidence for efficient human to human transmission of the virus *at this time*. However, even if efficient human to human is never established for this virus strain, H7N9 virus infection would nevertheless remain a potentially important threat to humans through routine exposure of the human population to infected but asymptomatic domestic poultry particularly in countries like China and Southeast Asian

nations. At present, there is no evidence for spread of H7N9 infection outside of China.

Susceptibility to infection and pattern of disease

Human infections with HPAI H5N1 virus were distributed across age ranges with a bias towards more severe lower respiratory tract infections in young adults. The very minimal information on the relationship between age of the affected individual and disease severity currently available suggest that severe and potentially fatal infections with H7N9 virus may be much more frequent in the elderly, that is >60 years old with infected young children displaying much more mild disease. Again, this impression awaits additional rigorous epidemiological analysis. However, an apparent increase in disease severity in the elderly, if true, may not necessarily reflect a unique or novel feature of H7N9 virus but simply reflect the presence of comorbidities in the elderly which would increase the potential for respiratory compromise and result in clinically more severe infections.

Autopsy results from fatal cases of H7N9 virus infection are not yet available. Consequently, it is not as yet possible to determine if the cause of fatal infections was primary viral pneumonia (as characteristically observed in human H5N1 infections) or a consequence of bacterial superinfection (as suggested for a significant fraction of lethal infections in the 1918 H1N1 Spanish influenza pandemic).

The clinical presentation of patients with severe H7N9 virus infection appears to be similar to severe H5N1 infection, that is, progressive diffuse lung inflammation resulting in progressive severe hypoxemia and the development of acute respiratory distress syndrome (ARDS) with multi-system (multi-organ) failure [1,2].

The virus

Sequence information is becoming available on several non-human H7N9 isolates (including avian) and on at least two of the human H7N9 isolates [2–4]. The human and nonhuman H7N9 isolates have identical sequences at the HA receptor binding pocket, suggesting preferential binding to the human cellular virus receptors: α2-6 linked sialic acids. The human H7N9 isolates also had the characteristic PB2-627K mutation linked to efficient virus growth in human cells while the non-human isolates sequenced so far, displayed the PB2-627E at this position. Whether the presence of the 627K residue in the PB2 and an HA sequence which confers preferential binding to the virus receptor on human cells is sufficient to facilitate transmissibility in mammals remains to be determined. The presence of these genomic alterations in the human H7N9 isolates sequenced so far suggests that these viruses have properties which would be conducive to adaptation to efficient mammalian transmission by respiratory droplets. In this connection it is worthwhile to point out that the transmission rate of the H7N9 virus from poultry to humans appears to date to be much faster than the rate of transmission of H5N1. This property may, in principle, increase the risk of selection of variant virus capable of efficient human to human transmission.

Preliminary evidence suggests that the human isolates of the H7N9 virus are sensitive to neuraminidase inhibitors. Consequently, early effective intervention and control of infection employing this class of antiviral drugs is feasible.

As noted the H7N9 is an LPAI virus for domestic poultry and appears to produce an asymptomatic infection. Thus, the epidemiology of virus spread and potential exposure of humans to infected poultry cannot be tracked based on the lethality of the virus in domestic poultry. As noted in Chapter 10, Pathogenesis, HPAI viruses of related subtypes, H7N3, H7N7 and LPAI H9N2 have been reported to infect humans at a low frequency with moderate to severe symptoms with H7 HPAI viruses and mild disease symptoms with H9N2.

The H9N2 LPAI virus circulating in avian species may prove to be of more than passing interest in the evolution of avian influenza viruses with the capacity to produce severe and widespread disease in humans. Emerging sequence information suggests that the H9N2 virus may have provided the genetic "backbone" in the generation of the H7N9 (and the H5N1) virus. In particular, the finding that six of the H7N9 genes (including the NP, M and polymerase genes) show extremely high sequence homology with that of the H9N2 virus [2–4] raises the possibility that H7N9 may be a triple reassortant using the H9N2 virus as a backbone with contribution of genes from other

virus strains. Therefore, even if the H7N9 LPAI virus proves to have limited potential for spread throughout the human population, it will be important to establish if the H9N2 can serve as a common template for the development of reassortant viruses with human pandemic potential and therefore to track the spread of H9N2 among avian species.

H7N9 and pandemic preparedness

The H7N9 avian influenza exhibits two of the properties required for pandemic spread: capacity for efficient replication in human cells and the lack of pre-existing immunity to this or related virus strains. If the emerging clinical, epidemiological and genome sequence data supports the view that this is an influenza A subtype prone to produce a variant capable of efficient human to human transmission then there must be concerted action globally by governments and health agencies to prevent as well as prepare for this potential outcome.

The effective elimination of H5N1 virus in Hong Kong by eliminating poultry markets and the destruction of infected or potentially infected poultry flocks in Hong Kong and South China points the way to effective control of H7N9 virus. However, as noted above, culling of infected poultry or an aggressive program of poultry vaccination is problematic when infection is produced by a virus strain with low pathogenicity for the likely immediate animal reservoir. In this regard, it should be emphasized that at present it is not certain whether transmission of the H7N9 virus to humans is primarily through contact with poultry, domesticated birds, or pigs and whether the H7N9 virus reservoir is avian or mammalian.

As with H5N1 infection, we now begin the long process of understanding the epidemiology and pathogenesis of the H7N9 virus as well as defining its host range and identifying the immediate and remote reservoirs.

An early perspective!

Are we witnessing the emergence of a truly novel influenza A virus with greater human pandemic potential than H5N1? For more than a century, human influenza pandemics have been confined to the

H1, H2, and H3 subtypes. However, the emerging evidence suggesting the potential for efficient human-to-human transmissibility of the H7N9 virus now appears capable of changing the historic record. The H7N9 combination has previously been isolated only rarely from wild birds or poultry, as a low-pathogenic avian influenza virus. Never before has it been isolated from gallinaceous poultry in a form highly pathogenic for either poultry or humans.

As mentioned above it is noteworthy that in the original H5N1 genotype and now in the H7N9 reassortant, H9N2 segments make up six of the eight 'backbone' genes. Although surveillance of live poultry markets quickly identified the source of the H5N1 virus, in this case initial surveillance of the markets has revealed a very low frequency of H7N9 viruses. Additionally, the H7N9 viruses isolated from the live poultry markets lack the 627K mutation in the PB2 gene [4], raising the possibility of a mammalian reservoir – if not swine, then perhaps an equivalent of the civet, which served as the intermediate host of the SARS virus. One such mammal that is common in China is the tree shrew (*Anathana ellioti*). The possible reservoir(s) at the time of writing remain an enigma. Consequently, there is no way of identifying the best strategies for control of this LPAI H7N9 virus at the animal-human interface.

As we are reminded by the experience of vaccine preparation for the H5N1 and 2009 pandemic H1N1 viruses, nearly six months are still required to prepare a new pandemic vaccine; further, for an avian antigen, adjuvants will most likely be required to achieve efficacy at an acceptable dose of antigen. Thus, antivirals will be the first line of defense until vaccines are ready.

Resistance to the adamantane drugs means that anti-neuraminidase drugs are the only currently approved option. Although the detection of an R294K mutation in the NA gene of A/Shanghai/1/2013 (H7N9) virus raises the possibility of eventual resistance, the H7N9 viruses, including A/Shanghai/1/2013 (H7N9), are currently sensitive to neuraminidase inhibitors.

Many of today's questions will have been answered by the time the second edition of the *Textbook of Influenza* has been published. In any case, the emergence of H7N9 serves to remind us that influenza is a continually evolving virus, and improved strategies for control remain of the essence.

References

1. Yang FWJ, Jiang L, Shao L, Zhang y, Zhang J, Weng X, Chen S, Zhang W. A fatal case caused by novel H7N9 avian influenza A virus in China. Emerging Microbes and Infection. 2013;2(e19):publised online. Epub 10 April 2013.
2. Gao R, Cao B, Hu Y, Feng Z, Wang D, Hu W, et al. Human Infection with a Novel Avian-Origin Influenza A (H7N9) Virus. The New England journal of Medicine. 2013 Apr 11. PubMed PMID: 23577628.
3. Wen Y, Klenk HD. H7N9 avian influenza virus – search and re-search. Emerging Microbes and Infection. 2013;2(e18): (published online). Epub 10 April 2013.
4. Kageyama T, Fujisaki S, Takashita E, Xu H, Yamada S, Uchida Y, et al. Genetic analysis of novel avian A(H7N9) influenza viruses isolated from patients in China, February to April 2013. Euro surveillance : bulletin europeen sur les maladies transmissibles; European Communicable Disease Bulletin. 2013;18(15). PubMed PMID: 2359 4575.

Index

Textbook of Influenza, Second Edition. Edited by Robert G. Webster, Arnold S. Monto, Thomas J. Braciale, and Robert A. Lamb.
© 2013 John Wiley & Sons, Ltd. Published 2013 by John Wiley & Sons, Ltd.